Acute Care Surgery in Geriatric Patients

Patrizio Petrone
Collin E.M. Brathwaite
Editors

Acute Care Surgery in Geriatric Patients

Springer

Editors
Patrizio Petrone
Department of Surgery
NYU Long Island School of Medicine
NYU Langone Hospital—Long Island
Mineola, New York, USA

Collin E.M. Brathwaite
Department of Surgery
NYU Long Island School of Medicine
NYU Langone Hospital—Long Island
Mineola, New York, USA

ISBN 978-3-031-30650-1 ISBN 978-3-031-30651-8 (eBook)
https://doi.org/10.1007/978-3-031-30651-8

This Springer imprint is published by the registered company Springer Nature Switzerland AG
The registered company address is: Gewerbestrasse 11, 6330 Cham, Switzerland

In loving memory of my mother Michelina Stella and
my father Giovanni Petrone who guided my steps
in life and never stopped believing in me.

Foreword

The elderly patient has limited physiological reserves due to the biological deterioration of all organ systems and the often-associated comorbid conditions and medications. Taking care of the trauma or non-trauma emergency surgery geriatric patient poses additional challenges. The acute stress of trauma and other emergency surgical conditions can cause rapid exhaustion of the already compromised physiological reserves, resulting in organ failure, increased need of hospital resources, and adverse outcomes. Good knowledge of the anatomical and physiological changes associated with aging, the patient response to an acute physical stress, the effects of the various medications on the clinical presentation and response to treatment, and the complexities of emergency resuscitation in the geriatric patient population are essential elements for optimal results.

This book by Dr. Patrizio Petrone provides an excellent and comprehensive resource for surgeons, emergency physicians, surgical intensivists, and nurses! It covers systematically all aspects of trauma and non-trauma surgical emergencies and can help improve outcomes and reduce the financial costs of caring of the elderly patient.

I am confident that this book will be a valuable companion for the healthcare provider taking care of the elderly patient.

Demetrios Demetriades
Department of Surgery
University of Southern California
Division of Acute Care Surgery
LAC+USC Medical Center
Los Angeles, CA, USA

Foreword

Aging is inevitable as I have discovered from a personal experience after retiring from clinical work recently at the age of 68. While still active supervising PhD students, research, etc. as well as trying to stay fit playing badminton, aging will bring obvious changes in what one does and what one should do. And with aging comes the increased risk of injuries; badminton is notorious for Achilles tendon injury.

Injuries to the elderly is a special field of trauma care. While the principles of managing specific injuries are the same in all adult age groups, the treating physician has to take into account the possibility of frailty and sarcopenia that might slow down the recovery of elderly patients, especially after major trauma and prolonged or extensive procedures. An elderly patient might also not tolerate complications as well as younger patients which implies that one has to play it safe and sometimes be more conservative. A colostomy might be a better option than risking an anastomotic leak and postoperative peritonitis.

Another important aspect in managing elderly trauma patients is to look at the overall picture and future quality of life. The best consultant here is the patient itself providing that he or she is able to communicate properly and understand the implications of treatment decisions. Unlike the children and other younger relatives of the patient, older folks are usually very clear about what to expect and how they want from their remaining life span. One must listen very carefully what the patient wants to say, and if needed, take the patient's side and not the relative's, even how well intended.

This book on geriatric trauma is timely and very important, since the proportion of elderly population is increasing at least in the developed countries, and more and more resources are needed to face this challenge. To make the most optimal use of the resources available and needed, understanding the special features of the trauma care of geriatric patients is highly relevant. This book is a clear step into that direction, and Dr. Patrizio Petrone is to be congratulated for this book that will be a milestone in its field.

Ari Leppäniemi
University of Helsinki
Helsinki, Finland

Aging is inevitable, as I have discovered from personal experience after retiring from clinical work recently at the age of 68. While still actively supervising child ... [illegible] ... as well as trying to stay in playing badminton, aging will bring obvious changes in what we do and what one should do. And with aging comes the increased risk of injuries; badminton is notorious for Achilles tendon injury.

... [illegible] ... is a special field of trauma care. While the principles of managing specific injuries are the same in all adult age groups, the treating physician has to take into account the possibility of frailty and accept that ... slow down the recovery of elderly patients, especially after ... prolonged or extensive procedures. An elderly patient might also not tolerate complications as well as younger patients would ... that one has to ... more conservative. A ... should ... [illegible] ...

... [illegible] ... important ... in managing elderly trauma patients is to look at the overall picture ... [illegible] ... other younger patients and ... [illegible] ... what to expect and how they want from their remaining life span ... [illegible] ...

This ... [illegible] ... book ... [illegible] ... and Dr. ... [illegible] ...

[illegible]
[illegible]
Helsinki, [illegible]

Prologue

The elderly population is the fastest-growing segment of the world's population. As they age, they are at an increased risk of developing acute surgical conditions, such as traumatic injuries, acute appendicitis, and perforated peptic ulcer disease, among others. These conditions require prompt diagnosis and intervention to ensure optimal outcomes. Acute care surgery in geriatric patients poses unique challenges for healthcare providers, including age-related physiologic changes, comorbidities, and cognitive impairment. The world-known authors, international leaders and experts in their field, draw on their extensive clinical experience and evidence-based practices to provide practical recommendations for managing these patients. This book will cover topics such as preoperative assessment and optimization, perioperative care, postoperative management, and the specific surgical procedures that are most common in geriatric patients.

In addition to practical guidance on clinical management, this book will also explore the broader issues that affect the care of geriatric patients in the acute care surgery setting. These include ethical considerations, communication strategies for working with patients and their families, and the importance of interdisciplinary collaboration in achieving the best possible outcomes. This book is an essential resource for surgeons, emergency medicine physicians, intensivists, anesthesiologists, physician assistants, nurses, and healthcare providers involved in the care of geriatric patients with acute surgical conditions.

This book aims not only to serve as a guide for the management of geriatric surgical patients but also to inspire further research and innovation in the field of acute care surgery.

Patrizio Petrone

Contents

Acute Care Surgery in the Geriatric Patient Population: General Principles

1

L.D. Britt and Michael Martyak

Acute Care Surgery Evolution

Dr. William Steward Halsted stated "... every important hospital should have on its resident staff of surgeons at least one who is well trained and able to deal with any emergency." The Acute Care Surgery model was designed to fulfill this need and has evolved into a robust specialty. The pillars of trauma surgery, emergency general surgery, surgical critical care, and surgical rescue are the backbone of acute care surgery. With our aging population, the acute care surgeon has also had to adapt to apply these principles to a growing geriatric population.

The evolution of acute care surgery did not occur de novo. On the contrary, several forces created an optimal environment for its birth and development. A precipitous decline in the surgical workforce involved in the management of emergencies along with the well-documented short supply of specialty support in the acute care setting provided the impetus for the development of the acute care surgery specialty. With an ever enlarging and aging population, a similar dilemma is presenting for ensuring adequate access to quality emergency care to our geriatric patient population.

L.D. Britt · M. Martyak (✉)
Department of Surgery, Eastern Virginia Medical School, Norfolk, VA, USA
e-mail: brittld@evms.edu; martyamt@evms.edu

The geriatric population, defined as those aged 65 and older, is the most rapidly growing segment of the US population. According to the US Census Bureau, it is expected that nearly one in five US residents will be aged 65 and older by the year 2030. This acceleration of the geriatric population is the result of the aging of the "baby boomer generation" and the increased longevity of the population. Life expectancy at age 65 has increased drastically over the past 30 years and a person aged 65 years can expect to live another 15 years. An ever-aging population not surprisingly has also resulted in a population with more comorbidities. An estimated 2 of every 3 geriatric patients have multiple chronic conditions. Almost half of the geriatric population has hypertension, nearly a quarter have coronary artery disease, and more than 8% report a history of stroke. This expansion of more medically complex elderly patients certainly complicates achieving quality outcomes in emergency scenarios.

Acute Care Surgery Principles

The overarching principle of acute care surgery is early and expedient medical/surgical intervention. Whether managing a patient with a perforated duodenal ulcer or a splenic laceration after a fall, early diagnosis, and prompt intervention make up the cornerstone of optimal management. These general principles are applicable to all

P. Petrone, C. E.M. Brathwaite (eds.), *Acute Care Surgery in Geriatric Patients*,
https://doi.org/10.1007/978-3-031-30651-8_1

patient populations with potential surgical emergencies and underscore the important role of surgical judgment and prioritization of patient management. Access to expeditious, quality, emergent surgical care is paramount to achieve the desired results for our elderly patients who lack many physiologic reserves.

The "4 E's" of the core management principles of acute care surgery are as follows:

- Expeditious initial assessment
- Endpoint-guided resuscitation
- Early intervention and definitive management (if possible)
- Essential physiological monitoring

With a wide range of pathologies encountered, acute care surgery is a time-sensitive discipline necessitating a rapid, methodical, and accurate evaluation process. When appropriate, a relevant history from the patient and possibly family members and/or healthcare providers caring for the patient should be obtained. Important details of the patient's chronic or acute conditions, medications, as well as wishes expressed in an advance directive are vital to ensure the patient receives the best possible care. While there is an array of possible presentations in acute care surgery, the core management principles remain the same.

Optimal resuscitation is imperative in the management of any patient in the acute care setting. It is a dynamic process that requires continual assessment, action, and reassessment to ensure target endpoints are achieved. Irrespective of the chosen endpoints, the overarching goal of the resuscitation efforts is to provide adequate tissue perfusion and oxygenation. Conventional markers such as blood pressure, heart rate, and urine output have been shown to exist in a normal state even while inadequate tissue perfusion prevails. Lactate levels, base deficit, and gastric intramucosal pH are all proposed markers for endpoints of resuscitation although the optimal marker remains debated. It is also prudent to recognize that pre-existing conditions, altered physiology, and the pharmacology of chronic medication use can alter the accuracy of these endpoints in the geriatric population.

Early intervention and definitive management are essential when dealing with emergent scenarios. Access to swift and effective care is the cornerstone of the acute care surgery model. Time is of the essence and limiting delays in care is paramount when dealing with the fragile geriatric patient. Many of the general principles of expedient trauma management can be translated to other acute care surgery situations. While each specific disease entity has its own unique diagnostic and management paradigm, the underlying core principles of emergent management remain.

Appropriate physiologic monitoring and prompt identification and resolution of complications is extremely important in ensuring quality outcomes. Various physiologic parameters become altered in the geriatric patient which can complicate the management. Derangements in the cardiovascular system are common. As the heart ages, we encounter a progressive loss of myocytes leading to myocardial dysfunction. Cardiac medication such as beta-blockers can blunt physiologic responses to stress. Atherosclerosis can lead to impaired organ perfusion. Respiratory function declines with age as the chest wall stiffens, the respiratory muscles weaken, and lung compliance decreases. Decreased glomerular filtration rate (GFR) and diminished renal tubule reabsorption and secretion results in dysfunction with fluid homeostasis, solute clearance, and acid-base balance. These and many other physiologic derangements in the elderly patient complicate the care of these patients.

Emergency General Surgery in Elderly Patients

It has been well documented in the literature that geriatric patients undergoing emergency general surgery (EGS) have disproportionally higher rates of complications, mortality, failure of surgical rescue, and increased length of stay. A study querying a large national database detected that seven EGS cases accounted for all EGS cases. These seven cases include partial colectomy, small bowel resection, cholecystectomy, appendectomy, lysis of adhesions, operative management of peptic ulcer disease, and laparotomy. These seven cases also accounted for 80.3% of all mortalities and 78.9% of complications. Ang et al. evaluated a large cohort of geriatric patients from the Centers for Medicare and Medicaid Services Dataset Files undergoing these most commonly performed emergency general surgery cases. They evaluated low volume centers compared to high volume centers and demonstrated large volume centers had significantly improved mortality rates in partial colectomy and small bowel resection cases. Mehta et al. identified that a hospital's proportion of geriatric emergency general surgery patients, rather than simply total hospital volume, may be more implicated in improvements in quality outcomes. The acute care surgery model is well positioned to fill this void of specialized emergency care to the geriatric patient population but further advancements are needed to ensure these results can be replicated more broadly in varying hospital settings.

Preoperative optimization is desired whenever possible, but often is not feasible in the emergency setting due to the constraints of time and need for expeditious surgical intervention. However, when appropriate, every effort should be made to ensure parameters are met to optimize perioperative outcomes especially in the complex geriatric patient with multiple comorbidities. The American College of Surgeons National Surgical Quality Improvement Program (ACS-NSQIP) and American Geriatrics Society collaborated to release best-practice guidelines for perioperative care in elderly patients. The aspects relevant to preoperative care emphasize assessing baseline functional status, screening for preoperative cognitive dysfunction, addressing polypharmacy, and modified goals of care discussions to reflect enhanced risk of complication. There are major limitations to implementing these optimization profiles in the acute setting, but when appropriate and feasible, care should be taken to maximize the patient's preparedness for surgical intervention. Furthermore, identifying factors that are unable to be optimized will help to better predict the expected outcomes for an emergent intervention.

Geriatric Trauma

The Acute Care Surgery specialty developed out of the need for emergency surgical services in the climate of a declining surgical workforce and increasing patient population. Similarly, the acute care surgeon has had to evolve to handle an ever-aging population. With advancements in medical therapies, patients are experiencing not only longevity but vitality. Trauma is no longer solely dominated by a youthful patient population. Injury is now the fifth leading cause of death in the elderly population. Numerous previous studies have identified age 65 and older as correlated with higher mortality rates and poorer functional outcomes after major trauma. Pre-existing medical conditions, frailty, and alterations in physiology and anatomy associated with the aging body all contribute to the higher morbidity and mortality associated with geriatric patients sustaining similar injury patterns to younger patients. Insults generally well tolerated by younger patients can be catastrophic for the geriatric trauma patient. This highlights the need for quality, expeditious, emergency care in this vulnerable patient population.

Blunt trauma predominates the injury pattern for elderly patients with a large proportion of injuries resulting from falls and motor vehicle accidents. Physical impairments, visual and cognitive disturbances, polypharmacy, as well as environmental factors that lead to trip hazards are some of the factors leading to a predominance of fall injuries in seniors. Traumatic brain injury is a common cause of mortality in falls in the elderly and hip fractures have been associated with loss of independence. Visual impairments, slower reaction times, and decreased hearing are known causative factors contributing to motor vehicle accidents in geriatric patients. Furthermore, medical conditions such as myocardial infarction and stroke can precipitate accidents in this vulnerable patient population. While penetrating trauma is not often thought of being synonymous with octogenarians, unfortunately the incidence of self-inflicted gunshot wounds for intended suicide remains a significant burden.

The initial trauma evaluation and work-up should follow the principles of the Advanced Trauma Life Support course. However, special attention should be paid to pre-existing medical conditions, chronic medication use and the effect on physiologic response to injury, and the underlying altered physiologic response in the elder trauma patient. Obtaining important medical history may be difficult or impossible to extract from the geriatric patient and so contacting family members to obtain this vital information early in the course is imperative. Furthermore, with the alterations of physiologic compensation that comes with the aging body, a heightened index of suspicion for early clinical deterioration is paramount when caring for this special patient population.

Surgical Rescue

Peitzman et al. identified that a critical service provided by the acute care surgeon is one of surgical rescue with timely recognition and management of complications. Data from the American College of Surgeon's National Surgery Quality Improvement Program (NSQIP) determined that there existed over a 10% failure to rescue rate in the surgical patient population and that 20% of the patients with the greatest risk for developing postoperative complications accounted for 90% of the failure to rescue. Early intervention by a high-performance surgical team provides the best opportunity to reduce failure to rescue rates, making it a key pillar in the acute care surgery model.

Goal Concordant Decision-Making

Frailty is a geriatric syndrome denoting loss of physical and cognitive reserve for which many scales and tools have been developed to assess. Lists of symptoms, disorders, and physical limitations such as involuntary weight loss, self-reported exhaustion, activity level, grip strength, and walking speed are used to help determine the level of frailty. While there are multiple metrics to assess frailty, regardless of how it is measured the presence of preoperative frailty has been correlated with increased length of stay, risk of complications, and postoperative mortality.

With the understanding of the constraints that increasing frailty has on favorable outcomes, specific care must be made to delineate the goals of care for the patient through the continuum of their care. Patients' desires for the types of therapies to receive may change as the patient transitions to the different phases of their care. It is essential to ensure the patient's values and preferences remain at the center of the decision-making process. Outcomes that need to be assessed, and re-assessed as the patient's condition evolves, are long-term symptoms, functional status, living location, and certainly likelihood of survival. It is incumbent on the acute care surgeon to align the treatment plan with the patient's overall health-care goals.

Undoubtedly the acute care surgeon will encounter patients with progressive, incurable, and terminal disease processes. Palliative care must be recognized as an essential component of the armamentarium when dealing with patients with surgical emergencies. Enhanced knowledge of this key component of care is vital when caring for elderly patients.

Summary

The aging population will continue to have wide-ranging implications for the Acute Care Surgery discipline. It is critical that this workforce expands to adequately address the expansion of our aging population. Furthermore, it is crucial that the evolution of this specialty persists to adapt to this ever-growing cohort of complex patients. This text provides the foundation to achieve the necessary transformation to better care for the geriatric patient requiring emergency surgical care.

References

1. Halaweish I, Alam HB. Changing demographics of the American population. Surg Clin North Am. 2015;95(1):1–10. https://doi.org/10.1016/j.suc.2014.09.002.
2. Menaker J, Scalea TM. Geriatric care in the surgical intensive care unit. Crit Care Med. 2010;38:S452–9.
3. Colloca G, Santoro M, Gambassi G. Age-related changes and perioperative management of elderly patients. Surg Oncol. 2010;19:124–30.
4. Havens JM, Olufajo OA, Cooper ZR, Haider AH, Shah AA, Salim A. Defining rates and risk factors for readmissions following emergency general surgery. JAMA Surg. 2016;151(4):330–6.
5. Mehta A, Efron DT, Canner JK, Dultz L, Xu T, Jones C, Haut ER, Higgins RSD, Sakran JV. Effect of surgeon and hospital volume on emergency general surgery outcomes. J Am Coll Surg. 2017;225(5):666–75.e662
6. Scott JW, Olufajo OA, Brat GA, et al. Use of national burden to define operative emergency general surgery. JAMA Surg. 2016;151(6):e160480.
7. Ang D, Sugimoto J, Richards W, Liu H, Kinslow K, McKenney M, Ziglar M, Elkbuli A. Hospital volume of emergency general surgery and its impact on inpatient mortality for geriatric patients: analysis from 3994 hospitals. Am Surg. 2021;11:31348211049251.
8. Mehta A, Varma S, Efron DT, Joseph BA, Lunardi N, Haut ER, Cooper Z, Sakran JV. Emergency general surgery in geriatric patients: how should we evaluate hospital experience? J Trauma Acute Care Surg. 2019;86(2):189–95.
9. Mohanty S, Rosenthal RA, Russell MM, Neuman MD, Ko CY, Esnaola NF. Optimal perioperative management of the geriatric patient: a best practices guideline from the American College of Surgeons NSQIP and the American Geriatrics Society. J Am Coll Surg. 2016;222(5):930–47.
10. Lehmann R, Beekley A, Casey L, et al. The impact of advanced age on trauma triage decisions and outcomes: a statewide analysis. Am J Surg. 2009;197:571e575.
11. Joseph B, Pandit V, Zangbar B, et al. Superiority of frailty over age in predicting outcomes among geriatric trauma patients. JAMA Surg. 2014;149(8):766–72.
12. Hashmi A, Ibrahim-Zada I, Rhee P, et al. Predictors of mortality in geriatric trauma patients: a systematic review and meta-analysis. J Trauma Acute Care Surg. 2014;76:894e901.
13. Pandit V, Rhee P, Hashmi A, et al. Shock index predicts mortality in geriatric trauma patients: an analysis of the National Trauma Data Bank. J Trauma Acute Care Surg. 2014;76:1111e1115.
14. Peitzman AB, Sperry JL, Kutcher ME, Zuckerbraun BS, Forsythe RM, Billiar TR, et al. Redefining acute care surgery: surgical rescue. J Trauma Acute Care Surg. 2015;79:327.
15. Lin HS, Watts JN, Peel NM, Hubbard RE. Frailty and post-operative outcomes in older surgical patients: a systematic review. BMC Geriatr. 2016;16(1):157.

Healthcare Economics and Aging

2

Jonathan Tamir

Population Trends

When Medicare coverage was initiated in 1965, the average life expectancy for a 65-year-old man was 78 and the life expectancy for a 65-year-old woman was 81. These figures anchored baseline calculations for the costs of the Medicare program. Today, average life expectancies are 83 and 85, respectively. This represents a significant increase in the number of years healthcare costs need to be covered by Medicare.

As of the 2020 Census, 10,000 baby boomers were aging into the program every day!

The US Census Bureau (2015) estimates that 20% of the US population will be older than 65 by 2030. This is a significant increase from the 17% of the population that is over 65 in 2020. The Census Bureau further estimates that the 62.3 million Medicare beneficiaries in 2020 are expected to increase to 77.5 million in 2030.

MedPAC, a group established by the Balanced Budget Act of 1997 which provides Congress with analysis and policy advice on the Medicare program, has a more pessimistic projection. In their June 2015 report to Congress, they projected that Medicare beneficiaries will grow to over 80 million by 2030. Medicare is extended to both people over 65 as well as younger people with disabilities and people with End Stage Renal Disease (ESRD).

Using the Future Elderly Model (FEM), funded by the Centers for Medicare and Medicaid Services (CMS), and developed by a number of high-profile research organizations and universities, to estimate the population and Medicare, it is expected that the US population aged 65 or older will be increasing from 40 million to 67 million between the years of 2010 and 2030. The largest increase in that population will occur among the so-called young elderly (aged 65 to 74). The young elderly cohort will comprise 15.5 million people compared to 12 million people in the 75 and older group. However, the most worrisome increase will come in the number of the very oldest Americans (aged 85+) which will more than double from about 400,000 in 2010 to about 850,000 in 2030. These oldest Americans are the ones that access the greatest number of medical services.

The model also predicts that the life expectancy for people over 65 will grow by 0.8 years between 2010 and 2030 while the expected lifespan of people with disabilities at age 65 will grow even more (1.2 years) from 7.4 years in 2010 to 8.6 years in 2030. Medicare beneficiaries with disabilities clearly have higher acuity and thus have a higher cost of care on average than non-disabled beneficiaries. Furthermore, the rate of obese (BMI ≥30) beneficiaries will rise to 47% compared to the 28% of elderly beneficiaries that

J. Tamir (✉)
NJ Brain and Spine, Hackensack, NJ, USA

P. Petrone, C. E.M. Brathwaite (eds.), *Acute Care Surgery in Geriatric Patients*,
https://doi.org/10.1007/978-3-031-30651-8_2

were classified as obese in 2010. Even more troubling is that the estimated number of people 65 or older that are considered extremely obese (BMI ≥40) will more than double between 2010 and 2030 from 3% to 7%. The rate of diabetes will also rise precipitously. In 2010, 24% of those age 65 or older were diabetic, and it is projected that almost 40% of these individuals will be diabetic in 2030. It is also expected that, by 2030, 40% of Medicare beneficiaries will have three or more chronic conditions. Almost 50% of Non-Hispanic Black beneficiaries will have three or more chronic conditions and that 80% of all Medicare beneficiaries will be hypertensive. In all, the 2030 cohort of elderly will perform worse on almost all health indicators. The only bright spot in these predictions of wellbeing will relate to smoking, as fewer people that will be turning 65 in 2030 will smoke or will have ever smoked.

How Medicare Rates Are Determined

Physician Charges (Medicare Part B)

Prior to 1990, physician charges were the basis of Medicare reimbursement levels. However, costs were rising much more quickly than expected so Congress enacted the Medicare Value Performance Standards (MPVS) program, which was in effect from 1990 to 1997, to contain costs. In 1997, congress enacted the Sustained Growth Rate (SGR) payment system. The SGR was meant to reduce physician fees if physician spending exceeded a target that had been established based on the country's overall economic growth. However, Congress overrode these decreases in all but one year. Finally in 2015, when the Affordable Care Act (ACA) was debated, the SGR was eliminated and replaced with the Merit-based Incentive Payment System (MIPS). The MIPS adjustment is annual and based on four performance categories: quality (30%), cost (30%), promoting interoperability (25%), and improvement activities (15%). Physicians get points based on performance in each of these areas. There is an opportunity to earn bonus points. The Centers for Medicare and Medicaid Services (CMS) determines scores necessary to avoid penalties or receive reimbursement bonuses. Adjusting factors used to modify payment to physicians are: RVUs (reflecting physician effort and complexity of care), PE (Practice Expenses), and PLI (Professional Liability Insurance). Nothing in this calculation reflects patient acuity. Patient acuity may be somewhat captured in the CPT (Current Procedural Terminology) codes that could be increased for more complicated patients, but many physicians are already appropriately billing high level codes as needed.

There is an opportunity for physicians to increase their reimbursement by participating in a quality program like MACRA (Medicare Access and CHIP Reauthorization Act), for providers participating in Alternative Payment Models, or MIPS (Merit-based Incentive Program System), for all other providers. The MIPS program adjusts payment to providers based on four areas: quality, resource use, advancing care information (interoperability of information systems), and clinical practice improvement. Again, there is no mention or consideration of patient acuity.

Facility Charges (Part A)

Hospitals (Inpatient Prospective Payment System IPPS) and long-term care hospitals (LTCH PPS) are still essentially paid under the DRG system modified by a growing number of performance standards and quality programs; Value Based Purchasing (VBP) program, Hospital Readmissions Reduction program, Hospital Inpatient Quality Reporting (IQR) Program, and Hospital Acquired Condition (HAC) program. Due to Covid, the VBP and HAC reduction programs may be suppressed. These programs require a tremendous amount of reporting but thus far are required if hospitals are to avoid their mandated 2% reduction to the base operating DRG payment amount. However, even if delayed, this shows that Congress is zealously cost conscious and is baking in an annual decrease in reimbursement for the Part A Medicare program.

The Inpatient Standardized Payment Amounts (ISPAs) are comprised of labor and supply cost portions as well as a capital (interest, depreciation, rent, property-related expenses) allocation. The labor piece is modified by geographical factors (an adjusted hospital wage index calculated by CMS). On the plus side, Part A payments can be adjusted in two ways for acuity/complexity. The first way is through a case mix adjustment that pays more for cases of higher complexity. While helpful, this is not an inter-condition acuity inflator. However, the second is a high-cost outlier payment. While this results in additional reimbursement, Medicare only pays 80% of the hospital's costs that exceed the expense threshold.

Medicare Budgets and Projected Payment Levels

The 2022 Continuing Resolution allocated $3,974,744,000 to the Medicare program. However, CMS is requesting $4,346,985,000 for FY2023. This request is an increase of over 9% in a single year!

Congress has a mandate and incentive to reduce the costs of the Medicare program. However, CMS will continue to request large increases as beneficiaries are added to the program, the cost of existing wages, supplies, and services continue to rise and the need to maintain or improve the service level to Medicare beneficiaries endures. This is a conundrum for Congress. Congress needs to hold the line on taxes and therefore, spending but cannot upset their constituents by reducing benefits for the elderly. The elderly vote counts!

Clearly, CMS' request will not be approved in its entirety. However, this shows the need for an increased federal allocation which can be satisfied by additional budgetary authorizations (increase taxes or take funds from other programs), reductions in service levels, decreased reimbursement to facilities and providers or a combination of these and other funding methods. Given such a wide divide between the existing and requested budget there is very little guidance to observers regarding the scale of future requests or at what level funding will be approved.

What is clear is that as the population ages, without modification to the elements of the rate calculations detailed above, the cost per enrollee will climb. In 2011, Medicare beneficiaries 80 years of age and older were 24% of the Medicare population but used 33% of total Medicare spending. Beneficiaries between the ages of 65 and 69 were 26% of the Medicare population but used only 15% of total Medicare spending.

The Kauffman Foundation reported that, in 2011, average per capita spending on 96-year-old beneficiaries ($16,145) is almost three times as much as average per capita spending on 66-year-old beneficiaries ($5562). In 2011, the average per capita Medicare spending was $9839 but by 2019, the average Medicare expenditure per enrollee was $13,276. While this figure is not necessarily remarkable, what is significant is how quickly these figures grow. A 35% increase in just 8 years!

Furthermore, this significant increase occurred before the anticipated population bump that will be caused by the baby boom generation aging into Medicare. These increases will only accelerate as the number of elderly grow and the ultra-elderly population grows even more rapidly if the program does not decrease service levels.

While it may appear that these increased payments will benefit institutions and providers, this increased volume will lead to a poorer financial situation for institutions and providers. Medicare does not reimburse sufficiently to cover the cost of the care that facilities and providers offer to Medicare beneficiaries. Therefore, providing increased Medicare services will further reduce net margins for facilities and providers.

Even if the Medicare beneficiary age cohorts will skew younger (young elderly) due to the baby boomers aging into Medicare, there will still be a very large inflow of patients and an increasing pressure to reduce the per patient expenditure so that the Medicare budget does not grow as quickly as it is forecasted to grow today. It is difficult to reduce services offered to seniors; however, it is also difficult to raise taxes to pay for services for an additional number of seniors. It affects fewer constituents to solve this funding shortfall by reducing payments to facilities and providers.

In the July 2021 MedPAC Databook, section 2, there are two telling data charts from 2018. The first shows that non-disabled Medicare beneficiaries make up 85% of the total people covered by Medicare but cost only 76.5% of the total outlays. Disabled beneficiaries make up 14% of the total number of people covered by Medicare but use almost 19% of Medicare's resources. Spending by age cohort increases with advancing age. Beneficiaries above the age of 85 make up 11% of the Medicare population but make up 15% of Medicare's spending. Beneficiaries who reported being in poor health regardless of age cohort and who make up 5.5% of the Medicare beneficiaries cost Medicare almost 14% of its total annual spending.

In 2010, there was a $131,000 estimated total lifetime spend for a typical Medicare beneficiary. In 2030, the estimated total lifetime spend for a typical Medicare beneficiary will go up to $223,000. The Congressional Budget Office (May 2022) documented that Medicare net outlays (gross outlays minus receipts) were $695 billion in 2021. They project these same net outlays will be $1.39 trillion in 2030. These significant increases in costs are going to challenge the Medicare system which, according to the Cabinet Secretaries for the Treasury, Health and Human Services, and Labor is forecasted to go bankrupt in 2026. CMS leadership assures us that this will not occur but revenues will need to be found to support this expense if the Medicare system is to continue in its current formulation.

In short, the growth in the elderly population will lead to an increase in acuity for the beneficiaries being cared for throughout the healthcare system. Ordinarily, an increase in acuity will lead to an increase in reimbursement. As discussed above, payments to institutions have case mix and outlier adjustments that will help increase revenues. However, as acuity goes up across the board, the average cost will go up while still reimbursing facilities at DRG-like levels. If acuity increases uniformly, it will push up the outlay which facilities will need to spend to achieve outlier status on cases and thus will decrease the reimbursement for Medicare patients on average. There is little that can be done to increase reimbursement for providers as many existing patients already require complex care and many providers already code at the highest CPT code levels.

Medicare Rates are Insufficient and not Keeping Up with Cost Inflation

The increasing number of people covered by Medicare may have been good news for institutions and providers if only Medicare covered the cost of the necessary treatment.

It does not.

Physician and Surgeon Reimbursement

Medicare's Conversion Factor, which is the major driver of the Medicare reimbursement for physicians, is clearly not keeping up with the inflation rate/Consumer Price Index (CPI). Below is a table generated by listing the Medicare Conversion factor from CMS and the CPI numbers from Labor Department's Bureau of Labor Statistics (BLS). The conversion rate is the number that the Relative Value Units (RVUs) get multiplied by to determine a physician's reimbursement for each CPT code billed.

Medicare conversion Rate vs. CPI

	Medicare			
	Conversion	percent		
Year	factor	change	Change in CPI	
2012	$34.04	0.18%	1.70%	
2013	$34.02	−0.04%	1.50%	
2014	$35.82	5.30%	0.80%	
2015	$35.93	0.31%	0.70%	
2016	$35.80	−0.36%	2.10%	
2017	$35.89	0.24%	2.10%	
2018	$36.00	0.31%	1.90%	
2019	$36.04	0.11%	2.30%	
2020	$36.09	0.14%	1.40%	
2021	$34.89	−3.30%	7.00%	
2022	$34.61	−0.80%		
Sum		2.09%	21.50%	CPI through 2021
Cumulative		1.91%	23.54%	

Clearly Medicare reimbursement rates are not keeping up with the growing expenses that physician practices face many of which are growing at rates exceeding the inflation rate (CPI). A 2020 paper by CD Lopez et al. in Arthroplasty Today documented the reimbursement trends for Total Joint Arthroplasty (TJA) between 2012 and 2017. They found that Medicare reimbursement to hospitals for TJA cases increased by 0.3% between 2012 and 2017. However, this resulted in a real decline of 7.7% when adjusted for inflation. Similarly, surgeon reimbursement increased by 4.9% which resulted in a 3.5% inflation adjusted decrease in reimbursement. This is further validation that despite reimbursement appearing to stay constant or even modestly increase, real reimbursement levels, when adjusted for inflation, are decreasing. A stark example of this decrease in real reimbursement rates for surgeries is offered by Hue et al. in a paper in the American Journal of surgery in 2021. He showed that while reimbursement rates for inguinal hernia repairs (6.5–7.2%), appendectomies (5.1–6.1%), and cholecystectomies (a decrease of 6.8–4.4%) increased in nominal rates, when adjusted for inflation, all showed significant declines with laparoscopic cholecystectomies declining by 19.8% Similarly, a paper by Haglin et al. researched reimbursement for the 10 most utilized CPT codes in both spinal and cranial neurosurgery. They found that adjusted for inflation, the average reimbursement for these procedures fell 25.8% from 2000 to 2018. A steady year by year decrease shows that the downward pressure on Medicare reimbursement is consistent and persistent.

Hospital Reimbursement

There is also much written about whether Medicare rates are sufficient to cover the expense of the care provided by institutions. The American Hospital Association (AHA), in a recent 2019 paper based on data from 1995–2016, found that Medicare reimbursement was $54 billion lower than the actual cost of care provided. They also reported that Medicare reimbursement only covered 86.8% (2016) of Hospital costs of care for Medicare beneficiaries. Private insurance paid 144.8% (2016) of Hospital costs of care for their enrollees. Therefore, the large shift of patients to Medicare will have a significant negative effect on Hospital financial viability. The AHA also reported that more than 30% of hospitals had negative operating margins. Even with this below cost reimbursement, Medicare's national health expenditures (2016) have never been higher at 17.9% of Gross Domestic Product (GDP). For 2019, MedPAC, reported that IPPS hospitals' overall Medicare margin remains a negative 8.7%.

An interesting comparison done by the Rand corporation, titled "Prices Paid to Hospitals by Private Health Plans Are High Relative to Medicare and Vary Widely," by White and Whaley, studied hospital reimbursement data and found that if private health plans had paid hospitals using Medicare's payment formulas, the total allowed amount (total hospital clinical revenues) over the 2015–2017 period would have been reduced by $7.7 billion. This is a clear example of the inadequacy of Medicare reimbursements.

Another significant pressure on the funding of the Medicare program is the rapid decline in the number of workers per Medicare beneficiary. In 2015, there were 3.1 workers per Medicare beneficiary and the projections show that in 2030 there will only be 2.3 workers per Medicare beneficiary. This is critical as worker payroll taxes are the primary funding mechanism for the Medicare program.

Tactics Medicare Uses to Decrease Reimbursements

Whenever Medicare costs are higher than expected and the budget is in danger of being exceeded, CMS looks to find alternative treatment methodologies or payment mechanisms to allow a reduction in expense.

In addition to the methods detailed above of reducing the conversion factor and instituting a 2% annual reduction for reimbursement to hospitals, among others, Medicare tried another tactic which was to move procedures out of inpatient hospitals and into ASCs. Medicare has an

Inpatient-only list. This is a list of procedures that must be performed in a hospital. ASCs get reimbursed at approximately 60% of hospitals for the same procedures. As Medicare removes procedures from the Inpatient-only list, these procedures get moved to ASCs and the overall reimbursement paid into the system for these procedures decreases. Medicare keeps removing procedures from the Inpatient-only list, and there has been significant confusion lately as it was announced that the Inpatient-only list was going to be discontinued in 2024 as part of a location independent reimbursement proposal which would have paid the same amount regardless of where the procedure was performed. Thankfully, this initiative was not successful. While this proposal may have reduced Medicare outlays, it would have devastated hospitals that rely on that procedural revenue to fund their infrastructure costs.

Another reduction strategy Medicare uses is called the productivity adjustment. Every year, Medicare calculates the increase in payments to hospitals and providers that should be offered to keep up with inflation. The productivity adjustment is just another element they add to the calculations after determining the hospital Market Basket increase detail in the "how rates are developed" section above. CMS assumes the healthcare productivity level increases the same amount as the economy-wide labor productivity rate. Regardless of the explanation, this is a reduction in the reimbursement Medicare pays to hospitals and is expected to average 0.5% through 2030. This reduction in reimbursement to keep up with economy-wide productivity gains would make sense if the reimbursement rate was also increased annually to keep up with the economy-wide inflation rate so that all economic factors would be included in the calculation of Medicare reimbursement levels. That is not the case.

As tax revenues decrease and the cost of care increases due to the increased number of elderly patients, increased acuity, and the cost of new technologies, substantial pressure will be put on the Medicare program to find additional methods or adjustments to increase funding or reduce costs.

Bundled Payments: A Major Medicare Cost Savings Initiative

In April 2015, the Comprehensive Care for Joint Replacement (CJR) program was introduced by CMS. It was a mandatory bundled payment model which essentially extended the hospital DRG payment model to all care involved in a total joint arthroplasty (TJA) course of treatment. This meant that all costs including hospital, physician (surgeon, physician, anesthesiologist, pathologist, etc.), ancillary, labs, rehab, home care, etc. would all be covered by one payment from CMS.

All hospitals in the 67 Metropolitan Service Areas (MSAs) selected by CMS were required to participate. Hospitals were held accountable for costs and quality metrics for patients receiving hip or knee replacements during the pre-procedure time as well as for the 90-day postoperative period. If the cost incurred by the hospital/providers exceeded the quality-adjusted spending benchmark set by CMS, hospitals were penalized. If the hospitals were able to bring costs below this quality-adjusted spending benchmark, they received part of the savings as a bonus.

Total joint replacements (knee and hip) were chosen because they are a common Medicare beneficiary procedure and volumes were growing quickly. The number of total hip arthroplasties was expected to reach 498,000 in 2020 while the number of total knee arthroplasty was expected to reach 1,065,000 in 2020. This volume prompted CMS to undertake this pilot project scheduled to run from 2015 to 2020.

While this program provided clear incentives to reduce costs, it also led to significant reimbursement uncertainty because CMS pays on a fee for service (FFS) basis and then reconciles the total cost of the services with the targeted expenditure level. Hospitals and providers could experience retrospective penalties (or bonuses) that were to be recouped in future years.

Aggregating all the TJA costs in one payment makes it that much easier to reduce the amount hospitals and providers are reimbursed as it is much clearer what the total budget line item is for the procedures individually as well as what the otal CMS spend is on these procedures for the ntire population.

This all seemed to be a precursor to CMS emoving Total Knee Arthroplasty (TKA) from he Inpatient-only list in 2018 and adding it to the Medicare ASC payable list in January of 2020. As mentioned above, ASC procedural reimbursement rates are approximately 60% of inpatient procedural reimbursement rates.

The bundled payment program, as proposed by CMS, originally had four sub-programs. These were the Comprehensive Care for Joint replacement (CJR) model, the Oncology Care Model (OCM), the Episode Payment Models (EPM) [which included the Acute Myocardial Infarction (AMI) model, the Coronary Artery Bypass Graft (CABG) model and the surgical hip and femur fracture treatment (SHFFT) model], and the Cardiac Rehabilitation (CR) incentive payment model. The only programs that got off the ground were the CJR model and the OCM model.

The CJR program for total knee and hip replacements was the only program that demonstrated significant savings. The two major components of savings for that program appeared to result from the decreased usage of Skilled Nursing Facilities (SNFs) and Inpatient Rehabilitation Facilities (IRFs). This may indicate that savings were achieved primarily by changing the location of after-procedure care and may result in only a one-time readjustment.

If this was only a one-time readjustment, it may prove impossible to increase savings further in future years once this change of service location savings created the new cost target. Apparently, hospitals and provider groups that participated in this program believed this to be the case as 73% of the hospitals that were able to leave the CJR program did so once it was made no longer mandatory.

While CMS has started a second round of the bundled payment program in 2020, there are no plans to extend the program further or expand it to other specialties or conditions. CMS will therefore need to look to other areas for additional cost savings. Additional cost savings measures will be developed and implemented. In all these cost savings programs, hospital and provider reimbursements shrink.

Impact on Facilities and Providers

While Medicare does not comprise most of the average hospital's revenue, it is a major share of it. Not accepting Medicare and Medicaid reimbursement, while increasing a hospitals net revenue per patient, would be very difficult, if not impossible, for hospitals to operationalize as government programs make up over a third of hospital revenue. Foregoing Medicare patients would cause a significant drop in reimbursement and a major difficulty in covering fixed institutional and practice costs.

While Medicare and Medicaid reimbursement rates are significantly less than the average reimbursement for private payers, as shown above, the financial argument for continuing to accept Medicare patients is the marginal profit argument. This marginal profit argument is a financial rationalization and puts hospitals in a dangerous situation if private health insurance were to decrease their reimbursement levels. The argument is that while Medicare and Medicaid pay less than cost, the private insurance pays more and can be used to cover the fixed expenses so that the Medicare and Medicaid revenues can be applied solely against the variable costs. This is helpful if you have an open slot in the OR schedule but not a way to maintain overall financial viability. This marginal profit analysis would have no legitimacy in a proper financial step-down analysis done to allocate cost to the appropriate revenue producing activity.

Another major issue stemming from this Medicare underpayment and projected larger underpayment in the future is that many private insurance fee schedules are denominated in multiples of the Medicare fee schedule. While specific citations for this are unavailable, private insurance fee schedules based on a multiple of the Medicare fee schedule have been the case in every institution and medical group at which I have worked for the past 30 years. Therefore, any reduction in Medicare fee schedules means a decrease across the board in reimbursement as private insurers will reduce their fee schedules proportionally.

One of the only ways to avoid this pricing pressure is to be in a strong negotiating position vis a vis your regional insurance payer. An article in Health Affairs (2011) showed that hospitals in concentrated markets can raise prices for private insurers because they have disproportionate market share, and therefore market power, while hospitals that are in competitive markets need to focus on cutting costs because their negotiating power is significantly less. The power in this situation lies with the insurers and they can suppress rate increases. Physicians have a much harder time with this as most groups are not large enough in and of themselves to pressure insurance companies to raise or maintain their reimbursement rates.

Therefore, not only will Medicare reimbursement fall in real terms in the future but private insurance reimbursement, which was relied upon to make up for the Medicare reimbursement shortfall, will fall as well, bringing multiple elements of negative cost pressure to bear on hospitals and providers.

A simple calculation using the relative payment to cost ratios above shows that there will be a 40% reduction in reimbursement when a patient moves from a private payer to Medicare. We can assume that people with no insurance, that age into Medicare, will be covered as well which would increase overall reimbursement to the system and that Medicaid enrollees would reduce reimbursement to the system slightly when they transition to Medicare (Medicare paying 86.8% of cost and Medicaid paying 88.1% of cost).

In 2020, 91.4% of the population had health insurance and 8.6% were uninsured. Of the 91% that had insurance, 66.5% had private health insurance coverage and 34.8% had public coverage. This adds up to more than 100% because some people had both private and public insurance (Medicare as a primary insurance with a private secondary insurance, for example). The 34.8% included 18.4% Medicare, 17.8% Medicaid, and VA of 0.9% (individual totals are more than the sum for the reason given before).

A quick calculation showing how insurance payments would change as more of the population enters Medicare follows. Of the 91.4% of insured, there would be only two components since Medicare patients are already in the program. The Private insurance vs. public (Medicaid and VA only) would proportionally be 78% (of 91.4%) private vs. 22% (of 91.4%) public less Medicare. There are approximately 8.6% uninsured individuals who would be receiving Medicare coverage and thus increasing payments into the system.

From above:

Payer class	Percent of population	
Uninsured	8.6%	+100%
Medicaid/VA	19.8% (22% of 91.4%)	−1.5% (88.1–86.8%)
Private	71.6% (78% of 91.4%)	−40% (144.8–86.8%)
Total	100%	−20.4%

This is a rough estimate of the increase/decrease per patient in reimbursement when moving from our current insurance payer mix to one where the population ages into Medicare. This does not consider the disabled or ESRD patients.

CMS in their National Health Expenditures Fact Sheet Data document that in 2020, Medicare spent $12,530 per beneficiary. So, for every patient that moves from our current payer mix into Medicare, we would expect a 20.4% decrease in reimbursement or, using CMS' 2021 per capita cost, a decrease in payments of $2553 per patient per year. As previously mentioned, the 2020 Census projected 10,000 patients will be moving into Medicare every day.

10,000 people a day moving to Medicare
365 days per year
3,650,000 people moving to Medicare per year
Per capita reduction of $2553 per year (20.4% decline)
Reduction in payments into the system of $9.3 billion per year

There will be regional differences. In regions where there are low medical services supply and high demand physicians and hospitals will have a disproportionate influence on reducing the decrease and on maintaining a reasonable reimbursement rate for services. Unfortunately, in many areas, most of which have large academic medical centers, there will be significantly more competition and therefore reimbursement from commercial payers will decrease more quickly as there are more people who are willing to service patients for even less.

Looking to the Future

Hospitals and surgeons will likely need to contend with lower reimbursement even if they do not accept Medicare as reimbursement trends developed by CMS seem to diffuse out to the commercial payers and result in reduced reimbursement throughout the healthcare system. Physicians and hospitals will need to continue to diversify their service offerings and rely less on Medicare and Medicare-multiplier-dependent reimbursing payers.

Value-based healthcare will continue to be a goal. It is highly likely that CMS, having developed the Bundled Payment for Care Improvement (BCPI) model, will continue to try to apply it in other treatment areas despite its less than stellar results to date.

The easiest sell would be model 2, which is a retrospective model where providers and hospitals are reimbursed in the usual FFS model (they get paid what they bill for). The total cost of care for the entire episode is compared to the agreed upon cost, developed by CMS. If the actual cost is higher than the agreed upon cost, then CMS is refunded. If the reimbursement paid is less than the agreed upon cost, CMS shares the savings. The danger in this model is that CMS keeps ratcheting down the agreed upon level of appropriate cost.

It is likely, however, that CMS will prefer BCPI model 4. Model 4 is a prospective reimbursement model where CMS will pay a lump sum to the hospital/provider, and they figure out how to divide the money and cover all costs over or under the paid amount. This will likely be attractive to CMS because the administration of this model is much simpler compared to the other models. A procedure is completed and one payment is sent. No follow-up evaluation is needed, and no additional payments or take-backs/offsets are necessary. Quality metrics need to be reported but that is a hospital/provider responsibility.

As in the CJR model, the success or failure of this initiative will be in how the target cost and quality metrics are set. Setting these too low or setting them at a reasonable level only to follow up by decreasing them every year will be detrimental to continued medical group and hospital solvency.

As more procedures are moving to ASCs, investing in ASCs, by hospitals and professionals, may be a viable revenue generating strategy. Conditions vary region to region and close attention to the specifics of payer dominance, number and patient recruitment strength of hospitals, number and patient recruitment strength of competing physician groups, and any existing hospital/ASC/physician group joint ventures or agreements is critical to the success of such a venture.

In less competitive markets, agreements with payers and with employers to ensure exclusive or semi-exclusive contracts to providing set, prospective reimbursement will allow hospitals and providers to increase efficiency and reduce costs through better resource planning. One example of this is Walmart's Centers of Excellence program. Clearly there would need to be some sort of acuity built into the model, and this would work for older patients who still had non-Medicare insurance.

Developing care plans/packages which would include transparent pricing (maybe with ranges) and quality indicators for the facility and the physician/surgeon performing the service is another option. This would advance the pay for quality argument and hopefully attract more patients. However, currently many patients needing a procedure decide that they will deal with the expense later, an approach which blinds them to the cost of the procedure when it is being scheduled. Quoting comprehensive costs clearly and completely (providers, ancillaries, facility, etc.) may result in a very large number and deter some patients, overwhelmed by the cost and the process, from getting the procedure at all. This would also be relevant for older patients that were still covered by commercial or managed care insurance with secondary responsibility.

New and innovative strategies will need to be developed to counter this pressure to reduce costs above and beyond what healthcare providers can tolerate.

References

1. Gaudette É, Tysinger B, Cassil A, Goldman DP. Health and health Care of Medicare Beneficiaries in 2030. Forum Health Econ Policy. 2015;18(2):75–96. https://doi.org/10.1515/fhep-2015-0037.
2. kff.org. https://www.kff.org/report-section/the-rising-cost-of-living-longer-section-1-medicare-per-capita-spending-by-age-among-traditional-medicare-beneficiaries-over-age-65-2011/.
3. cms. gov. 2021. https://www.cms.gov/Research-Statistics-Data-and-Systems/Statistics-Trends-and-Reports/NationalHealthExpendData/NHE-Fact-Sheet.
4. Congressional Budget office Baseline projections (2022). https://www.cbo.gov/system/files/2022-05/51302-2022-05-medicare.pdf.
5. Lopez CD, Boddapati V, Neuwirth AL, Shah RP, Cooper HJ, Geller JA. Hospital and surgeon Medicare reimbursement trends for total joint arthroplasty. Arthroplasty Today. 2020;6:437.
6. Hue JJ, Paukovits JL, Bingmer K, Sugumar K, Onders RP, Hardacre JM. Medicare reimbursement for common general surgery procedures has declined over the last decade. Am J Surg. 2022;223(3):550–3. https://doi.org/10.1016/j.amjsurg.2021.10.040.
7. Haglin JM, Richter KR, Patel NP. Trends in Medicare reimbursement for neurosurgical procedures: 2000 to 2018. J Neurosurg. 2019;132(2):649–55. https://doi.org/10.3171/2018.8.JNS181949.
8. American Hospital Association. 2018. https://www.aha.org/system/files/2018-07/2018-aha-chartbook.pdf.
9. RAND Corporation. https://www.rand.org/content/dam/rand/pubs/research_reports/RR3000/RR3033/RAND_RR3033.pdf.
10. https://www.beckersasc.com/asc-coding-billing-and-collections/doing-the-deal-understanding-the-key-differences-between-asc-and-hospital-rcm.html.
11. 2021 Annual Report of the Boards of Trustees of the Federal Hospital Insurance and Federal Supplementary Medical Insurance Trust Funds.
12. https://www.rheumatologyadvisor.com/home/topics/osteoarthritis/increased-rate-of-total-joint-replacements-predicted-from-2020-to-2040/.
13. https://www.modernhealthcare.com/finance/joint-replacement-bundled-payments-losing-their-appeal-bpci-advanced.
14. https://www.aha.org/system/files/2018-07/2018-aha-chartbook.pdf-Table-4-4.pdf. Aggregate hospital payment to cost ratios for private payers, Medicare and Medicaid 1995–2016.
15. Keisler-Starkey K, Bunch LN. Health insurance coverage in the United States: 2020, Current population reports. 2021.

A Rationale and Systems Impact for Geriatric Trauma and Acute Care Surgery

3

Alexandra Briggs and Lisa M. Kodadek

Introduction

By 2050, 22% of the American population will be over the age of 65, which will result in steady increases in the number of geriatric adults presenting with trauma and Emergency General Surgery (EGS) concerns. The burden and cost of both trauma and EGS is well established. EGS accounts for 7.1% of all hospitalizations nationally and costs over $28 billion, with higher costs in older adults. Costs of EGS are projected to increase by 45% by 2060 due in significant part to our aging population. Trauma in older adults already accounts for 8.5% of all Medicare hospitalizations and costs $32.9 billion and will continue to expand as our population ages. Perhaps even more important is the human cost, as the morbidity and mortality of trauma and EGS in geriatric adults is significant. In addition, older adults are at risk for loss of independence and function, as well as long-term morbidity and mortality from acute admissions.

In this chapter, we discuss the rationale for geriatric-focused care in trauma and acute care surgery, focusing on the physiologic and social challenges that arise in older adults. We review current prediction models in geriatric patients to inform shared decision-making discussions. Finally, we present current approaches to geriatric-centered care both on the individual institutional level and nationally with the American College of Surgeons Geriatric Surgery Verification program.

Rationale for Geriatric Trauma and Acute Care Surgery

Older adults with injuries and acute care surgical needs require a unique approach to medical care with thoughtful recognition and consideration of the features which contribute to increased risk of complication in this population. Older adults experience greater morbidity and mortality after surgery than their younger counterparts and are less likely to return to their baseline functional status after illness. Clinical presentation of disease may differ in older adults, and this may lead to delay in diagnosis or failure to rescue. The ability of this cohort to tolerate emergency operations or severe stress may be limited due to lack of organ system reserve. Attention to special considerations including medical comorbidities, frailty and sarcopenia, cognitive impairment and

A. Briggs (✉)
Division of Trauma and Acute Care Surgery, Dartmouth Hitchcock Medical Center, Lebanon, NH, USA
e-mail: Alexandra.Briggs@hitchcock.org

L. M. Kodadek
Division of General Surgery, Trauma and Surgical Critical Care, Yale School of Medicine, New Haven, CT, USA
e-mail: lisa.kodadek@yale.edu

P. Petrone, C. E.M. Brathwaite (eds.), *Acute Care Surgery in Geriatric Patients*,
https://doi.org/10.1007/978-3-031-30651-8_3

delirium, nutrition, polypharmacy, and geriatric vulnerabilities are critical in the geriatric trauma and acute care surgical population. Outcomes among older adults who sustain injury or experience acute care surgical conditions depend on a complex interplay between predisposing and precipitating factors. Predisposing factors may be related to factors including physiology, sociodemographic status, functional status, impairment, or genetics. Precipitating factors may include injury or surgical disease, but also behavioral, environmental, social, or psychological considerations. Thoughtful consideration of predisposing and precipitating factors is crucial to ensure optimal care for the geriatric surgical patient.

Medical Comorbidities and Surgical Risk

Aging is often accompanied by an increased burden of medical comorbid diseases. These pre-existing medical comorbidities may impair the older patient's ability to tolerate injury or an acute care surgical disease. In some cases, the medical comorbidity itself (vision loss or neuropathy due to diabetes, for example) may predispose to falls and subsequent injury. Likewise, sequelae of a medical problem or its treatment may lead to an emergency surgical condition. While the older person's organ function at rest may be preserved, the ability to respond appropriately in the event of physiologic stressors such as acute illness or surgical intervention may be limited. Comorbid disease is common among older adults and over two thirds of patients aged 65 and older have at least one comorbid disease. Common comorbid diseases among the elderly include hypertension, coronary artery disease, diabetes mellitus, and pulmonary conditions. A careful assessment of the patient's medical history, with particular attention to concomitant medical illness is imperative prior to surgical intervention in older adults. Optimization of medical comorbidities should be pursued when feasible prior to operation, although in the emergency setting, optimization needs to be pursued in an expedient manner and must be balanced with the time-sensitive need for surgical intervention.

Various prediction tools are available and may better prepare the surgeon to predict surgical risk based on factors including comorbid conditions. One readily available online tool is the American College of Surgeons (ACS) National Surgical Quality Improvement Program (NSQIP) Surgical Risk Calculator (riskcalculator.facs.org). This tool uses various patient-specific data including age, sex, functional status as well as comorbid conditions including malignancy, diabetes mellitus, hypertension, congestive heart failure, renal failure, and chronic obstructive pulmonary disease. Geriatric-specific outcomes may also be included in the prediction model including mobility aid use, fall history, dementia or cognitive impairment, palliative care or hospice use on admission, origin status on admission to hospital (i.e., home, not from home, supported at home), and whether consent for surgery was signed by a surrogate. The tool then provides specific predictions in percentages for various outcomes based on the type of operation proposed for the patient. These outcomes include risk of serious complication, any complication, death, postoperative delirium, functional decline, and new mobility aid use. Prediction tools such as the ACS NSQIP Surgical Risk Calculator may allow surgeons to counsel patients and families and participate in higher quality shared decision-making.

Frailty and Sarcopenia

Frailty is a syndrome prevalent in older adults which places these individuals at higher risk for falls, hospital stays, disability, and death. Prevalence of frailty in community dwelling older adults varies between 5% and nearly 30% based on the specific population. Frailty is a separate entity from disability and comorbidity although comorbidity may serve as a risk factor and disability may be an outcome of frailty. Preoperative frailty has been demonstrated to predict postoperative complications in patients aged 65 and older; frailty also predicts increased

Table 3.1 FRAIL scale—5-item questionnaire

Item	Question
Fatigue	Does the patient fatigue or get exhausted easily?
Resistance	Does the patient have difficulty walking up one flight of stairs on their own?
Ambulation	Does the patient have difficulty walking one block?
Illnesses	Does the patient have 5 or more illnesses?
Loss of weight	Has the patient lost 5 to 10% body weight over the last 6 months to 1 year?

Yes to 1–2 questions: consistent with pre-frailty
Yes to 3 or more questions: consistent with frailty

length of stay in the hospital and discharge to a skilled or assisted living facility. Frailty was originally defined as a syndrome present when three or more of the following criteria are met: unintentional weight loss (10 pounds in past year), exhaustion (self-reported), weakness (as measured by grip strength, lowest 20%), slow walking speed (slowest 20%), and low physical activity (lowest 20%).

The FRAIL scale (Table 3.1) has also been developed by Morley and colleagues as a rapid and simple screening tool for frailty. This is a 5-item questionnaire which queries Fatigue (Does the patient fatigue or get exhausted easily?), Resistance (Does the patient have difficulty walking up one flight of stairs on their own?), Ambulation (Does the patient have difficulty walking one block?), Illnesses (Does the patient have 5 or more illnesses?), and Loss of weight (Has the patient lost 5–10% body weight over the last 6 months to 1 year?). FRAIL serves as an apt mnemonic for the five areas of interest. If the answer to 3 or more of these questions is yes, this is consistent with frailty. An answer of yes to 1 or 2 of these questions is consistent with pre-frailty. The FRAIL scale has been validated in multiple populations and is a useful tool to identify patients who may benefit from dedicated preoperative efforts to decrease frailty prior to planned surgical intervention through prehabilitation programs. Complex interventions inclusive of exercise, nutrition, and social support have been shown to reverse frailty and improve outcomes.

Sarcopenia, a clinical entity associated with frailty, is similarly predictive of poor outcomes after surgery. Sarcopenia has been described as low muscle function or strength in the presence of low muscle mass. Sarcopenia may also be identified through computed tomography psoas index (psoas muscle area normalized for body surface area on computed tomography). Sarcopenia has been demonstrated to be an independent predictor of minor postoperative complications, prolonged hospital stay, and discharge to a skilled nursing facility or rehabilitation facility after emergency general surgery.

Cognitive Impairment and Postoperative Delirium

Pre-existing cognitive impairment is common among older adults and has been identified as an important risk factor for postoperative delirium. At least 20% of older adults who are 71 years of age or older have cognitive impairment without dementia. The Aging, Demographics, and Memory Study (ADAMS) established that cognitive impairment without dementia is more prevalent in the United States than dementia, with varying outcomes and prevalence based on subtype such as prodromal Alzheimer's disease and cerebrovascular disease. Cognitive impairment and postoperative delirium together have been found to have a synergistic and detrimental impact on outcomes; those with both risk factors have increased risk of long-term functional decline. Best Practice Guidelines from the American Geriatric Society and the American College of Surgeons recommend preoperative cognitive evaluation for those patients without a known history of cognitive impairment or dementia. Given that this group is at risk for poor postoperative outcomes, early recognition of cognitive impairment is crucial and early implementation of strategies to mitigate delirium are necessary. The Mini-Cog test, consisting of three item recall and a clock-drawing exercise, has been validated in geriatric surgical patients. Other prediction tools exist including the clinical prediction rule developed by Marcantonio and colleagues which stratifies patients into low, medium, or high delirium risk based on preoperative parameters. Risk factors considered in the Marcantonio rule include age, alcohol use disorder, cognitive impairment, activity level, electrolyte derangements, and type of surgical procedure.

Delirium prevention strategies have been identified and are recommended for postoperative patients, particularly those who require intensive care. The Intensive Care Unit (ICU) Liberation Bundle has been developed and promulgated by the Society of Critical Care Medicine (SCCM) and is available at sccm.org. The key elements of the bundle include assessment, prevention, and management of pain; coordination of both spontaneous awakening trials and spontaneous breathing trials; choice of analgesia and sedation; assessment, prevention, and management of delirium; early mobility and exercise; and family engagement and empowerment. Use of this bundle has been demonstrated to reduce delirium by 25–50%, decrease the likelihood of hospital death, prevent ICU readmission, and reduce discharges to rehabilitation facilities. The various elements of the ICU Liberation Bundle (Table 3.2) incidentally adhere to an alphabetical acronym familiar to the acute care surgeon.

Nutrition

Protein calorie malnutrition is common among older adults and associated with postoperative complications including infection, wound complications, readmissions, and falls. The prevalence of malnutrition may be as high as 50% in older patients who are residing in rehabilitation facilities although lower prevalence is seen among community-dwelling older adults (around 5%). Screening for malnutrition and interventions to improve nutritional status have been associated with decreased length of hospital stay and improved surgical outcomes. A simple screening tool supported by the American College of Surgeons Strong for Surgery quality improvement initiative recommends assessing preoperative patients for the following factors: Body Mass Index (BMI) <19, unintentional weight loss (>8 pounds in past 3 months), poor appetite or eating fewer than 2 meals per day or less than 50% of each meal, or inability to take oral nutrition. Albumin level may be a useful laboratory screening study to identify patients who may benefit from nutritional optimization.

Table 3.2 Society of critical care medicine ICU liberation bundle

Element	Strategy
A	Assess, prevent, and manage pain
B	Both spontaneous awakening trials and spontaneous breathing trials (for intubated patients)
C	Choice of analgesia and sedation
D	Delirium: Assess, prevent, and manage
E	Early mobility and Exercise
F	Family engagement and empowerment

Oropharyngeal dysphagia impairs normal swallowing mechanisms and places older adults at risk for aspiration and respiratory complications. Basic aspiration precautions include elevation of the head of bed, sitting upright when eating, avoidance of sedating medications, eating small pieces of food slowly and chewing well, and supervision/assistance with eating when needed. Patients who experience coughing or choking with drinking, difficulty initiating a swallow, regurgitation, difficulty managing oral secretions, or globus (sensation of something being stuck in the throat) should be formally evaluated by a speech and language pathologist. A fiberoptic endoscopic evaluation of swallowing (FEES) may be needed to assess for proper swallowing function and aspiration risk.

Supplemental nutrition may be considered for those patients who are appropriate candidates. The type of nutritional support (enteral versus parenteral) and route (e.g., oral, nasoenteric, percutaneous endoscopic gastrostomy tube) will depend on numerous patient specific factors. The American Society for Parenteral and Enteral Nutrition (ASPEN) provides resources for managing malnutrition in older adults. They recommend screening all older adult patients, assessing their nutritional status, diagnosing malnutrition when present, and intervening with supplemental nutrition when appropriate. Healthcare focused on diagnosis and treatment for malnutrition has been shown to reduce healthcare costs, improve outcomes and quality of care, and support healthy aging.

Polypharmacy

All acute care surgical patients require careful medication reconciliation at time of hospitalization and in the perioperative setting. Older adults more commonly experience polypharmacy, which has varying definitions, but is generally recognized as regular use of at least five different medications on a daily basis. Specific medications may need to be considered in the treatment plan for older surgical patients. Anticoagulant and antiplatelet agent use, for example, are very common among older adults for treatment of conditions such as atrial fibrillation, venous thromboembolism, and coronary artery disease. Use of these agents may predispose patients to increased bleeding risks after injury or in the setting of surgical interventions. Careful attention to use of anticoagulants and early reversal of these agents in cases of life-threatening hemorrhage or traumatic brain injury may be necessary.

The Beers Criteria for Potentially Inappropriate Medications have been developed by the American Geriatrics Society and are applicable to all older adult patients. These criteria highlight medications which should be avoided due to risk of adverse drug events and associated complications. Originally developed in 1991, the Beers Criteria were specifically developed for nursing home residents. However, over the years, multiple iterations of these criteria have been developed and they now serve as a resource for all older adult patients except those who are receiving palliative care or hospice services. Specific medication classes, which should be avoided, include benzodiazepines, anticholinergics, and anti-histamines. Clinical decision support tools embedded within the electronic medical record, daily review of inpatient medications by a pharmacist, and education of surgeons may improve care by avoidance of Beers Criteria medications.

Geriatric Vulnerabilities

In addition to the specific geriatric vulnerabilities already discussed including malnutrition, cognitive impairment, and delirium risk, additional vulnerabilities may include impaired functional status, problems with mobility, and frequent falls. Functional status, and specifically preoperative functional dependency, has been independently associated with postoperative mortality. It is important to inquire about a patient's Activities of Daily Living (ADL) and Instrumental Activities of Daily Living (IADL) in the preoperative setting. These measures were originally developed by Katz and colleagues through observing patients recovering from hip fracture. ADLs include bathing, dressing, toileting, transferring, and feeding. IADLs include shopping, food preparation, housework, using the telephone, using transportation, medication management, and finance management.

Difficulty with mobility and falls are not uncommon among older adults. About one in three adults aged 65 and older will fall each year. Use of mobility aid has been associated with poor outcomes following operation and increased mortality. The Timed Up and Go test (TUG) may be used to screen for mobility problems and risk of fall. The test involves observing the patient stand up from being seated in a chair, walk 10 ft., turn, and walk back to the chair and be seated. A patient who requires 12 or more seconds to complete the task is at increased risk for a fall. Interventions to prevent falls may include environmental changes such as removing rugs and other tripping hazards from the home. Early recognition and correction of vision loss may also decrease risk of falls and the associated burden of injury.

Care Planning and Shared Decision-Making

Shared decision-making and care planning with geriatric acute care surgical patients requires frequent communication and compassionate consideration of the unique goals, preferences, and values of the geriatric patient. The surgeon must also recognize that goals and preferences may change over the course of illness. Older patients may weigh risks, burdens, and benefits of medical treatments differently, particularly with respect to the relative values of quality and quantity of life. The general goals of clinical medicine are varied and include prevention of disease and untimely death, cure of disease when possible, care of illness and injuries, improvement and maintenance of functional status, patient education and counseling, relief of pain and suffering, and provision of comfort and dignity in all situations. Thoughtful consideration of each individual patient's goals is critical to ensure the care provided aligns with the patient's values and preferences.

Capacity

Capacity is a patient's ability in a specific medical situation to understand the relevant information about diagnosis and proposed treatment choices, reason and deliberate around the treatment choices, appreciate the risks, benefits, and burdens of the proposed treatment and alternative treatments, and communicate a choice (CURA Mnemonic, Table 3.3). Capacity is decision-specific and applies in the medical setting. There are different levels of complexity involved in various decisions pertaining to medical care. While a patient may have capacity to make decisions regarding a simple treatment or test, they may not have capacity to make decisions about more complex operative interventions. Competence is a legal term, applies globally, and should not be confused or interchanged with capacity. When a patient lacks capacity to participate in shared decision-making, a surrogate is sought to make decisions on behalf of the patient.

Table 3.3 Elements of decision-making capacity—**CURA** mnemonic

Communicate a choice
Understand the relevant information about diagnosis and proposed treatment choices
Reason and deliberate around the treatment choices
Appreciate the risks, benefits, and burdens of the proposed treatment and alternative treatments

Surrogates

A surrogate is sought when a patient lacks capacity to make their own medical decisions. Different types of surrogates have been described in terms of how they receive decision-making authority. The patient may formally designate a surrogate through advance directive or other documentation, or the patient may informally designate a surrogate by notifying their physician verbally. The physician may identify a surrogate based on hierarchy established by state law (e.g., spouse, adult child, parent, sibling). Some states do not adhere to a strict hierarchy and instead allow any adult individual who has demonstrated special care and concern for the patient to serve as surrogate, provided they are available, willing to serve, and familiar with the patient's values. The surrogate may be appointed by a court, particularly when the patient has no other individual who can serve as a surrogate. Court-appointed surrogates are usually referred to as guardians or conservators.

The surrogate should follow a hierarchy for optimal decision-making (Table 3.4). The expressed preferences of the patient may not be known if patients have not completed advance care planning documentation or discussed their wishes with the surrogate. Substituted judgment is the next best option and requires the surrogate to make a decision that is consistent with what they think the patient would decide for themselves based on the patient's values and preferences. When expressed preferences or substituted judgment is not possible, the best interest standard is used to make decisions that best promote the patient's well-being.

A number of concerns may impair decision-making by the surrogate. First, the surrogate may not know the patient's preferences and may strug-

Table 3.4 Hierarchy for clinical decision-making

Entity	Considerations
1. Expressed preferences	• The expressed preferences of a patient with capacity takes precedence in all clinical situations. • In some circumstances, prior to losing capacity, a patient may have directly addressed the treatment decision at hand through an advance directive, living will, or verbal conversation. In these cases, the surrogate should use the previously expressed preferences of the patient to guide decisions.
2. Substituted judgment	• A surrogate familiar with the patient's values and preferences makes the decision they think the patient would most likely make based on familiarity with the patient's prior statements, conduct, beliefs, ethics, religion and/or philosophy. • Advance care planning documentation may be used as a guide.
3. Best interest standard	• Based on ethical principle of beneficence. • In circumstances where expressed preferences and substituted judgment are not possible, decisions should be made to promote the patient's well-being with considerations of risks, burdens, and benefits of proposed treatments. • Utilized by a court-appointed guardian who does not personally know the patient. • Used for emergency situations (exception from informed consent) where consent is unable to be obtained for treatment (e.g., trauma laparotomy in unidentified unconscious patient with internal hemorrhage).

gle to infer what the patient would want in the exact clinical scenario they are facing. Second, the surrogate may have impaired capacity themselves, rendering their decision-making inappropriate. Finally, the surrogate may not follow the patient's preferences and instead make decisions based on their own values and preferences.

Palliative Care

Palliative care is defined by the World Health Organization as an approach that improves the quality of life of patients and their families facing the problems associated with life-threatening illness through the prevention and relief of suffering by means of early identification and treatment of pain and physical, psychosocial, and spiritual problems. Etymology stems from the Latin word *palliare* which means to cloak or to provide protection. Palliative care affirms life and regards dying as a normal process and intends neither to hasten nor to postpone death. Palliative care is appropriate for patients with potentially curable disease or for conditions with expected complete recovery in addition to patients at the end of life. Palliative care is not synonymous with hospice, which is a program of services for patients with life expectancy less than 6 months. All physicians are able to provide primary palliative care, which should incorporate treatment, plans to provide relief from pain and distressing symptoms and to enhance quality of life and positively influence course of illness.

The American College of Surgeons Palliative Care Best Practice Guidelines recommend palliative care screening and assessment within 24 h of admission to the hospital for traumatic injury. This process includes identifying the healthcare proxy or surrogate, obtaining any advance care planning documents, assessing prognosis, providing information and support for the patient and family, addressing any urgent decision-making needs, and screening for further palliative care needs. Patients who would screen positive for possible further palliative care needs include those with potentially life-threatening or disabling injuries, one or more serious illness, older age, frailty, or any patient who is identified by the clinician by an answer of "No" to the surprise question (i.e., Would you be surprised if this patient dies within the next 12 months?). Patients who screen positive should have a family meeting to address goals of care and potential palliative care needs within 72 h of admission to the hospital.

Advance Care Planning and Goals of Care

Establishing goals of care with patients and their families is a central component of primary palliative care. Goals of care differ from advance care planning in terms of acuity. Advance care planning addresses future hypothetical healthcare decisions whereas goals of care addresses current actual healthcare decisions. It is important to remember that patients may not conceptualize their goals of care in terms of medical treatments; for many patients, their goals may be individualized and focus instead on relationships, family events, or avoidance of distressing symptoms. Early goals of care discussions are important and should not be deferred until an acute decompensation or deterioration in the patient's status has occurred. Likewise, goals of care should not be limited to discussions about code status and intubation as this is an inappropriately narrow scope.

Establishing goals of care and engaging in shared decision-making are not unique to older patients nor to the discipline of acute care surgery. However, three challenges more commonly apply in the acute care surgical setting. First, treatment decisions often must be made in an urgent manner due to the time-sensitive nature of trauma and emergency surgical disease. Second, patients often lack capacity due to the acuity of their illness and surrogates must be identified. Third, there is usually no pre-existing relationship between the surgeon and patient and thus no foundational knowledge of the patient's values and preferences.

Withdrawing and Withholding Therapy

There is no ethical or moral difference between withdrawing and withholding medical therapy. However, a psychological difference is commonly perceived by physicians, patients, and families. While it may seem psychologically easier not to start treatment than to stop it, the decision to withhold therapy is just as much a willful decision as the decision to withdraw. There is no recognized ethical or moral difference between withdrawing and withholding therapy. However, the decision not to initiate treatment which may potentially help ought to require stronger substantiating reasons than the decision to withdraw treatment that clearly has not been of benefit. In cases of uncertainty where a potential therapy may offer benefit, time-limited trials of treatment may be pursued with intent to reevaluate the patient's progress after a specific amount of time (e.g., 72 h).

Futility is used to describe a rare circumstance where the intervention simply cannot accomplish the intended physiologic goal. Clinicians should not provide futile care. More commonly, a potentially inappropriate intervention describes a situation where there is no reasonable expectation that the patient will improve sufficiently to survive outside the acute care setting or that the patient's neurologic function will improve sufficiently to allow the patient to perceive the benefits of treatment. In these circumstances, the surgeon may recognize that the treatment has at least some chance of accomplishing the goal, but ethical considerations and competing interests may justify not providing the intervention.

Care at the End of Life

Acute care surgeons often have the opportunity and responsibility to provide excellent end of life care for their patients. Approximately one third of Medicare beneficiaries undergo an inpatient surgical procedure during their last year of life, and almost one in five undergo a procedure in their last month of life. It is important for the acute care surgeon to recognize the changes consistent with imminent death. These may include functional status decline (bed-bound state), changing respiratory patterns, incontinence, delirium, altered sleep/wake cycles, and difficulty with oropharyngeal secretions and swallowing. The dying patient may have little or no desire for food and liquid; while perhaps distressing for family members, preventing a dying person from consuming food and liquid may actually decrease distressing symptoms of dyspnea, air hunger, and fluid overload. Symptoms of the syndrome of imminent death may be treated with the goal of maintaining the patient's comfort and dignity. Dyspnea may be treated with opioid therapy such as continuous or as needed morphine injection (intravenous or subcutaneous). Excessive oral secretions or difficulty with clearing secretions may be managed by stopping artificial hydration and nutrition, and using antisecretory agents such as glycopyrrolate, scopolamine, or atropine. Hypoactive or hyperactive delirium may also be observed and can be treated as needed with agents such as haloperidol.

It is important to remember that the words we use when caring for patients matter, and these words may carry even more significance with bereaved family members and caregivers. The phrase "withdrawing care" does not have a place in discourse; healthcare professionals should *never* stop caring about patients and their families. The phrase "withdrawing life-sustaining therapies" or "focusing on the patient's comfort" are more appropriate language to consider using as they reflect the objectives of such efforts. Death is not purely a biological or physiological process; death is a social construct and for many a spiritual process as well. The way we care for our patients and families may help facilitate healing, grieving, and understanding, particularly when a patient dies from disease. How and why we do something as acute care surgeons is just as important as what we do; in this way, the physician's presence, particularly at the end of life, may afford patients and family members comfort, meaning, and solace.

Geriatric-Specific Prediction Models in Trauma and EGS

Given the observed significant morbidity and mortality in geriatric adults presenting with traumatic injuries or emergency surgery conditions, much focus has been placed on the development of geriatric-specific prediction models that can inform care. Development of reliable prediction models is contingent upon availability of high-quality data in a large patient population. For older adults, outcomes post hospitalization are of vital importance, as loss of function/mobility and loss of independence can be devastating. Prediction models could influence multiple aspects of a systems-based approach to geriatric care. Modeling could influence whether a patient should stay at the initial presenting hospital, or whether they should be transferred to a tertiary facility if they are high risk. If staying at the same institution, prediction models could influence the institutional system approach to care by informing the team of specific risk factors and areas of concern that merit additional team member involvement (such as nutrition, physical therapy, and geriatrics).

In trauma, one of the most commonly known prediction models is the Geriatric Trauma Outcome Score (GTOS), which includes age, injury severity score, and a correction factor for blood transfusion in the first 24 h to predict in-hospital mortality. The recently developed Elderly Mortality After Trauma (EMAT) score predicts in-hospital mortality in older adults after traumatic injury in both "quick" 8 factor and "full" 26 factor formats that are available in a free mobile-based application. This was created and validated using the National Trauma Data Bank (NTDB) with excellent performance (area under the receiving operating characteristic curve [AuROC]) of 0.84 and 0.86, respectively. While these models are focused on in-hospital mortality, efforts are also being made to identify factors affecting in-hospital morbidity. A recent publication demonstrates that the Geriatric Nutritional Risk Index is not only associated with mortality, but also inpatient infectious complications as well. There remain significant challenges to developing a more comprehensive prediction model that encompasses geriatric-focused outcomes including complications, non-home discharge, functional decline, and post-discharge morbidity/mortality. Both short- and long-term post-discharge data must be collected on a national scale in order to create such models that are essential for informed discussion between care teams and patients moving forward.

In the Emergency General Surgery population, the Predictive OpTimal Trees in Emergency Surgery Risk (POTTER) tool has been established as a predictor of both complications and mortality in EGS patients and has been validated in mortality prediction for patients 65 to 85, with the ability to predict some postoperative complications as well in this age group. The EGS-specific frailty index (EGSFI) is an established tool that predicts frailty of patients requiring EGS and correlates with postoperative complications, failure to rescue, and mortality. As discussed above, there remain challenges to predicting long-term outcomes in the geriatric population, and creation of a centralized databank for Emergency General Surgery outcomes is still needed in order to pursue such models.

Opportunities for Improvements in Geriatric Care

In order to optimize care in the older adult population, early identification of patients at risk and implementation of pathways to mitigate that risk is essential. One targeted area in trauma and EGS has been early frailty screening with subsequent interventions focused on this vulnerable population. Studies have demonstrated decreases in delirium, loss of independence, length of stay, and readmission rates through such processes. The actual intervention varies between institutions however all carry similar themes: careful attention to medication utilization, early ambulation and engagement with physical therapy/occupational therapy services, delirium prevention efforts, geriatric-focused assessments, evaluation of social determinants of health and utilization of social work resources, and geriatrician involvement when able.

An ongoing area of investigation in geriatric care is where older adults should receive trauma and emergency surgical care. Research demonstrates that older adults are more likely to suffer from undertriage that affects outcomes, even in robust trauma systems. This has driven discussions in how to adjust initial triage criteria for trauma activation and trauma transfers to adapt processes to the physiologic differences and risk profiles of older adults. For example, adjusting heart rate criteria for activation in older adults due to beta blockade use that could prevent tachycardia, or blood pressure criteria given that negative effects of hypotension in older adults may really start at a higher systolic blood pressure than in younger adults. Ultimately, further integration of new triage criteria as well as application of the geriatric-specific prediction models discussed previously could result in more patients being transferred to Level I or II trauma centers. With our nationally aging population, this could significantly stress EMS transport processes and trauma centers. Ongoing work to evaluate what patients can safely stay at level III/IV or even undesignated hospitals is required in order to not overstress trauma systems, while adaptation of EMS systems and Level I/II centers to accommodate higher volumes will be necessary.

Regionalization of Emergency General Surgery care has been discussed in recent years, with suggestions that EGS systems could benefit patients similarly to trauma systems, with theoretical mortality benefits shown in modeling studies. Given that evidence demonstrates significant variability in EGS outcome for geriatric patients at different centers, and that older adults have better outcomes at high volume centers, it follows that regionalization could be particularly beneficial in this population. However, the practicalities of such patterns also require further study to understand how such factors as rurality, resources, and transportation could affect care redistribution. As discussed with trauma management, further study of which patients truly require transfer will be essential to manage the volume increase anticipated with an aging population.

National Quality Programs for Geriatric Patients

In order to improve the quality of care provided to geriatric patients, care needs to be taken to implement a structured program that guides practice patterns and tracks quality to allow for ongoing improvement. While individual institutions can create programs of their own, a nationwide approach to such efforts can be beneficial in multiple ways: national standardization of care can allow for exchange of ideas and programs to benefit evolution of care over time, large-scale tracking of data and outcomes allows for research and quality that benefits patients broadly, and individual programs can follow a prescribed pathway to adapt programs to their institution rather than having to build from nothing.

The American College of Surgeons (ACS) Geriatric Surgery Verification (GSV) Quality Improvement Program was introduced in 2019, with the aim of improving surgical care of older adults aged 75 and older. The program encompasses all aspects of pre- and postoperative care through its 32 standards, detailing topics including goals of care conversations and documentation, preoperative vulnerability assessments, postoperative standardization of care, and education for patients, providers and facilities on geriatric syndromes. Patients requiring urgent/emergent surgical interventions are included in this program. Early data suggest that implementation of this program decreases length of stay compared to a matched cohort, which suggests clinical benefit to patients and families as well as financial benefit to institutions. This program was designed to be accessible to institutions of all types and sizes and provides support through online resources demonstrating how institutions have been able to achieve success. For surgeons aiming to create geriatric-centered processes at their program, utilization of an established process can provide both practical and data-driven evidence important for institutional buy-in and success.

Coinciding with the ACS GSV program, the ACS NSQIP also introduced four geriatric-focused domains (cognition, decision-making, function, and mobility) as well as geriatric-specific outcomes (pressure ulcer, functional decline, delirium, and new mobility aid use) to improve NSQIP Risk Calculator performance. Utilization of these tools is another important step in providing informed care to older adults, allowing for shared decision-making with data-driven models of potential outcomes. Furthermore, increasing awareness of baseline vulnerabilities and their risks can also inform postoperative care planning and interventions that could improve outcomes. Integration of these quality measures at individual programs can provide markers of success important for ongoing institutional support, while also identifying areas for continual process improvement.

Conclusions

More than 10,000 people turn 65 years old in the United States every day, and the percentage of the population age 65 and older is growing faster than ever before. Healthcare systems, and specifically acute care surgeons, must be prepared to care for this aging population. A thoughtful and unique approach to the care of geriatric trauma and acute care surgical patients is critical to provide the highest quality of care and to achieve optimal outcomes. Surgeons must be familiar with geriatric vulnerabilities including malnutrition, frailty, cognitive impairment, delirium, and impaired functional status. Shared decision-making with older patients requires careful assessment of the patient's goals, values, and priorities, with individual treatment plans designed to meet these goals. A working knowledge of approaches to advance care planning, goals of care, and end of life is critical for surgeons caring for the aging population. Prediction models and national efforts to improve the quality of care for geriatric surgical patients will help ensure that the care provided is of the highest quality, ensuring optimal outcomes for the aging population.

References

1. Gale SC, Shafi S, Dombrovskiy VY, Arumugam D, Crystal JS. The public health burden of emergency general surgery in the United States: A 10-year analysis of the Nationwide Inpatient Sample–2001 to 2010. J Trauma Acute Care Surg. 2014;77(2):202–8. https://doi.org/10.1097/TA.0000000000000362.
2. Fakhry SM, Shen Y, Biswas S, Duane TM, McBride KM, Elkbuli A, Wyse RJ, Wilson NY, Garland JM, Kurek SJ, Plurad DS, Banton KL, Fisher C, Gage A, Hunt DLS, Lieser MJ, Shillinglaw WRC, Watts

DD. The public health burden of geriatric trauma: analysis of 2,688,008 hospitalizations from Centers for Medicare and Medicaid Services inpatient claims. J Trauma Acute Care Surg. 2022;92(6):984–9. https://doi.org/10.1097/TA.0000000000003572.
3. Fried LP, Tangen CM, Walston J, Newman AB, Hirsch C, Gottdiener J, et al. Frailty in older adults: evidence for a phenotype. J Gerontol. 2001;56(3):M146–56.
4. Morley JE, Malmstrom TK, Miller DK. A simple frailty questionnaire (FRAIL) predicts outcomes in middle aged African Americans. J Nutr Health Aging. 2012;16(7):601–8.
5. Plassman BL, Langa KM, Fisher GG, Heeringa SG, Weir DR, Ofstedal MB, et al. Prevalence of cognitive impairment without dementia in the United States. Ann Intern Med. 2008;148(6):427–34.
6. Kaiser MJ, Bauer JM, Ramsch C, et al. Frequency of malnutrition in older adults: a multinational perspective using the mini nutritional assessment. J Am Geriatr Soc. 2010;58(9):1734–8.
7. Katz S, Ford AB, Moskowitz RW, Jackson BA, Jaffe MW. Studies of illness in the aged: the index of ADL: a standardized measure of biological and psychosocial function. JAMA. 1963;185(12):914–9.
8. Pope TM. Legal fundamentals of surrogate decision making. Chest. 2012;141(4):1074–81.
9. Kon AA, Shepard EK, Sederstrom NO, Swoboda SM, Marshall MF, Birriel B, Rincon F. Defining futile and potentially inappropriate interventions: a policy statement from the Society of Critical Care Medicine ethics committee. Crit Care Med. 2016;44:1769–74.
10. Kwok AC, Semel ME, Lipsitz SR, Bader AM, Barnato AE, Gawande AA, et al. The intensity and variation of surgical care at the end of life: a retrospective cohort study. Lancet. 2011;378:1408–13.
11. Morris RS, deRoon-Cassini TA, Duthie EH, Tignanelli CJ. Challenges in the development and implementation of older adult trauma prognostication tools to facilitate shared decision-making. J Surg Res. 2021;266:430–2. https://doi.org/10.1016/j.jss.2021.04.016.
12. Bryant EA, Tulebaev S, Castillo-Angeles M, Moberg E, Senglaub SS, O'Mara L, McDonald M, Salim A, Cooper Z. Frailty identification and care pathway: an interdisciplinary approach to Care for Older Trauma Patients. J Am Coll Surg. 2019;228(6):852–859.e1. https://doi.org/10.1016/j.jamcollsurg.2019.02.052.
13. Becher RD, DeWane MP, Sukumar N, Stolar MJ, Gill TM, Becher RM, Maung AA, Schuster KM, Davis KA. Hospital operative volume as a quality indicator for general surgery operations performed emergently in geriatric patients. J Am Coll Surg. 2019;228(6):910–23. https://doi.org/10.1016/j.jamcollsurg.2019.02.053. Erratum in: J Am Coll Surg 2020 Feb;230(2):263–268
14. Jones TS, Jones EL, Richardson V, Finley JB, Franklin JL, Gore DL, Horney CP, Kovar A, Morin TL, Robinson TN. Preliminary data demonstrate the geriatric surgery verification program reduces postoperative length of stay. J Am Geriatr Soc. 2021;69(7):1993–9. https://doi.org/10.1111/jgs.17154.
15. Berian JR, Zhou L, Hornor MA, Russell MM, Cohen ME, Finlayson E, Ko CY, Robinson TN, Rosenthal RA. Optimizing surgical quality datasets to care for older adults: lessons from the American College of Surgeons NSQIP geriatric surgery pilot. J Am Coll Surg. 2017;225(6):702–712.e1. https://doi.org/10.1016/j.jamcollsurg.2017.08.012.

Physiology of Aging

4

Thomas K. Duncan and Mattie Arseneaux

Introduction

The elderly population, people aged 65 years and older, is growing at a rate never seen before. By 2030, the elderly are expected to make up 21% of the population. This will affect all areas of medicine, including surgery. The elderly population is four times more likely to undergo surgery. Approximately 1.5 million Americans older than 60 years old are admitted with an acute care surgery (ACS) diagnosis. In a 2010 study, over a quarter of patients required surgery, and this estimated to an amount greater than the cost to care for many other common elderly conditions including myocardial infarction, pneumonia, chronic obstructive pulmonary disease (COPD), and diabetes. The aging population is at a much higher risk for mortality than the rest of the population. The reason for higher mortality amongst the elderly can be partially attributed to their comorbidities, but also due to normal physiology of the elderly patient. Aging can be defined as "progressive cellular decline that results in gradual deterioration of organ function. The physiological changes are inevitable and irreversible, and can lead to loss of viability and increase in vulnerability to disease and eventual death." Elderly people do have less ability to remain homeostatic in the face of stressors placed on the body. Understanding the physiology of the elderly patient is important so that they are treated properly in order to compensate for the inability of their physiology to compensate in face of stressors. This chapter will discuss the physiological changes of each major organ system due to aging and how this affects the outcomes of the elderly population undergoing acute care surgery. Though the focus of this chapter is physiology of aging in the geriatric patient and its impact on acute care surgery, there will be a brief discussion on how physiologic changes also affect the presentation of elderly trauma patients in general, and how management patterns may need to be modified due to such changes.

T. K. Duncan (✉) · M. Arseneaux
Ventura County Medical Center and Community Memorial Health Systems, Ventura, CA, USA
e-mail: thomas.duncan@ventura.org; marseneaux@cmhshealth.org

Various Issues Specific to the Elderly Population

Frailty

Frailty refers to the decreased physiologic reserve that makes a person less likely to respond to extrinsic and intrinsic stressors placed on the body. This specifically affects the elderly population, and women are more at risk for this than men. There is not one specific frailty assessment score, but the Fried frailty criteria is commonly used. It includes greater than or equal to 10

P. Petrone, C. E.M. Brathwaite (eds.), *Acute Care Surgery in Geriatric Patients*,
https://doi.org/10.1007/978-3-031-30651-8_4

pounds unintentional weight loss over the preceding 12 months, decreased grip strength, self-reported low energy and endurance, low weekly energy expenditure, and slow walking speed. If 3 of the 5 criteria are met, then the patient meets the definition of frailty. Frailty scores help predict 30-day and 6-month readmission and mortality. In fact, frailty index score was more important than age alone in predicting outcomes in trauma patients. Two other factors that should be considered when evaluating a patient for surgery are sarcopenia and cachexia, which should be thought of when a patient has more than 10 pounds or more than 10% of their body weight unintentionally lost in 1 year. For planned surgeries, these factors should be modified with things such as nutritional protein supplements and prehabilitation. For emergency general surgery (EGS) cases, this is not possible. However, frailty should be assessed quickly pre-operatively in order to help provide patients and their families what their postoperative course could look like, which may be helpful in decision-making.

Function

Functional status is defined as all the components needed to perform activities of daily life. Functional status can be broken up into independent, partially dependent, and totally dependent. Functional status includes cognitive components as well as physical components. However, the cognitive evaluation portions will be covered elsewhere in the chapter. One simple, in-office, test used to assist physical function is the Timed Up and Go (TUG) Test. This involves timing how long it takes a patient to stand up from a chair, walk 10 ft. away from the chair and back and sit down. If this takes more than 15 seconds, the patient is at higher risk for future functional decline. Impaired function is a predictor of poor postoperative outcomes. Some believe it may correlate with higher rates of morbidity and mortality than cardiac metabolic equivalents. Function, like frailty, is useful in identifying patients that would benefit from prehabilitation. While it is not an option for patients requiring acute care surgical services, it is helpful in discussing potential outcomes and discharge plans with patients and their family members. It is important to know that up to 30% of older adults develop a new functional impairment during an acute hospitalization, and even 1 year after surgery less than 50% of patients are back to their pre-operative functional status. A recently published study assessed the functional status of the elderly after emergency general surgery admission to the hospital. The study contained over 70,000 patients. They found that people's functional status fluctuated after discharge. Within the first 5 years after discharge, 32% required new chronic home care. However, 21% of those that required chronic home care required an intervention on two separate occasions with a time of independence within the said 5-year time period after discharge. 11 months was the average time that chronic home care was needed. Half of the patients requiring home care returned to full independence within 5 years after discharge.

Nutritional Status

Elderly patients are commonly malnourished. It is a known fact that 9–15% of elderly patients in the outpatient clinic setting are found to be malnourished. 12–50% of elderly patients in the acute hospital setting and 25–60% of elderly patients in chronic institutional settings are malnourished. Protein malnourishment is the most common nutritional deficiency found in the elderly population. Malnourishment is associated with higher risk of peri-operative complications. It increases risk for pneumonia, infection, sepsis, increased length of Intensive Care Unit (ICU) stay, and 30-day mortality rates. Much of a patient's nutritional status can be obtained from taking a detailed history about the patient's dietary habits, recent weight trends, and physical exam. Unintentional weight loss of 10 pounds or more in 1 year is a risk factor for cachexia and should cue a clinician to further consider a patient's nutritional status. Other nutritional indicators that correlate with increased mortality in geriatric populations include serum albumin, presence of decubitus ulcers, dysphagia, and decreased mid-arm muscle circumference. Given how intertwined nutritional status and morbidity and mortality outcomes are, it is imperative to get dieticians involved early in the inpatient setting whether it falls under the pre-operative or postoperative setting.

Medications/Polypharmacy

Elderly patients inherently have more medical comorbidities and thus take more medications. Although this is predominantly an issue that should be dealt with as an outpatient, it is of paramount importance and must be discussed regardless of which phase of care patients are in. Elderly patients should be seen by their primary care clinician periodically to perform a review of their medications with goals of limiting new medications and eliminating nonessential medications. During the intake of a new admit of an elderly patient, it is critical to have a complete and accurate medication reconciliation. If there is any concern for inaccurate information, it is important that someone from the care team calls the patient's pharmacy and/or primary care clinician's office to obtain a complete list. Excluding certain medications can have detrimental effects during their hospitalization. While it is important to not start benzodiazepines as an inpatient for agitation/anxiety because this can increase risk of delirium, it is crucial to not exclude home benzodiazepines as this can cause the patient to go through withdrawal. It is also beneficial to avoid anticholinergics and antihistamines in the elderly population for fear of delirium. Many elderly patients have impaired renal function, and it is important to remember to renally dose medications based on glomerular filtration rate and creatinine clearance, not just creatinine alone. Pharmacists play a key role in helping provide total care to the elderly population.

Medical Decision-Making in the Elderly Population

Many elderly patients have cognitive impairment which may limit their ability to make their own medical decisions. It is important to ensure a patient has capacity prior to having them make decisions. Capacity involves four components: understanding, appreciation, reasoning, and choice. Determining capacity involves the clinician describing the different treatment options (both surgical and medical) along with their possible benefits and complications. If the patient is able to recite the treatment options, possible benefits and complications back in their own words, then they are determined to have capacity to make their own medical decisions. However, if they are unable to do this, it is advisable to have their surrogate decision-maker formulate the best care plan for the patient. Sometimes it is difficult to determine if an individual has capacity, and it is important to obtain an evaluation for capacity in these circumstances. Although some elderly patients have cognitive impairments, this should not eliminate their involvement in the decision-making process. Many elderly patients with early cognitive impairments can still provide some insight into their personal values and wishes regarding the decision to operate or not.

Elder Abuse

The Centers for Disease Control and Prevention (CDC) defines elder abuse as any abuse or neglect of a person over the age of 60 by a caregiver or someone with a relationship with the elderly individual involving an expectation of trust. There are five types of elderly abuse, including physical, psychological, sexual, financial, and neglect. Elderly abuse is suspected to be largely underreported secondary to shame, ignorance, and fear of loss of independence. CDC reports more than 500,000 elderly adults are neglected each year. It is important to realize that one third of elderly patients living in assisted living or skilled nursing facilities have experienced some form of abuse.

Elderly patients who have been abused are three times more at risk for all-cause mortality. It is critical for clinicians to recognize signs of elderly abuse and is mandatory to report it if suspected.

Neuropsychiatric

Physiology

The structure, function, and metabolism of the brain changes over time. The volume of the brain starts decreasing at age 40 but rapidly increases at age 70. Volume loss of the brain starts earlier in men, but the changes are more rapid in females once they begin. Areas of the brain affected most include the pre-frontal cortex, medial temporal lobe, cerebellum, and hippocampus. The pre-frontal cortex affects cognitive control and thus influences attention, impulse inhibition, and memory. The medial temporal lobe contains the hippocampus, amygdala, and parahippocampal regions which is important for episodic and spatial memory. The cerebellum is very important for balance and postural changes. In addition to structural changes, cognitive changes also occur and begin in the fourth to fifth decade of life. Memory is one of the major cognitive changes that diminishes over time. Episodic memory is most commonly affected, which involves remembering how, when, and where information was picked up. The blood–brain barrier serves to protect the nervous system from insults through selective permeability. However, as people age, the blood–brain barrier becomes more permeable. It is theorized that the passage of certain modulators allows for an increased inflammatory response and structural changes to the brain as well. The vascular distribution in the brain also changes with time. Capillaries are denser in areas of higher processing. However, this decreases with age. In addition, the intima of the arteries starts to thicken, and these changes lead to atherosclerosis thus increasing vascular resistance and decreasing perfusion. As expected, this causes neurocognitive function to decline. All these changes lead to increased risk of delirium in the acute setting and long-term cognitive dysfunction.

Clinical Issues

The pre-operative evaluation from a neuropsychiatric perspective is important, as delirium is the most common postoperative complication in elderly patients with up to 50% of them being affected. The single most important risk factor for developing delirium is dementia. Delirium is associated with increased length of stay, increased costs, complications, poor recovery, and increased mortality. There are numerous risk factors for delirium including increased age, alcohol abuse, and poor physical function. The type of surgery can also be a contributing factor as certain surgeries invoke more physiological stress. The Mini-cog evaluation has been identified as a good screening tool for cognitive impairment. It is good for screening because it is easy to administer and has shown evidence of validity. Identifying people at risk for delirium based on their risk factors and screening tools is important. Some studies have shown that a pre-operative geriatric consultation reduces the incidence of delirium in patients who undergo surgery for hip fractures. However, if the patient does develop delirium, having a geriatric consultation does not decrease the severity or length of time delirium lasts. Some drug classes are associated with increased risk of delirium, including benzodiazepines and antihistamines, and these should be avoided in the elderly population. It is also beneficial to minimize all centrally acting medications. However, this is obviously a delicate balance in postoperative patients as poor pain control can be a cause of delirium.

Cognitive dysfunction includes deficits in areas like as attention, learning, short-term memory, visual and auditory processing, and motor functioning. The duration can be weeks to months. It is not always easy to identify. It is associated with more complications, increases mortality rates, long-term disability, and early retirement. Risk factors include metabolic problems, previous strokes, and lower educational level.

Depression is another important component regarding postoperative recovery. It is associated with worse prognosis, increased recovery time, and postoperative delirium. Depression is more prevalent in elderly women as opposed to men and is often missed in the elderly population. A useful screening tool is the Patient Health Questionnaire 2 (PHQ-2). Sometimes depression can appear as delirium in the acute postoperative phase. For this reason, it is nice to have a good baseline prior to surgery.

A large portion of the neuropsychiatric components are more effective to identify preoperatively, which is not always possible in the acute care surgery setting. However, not all cases are truly emergent and being able to at least recognize those at risk for deterioration from a neuro-psychologic perspective is important. It is still sometimes possible to have time to consult a medical or geriatric specialist to help decrease the risk for delirium pre-operatively which should help in the patient's overall prognosis. It is also essential to recognize those at risk for depression as this may only get worse after surgery, and this could require beginning treatment while patient is hospitalized and have an impact on overall prognosis.

Cardiovascular

Physiology

The physiological changes in the cardiovascular system start with changes in the connective tissues. Connective tissues stiffen within the vessels and myocardium, decreasing the compliance of the tissue. This is due to decreased production of elastin, which is then replaced with less flexible collagen fibers. These changes ultimately lead to hypertension, similar heart rates and ejection fractions with decreased left ventricular end-diastolic volume, stroke volume, and thus cardiac output. The stiffening of the aorta causes an increase in systolic blood pressure but a decrease in the diastolic blood pressure. The lowering in diastolic blood pressure leads to a reduction in coronary blood flow. The majority of the stroke volume remains within the thoracic aorta. Once the aorta begins to stiffen, the pressure to move this volume, which is equivalent to the afterload, increases. An increase in afterload causes left ventricular thickening. Elevated afterload and myocyte hypertrophy causes an increased time of contraction. This extended length of time needed for contraction leads to a delay in ventricular relaxation. This delayed relaxation decreases early diastolic filling rates. However, the end-diastolic volume is preserved as it becomes more dependent on the atrial filling pressures. This leads to diastolic heart failure.

Up to 80% of the blood can be stored in the venous network at one time, which is important in maintaining a constant preload. Venous stiffening leads to the inability to keep the preload constant.

Aging also increases sympathetic nervous activity with raised levels of norepinephrine. Increased levels of norepinephrine is a result of increased norepinephrine release from nerve terminals and decreased in the metabolism and reuptake. It ultimately leads to an increase in blood vessel constriction and systemic vascular resistance (SVR).

The heart's beta-receptor also changes with age. The response elicited from receptor stimulation is decreased. This ultimately leads to a decrease in heart rate and contractile response to hypotension and catecholamines. The heart becomes more dependent on Frank-Starling relationship to maintain cardiac output.

These overall physiological changes of aging to the cardiovascular system leads to more hypotension and an increase in blood pressure liability during anesthesia. This alters the depth of anesthesia needed resulting in an increase in the sympathetic response to surgical stimulus.

Clinical Context

The elderly population should be evaluated from a cardiac standpoint prior to surgery. There are a number of risk calculators for this. Major cardiac events are classified as: myocardial infarction, pulmonary edema, ventricular fibrillation, and complete heart block. Two models frequently used to calculate the rate of risk for major cardiac events are the Revised Cardiac Risk Index (RCRI) and National Surgical Quality Improvement Program (NSQIP). RCRI is quicker and easier to use and more focused on cardiovascular outcomes only. RCRI contains six components, each of which receives one point. The six components are: elevated-risk surgery, history of ischemic heart disease, history of congestive heart failure, history of cerebral vascular disease, pre-operative treatment with insulin, and pre-operative creatinine levels of >2 mg/dL. NSQIP uses Current Procedural Terminology (CPT) codes and 21 additional data points. It determines the risk of a cardiac event in addition to mortality, rate of deep vein thrombosis (DVT), and other outcomes.

A large portion of the elderly are on medications affecting the cardiovascular system. Beta-blockers should not be stopped during the peri-operative period, as stopping them increases the chance of a cardiac event. Interestingly, some studies have shown that prophylactic beta-blockers in the peri-operative period decrease the risk of mortality in patients with an RCRI score of 3 or more. It is also important to remember that beta-blockers mask changes in vital signs when the patient is in shock. It is imperative to evaluate hypoperfusion using other markers including base excess, lactate levels, and urine output. These will help guide resuscitation measures. Angiotensin Converting Enzyme (ACE)-inhibitors and Angiotensin Receptor Blockers (ARBs) before surgery reduces the risk of morbidity and mortality.

Pulmonary

Physiology

The lungs reach maximal functional status during the early portion of the third decade before their function begins to decline. The lungs change structurally with reduction in number of cross-links between elastin fibers which ultimately decreases the amount of elastic recoil of the lungs. There is a decrease in the compliance of the lung secondary to changes in the intercostal muscles and rib vertebral articulations. Chest wall muscular mass lessens over time and may lead to a decrease in force produced by respiratory muscles. However, the total lung capacity is largely unchanged as the lessening in chest wall muscular function decreases the outward force requirements. Although total lung capacity is unchanged over time, the functional residual capacity (FRC) increases over time which means there is a decrease in the vital capacity (VC) accordingly. This makes the geriatric population more vulnerable to infection and damage. Aging also affects the gas exchange. Arterial oxygenation declines over time likely secondary to decrease in alveolar surface area and premature closure of small airways. Increased ventilation is often required to compensate for the decreased efficiency of gas exchange.

In addition to changes in the structure and mechanics of the lungs, there are also alterations in the upper airway. There is a loss of muscular pharyngeal support making the elderly more likely to have upper airway obstruction. However, their respiratory effort in response to upper airway obstruction causes an increased risk of aspiration secondary to their decreased protective mechanisms of coughing and swallowing.

Clinical Context

Pulmonary complications are more frequent than cardiac complications, and they are associated with increased morbidity, increased length of stay, and increased costs. Postoperative pulmonary complications contribute to 40% of peri-operative deaths in the elderly population. Postoperative pulmonary complications include pneumonia, respiratory failure (requiring mechanical ventilation more than 48 hours (h) postoperatively), atelectasis, and exacerbation of chronic lung disease. A risk calculator for the pulmonary system provides the probability of postoperative respiratory failure based on five pre-operative predictors: type of surgery, emergency case, dependent functional status, pre-operative sepsis, and high American Society of Anesthesiologist (ASA) classification. There are several risks factors that contribute to pulmonary complications. Patient factors that increase risk of pulmonary complications include functional dependence, weight loss greater than 10% in the preceding 6 months, and albumin less than 3.5 g/dL. COPD, obstructive sleep apnea (OSA), and congestive heart failure (CHF) are disease processes that also increase the risk of pulmonary complications. Surgical risk factors that contribute to pulmonary complications include operations longer than 3 h, urgent operations, operations requiring general anesthesia, and surgical site location near the respiratory system. It is thought that type of surgery may be the largest contributor to postoperative pulmonary complications. Although we may be able to identify patients at risk for pulmonary complications, it is difficult to alter their outcomes. It takes more time than feasible to optimize a patient's pulmonary diseases, improve their functional status, and/or their nutritional status. This is especially true in the acute care setting. However, having the ability to recognize those at-risk for postoperative pulmonary complications, especially respiratory failure, may help guide patients and their families about postoperative recovery and discharge plans. It could ultimately help in discussions of goals of care.

Gastrointestinal

Physiology

The elderly population is more susceptible to slower gastric emptying. It can take twice as long for the stomach to empty after a standard meal. Gastric acid secretion decreases with age, which is a result of atrophic gastritis. However, this is not enough to cause clinical significance which would result in B-12 malabsorption. The pancreatic function does not decrease with age. There is a decrease in liver volume as we age, which results in a decrease in hepatic blood flow. This decreases the amount of endoplasmic reticulum, which can affect drug metabolism. Thus, the elderly are at higher risk for adverse medication reactions. However, this decline is variable per individual and can be different amongst different mediations. There is a decrease in synthetic function of the liver, which can alter levels of albumin and coagulation factors.

Clinical Context

The entire GI tract from stomach to colon has decreased motility in the elderly population. Slower gastric emptying results in increased risk of aspiration. Elderly patients should routinely have aspiration precautions in place. The use of nasogastric tubes is frequently necessary in the general surgery population. However, their use can increase risk of aspiration by keeping the lower esophageal sphincter open and thus important to not keep them in place longer than necessary especially in the elderly population, and not feed a patient by mouth with a nasogastric tube in place. A decrease in colonic motility leads to the elderly experiencing more constipation. It is crucial to keep the elderly population on a good bowel regimen. The elderly population's decreased gastric acidity and blood flow to the intestines results in diminished absorption of medications. The decreased hepatic function can also cause increased recovery time due to prolonged activity of anesthetics. The reduction in hepatic blood flow equates to a decline in clearance of medications with high hepatic extraction such as Fentanyl, Ketamine, and Morphine. It is important to keep track of labs such as prothrombin time, partial thromboplastin time, and fibrinogen levels in patient's where there is concern for bleeding given a decrease in synthetic liver function with aging.

Renal/Volume/Electrolytes

Physiology

Age-related kidney functional decline is well documented. Males are more affected than females in regard to renal dysfunction, and this is due to vascular changes and androgen production. Aging affects both creatinine clearance and glomerular filtration rate, which makes the elderly not only prone to chronic changes in the kidney but also more susceptible to acute kidney injury. These changes in the elderly happen due to alterations in the renal vasculature, which are due to intimal and medial hypertrophy. These shift leads to a decrease in actual blood flow and the proportion that reaches the kidneys. This decrease in blood flow to the kidneys results in a reduction in the elderly population's ability to autoregulate their volume status. Serum creatinine should not be used alone to assess kidney function as this can be influenced by non-kidney factors like total muscle mass, age, sex, and race. Kidney disease can go unnoticed in the elderly population because creatinine clearance can decrease without affecting serum creatinine levels.

The elderly population also has a slower responsiveness to sodium changes resulting in the ability to dilute or concentrate their urine which ultimately affects their volume status. Other electrolytes and ions are also affected in a similar manner. There are pharmacokinetic changes involving absorption, distribution, metabolism, and excretion of medications. There is overall decrease in the systemic clearance of medications that are eliminated unchanged by the kidney.

Clinical Context

In patients over the age of 70, pre-operative renal impairment has been proven to be an independent risk factor for 6-month mortality. Postoperative renal complications are also a predictor of long-term survival. Risk factors for postoperative acute kidney injury include age greater than 59 years, emergent surgery, liver disease, body mass index (BMI) of 32 or more, high risk surgery, peripheral arterial disease, and COPD requiring bronchodilators. Pre-operative management includes avoiding hypotension and hypovolemia, correcting electrolyte imbalances, and avoiding nephrotoxic medications. Under-resuscitation is seen in smaller hospitals and is associated with decreased survival and worsening chronic renal failure. It is also important to dose adjust medications that are renally cleared or metabolized. It is critical to record strict intake and output measurements both pre-operatively and postoperatively to help manage fluid status carefully.

Endocrine

Physiology

Over half of the population older than 80 years old have impaired glucose intolerance, secondary to a decrease in beta cell production of insulin and an increase in insulin resistance. Insulin resistance is a result of poor diet, increased amount of intra-abdominal fat, and a decrease in muscle mass.

Women typically go through menopause during the sixth decade of life when estrogen levels are lower and follicle-stimulating hormones (FSH) are higher. The drop in estrogen levels results in increased risk of cardiac events, loss of lean muscle mass, and psychological symptoms. In men, there is a decline in free testosterone levels as a result of an increase in sex hormone-binding globulin levels. These changes are fairly variable in men.

Clinical Context

Diabetes can affect multiple organ systems, and thus should be taken very seriously especially in the elderly population as they do not have much reserve. Uncontrolled diabetes can cause life-threatening issues including electrolyte derangements, dehydration, and wound infections. Hyperglycemia should be well controlled in the peri-operative setting but at levels safely achieved without causing significant hypoglycemia. A good target is to keep the glucose levels between 80–180 mg/dL peri-operatively. The elderly population are more susceptible to altered mental status and delirium as discussed previously, but this makes them less likely to be able to report symptoms of hypoglycemia. It is important to recognize that diabetes mellitus is a risk factor for postoperative congestive heart failure.

Common Emergency General Surgery Cases

Small Bowel Obstruction

Patients of all age groups have better outcomes if managed by a surgical team. Similar percentage of elderly patients and younger patients with small bowel obstruction (SBO) end up requiring surgical intervention. Elderly age alone is associated with higher rates of mortality after emergency laparotomy for bowel obstruction. Other predictors of morbidity in elderly patients with SBO include male gender, pre-operative functional status, chronic renal disease, COPD and need for peri-operative blood transfusions. When admitting a geriatric patient for small bowel obstruction, they should undergo pre-operative risk stratification and medical optimization as many of them undergo a period of non-operative management. Generally, there is also time for a clear goals of care discussion.

Acute Mesenteric Ischemia

The pathophysiology of mesenteric ischemia, including arterial or venous embolism or even non-occlusive pathologies occurs more frequently in the elderly population. This is not always an easy diagnosis to make especially early on in its course. However, it should be considered in those with low flow state, atrial arrythmias not on anticoagulation or new onset arrythmias with generalized abdominal pain. Some studies have suggested that a d-dimer can be used as a screening tool with 60–84.6% sensitivity rates. The initial treatment is with fluid resuscitation regardless of the pathophysiology. Patients with arterial thrombosis as the cause should be considered for surgical embolectomy and bowel resection if necessary. However, percutaneous endovascular approaches can be a successful means of treatment in some instances. The endovascular approach can be used if the problem is identified early with some studies showing decreased mortality, bowel resection, and need for total parenteral nutrition. Venous occlusive disease involves intravenous (IV) hydration, bowel rest, and anticoagulation with frequent monitoring for bowel necrosis that would require surgical intervention. Non-occlusive disease is treated with IV hydration and treatment of the underlying cause.

Diverticulitis

Diverticular disease is typically a disease of the elderly population. However, the mainstay of treatment is the same regardless of age. Frank perforation, sepsis, or failed medical management still results in sigmoidectomy, sigmoidectomy with diverting loop ileostomy, or classic Hartmann's procedure. The elderly population has worse outcomes after emergency operation with age being an independent risk factor. There is a 20% mortality rate for those undergoing a Hartmann's procedure after the age of 80. Elderly patients who undergo a Hartmann's procedure are more unlikely to be offered an ostomy reversal given the increased morbidity and mortality associated with it. This information can be useful in discussion with patients and their family members regarding treatment options and possible surgical intervention. It is also important to note that those aged 65 or older with end stage renal disease (ESRD) are at increased risk of morbidity and mortality postoperatively even if undergoing elective surgery for diverticular disease.

Trauma

Although this chapter focuses mostly on Acute Care Surgery and the elderly population, they also make a large portion of the trauma population and will continue to increase in proportion compared to other age groups. Thus, we decided to devote a short segment to some of the most common injuries the elderly population experiences.

Elderly trauma patients suffer worse outcomes in the immediate postinjury phase and long term than those with similar injuries but younger in age. Treating the injuries of the elderly trauma patients more frequently results in congestive heart failure exacerbations, respiratory failure, acute kidney injury, and infection. Elderly trauma patients are more likely to undergo reinjury and death for as long as 5 years from the time of initial injury. The more chronic medical conditions a patient has increases their risk of trauma-related mortality. Injury severity score (ISS) above 25 also increases the risk of fatality in elderly trauma patients. It is beneficial to remember elderly patients have less reserve, and thus higher suspicion for occult shock is imperative in their management. Also, because they have less physiologic reserve and some of their medications may mask signs such as tachycardia, it is important to consider early operative management when indicated as they may not tolerate failure of non-operative treatment. Consultation of medicine service to help manage comorbidities and end-of-life issues has proven to be beneficial.

Falls

Falls are the most common mechanism of injury in the elderly population. 55% of all unintentional injuries resulting in death in the elderly population are due to falls. Gait disturbances, worsening proprioception, and peripheral neuropathy are all part of aging and contribute to the increased rate of falls in the elderly population. There are a number of risk factors for falls; they can be extrinsic, intrinsic, and environmental. Old age, history of falls, functional impairment, use of walking assist device, dementia, and balance impairment all contribute to falls. Medications such as beta-blockers or sedatives can contribute to orthostatic hypotension or worsening proprioception/gait disturbances which leads to more falls as well. Some environmental factors include particular footwear, poor lighting, and rugs. Increasing number of elderly patients are on anticoagulation, and these are associated with increased mortality, morbidity, and increased length of stay in ICU for those who experience traumatic falls. Fall intervention programs have been shown to decrease falls by 19%. Physical strength and conditioning evidence-based exercise programs improve overall fitness which also reduces the rates of falls. Requiring trauma centers to screen and offer fall prevention interventions and developing best practices may prevent elderly falls.

Rib Fractures

Torso trauma is the second most common cause of mortality amongst elderly trauma patients. This includes blunt chest trauma and rib fractures which occur commonly in the elderly population. Treatment of blunt chest trauma including pneumothorax, hemothorax, and rib fractures remains the same amongst elderly and young patients. In people older than 65 years, mortality rate increases by 19% and the rate of pneumonia increases by 27% for each rib fracture. The strongest predictors of mortality after rib fractures in the elderly include admission to a trauma facility, intubations, increased age, increased ISS score, and preexisting congestive heart failure. There is evidence that admitting elderly patients with multiple rib fractures to the ICU has improved outcomes. In one study, they had a decreased length in-hospital mortality and more of them discharged to home from the hospital.

Traumatic Brain Injury

The highest mortality rate for elderly trauma patients is associated with head injuries. Their assessment can be difficult as they may already suffer from neurocognitive issues and more affected by opioids or other sedatives. Clinicians should maintain a high index of suspicion and obtain an early computerized tomography (CT) of the head if traumatic brain injury is suspected. As discussed previously in the chapter, elderly patients have decreased intracranial volume which can lead to vascular shearing injuries. More intracranial space due to decreased intracranial volume means larger intracranial hemorrhage is required to increase the intracranial pressure and cause a midline shift.

References

1. Nashi R, Misra D. Special considerations in geriatric populations. Arthritis Care Res. 2020;72(S10):731–7. https://doi.org/10.1002/acr.24342.
2. Dewan SK, Zheng SB, Xia SJ. Preoperative geriatric assessment: comprehensive, multidisciplinary and proactive. Eur J Intern Med. 2012;23(6):487–94. https://doi.org/10.1016/j.ejim.2012.06.009.
3. Katz M, Silverstein N, Coll P, et al. Erratum to ``surgical care of the geriatric patient'' Current Problems in Surgery. [YMSG 56(7) (2019) 260–329]. Curr Probl Surg. 2019;56(12):100647. https://doi.org/10.1016/j.cpsurg.2019.100647.
4. Nakhaie M, Tsai A. Preoperative assessment of geriatric patients. Anesthesiol Clin. 2015;33(3):471–80. https://doi.org/10.1016/j.anclin.2015.05.005.
5. Sharoky CE. Not all is lost: dynamic functional recovery in older adults following emergency general surgery. J Trauma Acute Care Surg. 2022;93(1):74. https://doi.org/10.1097/ta.0000000000003657.
6. CDC. Understanding elder abuse–centers for disease control and prevention. https://www.cdc.gov/violenceprevention/pdf/em-factsheet-a.pdf. Accessed 14 Aug 14 2022.

7. Alvis BD, Hughes CG. Physiology considerations in geriatric patients. Anesthesiol Clin. 2015;33(3):447–56. https://doi.org/10.1016/j.anclin.2015.05.003.
8. Asensio JA, Trunkey DD. Current therapy of trauma and surgical critical care. 2nd ed. Philadelphia: Elsevier; 2016.
9. Diaz G, Lamb A, Cahatol I, Frugoli A, Romero J, Duncan T. A comparative study on the effects of matter of balance and TaiChi on measures of balance in community-dwelling older adults. J Prev Med Healthc. 2021;3(1):1023.
10. Duncan TK, Waxman K, Faul M, Bilal M, Diaz G. An evaluation of a community fall prevention program to prevent recurrent falls among older adults. J Prev Med Healthc. 2021;3(1):1023.
11. Allee L, Faul M, Guntipalli P, Burke PA, Rao SR, Reed DN, Gross R, Duncan TK, Palmieri TL, Cooper Z, Bulger EM, Stewart RM, Kuhls DA. 2021. The role of the US trauma centers in older adult fall prevention: a national survey. Am Surg. 2021;102–109. https://doi.org/10.1177/00031348211047509.

5 Frailty in Geriatric Trauma and Emergency General Surgery

Khaled El-Qawaqzeh, Hamidreza Hosseinpour, Sai Krishna Bhogadi, and Bellal Joseph

Overview

Currently, in the United States, the fastest growing demographic is geriatric (age ≥65 years). In 2014, 15% of the population was geriatric, and by 2030, it will grow to 21%. Approximately 41% of all annual in-patient surgeries in the United States are already being performed in the older population subset. Geriatric trauma has increased as a proportion of trauma patients in trauma registries and is hypothesized to be underestimated because of care provided at lower level or non-trauma centers. Geriatric individuals report an increasing prevalence of chronic health conditions; thus, trauma/acute care surgeons will frequently be faced with the care of older patients who often present with unique diagnostic and therapeutic challenges.

Trauma is generally considered to affect primarily the young population, with the older population being perceived as sedentary and less active. However, the traditional norm is changing, and older adults are becoming better at maintaining their health, placing them at risk for trauma from an active lifestyle. These trends, in addition to falls, burns, and motor vehicle crashes that affect frail elders, result in trauma becoming a leading cause of morbidity and mortality in the elderly.

Those 65 years and older have higher rates of surgery compared with others. Consequently, the inherent risk of having an emergency procedure combined with older age results in worse outcomes and the utilization of more resources. Geriatric emergency general surgery includes a diverse range of disorders with distinct disease processes, presentations, and management issues. The most common conditions include acute diverticulitis, mesenteric ischemia, acute cholecystitis, and acute appendicitis.

Aging is associated with anatomical and physiological changes that further complicate the management of acute care surgery in the elderly population. Older adults also have distinct physical and social vulnerabilities, as well as unique goals for their care, that warrant a more thorough and individualized approach to surgery. However, factors besides age need to be considered when caring for geriatric acute care surgery patients. Prior research has shown that frailty is a better predictor of mortality and morbidity compared with chronological age in this population. Frailty is defined as a state of vulnerability to poor outcomes that is independent of age. Frailty is a combination of a multitude of age-associated factors, including extensive comorbidities, cognitive impairment, social isolation, functional impairment, sedentary behaviors, sarcopenia, and

K. El-Qawaqzeh · H. Hosseinpour · S. K. Bhogadi
B. Joseph (✉)
Department of Surgery, The University of Arizona, Tucson, AZ, USA
e-mail: bjoseph@surgery.arizona.edu

P. Petrone, C. E.M. Brathwaite (eds.), *Acute Care Surgery in Geriatric Patients*,
https://doi.org/10.1007/978-3-031-30651-8_5

weight loss, that leads to an "accelerated aging" and a decline in overall health and physiologic reserve. Thus, surgeons must first better identify the frailty syndrome and then adapt specific treatment strategies to decrease potential adverse effects and improve the care that they provide for their older patients.

Frailty in Geriatric Trauma

Over the last few decades, multiple health care disciplines, including the field of trauma surgery, have focused on the concept of frailty to identify the subset of the geriatric population at high risk for poor outcomes following illness. Frailty, an indicator of senescence, is clinically distinct from age, comorbidity, and functional disability. The frailty syndrome is broadly considered as decreased physiologic reserve across multiple organ systems leading to an impaired ability to withstand physiologic stress. The prevalence of frailty in the geriatric trauma population is high, and understanding it is relevant for trauma surgeons because frailty is associated with injury following falls, frail trauma patients are more likely to develop in-hospital complications, and more likely to have adverse discharge disposition than non-frail patients.

Measuring Frailty

In addition to the traditional ABCDE's of trauma in the elderly, frailty assessment is an extremely important consideration during the secondary evaluation, when possible. Identification of frailty in the ED can help guide decision-making about patient management and the prognosis, and to concentrate early resources to patients most at risk for iatrogenic harms, functional decline, progression of disease, and death.

There are multiple models for defining frailty. Two popular models are the deficit accumulation model, which considers frailty as a reflection of health deficits across several domains (disabilities, comorbidities, symptoms, signs, and laboratory data), and the phenotypic model of frailty, which is based on the concepts of physical disability and energy depletion as predictors of worse outcomes. Based on the many different models defining frailty syndrome, many measurement tools have been developed to measure frailty, each with varying degrees of success in defining the full spectrum of this condition in geriatric patients. Examples include the Rockwood and Fried frailty indices, and the American College of Surgeons Frailty calculator. However, these models lack feasibility in geriatric trauma patients because they require assessment of up to 30–70 variables, many of which (i.e., gait speed and handgrip strength) cannot be performed on geriatric trauma patients.

Limitations of the existing frailty measures prompted the development of the modified 15-variable Trauma-Specific Frailty Index (TSFI) (Table 5.1), a tool designed to be specific to the geriatric trauma population to accurately predict worse outcomes including major complications. The TSFI has been validated as an independent predictor of unfavorable discharge disposition in geriatric trauma patients. The TSFI is an effective tool that can aid clinicians in identifying high-risk patients and planning care and discharge disposition of vulnerable geriatric trauma patients. The 15-variable TSFI is an equally effective predictor of mortality, in-hospital complications, adverse discharge disposition, and 30-day readmission compared to the more comprehensive 50-variable Rockwood frailty score. However, the TSFI was also found to be a stronger and better predictor of worse outcomes compared to the modified frailty index (mFI) and frailty scale (FS) in trauma patients.

The TSFI only requires the assessment of 15 variables, which has been proven to be practical in assessing geriatric trauma patients. It is simple to use, trauma-specific, tied to delirium and other markers we identify for patient care and does not require the assessment of variables, such as gait speed and handgrip strength that are cumbersome to assess in the geriatric trauma patient. The TSFI is a 15-variable score derived from the Canadian Study of Health and Aging Frailty Index (CSHA-FI). As the CSHA-FI is an extensive and time-consuming questionnaire that is difficult to

Table 5.1 Fifteen variable Trauma-Specific Frailty Index (TSFI)

Comorbidities			
Cancer history	YES (1)	No (0)	
Coronary Heart Disease	MI (1)	CABG (0.75)	PCI (0.5)
	Medication (0.25)	None (0)	
Dementia	Severe (1)	Moderate (0.5)	Mild (0.25)
	No (0)		
Daily activities			
Help with grooming	Yes (1)	No (0)	
Help managing money	Yes (1)	No (0)	
Help doing housework	Yes (1)	No (0)	
Help toileting	Yes (1)	No (0)	
Help walking	Wheelchair (1)	Walker (0.75)	Cane (0.5)
	No (0)		
Health attitude			
Feel less useful	Most time (1)	Sometimes (0.5)	Never (0)
Feel Sad	Most time (1)	Sometimes (0.5)	Never (0)
Feel effort to do everything	Most time (1)	Sometimes (0.5)	Never (0)
Falls	Within last month (1)	Present not in last month (0.5)	None (0)
Feel lonely	Most time (1)	Sometimes (0.5)	Never (0)
Function			
Sexual active	Yes (0)	No (1)	
Nutrition			
Albumin	<3 (1)	>3 (0)	

implement in the acute setting of trauma, the TSFI was developed to facilitate the clinical implementation of frailty under such circumstances. Its components include five domains that account for comorbidities, daily activities, health attitude, functionality, and nutrition. The total score obtained from the questionnaire is divided by 15 to obtain the TSFI. Patients can also be stratified based on their TSFI into non-frail (TSFI <0.25) and frail (TSFI ≥0.25) groups.

Association Between Frailty and Outcomes Among Geriatric Trauma Patients

Recent data show that frailty is more predictive of in-hospital complications and adverse discharge disposition than age alone in geriatric trauma patients. This trend remains true of both short-term in-hospital complications such as failure to rescue, rates of acute kidney injury, delirium, infectious, venous thromboembolism, respiratory, cardiac complications, and in-hospital mortality, as well as long-term outcomes, including long-term functional independence, trauma-related readmissions, and long-term mortality and health-related quality of life. Multiple studies have identified frailty as an independent predictor of worse outcomes among the elderly, and especially within the geriatric trauma population. It is imperative then, to accurately identify this high-risk patient population early in the course of management, to tailor care specifically toward preventing complications and achieving optimal short- and long-term outcomes. Indeed, adhering to frailty screening and multidisciplinary care pathways in the care of geriatric trauma patients has been found to be accompanied by a significant improvement in outcomes and quality of care. Hence, early assessment and identification of these vulnerable patients are critical in optimizing outcomes in geriatric trauma patients.

Optimization of Frail Trauma Patients

In surgery, frailty receives considerable attention because proactive intervention has the potential to positively impact surgical outcomes. Early assessment and identification of these frail patients is critical in optimizing their care by involving interprofessional teams and the implementation of focused and standardized management plans. The development of multidisciplinary frailty pathways for trauma and acute care surgery patients helps reduce length of stay, delirium, and 30-day readmission rates. Frailty pathways are multimodal, multidisciplinary, and successfully improve outcomes. See Table 5.2 for a possible model multidisciplinary frailty pathway.

Table 5.2 Possible Model Frailty Pathway (TSFI)

Intervention	Action plan
Physical and occupational therapy services	• Fall prevention education • Early ambulation • Meals out of bed
Nutrition; speech and language pathology	• Early nutrition • Vitamin D screening • Aspiration precautions (head of bed elevation, meals out of bed, and hydrogen peroxide mouth swab) • Bowel regimen to avoid constipation (nurse stool assessments every shift and avoidance of stool softeners)
Use of a standardized admission order set	• Avoid polypharmacy • Avoid treatments that can lead to confusion and delirium
Multimodal pain management	• Provide adequate pain control • Use opioid-sparing agents • Improve functional status
Cautious use of fluids	• Initiate timely de-resuscitation • Avoid fluid overload
Early engagement of social workers	• Identify a health care proxy (within 24 h) • Establish code status (within 24 h) • Discuss potential placement options after surgery • Family meeting
Proactive geriatric consultation/comprehensive geriatric assessment	• Comprehensive geriatric assessment • Engage inpatient multidisciplinary care teams • Address chronic concurrent illnesses • Medication management/prognostic assessment • Improve documentation of delirium • Nonpharmacologic management of delirium • Perform medication adjustment • Address goals of care • Trigger early palliative care consultations
Geriatric verified nursing care	• Have a geriatric surgery nurse champion • Promote evidence-based best practices for the nursing care of older surgical patients • Improve adherence and compliance with evidence-based best geriatric practices • Nurse bedside speech and swallow screen • Avoid overnight vital signs
Multimodal prehabilitation	• Nutritional supplementation • Feedback-based exercise regimens • Pulmonary optimization
Rigorous post-discharge follow-up	• Improve surgeon communication with the primary care provider for elective high-risk patients • Help facilitate the transition both into and out of the hospital

There is also significant interplay between patient-related factors in their contribution toward worsened outcomes in geriatric trauma patients. For example, frailty is independently associated with both worsened outcomes and with the development of delirium, which is in turn linked to worsened outcomes on its own. In-hospital delirium in geriatric trauma patients is common and is associated with increased morbidity and mortality in geriatric trauma patients and may even precipitate the injury, to begin with. Delirium is significantly underdiagnosed, especially in the elderly and more importantly, delirium is a predictor of threefold higher mortality and a higher cost of care. The presence of delirium should be routinely monitored and aggressively treated with a standard protocol to achieve optimal outcomes. Programs such as the Hospital Elder Life Program (HELP), which consists of multicomponent nonpharmacological interventions, and the Nursing Improving Care of Health System Elders (NICHE), which encourages a multidisciplinary approach to the care of older patients, demonstrated effectiveness in reducing incidence of delirium, complications, and rate of falls, with a trend toward decreasing length of stay and preventing institutionalization.

Frailty in Geriatric Emergency General Surgery

Approximately 41% of all annual in-patient surgeries in the United States are already being performed on the older population. As a result, acute care surgeons will frequently be faced with the care of older patients who often present with unique diagnostic and therapeutic challenges. Patients undergoing emergency general surgery (EGS) are more likely to die and to have postoperative complications compared with those undergoing elective surgery. Consequently, the inherent risk of having an emergency procedure combined with older age results in worse outcomes and the utilization of more resources. However, other factors besides age need to be considered. Prior research has shown that frailty is a better predictor of mortality and morbidity compared with chronological age alone in this population. The procedural risk level is associated with frailty and mortality in emergency general surgery patients, and preoperative frailty assessment should be strongly considered even within low-risk procedures (appendectomy and cholecystectomy).

Measuring Frailty

During the past few decades, quality of health care has become an important focus of outcomes research. Countless studies have examined outcomes after emergency general surgery in older adults. Predominantly, these studies have looked at mortality and complications as outcomes. The association between age and adverse outcomes is well established and validated, and several surgical risk calculators take age into account when assigning operative risk to patients. However, more recently the focus has shifted from age to functional status, and thus, frailty, as a predictor of postoperative outcomes in patients undergoing general surgery. Studies have also shown that for patients undergoing emergency general surgery, the frailty index better predicts complications and the addition of these additional variables to such surgical risk calculators may significantly improve their predictability.

Several models exist for the calculation of frailty index, as previously mentioned. The most comprehensive frailty questionnaire is the Rockwood frailty model based on 70 variables that assess the cognitive, physiological, physical, and social wellbeing of the individual. The Rockwood frailty index has been validated in patients undergoing elective surgery. More recently, a modified 50-variable Rockwood frailty index has been shown to reliably predict morbidity in patients undergoing emergency general surgery. Interestingly, using just the 15 strongest predictors out of the 50 variables, a similar pre-

Table 5.3 Fifteen Variable EGS-Specific Frailty Index (EGSFI)

Comorbidities			
Cancer history	YES (1)	No (0)	
Hypertension	YES (1)	No (0)	
Coronary Heart Disease	MI (1)	CABG (0.75)	PCI (0.5)
	Medication (0.25)	None (0)	
Dementia	Severe (1)	Moderate (0.5)	Mild (0.25)
	No (0)		
Daily activities			
Help with grooming	Yes (1)	No (0)	
Help managing money	Yes (1)	No (0)	
Help doing housework	Yes (1)	No (0)	
Help toileting	Yes (1)	No (0)	
Help walking	Wheelchair (1)	Walker (0.75)	Cane (0.5)
	No (0)		
Health attitude			
Feel less useful	Most time (1)	Sometimes (0.5)	Never (0)
Feel Sad	Most time (1)	Sometimes (0.5)	Never (0)
Feel effort to do everything	Most time (1)	Sometimes (0.5)	Never (0)
Feel lonely	Most time (1)	Sometimes (0.5)	Never (0)
Function			
Sexual active	Yes (0)	No (1)	
Nutrition			
Albumin	<3 (1)	>3 (0)	

dictive power can be achieved. The use of this 15-variable EGS-specific frailty index allows for a more rapid yet accurate assessment of frailty status of patients undergoing emergency general surgery (Table 5.3). For each question in the frailty index, a patient receives a score varying from 0 to 1. The sum of the final score is then divided by 15 to calculate the frailty index of the patients. Patients with a frailty index of >0.325 are considered frail and are at high risk for morbidity following emergency general surgery. This new EGSFI was found to be a strong and reliable predictor of postoperative complications and mortality among frail patients, proving it to be a simple and reliable bedside tool to determine the frailty status of patients undergoing EGS. A study compared the predictive validity of the EGSFI to other frailty indices and found it to have increased practicality while having superior predictive validity for adverse discharge disposition.

Association Between Frailty and Outcomes Among Geriatric EGS Patients

Frailty has been extensively studied in the geriatric EGS patient population. Frailty syndrome was found to be significantly associated with higher rates of worse in-hospital outcomes, including postoperative complications, failure-to-rescue (defined as death of a patient after suffering a complication), and in-hospital mortality. Frail patients have also been found to be at higher risk of non-home discharge disposition, such as discharge to a skilled nursing facility and in-patient rehabilitation. Interestingly, frailty was also independently associated with the development of postoperative delirium even in the EGS patient population, an alarming finding considering the prevalence, morbidity, and overall health decline associated with delirium.

Finally, frailty has also been associated with worse long-term post-discharge outcomes. Frail EGS patients had higher overall 30-day mortality after discharge, with an even greater association in low-risk procedures. Patients with mild frailty experienced a higher risk of 1-year mortality compared with non-frail patients (hazard ratio 1.97). In the year after discharge, patients with mild and moderate to severe frailty had more hospital encounters compared with non-frail patients (7.8 and 11.5 vs 2.0 per person-year; incidence rate ratio [IRR] 4.01 vs IRR 5.89). Patients with mild and moderate to severe frailty also had fewer days at home in the year after discharge compared with non-frail patients. Considering the worse pre-, peri-, and postoperative outcomes attributed to frailty syndrome, it is vital that we identify and address frailty at every point of intervention possible.

It is also worth noting that frailty may have implications for operative decision-making as well. Frail geriatric acute uncomplicated appendicitis patients were found to have significantly higher rates of mortality, complications, Clostridium Difficile infections, and total hospital costs when managed with delayed appendectomy versus those managed operatively on index admission. Similarly, frail geriatric patients with acute calculous cholecystitis who were managed nonoperatively on index admission were found to have worse 6-month outcomes compared to those who were managed with early cholecystectomy on index admission, including longer lengths of stay, increased mortality, a 19% rate of failure of nonoperative management, and higher rates of emergency operations and postoperative complications among those managed with a delayed emergent cholecystectomy. These findings highlight the need for further research into the optimal management approaches of common EGS procedures among frail geriatric patients.

Optimization of Frail EGS Patients

When possible, modifiable factors should be optimized if frailty is identified prior to elective surgery to improve the likelihood of favorable outcomes. Preoperative optimization can include attention to prehabilitation, nutrition, psychosocial factors, and possibly drug therapy.

Prehabilitation, consisting of nutritional supplementation, feedback-based exercise regimens, and pulmonary optimization, and exercise therapy can improve frailty and may be particularly important for frail patients with cardiac disorders. A reconditioning program for elderly abdominal surgery patients was found to improve both sit-to-stand time and timed up-and-go time compared to usual care. Improving nutritional deficiencies, including attention to vitamin replacement, protein supplementation, and iron supplement when indicated, may also be of value though more research is needed to explore the benefit of these interventions. Screening with a depression instrument such as the PHQ-9, and dealing with other psychosocial factors, including social support, and "will to improve" should also be addressed. Additionally, although the safety, benefit, and mechanism of "performance-enhancing drugs" (e.g., anabolic steroids) are unclear, it is thought that they are helpful.

Finally, a frailty identification and care pathway implemented at a hospital may be the ideal method of both identifying at-risk patients as well as reversing and optimizing their frailty status preoperatively. An example of a frailty identification pathway would use a validated frailty index such as the EGSFI as a screening tool for all elderly EGS patients. The frailty care pathway would then employ a combination of hospitalist/geriatrician consultations, nutritional/speech/physical/occupational/language therapist consultations, early family and social support engagement, social worker involvement for identifying social needs and goals of care, a specialized geriatric-specific order set, and thorough post-discharge follow-up plans in order to holistically and comprehensively attend to all of the unique challenges faced by a frail geriatric EGS patient. Such a screening and care pathway has already been implemented and was found to lead to reduced length of stay, 30-day emergency readmissions, and loss-of-functional independence. Similarly, specialized enhanced recovery after surgery (ERAS) pathways for geriatric EGS patients consisting of recommendations on perioperative glycemic and fluid management, temperature control, pain, nausea, and vomiting management, and mobilization and diet have also been found to result in shorter hospital lengths of stay as well as fewer postoperative complications. Likewise, prospectively implementing a quality improvement project called the Frailty Screening Initiative in patients who underwent surgery, decreased postoperative mortality significantly at 30, 180, and 365 days. Frail patients were flagged for administrative review by the chief of surgery (or designee) before the scheduled operation. Based on this review, clinicians from surgery, anesthesia, critical care, and palliative care were notified of the patient's frailty and associated surgical risks; if indicated, perioperative plans were modified based on team input.

Geriatric Specialists and Multidisciplinary Care

The sheer volume of geriatric patients demands that those caring for them, including trauma surgeons, become familiar with their special needs and requirements to provide optimal care. A multidisciplinary team approach (geriatricians, social workers, pharmacists, nursing, etc.) to the care of the hospitalized elderly patient has been shown in the geriatric literature to work best. Multidisciplinary care improves the quality of care because it addresses the associated comorbidities, improves processes and outcomes for geriatric syndromes, and provides value for the health care system.

Geriatrics has matured as a specialty and the geriatric patient population is now being recognized as a specialized population that should receive care in the hands of specialists trained in taking care of these patients and at specialized geriatric centers dedicated to geriatric care. There is emerging evidence that suggests that centers that handle higher volumes and a higher proportion of geriatric patients have better outcomes. Geriatric consultation improves trauma care by identifying additional diagnoses not readily assessed by the acute care surgery service, assisting with advanced care planning, managing medication changes, improving pain management, decreasing the length of stay, and reducing discharges to long-term care. Any significantly injured patient should be admitted by the acute care surgeon with appropriate consultation and multidisciplinary input as the initiation of mandatory geriatric consults is associated with improved advance care planning, shorter in-hospital length of stay, and increased multidisciplinary care. Ensuring the involvement of geriatricians aids in reducing adverse outcomes among geriatric acute care surgery patients. Additionally, geriatric nursing, using an acute care elderly unit model, has also led to improved care.

Acute care elderly units incorporate a patient-centered, homelike environment that includes plans for preventing disability and iatrogenic illness as well as providing comprehensive discharge planning and management. Some centers have dedicated geriatric units to provide care for elderly patients transferred from other services. Along with the inpatient care of elderly patients, these geriatric programs also emphasize and provide early rehabilitation services for these patients. The effectiveness of these geriatric programs has been evaluated in several randomized controlled trials. The largest trial randomized over 1300 frail patients to receive geriatric inpatient care or usual inpatient care. Patients who received geriatric inpatient care had significantly reduced morbidity and improved functional recovery quality of life at the time of discharge compared to the patients who received usual inpatient care. The overall 1-year mortality and total costs were similar between the two groups.

There are no conflicts of interests to report. The authors have no financial or proprietary interest in the subject matter or materials discussed in the manuscript.

References

1. Bonne S, Schuerer DJ. Trauma in the older adult: epidemiology and evolving geriatric trauma principles. Clin Geriatr Med. 2013;29(1):137–50.
2. Cooper Z, Scott JW, Rosenthal RA, Mitchell SL. Emergency major abdominal surgical procedures in older adults: a systematic review of mor-

tality and functional outcomes. J Am Geriatr Soc. 2015;63(12):2563–71.
3. Joseph B, Pandit V, Zangbar B, Kulvatunyou N, Hashmi A, Green DJ, et al. Superiority of frailty over age in predicting outcomes among geriatric trauma patients: a prospective analysis. JAMA Surg. 2014;149(8):766–72.
4. Joseph B, Pandit V, Zangbar B, Kulvatunyou N, Tang A, O'Keeffe T, et al. Validating trauma-specific frailty index for geriatric trauma patients: a prospective analysis. J Am Coll Surg. 2014;219(1):10–7.e1.
5. Hamidi M, Haddadin Z, Zeeshan M, Saljuqi AT, Hanna K, Tang A, et al. Prospective evaluation and comparison of the predictive ability of different frailty scores to predict outcomes in geriatric trauma patients. J Trauma Acute Care Surg. 2019;87(5):1172–80.
6. Joseph B, Phelan H, Hassan A, Jokar TO, O'Keeffe T, Azim A, et al. The impact of frailty on failure-to-rescue in geriatric trauma patients: a prospective study. J Trauma Acute Care Surg. 2016;81(6):1150–5.
7. Hamidi M, Zeeshan M, Leon-Risemberg V, Nikolich-Zugich J, Hanna K, Kulvatunyou N, et al. Frailty as a prognostic factor for the critically ill older adult trauma patients. Am J Surg. 2019;218(3):484–9.
8. Engelhardt KE, Reuter Q, Liu J, Bean JF, Barnum J, Shapiro MB, et al. Frailty screening and a frailty pathway decrease length of stay, loss of independence, and 30-day readmission rates in frail geriatric trauma and emergency general surgery patients. J Trauma Acute Care Surg. 2018;85(1):167–73.
9. Persico I, Cesari M, Morandi A, Haas J, Mazzola P, Zambon A, et al. Frailty and delirium in older adults: a systematic review and meta-analysis of the literature. J Am Geriatr Soc. 2018;66(10):2022–30.
10. Hshieh TT, Yang T, Gartaganis SL, Yue J, Inouye SK. Hospital elder life program: systematic review and meta-analysis of effectiveness. Am J Geriatr Psychiatry. 2018;26(10):1015–33.
11. Castillo-Angeles M, Cooper Z, Jarman MP, Sturgeon D, Salim A, Havens JM. Association of frailty with morbidity and mortality in emergency general surgery by procedural risk level. JAMA Surg. 2021;156(1):68–74.
12. Moutamn S, Bardiya Z, Peter MR, Narong K, Mazhar K, Terence OK, et al. NSQIP surgical risk calculator and frailty in emergency general surgery: a measure of surgical resilience. J Am Coll Surg. 2015;221:S130. https://doi.org/10.1016/j.jamcollsurg.2015.07.307.
13. Jokar TO, Ibraheem K, Rhee P, Kulavatunyou N, Haider A, Phelan HA, et al. Emergency general surgery specific frailty index: a validation study. J Trauma Acute Care Surg. 2016;81(2):254–60.
14. McComb A, Warkentin LM, McNeely ML, Khadaroo RG. Development of a reconditioning program for elderly abdominal surgery patients: the Elder-friendly Approaches to the Surgical Environment–BEdside reconditioning for Functional ImprovemenTs (EASE-BE FIT) pilot study. World J Emerg Surg. 2018;13(1):1–6.
15. Hall DE, Arya S, Schmid KK, Carlson MA, Lavedan P, Bailey TL, et al. Association of a frailty screening initiative with postoperative survival at 30, 180, and 365 days. JAMA Surg. 2017;152(3):233–40.

Hematologic Changes with Aging

6

Mark T. Friedman

Overview of the Hematologic System

Aging, generally defined as system deterioration over time, is a process that affects all cells, tissues, and organ systems, including the hematologic system. The hematologic system, in turn, is comprised of the blood and blood forming tissues, including the bone marrow, liver, spleen, endothelium, thymus, and the lymphatic system. Blood, itself, has important functions in: (1) transporting oxygen, carbon dioxide, nutrients, hormones, and waste products; (2) regulating body temperature; (3) regulating fluid, electrolyte, and acid-base balances; (4) coagulation; and (5) inflammatory and immune functions to fight infections. Bone marrow is important as the site of hematopoiesis whereby red blood cells (RBCs), white blood cells (WBCs), and platelets are produced. The liver has important hematologic functions in that it produces the majority of coagulation factors, natural anticoagulants (i.e., antithrombin, proteins C and S), and fibrinolytic system factors as well as albumin, a blood plasma protein that maintains fluid balance and transports hormones, vitamins, and enzymes. The liver also houses macrophages (Kupffer cells) and other immune cells (e.g., T cells) and acts to clear damaged RBCs from the circulation along with the spleen. In addition, the hepatic and splenic reticuloendothelial systems are paramount for recycling iron necessary for maintaining erythropoiesis. The liver also produces hepcidin, a hormone that is involved in iron regulation and, along with bone marrow, is involved in heme (a ring-shaped porphyrin structure containing a central iron molecule) synthesis. Both the liver and the spleen serve as sites of erythropoiesis during fetal development in the first trimester of pregnancy. Aside from blood filtration, the spleen, the largest peripheral lymphoid organ in the human body, plays an important role in the immune response and acts as an important reservoir of lymphocytes and platelets. Endothelium produces and stores coagulation factors, namely von Willebrand factor (vWF) and factor (F)VIII, and regulates the blood clotting process, both through inhibition and activation of clotting factors. Endothelial activation of clotting occurs through vasoconstriction and platelet activation via expression of vWF in addition to promotion of thrombosis via expression of tissue factor. Finally, the thymus and lymphatic system play key immunological roles.

M. T. Friedman (✉)
NYU Langone Health System, NYU Long Island School of Medicine, Mineola, NY, USA

Department of Pathology, Blood Bank and Transfusion Medicine Service, Mineola, New York, NY, USA
e-mail: mark.friedman@nyulangone.org

P. Petrone, C. E.M. Brathwaite (eds.), *Acute Care Surgery in Geriatric Patients*,
https://doi.org/10.1007/978-3-031-30651-8_6

Effects of Aging on the Hematologic system

Anemia is common in the geriatric population with an overall prevalence approaching 20% and rising to 40% and nearly 50% in hospitalized and nursing home patients, respectively. Although anemia in this population is often asymptomatic and discovered incidentally on laboratory testing, it is associated with increased morbidity and mortality in older adults. Common causes of anemia include nutritional deficiency (i.e., iron deficiency anemia), chronic kidney disease, chronic inflammatory conditions, and gastrointestinal blood loss, although, in many cases the etiology remains undetermined. Bone marrow age-related changes are marked by decreasing cellularity, from 90% at birth to 50% by age 30 and further reduction to 30% by age 65–70 years, and an increased risk of myeloproliferative disease and anemia. Fat infiltration of bone marrow contributes to these changes, which also affects the thymus, an important site of T cell production, leading to a decline in adaptive immunity in the elderly. Thymic mass notably declines 3% annually up until age 45 years and 1% thereafter, with approximately 10% remaining by age 70 years. However, it is unclear whether or not fat infiltration of bone marrow is an effect or cause of aging and whether the bone marrow and thymic changes are related. Nevertheless, elderly patients are less able to compensate for their anemia owing to the diminished volume of hematopoietic tissue. Furthermore, there is evidence to show an inverse relationship between marrow adiposity and bone strength, with increased risk of osteoporosis and fractures in the elderly. Declining growth hormone with advanced age also contributes to marrow fat deposition. Furthermore, hematopoietic stem cells (HSCs), once thought to be capable of endless self-renewal, have been shown to be considerably affected by the aging process, with shortening of telomeric deoxyribonucleic acid (DNA) length at the molecular level and corresponding cellular senescence with loss of CD34+ progenitor cell proliferative capability. The functional decline in HSCs also leads to myeloproliferative and immune deficiency-related diseases in older adults.

Liver aging is associated with impaired proliferative and metabolic functions with increasing susceptibility to nonalcoholic fatty liver disease and other chronic liver diseases such as primary biliary and primary sclerosing cholangitis. Intuitively, one might conclude that liver aging is associated with functional decline in coagulation (i.e., hypocoagulability and increased bleeding risk) considering the liver's role in coagulation factor synthesis. Yet, quite the opposite is true. This is because plasma concentrations of clotting factors, namely fibrinogen, FVII, FVIII, FIX, and vWF, progressively increase in otherwise healthy adults, some attributable to being acute-phase reactants (i.e., fibrinogen, FVIII, and vWF), while levels of natural anticoagulants produced by the liver are more variable. Rises in interleukin (IL)-6 in the elderly contribute to a proinflammatory state and rise of acute-phase reactants although it should be noted that IL-6 also has anti-inflammatory properties. Meanwhile, fibrinolytic activity is impaired in the elderly, mainly due to an increase in plasminogen activator inhibitor 1 (PAI-1) levels. PAI-1 is an acute-phase reactant but increased levels have also correlated with increasing obesity rates in the older population. Alteration in platelet activation also occurs with advanced age. Although the net effect is a state of biochemical hypercoagulability, this does not necessarily result in a high risk of arterial or venous thrombosis in the absence of other risk factors such as obesity, reduced mobility, atherosclerotic cardiovascular disease, and cancer. Nevertheless, the risk of serious bleeding, such as intracranial hemorrhage, does increase with advanced age because of increased risk of falls and use of antiplatelet and anticoagulant agents owing to high rates of cardiovascular disease and atrial fibrillation in this population.

Elderly adults progressively undergo a process known as immunosenescence, the decline of the immune system as one ages. Both the spleen and the lymph nodes, centers of innate and adaptive immunity, undergo age-related changes with loss of splenic marginal zone B cells and follicular dendritic cells and reduction of lymph nodes throughout the human body. Both B and T cells lose their ability to proliferate with loss of naïve peripheral lymphocytes and gain of memory cells. Furthermore, defects in B cell development lead to a decrease in antibody diversity and affinity. As a result, older adults have weakened immune systems, affecting both humoral and cellular immunity, with diminished ability to mount antibody responses to pathogens and develop effective immunity after vaccinations. In particular, there is an increased risk of pneumococcal infection because of a weakened antibody response to microbial capsular polysaccharides. Both neutrophils and macrophages have diminishing ability to phagocytose and clear infections over time. Macrophages have diminishing ability to produce pro-inflammatory cytokines, important signaling molecules, such as tumor necrosis factor, IL-1, IL-6, IL-8, and IL-12. Increased cancer incidence in the elderly is also linked to declines of immune surveillance and the removal of precancerous and cancerous cells.

Although endothelium is typically linked to the cardiovascular system, it has important functional roles in regulating blood flow, vascular homeostasis, and coagulation and, therefore, is integrally tied to the hematologic system. Endothelium lines the inner blood vessels, creating a barrier that separates clotting factors from the prothrombotic extracellular matrix components. Furthermore, endothelium secretes or expresses factors, including nitric oxide, vWF, thrombomodulin, tissue factor pathway inhibitor, and endothelin (a potent vasoconstrictor agent), that modulate platelet reactivity, coagulation, and fibrinolysis. Although coagulation has traditionally been viewed in two stages, primary (i.e., platelet adhesion, activation, and aggregation) and secondary (coagulation system activation leading to cross-linked fibrin clot formation), the essential role of endothelium in coagulation has only been more recently appreciated. As aging occurs, endothelial cells undergo senescence, a process by which cell-cycle arrest and pro-inflammatory changes occur, ultimately leading to impaired angiogenesis and endothelial dysfunction. Such changes, in turn, promote atherosclerosis, a disease involving lipid accumulation and inflammation in the arterial wall that is additionally triggered by risk factors such as dyslipidemia, arterial hypertension, diabetes mellitus, and smoking. Cardiovascular disease (e.g., myocardial infarction and stroke) is a leading cause of death and disability among elderly in Western nations, with approximately two-thirds of cardiovascular disease occurring in patients 75 years or older. As atherosclerosis progresses, with endothelial plaque build-up and greater degrees of inflammation, plaque rupture occurs, resulting in damaged endothelium, exposure to prothrombotic subendothelial matrix, and promotion of occlusive clot formation leading to adverse cardiovascular events, such as myocardial infarction and stroke.

Anticlotting Medications in the Geriatric Population

Elderly patients are frequently prescribed anticlotting medications, given their risk factors for venous and arterial thrombotic complications. Although these agents are not a natural part of the aging process, trauma surgeons do need to be aware of these medications and measures to counteract them as they increase the risks for serious bleeding events and complicate surgical management in the acute care setting. Table 6.1 lists antiplatelet and anticoagulant agents and their reversal agents in case of significant hemorrhage. Antiplatelet medications include aspirin (acetylsalicylic acid), a cyclooxygenase-1 (COX-1) inhibitor that blocks thromboxane A_2 production, and the thienopyridine (clopidogrel and prasugrel) and non-thienopyridine (ticagrelor) $P2Y_{12}$ inhibitors that target the adenosine diphosphate (ADP) receptor. Aspirin and clopidogrel are commonly prescribed in a combination known as dual antiplatelet therapy (DAPT) for high-risk cardiovascular patients. As these agents are irreversible, platelet transfusion (one apheresis unit) is the main intervention for control of significant bleeding. Guidelines put forth by the Neurocritical Care Society and Society of Critical Care Medicine also recommend a single intravenous dose (0.4 μg/kg) of desmopressin (1-desam ino-8-D-arginine-vasopressin, DDAVP) for con-

Table 6.1 Anticlotting agents by class

Therapeutic class	Drug	Administration route	Reversal
Antiplatelet agents			
Cyclo-oxygenase (COX)-1 inhibitor	Aspirin	Oral	Platelet transfusion DDAVP 0.3–0.4 mg/kg
Phosphodiesterase inhibitors	Cilostazol	Oral	
	Dipyridamole[a]		
$P2Y_{12}$/ADP receptor inhibitors	Clopidogrel	Oral	
	Prasugrel		
	Ticagrelor		
	Cangrelor	Intravenous	
Glycoprotein IIb/IIIa inhibitors	Abciximab	Intravenous	
	Eptifibatide		
	Tirofiban		
Vitamin K antagonist	Warfarin	Oral	Nonactivated four-factor PCC[b] plus vitamin K
Heparin			
Unfractionated heparin (UFH)		Intravenous, subcutaneous	Protamine sulfate[b]: Complete reversal Max dose 50 mg 1 mg neutralizes 100 units UFH Reduce dose based on timing of last UFH dose (i.e., full dose if <30 min; 3/4-dose if 30–60 min; half-dose if 60–120 min; 1/3-dose if >120 min)
Low-molecular weight heparin (LMWH)	Dalteparin	Subcutaneous	Protamine sulfate[b]: 60–70% reversal 1 mg neutralizes 1 mg enoxaparin or 100 units dalteparin/tinzeparin Max dose 50 mg Repeat half dose in 4 h Reduce dose by half if last LMWH dose 4–8 h prior
	Tinzeparin		
	Enoxaparin		
Synthetic pentasaccharide	Fondaparinux	Oral	Recombinant FVIIa 90 mcg/kg: Incomplete reversal Activated PCC 20 IU/kg: Incomplete reversal
Direct thrombin inhibitors	Dabigatran	Oral	Idarucizumab[b]
	Argatroban	Intravenous	No specific recommendations; short half-life
	Bivalirudin		
	Desirudin	Subcutaneous	Four-factor PCC 50 IU/kg (max 5000 IU): Incomplete reversal DDAVP 0.3–0.4 IU/kg
	Lepirudin	Intravenous	
Direct Xa inhibitors	Apixaban	Oral	Andexanet alfa[b] (off-label for betrixaban and edoxaban) Nonactivated four-factor PCC 50 IU/kg (max 5000 IU)[c]: Incomplete reversal
	Rivaroxaban		
	Betrixaban		
	Edoxaban		

DDAVP desmopressin, *FVIIa* factor VIIa, *PCC* prothrombin complex concentrate
[a] extended release preparation available in combination with aspirin
[b] follow manufacturer prescriber insert
[c] substitute if andexanet alfa not on formulary

trol of intracranial hemorrhage, which can improve platelet function through its mechanism of endothelial vWF release. Hyponatremia and fluid retention may occur, though, when administering this medication. Nevertheless, variable response to antiplatelet medications is a well-known phenomenon, in part because of medication compliance issues, but also because of polymorphisms in the *CYP2C19* gene, responsible for hepatic cytochrome P450 enzymes which convert clopidogrel to its active metabolite, contributing to clopidogrel resistance (notably, one-third of patients taking the drug may exhibit resistance). Platelet function analyzers, using assays such as thromboelastography (TEG®5000/TEG®6 s Hemostasis Analyzer, Haemonetics Corp., Boston, MA, USA) and VerifyNow™ (Werfen, Bedford, MA, USA), can be helpful although turnaround time (in the range of 30 min to 1 h, though may be longer depending on laboratory set up) can be prohibitive in the setting of severe acute bleeding.

Warfarin, an oral vitamin K antagonist, is a commonly prescribed anticoagulant medication for high-risk patients. Its anticoagulant effect is monitored via the international normalized ratio (INR), a calculated measurement derived from the prothrombin time (PT) and the international sensitivity index (ISI) of the thromboplastin testing reagent as well as the geometric mean of the PT control range of the testing laboratory. Warfarin is rapidly reversed using nonactivated four-factor prothrombin complex concentrate (PCC containing nonactivated FVII) in combination with intravenous vitamin K. Plasma transfusion may also reverse warfarin anticoagulation but is inefficient due to the time it takes to thaw frozen plasma (although some hospital blood banks may bypass this by maintaining thawed plasma at all times, depending on their policy) and transfuse multiple plasma units (10–20 mL/kg is the recommended dose; thus, at least two units of plasma are required for an average size adult patient). In addition, there is increased risk of volume overload with plasma transfusion in debilitated elderly patients. Direct oral anticoagulants (DOACs) are also commonly used nowadays, given their predictable pharmacokinetics without the need for routine laboratory monitoring. These agents include dabigatran, a direct thrombin inhibitor, and the direct factor Xa inhibitors, apixaban, betrixaban, edoxaban, and rivaroxaban. Unfortunately, routine coagulation tests, including the activated partial thromboplastin time (aPTT), PT/INR, and the thrombin time (TT), are relatively insensitive for measuring DOAC anticoagulation levels. There is some limited evidence that viscoelastic testing (TEG® and ROTEM® [Werfen, Bedford, MA, USA]) may be useful for measuring these agents. The chromogenic anti-Xa assay may also be useful for anti-Xa inhibitors, at least for rivaroxaban and/or apixaban, particularly if calibrated for these agents. Reversal antidotes have been approved by the United States Food and Drug Administration (FDA), idarucizumab for dabigatran reversal and andexanet alfa for reversal of apixaban and rivaroxaban. However, owing to the high cost of andexanet alfa (reportedly over $22,000 per patient or roughly 3–4 times the cost of PCC), many healthcare facilities have reverted to using nonactivated four-factor PCC for anti-Xa inhibitor reversal, which may have partial effect in this capacity.

Low-molecular-weight heparin (LMWH, for example, ardeparin, dalteparin, enoxaparin, tinzaparin, nadroparin [Canada]) and related synthetic anticoagulant (i.e., fondaparinux, a synthetic pentasaccharide-specific inhibitor of FXa) are available for subcutaneous injection for outpatient acute deep venous thrombosis (DVT)/pulmonary embolism treatment and/or DVT prophylaxis as well as for prophylaxis of ischemic complications of unstable angina or non-Q wave/non-ST segment elevation myocardial infarction (NSTEMI). The latter agent (fondaparinux) has the advantage over LMWH in that it has reduced risk of heparin-induced thrombocytopenia (HIT). Unlike unfractionated heparin, the aPTT cannot be used for routine anticoagulation monitoring of these agents although such monitoring is not typically necessary. Measurement of FXa activity via the chromogenic anti-Xa assay; however, is more reliable for measuring the anticoagulant level. LMWHs have a much shorter half-life (4–6 h) than fondaparinux, which can exceed 20 h in elderly individuals. Protamine sulfate partially reverses the anticoagulant effect of LMWH while there is no specific reversal agent for fondaparinux; recombinant FVIIa or activated PCC (PCC containing FVIIa) may lessen the bleeding associated with fondaparinux.

Aside from over-the-counter and prescription medications, dietary supplement use in the United States is high among older adults, many of which may interfere with coagulation and platelet function. Notably, bleeding risks are associated with use of garlic, ginkgo, ginseng, green tea, saw palmetto, St. John's wort, and fish oil, among others.

Anti fibrinolytic agents (tranexamic acid [TXA] and epsilon-aminocaproic acid) are often used in the trauma setting to stabilize hemorrhaging patients. In this regard, the CRASH-2 and CRASH-3 trials demonstrated that early (i.e., within 3 h) administration of TXA safely reduced the risk of death in bleeding trauma patients and head injury-related death, respectively, and is cost effective. Thrombolytic agents (streptokinase, tissue plasminogen activator [tPA, alteplase], urokinase) are also administered in the acute setting for the treatment of ischemic stroke, myocardial infarction, and massive pulmonary embolism. Bleeding is a major risk of thrombolytic agents, particularly symptomatic intracranial hemorrhage (ICH). Transfusion of cryoprecipitate (ten units, typically given as two pools of five units) is the main recommendation for management of post-tPA ICH, although anti fibrinolytic agents may also be of benefit. There is less evidence for the use of platelet, plasma, PCC, or recombinant FVIIa administration.

Conclusion

Geriatric patients in need of acute surgical care present challenges and are at higher risk compared with younger patient populations because of increased frailty, polypharmacy, and other comorbidities, including increased rates of hypertension, hyperlipidemia, diabetes mellitus, osteoporosis, inactivity, obesity, and cardiovascular disease. Hematologic senescence contributes to worse outcomes in the elderly. Geriatric patients have increased rates of anemia with reduced capacity to respond because of reduced bone marrow cellularity and increasing hematopoietic stem cell senescence. Immunosenescence and immune dysfunction are also problematic in this age group. Pro-inflammatory alterations in platelet activation, coagulation, and fibrinolytic capability may promote a prothrombotic state, particularly when other risk factors are present, including endothelial senescence resulting in atherosclerotic changes that can lead to occlusive thrombosis and adverse cardiovascular events. However, elderly patients commonly take antiplatelet and anticoagulant agents that increase the rate and severity of hemorrhagic events. Trauma surgeons need to be familiar with these agents and measures to counteract their effects.

References

1. Lanier JB, Park JJ, Callahan RC. Anemia in older adults. Am Fam Physician. 2018;98(7):437–42. PMID: 30252420
2. Prabhakar M, Ershler WB, Longo DL. Bone marrow, thymus and blood: changes across the lifespan. Aging Health. 2009;5(3):385–93. https://doi.org/10.2217/ahe.09.31.
3. Wilkerson WR, Sane DC. Aging and thrombosis. Semin Thromb Hemost. 2002;28(6):555–67. https://doi.org/10.1055/s-2002-36700.
4. Yu Y, Zheng S. Research progress on immune aging and its mechanisms affecting geriatric diseases. Aging Med. 2019;2:216–22. https://doi.org/10.1002/agm2.12089.
5. El-naseery NI, Mousa HSE, Noreldin AE, El-Far AH, Elewa YHA. Aging-associated immunosenescence via alterations in splenic immune cell populations in rat. Life Sci. 2020;2020(241):117168. https://doi.org/10.1016/j.lfs.2019.117168.
6. Frontera JA, Lewin JJ III, Rabinstein AA, et al. Guideline for reversal of antithrombotics in intracranial hemorrhage: executive summary. A statement for healthcare professionals from the Neurocritical care society and the Society of Critical Care Medicine. Crit Care Med. 2016;44(12):2251–7. https://doi.org/10.1097/CCM.0000000000002057.
7. Ford NF. Clopidogrel resistance: pharmacokinetic or pharmacogenetic? J Clin Pharmacol. 2009;49(5):506–12. https://doi.org/10.1177/0091270009332433. Epub 2009 Feb 26. PMID: 19246723
8. Henskins YM, Gulpen AJW, van Oerle R, et al. Detecting clinically relevant rivaroxaban or dabigatran levels by routine coagulation tests or thromboelastography in a cohort of patients with atrial fibrillation. Thromb J. 2018;16:3. https://doi.org/10.1186/s12959-017-0160-2.
9. Derogis PBM, Sanches LR, de Aranda VF, et al. Determination of rivaroxaban in patient's plasma samples by anti-Xa chromogenic test associated to High Performance Liquid Chromatography tandem Mass Spectrometry (HPLC-MS/MS). PLoS One.

2017;12(2):e0171272. https://doi.org/10.1371/journal.pone.0171272.
10. Frontera JA, Bhatt P, Lalchan R, et al. Cost comparison of andexanet versus prothrombin complex concentrates for direct factor Xa inhibitor reversal after hemorrhage. J Thromb Thrombolysis. 2020;49(1):121–31. https://doi.org/10.1007/s11239-019-01973-z. PMID: 31664662
11. Yee J, Kaide CG. Emergency reversal of anticoagulation. West J Emerg Med. 2019;20(5):770–83. Published 2019 Aug 6. https://doi.org/10.5811/westjem.2018.5.38235.
12. Wang CZ, Moss J, Yuan CS. Commonly used dietary supplements on coagulation function during surgery. Medicines (Basel). 2015;2(3):157–85. https://doi.org/10.3390/medicines2030157.
13. Roberts I, Shakur H, Coats T, et al. The CRASH-2 trial: a randomised controlled trial and economic evaluation of the effects of tranexamic acid on death, vascular occlusive events and transfusion requirement in bleeding trauma patients. Health Technol Assess. 2013;17(10):1–79. https://doi.org/10.3310/hta17100. PMID: 23477634; PMCID: PMC4780956
14. Dewan Y, Komolafe EO, Mejía-Mantilla JH, et al. CRASH-3 collaborators. Effects of tranexamic acid on death, disability, vascular occlusive events and other morbidities in patients with acute traumatic brain injury (CRASH-3): a randomised, placebo-controlled trial. Lancet. 2019;394(10210):1713–23. https://doi.org/10.1016/S0140-6736(19)32233-0.
15. Yaghi S, Willey JZ, Cucchiara B, et al. Treatment and outcome of hemorrhagic transformation after intravenous alteplase in acute ischemic stroke. A scientific statement for healthcare professionals from the American Heart Association/American Stroke Association. Stroke. 2017;48:e343–61. https://doi.org/10.1161/STR.0000000000000152.

7 Sarcopenia

Christopher A. Butts, M. Victoria P. Miles, and D. Dante Yeh

Introduction

Background

The word *sarcopenia* is derived from the Greek *sarx*, for flesh, and *penia*, for lack, deficiency, or poverty. Broadly defined as a reduction in both muscle mass and function, sarcopenia is a syndrome, which results in a precipitous decline in functional status. Sarcopenia associated with aging is a recognized precursor to frailty and greatly impacts geriatric surgical decision-making as well as pre- and postoperative care.

While sarcopenia may develop acutely (usually within 6 months of a traumatic event), chronic sarcopenia is also common due to muscle quality degradation and fat infiltration of the growing elderly population. The prevalence of sarcopenia in the geriatric population is dependent on living situation, with higher prevalence observed in the institutionalized and hospitalized. When stratified according to mobility status, sarcopenia is found most commonly in those who are immobile and confined to wheelchairs as compared to independent ambulators and those who ambulate with assist devices. Not surprisingly, sarcopenic geriatric patients experience worse postoperative outcomes including increased need for ventilatory support, longer Intensive Care Unit (ICU) length of stay, loss of independence on discharge, worsened quality of life, and increased mortality. However, knowing the prevalence of sarcopenia in various populations alone does not allow for identification of individual, at-risk patients. Given the prevalence of sarcopenia and the postoperative risks associated with this syndrome, the following chapter will discuss the identification, treatment, and impact of geriatric sarcopenia, including strategies for perioperative optimization.

Relation to Frailty

Although age has traditionally been used to stratify risk in surgical, trauma, and critical care patients, chronologic age alone does not adequately define nor predict the true physiologic reserve and functional status of a patient. Recently, frailty has replaced age as a more accu-

C. A. Butts (✉)
Department of Surgery, Division of Trauma, Acute Care Surgery & Surgical Critical Care, Reading Hospital-Tower Health, West Reading, PA, USA
e-mail: Christopher.butts@towerhealth.org

M. V. P. Miles
Department of Surgery, University of Tennessee College of Medicine Chattanooga, Chattanooga, TN, USA

D. D. Yeh
Department of Surgery, Division of Trauma, Emergency General Surgery, and Surgical Critical Care, Denver Health Medical Center, Denver, CO, USA
e-mail: Daniel.Yeh@dhha.org

P. Petrone, C. E.M. Brathwaite (eds.), *Acute Care Surgery in Geriatric Patients*,
https://doi.org/10.1007/978-3-031-30651-8_7

rate measure to better predict postoperative outcomes. Various frailty scoring systems such as the Five Item Modified Frailty Index exist, but their universal applicability across patient populations is currently being evaluated. Previous studies have shown that muscle mass, often measured by psoas muscle cross-sectional area, correlates well to patient age, weight, and comorbid status, making it a robust surrogate for frailty. Psoas muscle cross-sectional area measurement is especially beneficial in patients who are unable to communicate their functional status or may not be able to perform an ambulatory exam.

Given the significant association of patient frailty with postoperative morbidity and mortality, many have sought to identify modifiable risk factors in the preoperative setting. Improving preprocedural frailty makes the identification and treatment of sarcopenia a potentially significant avenue for improving surgical patient outcomes.

Diagnostic Modalities

The last two decades were punctuated by several attempts to diagnose sarcopenia. Contemporary studies have expended much effort to develop optimal tools for diagnosing sarcopenia independent of the more traditional use of serum albumin level, body mass index (BMI), and weight fluctuations. Diagnostic modalities for sarcopenia most often rely on measures of muscle mass, self-reported exhaustion, handgrip strength, and gait speed. Below, the imaging and functional techniques commonly used to diagnose sarcopenia are discussed (Table 7.1).

Table 7.1 Summary of sarcopenia diagnostic modalities

Sarcopenia diagnostic modality	Description
Imaging modalities	
Psoas muscle index	Inferior lumbar vertebral level 3 psoas index on computed tomography scan, calculated as (right psoas muscle area + left psoas muscle area)/height^2
Psoas muscle density	Psoas muscle average density in Hounsfield Units (HU) is traced on computer tomography scan at the lumbar vertebral level 3. Calculated as [(right psoas HU x right psoas area) + (left psoas HU x left psoas area)]/total psoas area
Ultrasound measurement of cross-sectional muscle thickness	Using a linear probe ultrasound with minimal pressure at end exhalation, the muscle mass of the gastrocnemius, rectus femoris, rectus abdominis, and internal and/or external oblique muscle groups may be calculated
Dual energy X-ray absorptiometry	By dividing the body into bone, muscle and lean components, software may be used to differentiate lean muscle and determine limb skeletal muscle mass. Dependent on patient hydration status
Functional assessments	
Hand grip strength	Hand strength dynamometer is used the measure the static force exerted as a patient squeezes. Well established guidelines define sarcopenia as a hand grip strength less than 27 kg in males and 16 kg in females
Stair climbing	Timed stair-climb of standard 12-step flight of stairs
SARC-F questionnaire	Self-reported screening tool. Five components: (1) lifting/carrying 10 pounds, (2) walking across a room, (3) transferring from bed/chair, (4) climbing a flight of 10 stairs, and (5) falls in the last year.

Imaging

Computed Tomography (CT)

Given the relative ease of procurement, CT has become the gold standard diagnostic modality for many common medical issues. Using CT to diagnose sarcopenia proves beneficial for patients when CT imaging is routinely obtained during the initial evaluation of surgical patients, allowing for sarcopenia diagnosis without additional testing, radiation, or cost.

CT evaluation of the psoas muscle group is routinely used for evaluation of frailty and sarcopenia. Measurement of psoas muscle cross-sectional area has been shown to serve as a reasonable surrogate to approximate lean core muscle mass and is used for stratification of sarcopenia in a variety of patient populations (Fig. 7.1). Often, the skeletal muscle index is calculated to normalize muscle area for the height of the patient. Psoas muscle cross-sectional area has been proven useful to predict mortality in liver transplant, abdominal aortic aneurysm repair, and pancreatic adenocarcinoma resection and to predict morbidity in geriatric emergency surgery patients and patients undergoing colorectal cancer resection.

In addition to cross-sectional area using CT Hounsfield Units to measure skeletal muscle density has also been used to detect sarcopenia. Fat exhibits a less dense appearance when compared to skeletal muscle. Patients with poorer muscle quality will demonstrate less-dense appearing muscle due to fatty infiltration (Fig. 7.1). Multiple studies have reported that skeletal muscle density measurements at the third lumbar level correlate to total body skeletal muscle mass.

Ultrasonography (US)

US is a commonly utilized diagnostic technique spanning all facets of acute care surgery. For experienced users, US is portable, simple to interpret, allows for imaging without ionizing radiation, and is low cost, making US a convenient, practical, and easily employable bedside imaging tool for clinicians. In terms of sarcopenia, US diagnostics most commonly involve measuring the cross-sectional thickness of a muscle group at one or more anatomical sites to

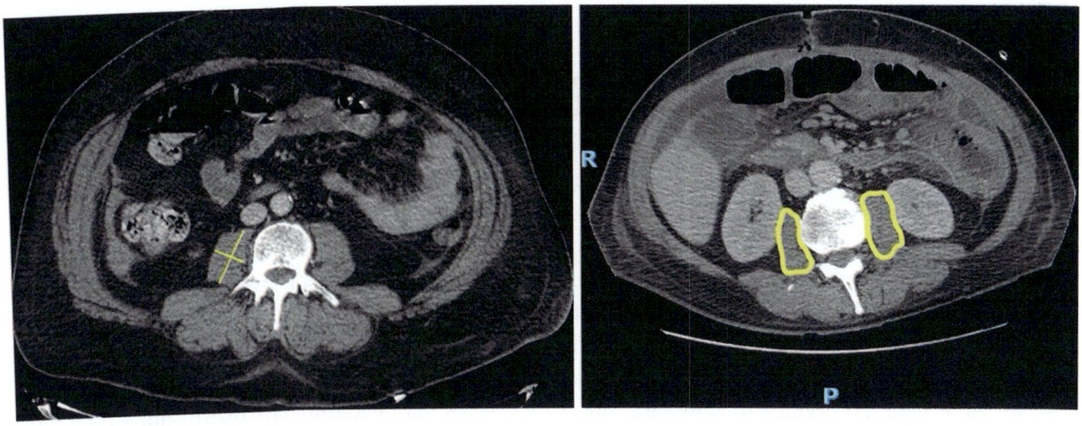

Fig. 7.1 Left: Psoas muscle area measurement in sarcopenic surgical patient at lumbar vertebral 3 level. Yellow lines represent the anterior-posterior and transverse measurements. Right: Using accessory software, the right and left psoas muscle density may be calculated as a Hounsfield Unit average at lumbar vertebral 3 level

obtain a corresponding muscle thickness. Superficial skeletal muscles are chosen as proxies for deeper muscle groups, which are often more challenging to visualize and suffer from inaccuracies relating to the scattering effect of sound wave absorption and reflection from overlying tissue. US provides an accurate measurement of muscle mass by providing both qualitative and quantitative data and previous studies utilizing the rectus abdominis, external and internal abdominal obliques, rectus femoris, and gastrocnemius muscles have confirmed that US is a reliable method for determination of sarcopenia.

Magnetic Resonance Imaging (MRI)

MRI is advantageous in that it provides high resolution of soft tissue structures without the ionizing radiation required for CT. Unlike CT imaging, however, MRI is more costly and less time-efficient. Given these drawbacks, literature on the use of MRI in sarcopenia is often limited to research-based studies rather than clinical utility evaluations.

Dual Energy X-Ray Absorptiometry (DEXA)

DEXA is a technique which utilizes varying energy X-rays to pass through tissue which are then recorded to allow for differentiation of bone, fat, and lean components. Its low cost, ease of availability, and minimal radiation exposure make DEXA an attractive modality to define sarcopenia in geriatric individuals. To diagnose sarcopenia, DEXA has been to be shown to be both highly accurate and reproducible in clinical and research studies. By dividing the body into bone, muscle, and lean components, software algorithms are then able to differentiate lean muscle and determine limb skeletal muscle mass. DEXA is not without limitations, however. DEXA imaging relies on the assumption that the body is composed of 73% water. Alterations in the hydration status of a patient are dynamic over time and are often affected by variables such as age, gender, level of activity, and overall health. Given the reliance of DEXA on a standard constant for body water, calculated skeletal muscle mass has the potential to vary in overall accuracy.

Functional Assessments

Functional assessments are commonly used metrics for the evaluation of sarcopenia in surgical patients. Unlike imaging modalities, these tests do not expose patients to ionizing radiation and, in most cases, are easily and readily performed bedside. However, functional assessments do rely on the ability of a patient to perform specific tasks and, therefore, are often limited to patients without decreased cognition or neurologic/musculoskeletal diagnoses that would preclude full assessment participation.

Hand Grip Strength

Hand grip strength (HGS) is the gold standard for functional-based assessments to diagnose sarcopenia. HGS is determined by using a hand strength dynamometer to measure the force exerted as a patient squeezes the device with maximal effort. According to the European Working Group on Sarcopenia in Older People, sarcopenia is defined as patients with HGS less than 27 kilograms (kg) for men and 16 kg for women. HGS has been clinically evaluated in a variety of patient population and has been shown to correlate with nutritional status, increasing age, sarcopenia, and frailty and is believed to be a reliable measure of overall muscle strength. HGS demonstrates acceptable inter-tester reliability making it a simple and practical mode of evaluation.

HGS, while a clinically useful functional metric, still has its limitations. HGS assessment relies on the cognitive and neuromuscular status of a patient for accuracy. The findings of the exam may be affected by elbow and wrist position, the hand used by the patient, and the calibration of the dynamometer. To mitigate error based on performance variation, the American Society of Hand Therapists recommends the patient be seated with shoulders adducted and elbows at 90° flexion. The forearms should lie in a neutral position, and a Jamar dynamometer should be used. However, these recommendations have undergone multiple revisions and a lack of protocol consistency still exists within the literature.

Stair Climbing

Stair climbing is a functional assessment that has been extensively studied. Baker et al. timed patients on their ability to walk up and down a 12-step flight of stairs, a standard height staircase. In this study, a correlation was demonstrated between timed stair climbing and rate of postoperative complications. When the psoas muscle density was compared to stair climb, the time it took to complete the stair climbing assessment was inversely correlated to psoas muscle density. Given the direct correlation of outcomes with imaged-based psoas muscle density, Baker et al. were able to show that in the absence of imaging, timed stair climbing was an accurate predictor of postoperative morbidity in geriatric patients.

SARC-F Questionnaire

The SARC-F questionnaire differs from the prior functional assessments described as this form requires no direct functional examination of the patient. SARC-F is a self-reported screening tool, which consists of five questions that can be both easily and rapidly obtained. The five components of SARC-F are (1) lifting/carrying 10 pounds, (2) walking across a room, (3) transferring from bed/chair, (4) climbing a flight of 10 stairs, and (5) falls in the last year. The questionnaire has a reported sensitivity ranging from 29 to 55% and specificity ranging from 69 to 89%. Given these ranges, several modified scores have also been developed using SARC-F with incorporation of additional variables such as age, BMI, and muscle measurement to increase both sensitivity and specificity.

Although sensitivity and specificity vary, SARC-F holds several advantages compared to other sarcopenia screening modalities. SARC-F does not require costly imaging, expose patients to radiation, or rely on the ability of a patient to perform a functional task. Instead, SARC-F relies on a small set of survey questions, which may be answered by the patient or a caregiver on the patient's behalf.

Outcomes

Trauma

Trauma patients are a complex and challenging population. Especially in the aging population, practitioners must treat traumatic injuries while managing multiple medical comorbidities. One of the most common geriatric trauma mechanisms is ground level falls. Landi et al. found that sarcopenic patients were over three times more likely to fall over a 2-year follow-up period when compared to non-sarcopenic patients. Recently, Chen et al. examined the correlation between sarcopenic status and hip fracture, reported that sarcopenia was an independent predictor of poor functional outcomes, and decreased quality of life after hip fixation. The authors further demonstrated that sarcopenia was associated with a 10% decrease in muscle mass (compared to 1% in non-sarcopenic patients) and a 2.8-fold higher risk of mortality in the first year after operative hip fixation. One possible way to mitigate these risks is through high intensity strength training; geriatric patients who undergo high intensity strength training for 12 weeks postoperatively had longitudinal improvement in both muscle performance and physical function.

General Surgery

Sarcopenia is an important modifiable factor in geriatric general surgery patients. A plethora of literature exists spanning multiple subspecialty surgical populations demonstrating the association of sarcopenia with poor surgical outcomes in colorectal, hepatobiliary, orthopedic, and vascular surgery patients. In addition to effecting discharge disposition, sarcopenia has also been associated with morbidity, long-term mortality, and length of stay in a variety of surgical cohorts.

Although many studies have examined elective surgical cohorts, newer research efforts have begun to examine the effects of sarcopenia on emergency general surgery outcomes. Rangel et al. found that sarcopenic patients undergoing emergency abdominal surgery demonstrated a mortality risk ratio of 2.6 compared to non-sarcopenic patients within 1 month of surgery. Given its chronic nature, sarcopenia has become a more appealing metric of chronic health status compared to BMI which has long functioned as a more rudimentary measure of nutritional status and health.

Taking advantage of the preponderance of CT imaging obtained to diagnose surgical pathology, a surgeon may then assess psoas muscle cross-sectional area and density and determine, acutely, the sarcopenic status of a patient undergoing emergent surgical intervention. Even in emergent scenarios, this valuable tool can be utilized during preoperative discussion with both patients and families, to fully inform, counsel, and provide more realistic outcome expectations.

Critical Care

Critically ill sarcopenic patients present significant challenges to ICU physicians. One challenge is the skeletal muscle wasting that occurs during a patient's ICU course, which can be up to 1% per day. Additionally, sarcopenia has been shown to be an important risk factor for mortality in ventilated patients.

Paris and Mourtzakis demonstrated that approximately 70% of patients over the age of 65 suffer from decreased muscularity on admission to the ICU. At baseline, geriatric patients can lose up to 0.5% of their muscle mass annually but may lose the same amount *per day* during an ICU hospitalization. The vast majority, over 90%, of ICU patients suffer muscle loss during the first 10 days of critical illness and the degree of muscle loss ranges between 17 and 30%. The reason for the substantial muscle wasting seen, particularly in geriatric patients, is a catabolic state, which results from acute inflammation, prolonged immobility, decreased protein synthesis, and insufficient nutrition.

Much research has focused on the determination of methods to diagnose and mitigate sarcopenia in the ICU population. Much of this work has sought to improve muscle loss and function through nutrition, pharmacologic agents, early infection source control, inflammatory response attenuation, and physical therapy. Increasing protein and amino acid supplementation has been shown to improve muscle preservation; however, this data is heterogenous and optimal supplementation and timing remains elusive. Overall, for geriatric patients, it has been proposed that daily protein intake should range from 1.2–1.5 g/kg/day in patients with both acute and chronic disease.

To better identify those individuals at risk for complications related to sarcopenia, several scoring systems such as the Modified Nutrition Risk in the Critically Ill (mNUTRIC), SARC-F, and Clinical Frailty Scale (CFS) have helped identify critically ill patients at highest risk for adverse outcomes secondary to sarcopenia. Through construction of a composite scoring system utilizing all three of the previously listed scoring systems into a single modified scoring system, Lee et al. showed that patients with an elevated NUTRIC-SF score of ≥ 2 experienced both a higher 60-day mortality as well as lower survival to discharge at 60 days. The NUTRIC-SF was also shown to outperform each of the individual component scoring systems.

Through the utilization of sensitive and specific scoring modalities coupled with aggressive physical and nutritional rehabilitation, critically ill sarcopenic patients may be more rapidly identified and expeditiously treated to minimize in-hospital ICU complications and long-term outcomes.

Financial Impact

Given the susceptibility of a sarcopenic patient to potential postoperative complications, the significant associated economic impact to the health-care system cannot be understated. Sheetz et al. found that mean unadjusted payor costs were higher in general surgery patients with sarcopenia when compared to both average and non-sarcopenic patients by $7680.53 and $13,416.30, respectively. Given the ability practitioners often have to modify and optimize a sarcopenic patient preoperatively, treating sarcopenia offers a potentially intervenable target for surgeons to minimize postoperative morbidity while decreasing overall healthcare expenditure.

Conclusions

Sarcopenia commonly occurs across a range of patient populations managed by acute care surgeons, with a high prevalence amongst the geriatric subgroup. A variety of imaging modalities and functional assessments are available to provide a timely diagnosis of sarcopenia. Many of these diagnostic and functional modalities are available either from index imaging studies or easily obtainable at bedside prior to procedural intervention. Given its modifiable nature, sarcopenia provides an optimizable target to enhance critical care and postoperative outcomes. Armed with the knowledge that sarcopenia may greatly impact operative outcomes, surgeons should focus on both diagnosing sarcopenia and modulating its deleterious effects in the geriatric acute care surgery population.

References

1. Dirks RC, Edwards BL, Tong E, Schaheen B, Turrentine FE, Shada A, et al. Sarcopenia in emergency abdominal surgery. J Surg Res. 2017;207:13–21.
2. Sheetz KH, Waits SA, Terjimanian MN, Sullivan J, Campbell DA, Wang SC, et al. Cost of major surgery in the sarcopenic patient. J Am Coll Surg. 2013;217(5):813–8.
3. Rangel EL, Rios-Diaz AJ, Uyeda JW, Castillo-Angeles M, Cooper Z, Olufajo OA, et al. Sarcopenia increases risk of long-term mortality in elderly patients undergoing emergency abdominal surgery. J Trauma Acute Care Surg. 2017;83(6):1179–86.
4. Yeh DD, Ortiz-Reyes LA, Quraishi SA, Chokengarmwong N, Avery L, Kaafarani HMA, et al. Early nutritional inadequacy is associated with psoas muscle deterioration and worse clinical outcomes in critically ill surgical patients. J Crit Care. 2018;45:7–13.
5. Salim SY, Al-Khathiri O, Tandon P, Baracos VE, Churchill TA, Warkentin LM, et al. Thigh ultrasound used to identify frail elderly patients with sarcopenia undergoing surgery: a pilot study. J Surg Res. 2020;256:422–32.
6. Paris M, Mourtzakis M. Assessment of skeletal muscle mass in critically ill patients: considerations for the utility of computed tomography imaging and ultrasonography. Curr Opin Clin Nutr Metab Care. 2016;19(2):125–30.
7. Minetto MA, Busso C, Gamerro G, Lalli P, Massazza G, Invernizzi M. Quantitative assessment of volumetric muscle loss: dual-energy X-ray absorptiometry and ultrasonography. Curr Opin Pharmacol. 2021;57:148–56.
8. Sousa-Santos AR, Amaral TF. Differences in handgrip strength protocols to identify sarcopenia and frailty - a systematic review. BMC Geriatr. 2017;17(1):238.
9. Baker S, Waldrop MG, Swords J, Wang T, Heslin M, Contreras C, et al. Timed stair-climbing as a surrogate marker for sarcopenia measurements in predicting surgical outcomes. J Gastrointest Surg. 2019;23(12):2459–65.
10. Bahat G, Erdogan T, Ilhan B. SARC-F and other screening tests for sarcopenia. Curr Opin Clin Nutr Metab Care. 2022;25(1):37–42.
11. Landi F, Liperoti R, Russo A, Giovannini S, Tosato M, Capoluongo E, et al. Sarcopenia as a risk factor for falls in elderly individuals: results from the ilSIRENTE study. Clin Nutr. 2012;31(5):652–8.
12. Chen YP, Kuo YJ, Hung SW, Wen TW, Chien PC, Chiang MH, et al. Loss of skeletal muscle mass can be predicted by sarcopenia and reflects poor functional recovery at one year after surgery for geriatric hip fractures. Injury. 2021;52(11):3446–52.
13. Briggs RA, Houck JR, LaStayo PC, Fritz JM, Drummond MJ, Marcus RL. High-intensity multimodal resistance training improves muscle function, symmetry during a sit-to-stand task, and physical function following hip fracture. J Nutr Health Aging. 2018;22(3):431–8.
14. Tieland M, van Dronkelaar C, Boirie Y. Sarcopenic obesity in the ICU. Curr Opin Clin Nutr Metab Care. 2019;22(2):162–6.
15. Lee ZY, Hasan MS, Day AG, Ng CC, Ong SP, Yap CSL, et al. Initial development and validation of a novel nutrition risk, sarcopenia, and frailty assessment tool in mechanically ventilated critically ill patients: the NUTRIC-SF score. JPEN J Parenter Enteral Nutr. 2022;46(3):499–507.

Immunology: Features of Immunesenescence

8

Niharika A. Duggal

Introduction

Human life expectancy has risen drastically over the last century. During the period 2016–2018, the life expectancy increased by 0.8 years and 0.6 years for males and females, respectively. Unfortunately, health span (healthy life expectancy) has not kept pace with increases in lifespan in recent years and older adults are spending these additional years of life in ill health, healthy life expectancy for males increased by 0.4 years and for females by only 0.2 years during this period. Advancing ageing is accompanied by functional deterioration across multiple systems that culminates into an increased susceptibility, risk of hospitalisation and mortality from infections such as influenza, and increased risk of chronic inflammatory diseases such as rheumatoid arthritis, and other chronic illnesses; together making older adults a vulnerable population. Thus, developing an understanding of underlying biogerontological processes is vital for maintaining good health by reducing the risk of multimorbidity in old age.

As the population ages, the rate of surgical procedures in the older population is rising. In recent years in England, aged individuals undergoing surgery is on an exponential rise. In this book chapter, we discuss age-related changes in the immune system and their contribution towards inflammatory processes and how this contributes towards poor outcomes post-surgery in geriatric patients. Lastly, focussing on therapeutic targets to boost immunity and combat immunesenescence, which may translate into significant improvements in the quality of life for the vulnerable geriatric population post-surgery.

Immunesenescence and Inflammaging

Advancing age is accompanied by profound remodelling of the innate and adaptive arms of the immune system, accompanied by an impaired functional response to an antigenic challenge, termed immunesenescence, which has been viewed as a major contributory factor towards the increased susceptibility of older adults to bacterial and viral infections, poor vaccination responses, increased risk of chronic inflammatory conditions, such as rheumatoid arthritis and multimorbidity (Fig. 8.1).

Impact of Ageing on Innate Immunity

Neutrophils are the first innate immune cell that leaves circulation (extravasation) and migrate

N. A. Duggal (✉)
MRC-Versus Arthritis Centre for Musculoskeletal Ageing Research, Institute of Inflammation and Ageing, University of Birmingham, Birmingham, UK
e-mail: n.arora@bham.ac.uk

P. Petrone, C. E.M. Brathwaite (eds.), *Acute Care Surgery in Geriatric Patients*,
https://doi.org/10.1007/978-3-031-30651-8_8

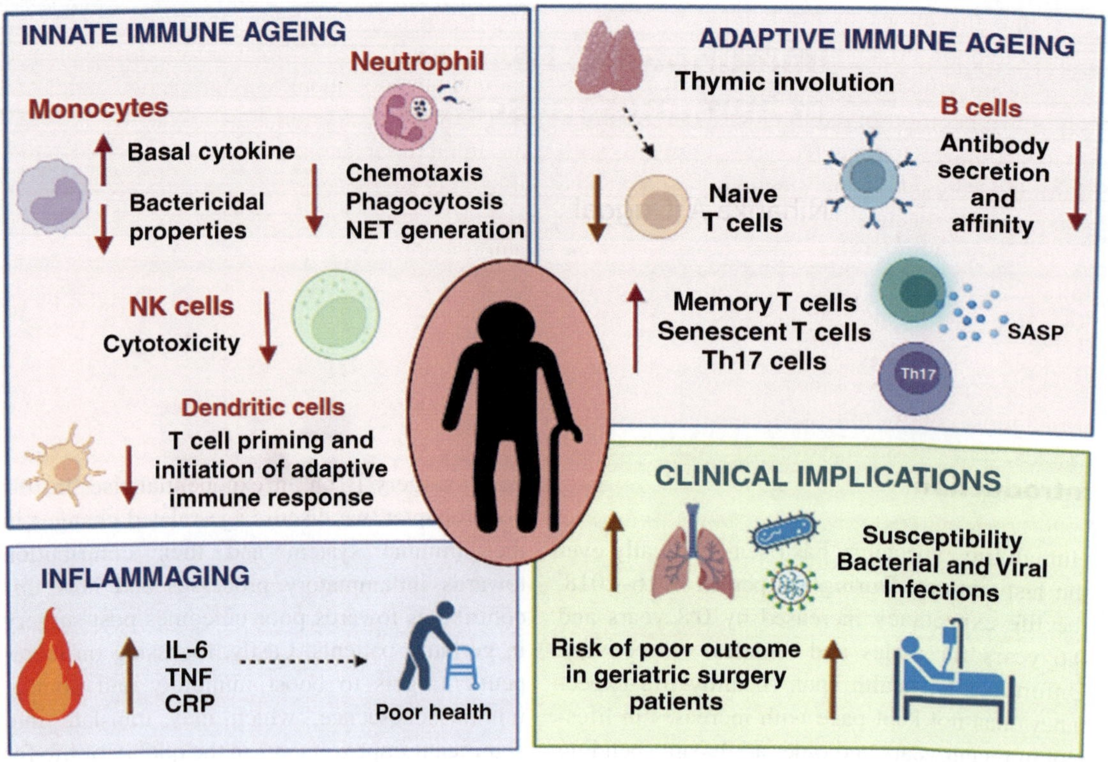

Fig. 8.1 Immunesenescence and Inflammaging with advancing age. Advancing age is accompanied by remodelling of the immune system, known as immunesenescence. Key hallmarks of and adaptive immune ageing which has implications on health of older adults. Another universal feature of physiological ageing is a low-grade increase in systemic levels of pro-inflammatory cytokines, termed Inflammaging. which is a contributor towards elevated mortality in older adults

towards the site of infection (chemotaxis), and these cells are equipped with several defence strategies to engulf (phagocytose) and kill the invading pathogens. Circulating numbers of neutrophils and the ability of the host to upregulate neutrophil production during an infection (neutrophilia) are preserved with advancing age. Neutrophil adhesion receptors CD15 and CD11a/CD11b which bind to E-selectin and β_2-integrins on the endothelium, their expression is preserved in aged neutrophils; thus, reduced extravasation of neutrophils is not a significant factor contributing to increased risk of infection in the older adults. Key features of neutrophil ageing include compromised neutrophil chemotaxis towards the site of infection making migration inefficient, resulting in tissue damage and secondary systemic inflammation. Neutrophils have reduced phagocytosis ability towards opsonised pathogens in older individuals due to decreased expression of the CD16 receptor to form phagosome into which reactive oxygen species generation in response to *S. aureus,* whereas no decrease in response to *E. coli*. Lastly, ageing is accompanied by a reduced ability to extrude neutrophil extracellular traps to entrap bacteria extracellularly; together contributing towards the age-associated increased vulnerability towards bacterial infections and elevated mortality.

Monocytes are a heterogenous population of circulating leukocytes that can be classified into three subsets depending on the combination of cell surface expression of CD14 and CD16 membrane receptors; classical monocytes ($CD14^+CD16^-$), intermediate monocytes ($CD14^+CD16^+$), and non-classical monocytes ($CD14^-CD16^+$). No age-associated changes have been observed in total circulating monocyte numbers, but alterations in the composition of the monocyte pool, driven by an increased frequency of both intermediate and non-classical monocytes have been observed in older adults. Similar to neutrophils, monocytes are equipped with multiple strategies, which include phagocytosis, generation of reactive oxygen species (ROS) and cytokine production for host defence against pathogens. Age-associated alterations in monocyte functional capacity include a decline in phagocytosis, ROS production, and generation of pro-inflammatory cytokines by monocytes post-stimulation with toll-like receptors (TLRs) ligands, but an increase in pro-inflammatory cytokine production has been observed in basal conditions. In response to local environmental cues during infection, monocytes migrate into lymphoid organs and can polarise into two key subsets; M1 (induced by IFNγ) with a high microbicidal activity and M2 cells (induced by IL4) that participate in the immunoregulatory function and tissue repair; a skewing towards M2 macrophages has been observed in old mice.

Dendritic cells (DC) play a central role in orchestrating the onset and regulation of adaptive immune response. DCs are comprised of two subsets: known as myeloid DCs (mDCs) and plasmacytoid DCs (pDCs) that possess anti-viral properties. The circulating number of mDCs decreases whilst pDC numbers remain unchanged with age. Immature dendritic cells in circulation monitor the extracellular environment for foreign pathogens and post phagocytosis of the pathogen, resulting in DCs activation they undergo maturation and migrate to the lymph nodes to present antigens to T cells and secrete a range of cytokines and chemokines for priming an adaptive immune response. DCs from aged individuals display a state of basal activation, defective migratory ability capacity, impairment of antigen uptake potential of DCs, and subsequent T cell priming; together resulting in an age-associated impairment in the initiation of the adaptive immune response. Furthermore, aged DCs secrete higher basal levels of pro-inflammatory cytokines (IL-6 and TNF-a), but similar to monocytes impaired cytokine secretion is observed upon TLR stimulation. The reduction in type I interferon and TNF-α production by aged DCs has been linked with the impaired ability of aged individuals to mount a protective antibody response to vaccination. Lastly, aged DCs display an impaired clearance of apoptotic cells and impaired tolerance to self-antigens, which have been linked to the development of autoimmunity.

Natural killer (NK) cells are a vital component of the innate immune system that produce cytokines and chemokines in the early stages of viral infections and are responsible for the elimination of virus-infected and malignant cells. They are a heterogeneous population that can be categorised into two different subsets based upon CD56 expression; cytotoxic $CD56^{bright}$ (90% of NKs) or immune-regulatory $CD56^{dim}$ (10% of NKs). Aged hosts display an increase in circulating numbers of NK cells, driven by an accumulation of $CD56^{dim}$ NK cells and CD57-expressing senescent NK cells. The predominant mechanism by which NK cells eliminate viral or tumour-infected cells involves the secretion of cytolytic effector molecules, such as the pore-forming protein perforin and apoptosis-inducing granzyme B onto the target cell surface. A reduction in NK cell cytotoxicity mediated by granule exocytosis has been reported with age; mediated via defects in the polarisation of lytic granules to the NK target cell interface and reduced release of perforin into the NK-target cell synapse. Importantly, a longitudinal study has reported that low NK cell cytotoxicity is associated with an increased risk of developing infection and is also a predictor of infectious morbidity in old individuals. In addition to their cytotoxic potential NK cells are also a key source of immunoregulatory cytokines (TNF-a, IFN-γ, IL-8) and aged NK cells display impaired secretion of anti-viral cytokine IFN-γ but not TNF-α upon target cell stimulation. Recent evidence suggests that NK cells play a key role in the resolution of inflammation via clearance of senescent cells, although unexplored it can be postulated that age-associated impairments in NK cell clearance of senescent cells, contribute towards the age-associated accumulation of senescent cells and NK cell ageing may have more far-reaching consequences on the health of older adults than simply increasing their risk of cancer and viral infection.

Impact of Ageing on Adaptive Immunity

The thymus is a primary lymphoid organ consisting of a cellular network of various cell types including thymic epithelial cells (TECs), DCs, and mesenchymal cells creating a microenvironment that is devoted to the development of T cell progenitors into mature T cells. One of the most documented changes in the immune system during ageing is thymic involution; involving a reduction in thymic mass, loss of tissue architecture and cellularity, accompanied by infiltration of adipocytes and an altered thymic microenvironment, resulting in a decline in the net thymic output of naïve antigen-inexperienced T cells. This contributes to an age-associated increased vulnerability of older adults towards novel pathogens such as severe acute respiratory syndrome (SARS)-CoV-2 virus. Alongside the contraction of the naïve T cell pool, a compensatory accumulation of highly differentiated memory T cells that acquire a senescent phenotype that secrete abundant proinflammatory factors, such as tumour necrosis factor (TNFα) have been observed in aged hosts, possibly a result of lifelong antigenic stimulation.

Differentiated helper CD4 T lymphocytes have been classified into distinct subtypes, including Th1, Th2, Th17, and T_{reg}. Importantly, age-associated defects in CD4 T cell helper functions and a skewing towards a pro-inflammatory Th17 cell polarisation have been observed in aged hosts. Regulatory T cells (T_{reg}) play a pivotal role in maintaining immune homeostasis. An expansion of circulating Tregs has also been observed in with age, but these cells display an impaired suppressive functional capacity; shifting the Th17/T_{reg} balance towards a pro-inflammatory environment with age which has been associated with an increased risk of autoimmunity.

B cells have a variety of effector functions including antigen presentation and most importantly antibody production. Ageing is accompanied by impairments in B cell haematopoiesis in the bone marrow attributed to age-related changes in the microenvironment of the bone marrow, including diminished levels of the pro-B cell-survival cytokine IL-7; as a result, the circulating number of B cells declines with age in humans. Functional impairments including reduced antibody production and secretion of antibodies with a poor affinity that provide less protection have been reported by aged B cells; resulting in poor vaccination efficacy in older people, making protecting the aged population from infectious diseases even more challenging. Thus, it is no surprise that the World Health Organization has included the development of vaccines targeting older adults as a future research priority. Furthermore, dysfunctional B cell responses in older adults, such as an accumulation of Age-Associated B cells (ABC) that secrete pro-inflammatory cytokines (TNFα) and autoantibodies secretion and numerical and functional loss in immunoregulatory B cells (B_{regs}); a potential contributor towards the increased risk for autoimmune diseases.

Inflammaging

Another hallmark of ageing is a state of basal elevation of circulating pro-inflammatory cytokines (IL6, TNFα, CRP) termed inflammaging. Importantly, a recent study has created a metric for systemic inflammation (iAge), which is recognised as a robust predictor of the ageing trajectory. Expanding evidence highlights how inflammaging is being increasingly recognised as a risk factor for cardiovascular diseases, loss of muscle mass and strength, poor physical performance, together driving age-related frailty and development of neurodegenerative diseases, cognitive defects, and impaired memory with advancing age. Furthermore, inflammaging has recently been recognised as a predisposing risk factor for poor outcomes towards COVID-19 infections and other viral infections in older adults. Together these studies provide strong evidence of the role of inflammaging in the development of multiple age-related conditions making it a powerful predictor of mortality and morbidity with advancing age. Multiple factors have gained attention as potential drivers of inflammaging, including lifelong exposure to antigen stressors, immunesenescence, oxidative stress, the accumulation of senescent cells, intestinal barrier dysfunction, an unbalanced diet, increased central adiposity, and physical inactivity. Together, making it clear that the immune system does not operate in isolation and can be modified by a broad range of signals, we now need to consider how we boost the reduced immune responses of older adults.

Accelerating Immunesenescence in a Geriatric patient's Post-Surgery

Critical illness and surgical stress can elicit an inflammatory response and redistribution of systemic immunity. One such example is hip fracture, which is a devastating condition and a major health issue in old age, even though treatable the surgical procedure acts as a severe physical stressor for older individuals accompanied by increased physical disability, impaired quality of life, and increased mortality. We are only beginning to understand factors contributing towards poor outcomes after hip fracture and to test our hypothesis that the effects of surgical stress and age are interactive, we conducted a research study recruiting one hundred and one older hip fracture patients, 30% of whom developed depression post-surgery and we observed persistent elevation of systemic inflammation (IL6) levels in older hip fracture patients even 6 months post-surgery which was even higher in those patients who developed depressive symptoms. We have observed a further acceleration of key hallmarks of immunesenescence discussed in the section above including impairments in neutrophil and monocyte bactericidal functioning, NK cell cytotoxicity and accumulation of senescent T cells in hip fracture patients that persist even 6 months post-surgery, particularly in those that develop depression compared to healthy older adults. One potential mechanism mediating accelerated immunesenescence in depressed hip fracture patients could be altered activity of adrenal hormones, specifically elevated Cortisol (immune suppressive) and a loss of Dehydroepiandrosterone DHEAS (immune enhancing) levels. Importantly, our findings suggest an acceleration of immunesenescence could be a potential driver of poor post-surgical outcomes; such as the increased risk of infections; supporting the need for the development of strategies that boost immune health in vulnerable post-surgery aged individuals to improve clinical outcomes.

In the past decade, there has been an increasing number of studies aiming at the identification of clinically relevant biomarkers for geriatric patient stratification for a desirable outcome (low infection and mortality risk), and we hypothesise that features of immunesenescence have the potential to serve as clinically meaningful biomarkers. Our own work done in critically ill patients and traumatic injury patients has reported a state of accelerated immunesenescence as early as a few days post-injury in biologically young individuals and more importantly, these features of immunesenescence predict the risk of developing sepsis. The first evidence in older adults supporting our hypothesis comes from a study analysing monocyte subset distribution prior to mechanical circulatory support device implantation surgery reporting an overlap between features of inflammaging and monocyte ageing and prediction of adverse outcomes post-surgery such as the unfavourable development of multiple-organ failure, highlighting the potential of immunological assessment as a potential non-invasive test to predict outcomes in other cohorts of geriatric patients elective surgery in a future multicentre study to evaluate whether the assessment of immunesenescence may prove as an important tool for geriatric patient stratification.

Prevention of Accelerated Immunesenescene Post-Surgery in Older Patients

Recovery after surgery is a long process, and this process is even longer in the geriatric population. This section will explore anti-inflammatory and immune-boosting intervention strategies that could boost clinical outcomes post-surgery in a geriatric population.

Statins

Statins are lipid-lowering compounds that have gained considerable attention for their anti-atherosclerotic properties and are widely prescribed in patients with cardiovascular diseases (CVD). Several biological properties of statins are being recognised including, anti-inflammatory response mediated via reductions in CD28^{-ve} senescent T cells. Importantly, in vitro studies have reported that statin induces T cell skewing towards an anti-inflammatory regulatory T cell phenotype and suppression of Th17 cell polarisation. Although the anti-inflammatory and anti-immunosenescent properties have not been tested in geriatric surgery patients, a previous study has reported reduced mortality in patients consuming statins when admitted to the hospital with pneumonia.

Senolytics

Therapeutically targeting senescent cells that express a senescence-associated secretory phenotype (SASP) using senolytics (dasatinib and quercetin) has been shown to reduce the production of pro-inflammatory cytokines such as IL-6 and other SASP-related cytokines such as IL-8, GM-CSF, and MCP-1 in human adipose tissue. A pilot clinical trial in human diabetic kidney disease using senolytics has reported anti-inflammatory effects. Importantly, a recent study in aged mice has reported for the first time a beneficial effect of senolytics on CD4 T cell differentiation, which in turn boosts viral clearance during an influenza infection challenge. Taken together, evidence in mice and some pilot data in humans suggest that senolytics possess the ability to ameliorate inflammaging and boost immune responses in aged hosts, everting an overall beneficial effect on host health. However, it is unclear whether it would yield a beneficial impact post-surgery in aged hosts via modulating the micro-environment, which could be tested in future clinical trials.

Caloric Restriction Mimetics

Caloric restriction mimetics exert a beneficial effect on the aged host via positive effects on the biochemical and functional effects similar to caloric restriction which is recognised as a gero-protective strategy. Metformin, an antidiabetic drug, which regulates cellular autophagy and mitochondrial dynamics, inhibition of the mTOR pathway known mechanisms of blocking inflammatory cytokine signalling pathways and thus it is not surprising that anti-inflammatory effects of metformin have been observed in patients with immune-mediated and so is its ability to boost immunity in older adults. Rapamycin is another mTOR inhibitor with anti-inflammatory properties.

P38 MAPK Inhibitors

Mitogen-activated protein kinase (MAPK) pathways regulate a range of biological processes, such as cellular senescence and inflammation. Multiple studies have reported an immunomodulatory potential mediated via suppression of p38 MAPK inhibitors such as the reduction of SASP phenotype in senescent CD8 T cells and the ability to rejuvenate the resolution ability of aged macrophages to clear apoptotic bodies together possibly driving its anti-inflammatory properties. Importantly, a pilot study on a small cohort of healthy older adults reported that short-term treatment with the oral p38 MAPK inhibitor Losmapimod resulted in a decline in systemic levels of inflammation; providing the evidence base for future trial testing Losmapimod in vulnerable older adults such as those undergoing surgery to combat inflammation and boost clinical outcome.

Probiotics

Advancing age is accompanied by changes in microbiota composition (i.e. microbial dysbiosis) driven by a loss of core commensals alongside an increase in intestinal barrier permeability and translocation of bacterial products into circulation with ageing; that has been recently recognised as a contributing factor towards inflammaging and macrophage ageing; making therapies that restore microbiome homeostasis a promising intervention strategy to reverse the immune ageing clock. Probiotics consisting of live bacterial commensals (e.g. *Lactobacilli casei, Bifidobacterium*) confer multiple immune health-promoting benefits via increasing production of beneficial short-chain fatty acids (SCFAs) levels, which in turn induce the expansion of IL-10-secreting regulatory T cells, downregulate Th17 responses, and production of pro-inflammatory cytokines. Thus, it is no surprise that probiotics are gaining recognition as a safe treatment choice for chronic inflammatory conditions beyond the gastrointestinal tract.

Conclusion Remarks

The global expansion of the ageing population has highlighted the urgent need to identify novel targets that help increase health span in older adults and relieve the burden of poor post-surgical outcomes observed in geriatric patients, potentially via boosting the aged immune system and combating inflammaging. We are only beginning to understand the importance of immune responses in predicting post-surgical recovery, and there remain open questions that require investigation in future studies. Particularly, the hypothesis that boosting immune health in geriatric surgical patients is of utmost importance needs to be strengthened, and there is room for future well-planned studies in humans to help increase the translational potential of these findings. We are currently conducting one such study in which we are investigating the potential of DHEA supplementation, which has yielded promising results during in vitro studies in improving neutrophil superoxide generation to boost neutrophil function in geriatric hip fracture patients to reduce the risk of post-surgery infections. In conclusion, we propose the exploitation of the modifiable nature of the immune system and the development of translational interventional strategies to improve immune health and exert a positive impact on the health of the geriatric surgical population.

References

1. Agrawal A, Gupta S. Impact of aging on dendritic cell functions in humans. Ageing Res Rev. 2011;10:336–45. https://doi.org/10.1016/j.arr.2010.06.004.
2. Brugaletta S, Biasucci LM, Pinnelli M, Biondi-Zoccai G, Di Giannuario G, Trotta G, et al. Novel anti-inflammatory effects of statins: reductions of CD4^{+} CD28^{null} T lymphocyte frequency in patients with unstable angina. Heart. 2006;92(2):249–50. https://doi.org/10.1136/hrt.2004.052282.
3. Caruso R, Campolo J, Verde A, Botta L, Cozzi L, Parolini M, et al. Research article relationship between early inflammatory response and clinical evolution of the severe multiorgan failure in mechanical circulatory support-treated patients. Mediat Inflamm. 2014;2014:126. https://doi.org/10.1016/j.humimm.2018.11.004.
4. De Mol J, Kuiper J, Tsiantoulas D, Foks AC. The dynamics of B cell aging in health and disease. Front Immunol. 2021;12:733566. https://doi.org/10.3389/fimmu.2021.733566.
5. Dorshkind K, Montecino-Rodriguez E, Signer RA. The ageing immune system: is it ever too old to become young again? Nat Rev Immunol. 2009;9:57–62. https://doi.org/10.1038/nri2471.
6. Duggal NA, Upton J, Phillips AC, Hampson P, Lord JM. Depressive symptoms are associated with reduced neutrophil function in hip fracture patients. Brain Behav Immun. 2013;33:173–82. https://doi.org/10.1016/j.bbi.2013.07.004.
7. Duggal NA. Reversing the immune aging clock: lifestyle modifications and pharmacological interventions. Biogerontology. 2018;19(16):481–96. https://doi.org/10.1007/s10522-018-9771-7.
8. Dugan B, Conway J, Duggal NA. Inflammaging as a target for healthy ageing. Age Ageing. 2023;52(2):afac328. https://doi.org/10.1093/ageing/afac328.
9. Grudzinska FS, Dosanjh DP, Parekh D, Dancer RC, Patel J, Nightingale P, et al. Statin therapy in patients with community-acquired pneumonia. Clin Med (Lond). 2017;17(5):403–7. https://doi.org/10.7861/clinmedicine.17-5-403.
10. Hazeldine J, Lord JM. The impact of ageing on natural killer cell function and potential conse-

quences for health in older adults. Ageing Res Rev. 2013;12(4):1069–78. https://doi.org/10.1016/j.arr.2013.04.003.
11. Lorenzo EC, Torrance BL, Keilich SR, Al-Naggar I, Harrison A, Xu M, et al. Senescence-induced changes in CD4 T cell differentiation can be alleviated by treatment with senolytics. Ageing Cell. 2022;21(1):e13525. https://doi.org/10.1111/acel.13525.
12. De Maeyer RPH, van de Merwe RC, Louie R, Bracken OV, Devine OP, Goldstein DR, et al. Blocking elevated p38 MAPK restores efferocytosis and inflammatory resolution in the elderly. Nat Immunol. 2020;21(6):615–25. https://doi.org/10.1038/s41590-020-0646-0.
13. Mannick JB, Giudice GD, Lattanzi M, Valiante NM, Praestgaard J, Huang B, et al. mTOR inhibition improves immune function in the elderly. Sci Transl Med. 2014;6:268ra179. https://doi.org/10.1126/scitranslmed.3009892.
14. Panda A, Arjona A, Sapey E, Bai F, Fikrig E, Montgomery RR, et al. Human innate immunesenescence: causes and consequences for immunity in old age. Trends Immunol. 2009;30(7):325–33. https://doi.org/10.1016/j.it.2009.05.004.
15. Vukmanovic-Stejic M, Chambers ES, Suarez-Fariñas M, Sandhu D, Fuentes-Duculan J, Patel N, et al. Enhancement of cutaneous immunity during aging by blocking p 38 mitogen-activated protein (MAP) kinase-induced inflammation. J Allergy Clin Immunol. 2018;142(3):844–56. https://doi.org/10.1016/j.jaci.2017.10.032.

9 Epidemiology of Injury in the Elderly: Use of DOACs

Amanda Hambrecht, Natalie Escobar, and Cherisse Berry

Introduction

The geriatric population is one of the fastest growing demographics in the United States. It is estimated that there will be 77 million adults aged 65 years or older by the year 2034, projected to be more than the number of children for the first time in US history. Trauma is one of the leading causes of morbidity and mortality among this older age group. Falls and motor vehicle collisions are the first and second most common mechanisms of injury, respectively, with the highest mortality rate among pedestrians struck by vehicles. There are specific injury patterns unique to this age cohort as well as increased morbidity and mortality for the same injuries when compared with younger adults. The physiologic changes that accompany aging affect all organ systems; thus, a trauma evaluation among the elderly requires a high level of suspicion for serious injury. The medication list for the geriatric trauma patient should be thoroughly examined, with special attention to the presence of antiplatelets or anticoagulants. A multidisciplinary team is essential to care for the geriatric trauma patient and ensure a safe and successful discharge from the hospital.

Epidemiology of Injury

Traumatic injury is increasingly common in the elderly population, accounting for nearly one-quarter of hospitalizations each year. Trauma is the fifth leading cause of death in this age cohort, with mortality increasing after age 70 even after adjusting for severity score. Falls are the most common type of traumatic injury in the elderly population. According to the Centers for Disease Control, there were 36 million falls in 2018, with 8 million injuries and over 34,000 deaths. Motor vehicle collisions are the second most common mechanism of injury and leading cause of traumatic mortality in the geriatric population, with the highest mortality rate seen in pedestrians struck by a motor vehicle. Compared to younger adults, elderly patients are more likely to sustain serious injuries after falls or motor vehicle collisions with increased rates of traumatic brain injury.

A. Hambrecht
New York University Grossman School of Medicine-Department of Surgery, NYC Health & Hospitals-Bellevue-Department of Surgery,
New York, NY, USA

N. Escobar
New York University Grossman School of Medicine,
New York, NY, USA
e-mail: natalie.escobar@nyulangone.org

C. Berry (✉)
NYU Grossman School of Medicine, Department of Surgery, Division of Acute Care Surgery,
New York, NY, USA
e-mail: cherisse.berry@nyulangone.org

P. Petrone, C. E.M. Brathwaite (eds.), *Acute Care Surgery in Geriatric Patients*,
https://doi.org/10.1007/978-3-031-30651-8_9

Table 9.1 Characteristics of direct oral anticoagulants

Agent	Mechanism	Renal excretion (%)	Half-life (h)[a]	Reversal agent	Dialyzable
Apixaban (Eliquis)	Direct factor Xa inhibitor	25	12	Andexanet alfa or 4-factor PCC	No
Dabigatran (Pradaxa)	Direct thrombin inhibitor	80–85	12–17 (up to 34 h if on dialysis)	Idarucizumab, 4-factor PCC, or FEIBA	Yes
Edoxaban (Lixiana, Savaysa)	Direct factor Xa inhibitor	35	10–14	Andexanet alfa or 4-factor PCC	No
Rivaroxaban (Xarelto)	Direct factor Xa inhibitor	35	5–9 (11–13 h if elderly)	Andexanet alfa or 4-factor PCC	No

[a]In patients with normal creatinine clearance (half-life is extended if CrCl is reduced)
PCC prothrombin complex concentrate; *FEIBA* factor eight inhibitor bypassing activity (contains factor II, VII, IX, and X + activated VII)

Trauma Assessment

There are many physiologic changes that occur with age, affecting all organ systems ranging from cardiovascular, audiovisual, musculoskeletal, vestibular, and gait. These age-related changes result in hearing and vision impairment with decreased peripheral vision, visual motion perception, and hearing. Loss of subcutaneous tissue and increased muscle atrophy result in changes to posture with gait instability.

Thorough head-to-toe examinations are essential to ensure injuries are not missed. With increased rates of polypharmacy in the elderly population, many patients taking beta-blockers and antihypertensives may present with vital signs that are misleadingly "normal" due to a blunted physiologic response. Elderly patients are less sensitive to catecholamines and may not have the same response to hemorrhage after a trauma. Without such vital sign derangements, patients may be under-triaged and the diagnosis of their traumatic injuries delayed. Unsurprisingly, under-triage has been associated with increased risk of death in elderly patients; therefore, one must have a high level of suspicion for significant injury when there are no obvious external signs or manifestations of trauma. With concomitant dementia or delirium accompanying pneumonia, stroke, or sepsis from a urinary tract infection, these additional diagnoses may complicate the presentation of the geriatric trauma patient, leading to a delay in the recognition of shock or traumatic brain injury (TBI). Older patients are more susceptible to injury from minor mechanisms compared to younger patients and have a higher risk for severe disability or death after traumatic injury. Identifying occult shock early is paramount to prevent morbidity and improve patient survival. Elevated base deficits, greater than −6, are associated with increased mortality in elderly trauma patients. Clearance of base deficits and lactic acidosis should guide resuscitative efforts for this patient population.

Direct Oral Anticoagulants (DOACs)

With the increasing prevalence of atrial fibrillation, more patients are being treated with direct oral anticoagulants (DOACs) instead of the previously used warfarin. The first clinically available DOAC, dabigatran, was approved in 2010. Since that time, additional agents such as rivaroxaban, apixaban, and edoxaban have been developed for the treatment of non-valvular atrial fibrillation, venous thromboembolism or pulmonary embolism, and heparin-induced thrombocytopenia. These agents inhibit thrombin or factor Xa directly and do not require patients to have regular monitoring of therapeutic levels as is required with warfarin. All DOACs have some degree of renal excretion and have different half-lives depending on a patient's creatinine clearance (Table 9.1). A thorough review of a trauma patient's medication list including DOACS, warfarin, and antiplatelet agents is critical. Patients taking DOACs may have increased risk of bleed-

Table 9.2 Features of direct oral anticoagulant reversal agents

Reversal agent	Peak onset of action	Duration of infusion	Infusion volume (mL)	Risk of venous thromboembolism	Cost ($)
Andexanet alfa	4 h	30 min bolus, then 120 min infusion	100	Yes	$24,750–$49,500
4-factor PCC	1–6 h	17 min	100	Yes	$4000–$8000
FEIBA	15–30 min	25 min[a]	20	No	>$50,000
Idarucizumab	<1 min (ms)	5–10 min (two infusions)	100	Yes	$3600–$4700

[a] 10-min infusion time, 15 min to warm to room temperature

PCC prothrombin complex concentrate, *FEIBA* factor VIII inhibitor bypassing activity

ing with minor trauma and minimal to no laboratory abnormalities on routine coagulation studies.

Certain injury patterns, such as subdural hematomas or intra-abdominal hemorrhage, may require early reversal of these anticoagulants. The direct and indirect factor Xa inhibitors can be reversed with andexanet alfa, a recombinant modified factor Xa decoy protein that binds the active site of factor Xa inhibitors. Dabigatran, the only direct thrombin inhibitor, can be reversed with idarucizumab, a monoclonal antibody fragment that binds and neutralizes free and thrombin-bound dabigatran. All the direct oral anticoagulants can be reversed with 4-factor prothrombin complex concentrate (4F-PCC), a mixture of human factors II (thrombin), VII, IX, and X with endogenous inhibitor proteins C and S. Dabigatran is the only oral anticoagulant medication that is dialyzable. Specific testing of total thrombin and anti-factor Xa assays can be obtained to ensure adequate reversal.

There are limited data and studies available comparing the efficacy and side effect profiles of 4-factor PCC with andexanet alfa or idarucizumab, and there is a risk of venous thromboembolism with all agents. Andexanet alfa and 4-factor PCC have similar peak onsets of action (between 1–6 h for 4-factor PCC and 4 h for andexanet alfa), while idarucizumab has an onset of milliseconds with peak effect at the completion of its five-minute infusion. Both andexanet alfa and idaruzicumab require two infusions, with andexanet alfa composed of a bolus that takes almost 30 min followed by an infusion that lasts up to 2 h. Idaruzicumab, on the other hand, is composed of two back-to-back infusions that take 5–10 min each. The median infusion time for 4-factor PCC is 17 min. All three agents require an approximately 100 mL infusion volume, which is considerably less than the over 800 mL volume needed for the same concentration of clotting factors in fresh frozen plasma. Andexanet alfa reportedly costs between 5–10 times the amount of 4-factor PCC, which is more readily available given its more accessible price. The cost of idarucuzimab is reportedly similar to that of 4-factor PCC (Table 9.2).

Initially developed for the treatment of hemophilia-associated coagulopathy, Factor VIII Inhibitor Bypassing Activity (FEIBA), has been used off-label for reversal of oral anticoagulants. It is similar to 4-factor PCC in composition, though also contains activated factor VII. FEIBA requires 20 mL of infusion volume and can be infused over 10 min, though requires 15 min to first warm to room temperature. In small retrospective and prospective studies, use of FEIBA was not associated with any thrombotic complications. It is, however, more expensive than andexanet alfa, likely limiting its more widespread study and use. Further randomized trials are needed to compare the safety and efficacy profiles of these reversal agents.

Organ-Specific Injury

Traumatic Brain Injury

Traumatic brain injury (TBI) in the elderly is associated with increased morbidity and mortality for the same injury patterns when compared with younger adults. With age, the brain atrophies and its volume reduces, stretching the bridging dural veins. Older patients are at greater risk of subdural hematomas (SDH) from shearing or tearing these bridging veins, leading to intracranial hemorrhage after even minimal trauma. With the reduction in volume, there is increased space in which blood can accumulate, often resulting in delayed onset of symptoms and therefore, diagnosis. While the risk of epidural hematoma (EDH) decreases with age, the risk of SDH and associated midline shift after traumatic injury increases. Elderly patients are four times more likely to have evidence of intracranial trauma on cross-sectional imaging despite normal or only mild alterations in their Glasgow Coma Scale (GCS) score. To address the potential diagnostic delay, the American College of Surgeons Trauma Quality Improvement Program (ACS TQIP) released TBI best practice guidelines in 2015 recommending noncontrast head computed tomography (CT) for all patients aged 65 years and older with head trauma without loss of consciousness and all patients older than 60 years with head trauma in the setting of loss of consciousness. Additionally, patients with evidence of intracranial hemorrhage on oral anticoagulants should undergo reversal as soon as possible. The choice of reversal agent depends on several factors including the specific anticoagulant used and pharmacy or blood bank availability of reversal agents. Patients on anticoagulants are considered moderate-to-high risk for progression of their TBI. The Brain Trauma Foundation recommends repeat head CT imaging 6 h after the index scan in these patients for further monitoring and evaluation, or sooner, if there is a change in neurologic exam or clinical status. Compared to younger adults, geriatric patients have an increased risk of death or major disability requiring long-term care facility placement after severe TBI.

Cervical Spine Injury

With increasing age, geriatric patients have an increased risk of cervical spine and spinal cord injury after trauma. Due to underlying degenerative osteoarthritis leading to cervical stenosis, in addition to hyperostosis of the cervical ligaments, geriatric patients are predisposed to cervical fractures from minor mechanisms, such as a fall from standing or after a low velocity motor vehicle collision. Elderly patients are more sensitive to hyperextension injuries in the setting of cervical spondylosis that can result in central cord syndrome, the most common incomplete spinal cord injury, that manifests as extremity weakness, disproportionately affecting the upper extremities. This age cohort is also susceptible to odontoid fractures. Of the three types of odontoid fractures, type II fractures, which occur at the base of the odontoid, are the most common in older adults and considered unstable. Treatment options include surgical stabilization or external immobilization with a hard cervical collar. The optimal treatment depends on the presence of medical comorbidities, other associated injuries, overall functional status, and patient wishes. Elderly patients are at increased risk of complications related to prolonged immobilization, including continued loss of mobility and pressure ulcers, and extra care must be taken to ensure they do not become more deconditioned and that skin integrity is maintained.

Chest Trauma/Rib Fractures

Rib fractures are the most common chest injury after trauma in the geriatric population. An epidemiological study from Bonne and Schuerer noted one quarter of older patients involved in a motor vehicle crash sustained a chest injury. Due to decreased bone density that occurs with age, geriatric patients are more susceptible to fractures from minor mechanisms, such as a fall from standing. Age-related changes to the cardiopulmonary system place elderly patients at increased risk for morbidity and mortality after chest injuries. They have reduced vital capacity and functional residual capacity ultimately leading to decreased respiratory reserve, as well as a blunted physiologic response to hypercarbia and hypoxia, limiting their ability to adequately compensate after rib fractures. Geriatric patients are also at increased risk for complications after rib fractures including pneumonia and pulmonary contusions. Bulger et al. found mortality increases approximately 19% for each rib fracture sustained in patients over 65 years old. Intensive care unit admission should be strongly considered for patients over age 50 with 3 or more rib fractures. Multimodal pain control, including neuraxial blockade, with aggressive pulmonary toilet and intensive care admission have been associated with reduced mortality in older patients.

Abdominal Trauma

Elderly patients have similar intra-abdominal injury patterns after trauma when compared to younger adults. Their decreased pain sensation and misleadingly "normal" vital signs, as previously described, may lead to delay in diagnosis of intraperitoneal hemorrhage or hemorrhagic shock. Initial assessment of all elderly blunt trauma patients should include a focused assessment with sonography in trauma (FAST) examination. There should be a low threshold to obtain CT imaging in stable geriatric trauma patients, particularly after motor vehicle collisions or pedestrians struck by vehicles. It is important to consider the risk of contrast-induced nephropathy in this patient cohort, which can be superimposed on baseline chronic kidney disease or acute kidney injury in the setting of admission hypovolemia. Intravenous hydration and monitoring of creatinine levels after contrast imaging are crucial.

Musculoskeletal Injuries: Hip and Pelvic Fractures

Musculoskeletal injures, including pelvic and hip fractures, are the most common traumatic injuries in the geriatric population. Compared to younger adults, elderly patients have increased morbidity and mortality after pelvic fractures, with increased risk of major hemorrhage after injury. An aggressive approach should be taken to control bleeding in this patient population and may include reversing direct oral anticoagulant medications, advanced imaging with angiography, and Interventional Radiology consultation for possible intervention. Hip fractures are the most common injury requiring admission in this age cohort. Once admitted, multidisciplinary care teams including physiatry, physical and occupational therapy, nutrition and social work are essential for assessing a patient's functional status, improving their rehabilitation and recovery, and ensuring a safe discharge plan.

Skin

As elderly patients age, so too, does their skin. The composition changes with less elastin and collagen, leading to wrinkling and dryness. The epidermis becomes thinner and more susceptible to friction or shearing forces leading to skin tears. Skin injuries as defined by Payne and Martin can range from minor with no tissue loss to complete loss of an epidermal flap to cover the injury. These wounds can take longer to heal than in younger patients. Modifying risk factors such as control of diabetes, treatment of anemia and adequate nutrition, are essential to deter poor wound healing. A thorough skin assessment on initial presentation to the hospital and throughout the patient's hospital stay to document any skin tears or injuries and assess surrounding skin integrity is of paramount importance. These wounds can be painful and breaks in the skin serve as a nidus for infection. Meticulous wound care should be undertaken to prevent further injuries.

Multidisciplinary Hospital Care/ Disposition Planning

Treating the elderly trauma patient requires a multidisciplinary team approach with a geriatric-focused care plan. Such elderly-specific protocols can increase the likelihood of survival after discharge from the hospital. Nowak and Berry outlined these comprehensive geriatric evaluations to assess medical comorbidities, psychosocial factors, and pre-admission functional status and limitations. Multidisciplinary teams can include members from physiatry, physical and occupational therapy, pharmacy, nutrition services, social workers, and even palliative care specialists. An often-underutilized specialty, palliative care consultants can assist with establishing surrogate decision-makers, defining code status, and delineating advanced directives in-line with the patient's desired goals of care.

Early mobilization is essential to prevent functional decline and other hospital associated morbidities such as pneumonia or pressure ulcers. Coordinated efforts with respiratory therapy, occupational and physical therapy, and nursing can provide the patients with chest physiotherapy and deep breathing exercises, assess their fall risk, maintain aspiration precautions, and perform daily skin integrity checks with pressure ulcer screenings.

Pain control is essential for postinjury care. Inadequate pain control is associated with delirium in older patients. Multimodal pain management strategies utilize non-opiate adjuncts and dose adjust narcotic medications for the reduced renal and hepatic clearance, and changes in body fat distribution, associated with advanced age. Delirium in hospitalized elderly patients has been associated with increased morbidity and mortality. Daily efforts to reduce delirium and to assess for and treat reversible causes are critical. Addressing sleep-wake disturbances, managing urinary retention or constipation, and treating infection or electrolytes abnormalities can all reduce delirium.

Early discharge planning is a crucial element of hospital care plans. Screening tools have been developed to identify those at risk of functional decline during their hospitalization or with a greater likelihood of being discharged to a nursing home. The ACS TQIP released guidelines in 2013 outlining recommendations for geriatric trauma management. The report describes an Identification of Seniors at Risk (ISAR) questionnaire, which focuses on a patient's psychosocial functional status, including need for help with activities of daily living, memory issues and vision changes, and the presence of polypharmacy. The majority of seriously injured elderly patients do not return to their previous level of independence and function after discharge. A thorough assessment of the safety of their home environment and evaluation of the need for social support, equipment or home health services should be performed. Disposition planning should be initiated within 48 h of admission.

Dementia after Traumatic Brain Injury

It is well recognized that the sequelae from head trauma are long-lasting in the elderly population. Compared to younger adults, older patients have a slower recovery of cognitive function during rehabilitation after TBI. The estimated costs of dementia care in the United States are projected to be over one trillion dollars by 2050, with a large portion of care costs resulting from utilization of healthcare resources, including care facilities and nursing homes.

Several studies have posited a risk of developing dementia in geriatric patients after TBI. A 25-year study from Schneider and colleagues of over 15,000 Black and White patients from varied communities across the United States found a dose-dependent association between head trauma and dementia risk. A single prior head injury was associated with a 1.25-times risk while two or more prior head injuries were associated with an over 2-times risk. Overall, they found a 1.44-times risk of dementia after head trauma over 25 years. A 6-year longitudinal cohort study from Gardner et al. found a significant risk ranging from 1.2 to 1.5 times for developing dementia after mild, moderate, and severe TBIs in older adults, while moderate to severe TBI was associated with developing dementia in the 55–64-year-old cohort.

Given the association with even mild TBI and dementia in geriatric patients, and the increased likelihood of developing a TBI after a minor mechanism, risk-reducing strategies should be employed to prevent falls in this advanced age group.

Conclusion

Geriatric patients have increased morbidity and mortality after traumatic injuries compared to their younger counterparts. They typically have a myriad of medical comorbidities and extensive medication lists that increase the risk of poor outcomes after injury. The widespread use of anticoagulants increases the likelihood of postinjury hemorrhage and certain injury patterns, particularly traumatic brain injuries, require pharmacologic reversal. Elderly patients benefit from being triaged in and receiving care at designed trauma centers, with decreased rates of postinjury complications and mortality. Once admitted, a comprehensive and multidisciplinary team is essential to providing the high-quality, nuanced care for this special population. Early consultation with palliative care can provide critical assistance in establishing goals of care. Given the associated risks of developing dementia after TBI, elderly patients may continue to experience the complications and consequences of their injuries. With variable long-term outcomes after traumatic injury and the majority of patients often not returning to their baseline level of activity or functional status, early engagement of physiatry services is critical for developing a safe discharge plan.

References

1. Iriondo J, Jordan J. United States Census Bureau. Older people projected to outnumber children for the first time in U.S. history. Last updated 8 Oct 2021. https://www.census.gov/newsroom/press-releases/2018/cb18-41-population-projections.html.
2. Centers for Disease Control and Prevention. Older adult fall prevention. Last updated 14 Jul 2021. https://www.cdc.gov/falls/index.html.
3. Callaway DW, Shapiro NI, Donnino MW, Baker C, Rosen CL. Serum lactate and base deficit as predictors of mortality in normotensive elderly blunt trauma patients. J Trauma. 2009;66(4):1040.
4. Leung L. Direct oral anticoagulants (DOACs) and parental direct-acting anticoagulants: dosing and adverse effects. In: Mannucci PM and Tirnauer JS. UpToDate. last updated 12 May 2022.
5. Quinlan DJ, Eikelboom JW, Weitz JI. Four-factor prothrombin complex concentrate for urgent reversal of vitamin K antagonists in patients with major bleeding. Circulation. 2013;128(11):1179–81.
6. Shaw JR, Siegal DM. Pharmacological reversal of the direct oral anticoagulants–a comprehensive review of the literature. RPTH. 2018;2(2):251–65.
7. Colwell C. Geriatric trauma: initial evaluation and management. In: Moreira ME and Grayzel J. UpToDate. Last updated 16 Jul 2021.
8. Gardner RC, Dams-O'Connor K, Morrissey MR, Manley GT. Geriatric traumatic brain injury: epidemiology, outcomes, knowledge gaps, and directions. J Neurotrauma. 2018;35(7):889–906.
9. Bulger EM, Arneson MA, Mock CN, Jurkovich GJ. Rib fractures in the elderly. J Trauma. 2000;48(6):1040.
10. Victorino GP, Chong TJ, Pal JD. Trauma in the elderly patient. JAMA. 2003;138:1093–8.
11. Payne RL, Martin ML. Defining and classifying skin tears: need for a common language. Ostomy Wound Manage. 1993;39:16–22.
12. Tapper CX, Curseen K. Rehabilitation concerns in the geriatric critically ill and injured–part 1. Crit Care Clin. 2021;37:117–34.
13. Wong W. Economic burden of Alzheimer disease and managed care considerations. Am J Manag Care. 2020;26(8):S177–83.
14. Shively S, Scher AI, Perl DP, Diaz-Arrastia R. Dementia resulting from traumatic brain injury. Arch Neurol. 2012;69(10):1245–51.
15. Calland JF, Ingraham A, Martin N, Marshall GT, Schulman CI, Stapleton T, Barraco RD. Evaluation and management of geriatric trauma. J Trauma. 2012;73(5):S345–50.

Injury Prevention in the Geriatric Population

10

Yesha Maniar and D'Andrea K. Joseph

Introduction

Patients 65 and older are more likely to suffer traumatic injuries from falls and motor vehicle collisions. It is expected that by 2050 geriatric patients, defined as patients ≥65 years of age, will consist of 39% of trauma admissions across systems. Due to their increased age and altered physiology, elderly patients have worse outcomes after traumatic injury compared to younger patients. Changes in physiology such as decreased GFR, osteoporosis, reduced cough and pulmonary compliance, and comorbidities such as dementia, stroke, and hypertension, place elderly patients at higher risk of mortality and disability. Lower impact injuries result in higher injury severity scores, longer hospital length of stay and increased cost to the healthcare system.

Injury prevention in the geriatric population focuses on the most common causes of traumatic injuries. In 2020, unintentional injury contributed to more years of life lost than any other causes, according to the CDC. In the older population, unintentional injury was the fourth leading cause of death in patients 55–64, and eighth leading cause of death in patients 65 and older, dropping from third and seventh place in 2018 due to COVID.

Elderly patients suffer falls and motor vehicle collisions due to hearing loss, vision loss, gait instability, environmental conditions, cognitive deficits, drug and alcohol intoxication, polypharmacy, medical comorbidities, and postural hypotension. This chapter will discuss the specific contributors to injury and various prevention methods.

Physiology

Hearing Loss

Hearing loss in the geriatric population has been associated with increased risk of falls and injuries. Possible reasons include vestibular dysfunction affecting gait and balance, and poor awareness of spatial environment due to loss of auditory cues. In motor vehicle crashes, patients with hearing loss are unable to listen for changes in traffic. Most geriatric patients experience presbycusis, making it difficult for them to communicate effectively.

Currently, there are no guidelines for routine screening for hearing loss in asymptomatic patients age >50 years old or for when hearing aids are recommended. Routine screening at primary care visits or patients that present to the hospital after a traumatic injury could be consid-

Y. Maniar · D. K. Joseph (✉)
NYU Long Island School of Medicine, NYU Langone Hospital–Long Island, Mineola, NY, USA
e-mail: yesha.Maniar@nyulangone.org; d'andrea.Joseph@nyulangone.org

P. Petrone, C. E.M. Brathwaite (eds.), *Acute Care Surgery in Geriatric Patients*,
https://doi.org/10.1007/978-3-031-30651-8_10

ered to prevent future injuries. Screening tests include whispered voice, finger rub, and patient questionnaires. The gold standard for diagnosis remains pure-tone audiometry. Patients with hearing loss face significant barriers to obtaining hearing aids and audiology services due to cost, and lack of understanding.

Vision Loss

Most common causes for vision loss in the elderly population include age-related macular degeneration, cataract, glaucoma, diabetic retinopathy, and presbyopia. As patients age, changes in vision specific to the elderly population places them at higher risk of falls and traumatic injuries. These include poor contrast sensitivity, reduced depth perception, and visual field loss. Studies have shown that 46.7% of patients that fall age 65 years or older have severe vision impairment. In another study, it was shown that in frail elderly patients admitted with a hip fracture, 46% had vision impairment. These patients most commonly had uncorrected eyesight, or untreated cataract. Vision loss and impairment is a contributing factor to traumatic injuries in the geriatric population. Patients that fall are more likely to have untreated vision impairments. Through education aimed towards the elderly population regarding vision loss and falls, patients can change their home environment to prevent falls and recognize symptoms of worsening vision impairment. Yearly vision assessment at primary care visits can aid in identifying untreated vision impairments. Lastly, attending functional training programs focused on teaching patients with vision impairments to navigate mobility and the surrounding environment could help prevent falls in this patient population.

Environment

As health and functionality change with age, the surrounding home environment can be accommodated to prevent traumatic injuries from falls. Home assessments for patients with previous falls or increased risk of falls due to functional impairment or comorbidities can help identify necessary changes in their environment. Examples of home assessments include Check for Safety: A home prevention Checklist for Older Adults from the CDC, Westmead Home Safety Assessment, Falls home Assessment from the Fall Prevention Center of Excellence or Comprehensive Assessment and Solution Process for Aging Residents.

Home assessments focus on both the static home environment and the interaction of the patient with their home environment to determine fall risks. These checklists assess for the presence of objects on the floor blocking a path for walking, throw rugs, lighting, handrails on stairs, slippery floors in the bathroom, etc. Some solutions provided include placing objects in other locations, removing throw rugs, placing lamps at bedside, installing handrails and grab handles along stairs and in the shower, and using no-slip mats. Home assessments are conducted by social workers, healthcare providers, occupational therapists, or other trained staff. Most of these programs include multiple follow-up visits to assess changes that are made and to continue to evaluate the home environment. Home visits are usually coupled with general education regarding fall prevention. Some programs provide vision or hearing loss assessments along with home visits.

It has been shown that targeted home safety assessments to prevent falls are cost-effective and reduce rate of falls and risk of falling. These interventions are most effective in older patients, those with a prior history of falls, or vision impairment. Additionally, it was found that these interventions were most effective when conducted by an occupational therapist.

Significant challenges exist in implementing home assessments. Due to personnel cost and feasibility of conducting home visits, home safety assessments are difficult to implement. Patients living in rural areas are harder to reach and assess. Implementing changes once the home environment is assessed can also be costly for patients.

Gait and Mobility

In the elderly, gait impairment usually is a result of decreased gait velocity, increased double stance time, stooped posture, widened gait base, and less lift during the swing phase of walking. Prevalence of gait disorders increases from 10% in people aged 60–69 to >60% in people >80. Gait impairment is a result of neurological or musculoskeletal disease. Most common neurological conditions in the elderly that cause gait impairment are sensory ataxia due to polyneuropathy, and Parkinson's disease, and the most common musculoskeletal condition is hip and knee osteoarthritis. Gait impairment limits mobility and increases traumatic injury risk in elderly patients due to falls and pedestrian injuries. In a study conducted in Sao Paolo, Brazil, it was found that the time required to cross a street before the traffic light changes is 1.2 m/s, however, elderly patients walk at a slower rate.

Injury prevention focuses on recognizing gait impairment and limited mobility in elderly patients. Performing a thorough history and physical and focusing on patient's history of prior falls can aid in diagnosis. Additionally, clinical gait exam and neurological exam should be performed. The timed up and go test, which measures the time it takes a patient to get up from a chair, walk 3 m, and return to a sitting position in the chair, is a standardized method to assess fall risk. Currently, there are no guidelines on when to start screening and examining elderly patients for gait impairment and mobility. However, patients that have a history of prior falls are at greater risk for falls in the future, and these patients should undergo further evaluation.

Interventions to improve gait impairment and mobility in the elderly focus on exercise and physical therapy. Exercise has been the only intervention shown to decrease patients experiencing a fall, while other interventions such as Vitamin D supplementation, changes to the environment, vision and hearing assessments have reduced the number of falls patients experience. There exists no standard exercise or physical therapy regimen that has shown benefit or been studied in a large population. At this time, interventions focus on patient's specific needs after an evaluation by a physical therapist. Exercise in the elderly includes walking, aerobic condition, and resistance training to improve muscle strength, and posture. As with most interventions, limitations exist due to cost, insurance coverage, and transportation services. Systems-based interventions to decreased traumatic injury in elderly patients can address traffic light times to allow for increased time for elderly patients to cross streets and improvements in the built environment such as increased green spaces and parks to promote walking.

Cognition

Changes in cognition and memory in the elderly make them susceptible to traumatic injuries, particularly decrease in "nonverbal and abstract reasoning," "information processing speed," and "immediate memory." Elderly patients are less likely to quickly interpret changes in the environment and react accordingly to remember recent events and to analyze nonverbal information or recognize patterns. Cognition is also closely related to physical function in the elderly. Patients that have worse cognition, and memory deficits, such as patients with dementia, have muscle atrophy and deconditioning. These patients are at a higher risk for falls and other traumatic injuries.

Most commonly, the Mini-Mental State Exam (MMSE) is used to assess patients for worsening cognition. Based off this evaluation, more detailed assessments can be performed to diagnose patients with cognitive impairments. There are no direct interventions or treatment for cognitive impairment other than recognition and diagnosis. Previously, studies on preventing traumatic injuries in elderly patients excluded patients with cognitive impairment. However, there has been some benefit shown to physical exercise preventing falls in cognitively impaired patients.

Substance and Alcohol Abuse

When considering the elderly population and causes for traumatic injury, alcohol and drug intoxication is typically thought to be less likely. However, a study conducted in patients >65 admitted at a Level I trauma center showed that of those that underwent a urine drug screen (UDS) and blood alcohol content (BAC), 48.3% had a positive UDS, and 11.5% of patients had a positive BAC. Substance use in the elderly has been shown to lead to increased risk of motor vehicle crashes and increased readmissions for traumatic injuries.

While the prevalence of alcohol and substance use is less in the elderly compared to younger populations, the adverse effects are greater. Small amounts of alcohol and substance use can lead to greater impairments. Pre-existing medical conditions such as dementia or Parkinson's disease when combined with alcohol or substance use place elderly patients at greater risk of injury. Similarly, prescription medication used in the elderly population such as antidepressants or sleeping aids, and limited physiological reserve such as decreased metabolism and increased creatinine clearance, also place elderly patients at higher risk of injury when combined with substance or alcohol use.

Intervention in the elderly population is similar to those provided to younger populations. Screening should be performed regardless of age for all patients that present with a traumatic injury via validated questionnaires for assessing substance and alcohol use history, BAC and UDS. Limited research has been conducted on interventions tailored to the elderly population.

Polypharmacy

Polypharmacy is defined as the use of five or more medications, and associated with increased risk of falls, disability, and mortality in the elderly. However, it is not the number of medications but certain types of medications that are associated with increased falls.

Polypharmacy can be beneficial in managing multiple comorbidities, but inappropriate polypharmacy is when medications are prescribed that are not clinically indicated leading to adverse outcomes.

Elderly patients also have changes in physiology that impact pharmacokinetics. They have increased fat, and less lean mass. Lipophilic medications such as benzodiazepines and trazodone have increased duration of effect in the elderly leading to prolonged sedative effects. Lower creatinine clearance and slower elimination of medications can lead to increased effects of medications that are cleared by the kidneys such as oxycodone. The inability to clear metabolites of oxycodone can lead to lethargy, confusion, and respiratory depression. Decreased hepatic flow also leads to a decrease in hepatic clearance of medications such as benzodiazepines prolonging their effect in the elderly. Additionally, side effects of anticholinergic medications compound already existing physiological changes in the elderly. Side effects of dry mouth, blurred vision, urinary retention, constipation, and confusion, exacerbate already existing medical issues. Medications with anticholinergic properties, opiates, and benzodiazepines were associated with an increased probability of hip fractures in the elderly.

Prevention of inappropriate polypharmacy requires a multidisciplinary approach with coordination of care between a patient's different specialists. Reviewing medications frequently at outpatient visits and hospital admissions can lead to identification of unnecessary medications. Evaluating for adverse drug–drug interactions, starting medications at the lowest dose possible, and using the Beers criteria as outlined by the American Geriatric Society can also aid in preventing inappropriate polypharmacy. The Beers criteria identifies medications that can have harmful side effects in the elderly. Involving pharmacists in the care of elderly patients when admitted to the hospital after a traumatic injury to review medications could be a possible intervention to prevent polypharmacy and future falls.

Comorbidities

Elderly patients have more chronic health conditions compared to younger patients that place them at a higher risk of falls. There are chronic health conditions that have previously been mentioned in this chapter such as vision and hearing impairments, Parkinson's disease, dementia, and substance use disorder that are associated with falls in the elderly. Additionally, studies have shown that patients with conditions that limit gait and mobility such as arthritis, COPD, and history of stroke are associated with increased risk of falls.

However, there are other chronic health conditions that are associated with falls and traumatic injuries that may be less obvious. For example, depression was found to be associated with first falls and recurrent falls in the elderly. Surprisingly, other conditions such as diabetes, and CKD were also associated with falls. None of these conditions directly affect gait and mobility, but patients with these conditions are more likely to experience a traumatic injury. Studies have also shown that patients with greater than five comorbidities are also at risk of falls, and there are combinations of comorbidities such as osteoporosis and hypertension that are associated with increased risk of falls.

Screening patients that are at risk of falls usually focuses on conditions that directly affect gait and mobility. However, screening patients in this way could miss other patients that are also at risk such as patients with depression, diabetes, CKD, and patients with greater than five comorbidities. Interventions in injury prevention in the elderly should also include these patients.

Orthostatic Hypotension

Orthostatic hypotension is defined as a decrease in systolic blood pressure of at least 20 mmHg or diastolic blood pressure of at least 10 mmHg within 3 min of standing. While orthostatic hypotension present in the acute setting may be due to causes such as hypovolemia, or medications, chronic orthostatic hypotension is due to autonomic dysfunction. This condition is prevalent in the elderly, and approximately 20% of patients >65 years of age and 30% of patients >75 years of age have this condition. In frail elderly individuals, the prevalence is 50% or more. As people age, baroreceptors become less sensitive to sympathetic activation and the response of increased heart rate and vasoconstriction to assuming a standing position is diminished. In the elderly, the heart is less compliant, and diastolic dysfunction is common. This leads to a reduced stroke volume when moving from a sitting to standing position. Prolonged bedrest and immobility also contribute to deconditioning and orthostatic hypotension. Pathological causes of orthostatic hypotension include Lewy body dementia, Parkinson's disease, multiple cerebral infarctions, diabetes, alcohol use disorder, paraneoplastic syndrome, and pure autonomic failure. Orthostatic hypotension causes significant morbidity and is associated with falls and traumatic injuries in the elderly.

Unfortunately, treatment and prevention of orthostatic hypotension is challenging.

Non-pharmacologic interventions include discontinuing medications such as nitrates, tricyclic antidepressants, neuroleptics, and alpha-blockers that can cause orthostatic hypotension. Other interventions include compression stockings, abdominal binder, standing up gradually, lying in bed with head at 30° and increased intake of salt and water. Pharmacologic options include fludrocortisone and midodrine. These medications used in conjunction at lower doses can help with symptomatic orthostatic hypotension. However, there are many side effects such as hypokalemia, fluid overload, and supine hypertension. Other medications include droxidopa, a noradrenaline prodrug that can improve orthostatic hypotension without supine hypertension; however, there is limited research demonstrating its benefit. Atomoxetine has been shown to be as effective as midodrine and superior in ameliorating symptoms associated with orthostatic hypotension.

Recognizing orthostatic hypotension in elderly patients can prevent traumatic injuries.

Patients that are admitted to the hospital after a syncopal fall should undergo evaluation of orthostatic hypotension prior to discharge. Similarly, patients should be screened at primary care visits for orthostatic hypotension. Patients with Lewy body dementia or Parkinson's disease should especially be screened and recognized as higher risk for developing this condition.

Environment

Other interventions aimed at reducing the major risk factors for injury in the elderly include home safety assessments by occupational therapists have been shown to decrease the incidence of falls. Older persons may benefit from adjusting their living spaces by removing falling hazards, improving lighting, and securing rugs. Smart vehicles with rear cameras and ABS can help with elderly patients who drive.

Types of Injury

Falls

Of the most common mechanisms of injury experienced by the older population, falls top the list with highest frequency. It is one of the leading causes of death by unintentional injury and is a source of significant morbidity. Most commonly, patients suffer ground level falls with resulting hip fractures. Multiple factors contribute to the incidence of falls as listed previously, such that directed injury prevention with increasing strength and activity, reducing obstacles, and maintaining safe spaces will assist in changing that outcome. Improvement in bone health has also been shown to decrease the likelihood of fracture after fall. In a recent study by Anam and Insogna, well-balanced diet with calcium and vitamin D with exercise, limited alcohol and no smoking, decreased the incidence of fragility fractures in older patients. Therefore, the addition of exercise and healthy diet should be considered in injury prevention when addressing falls in the elderly.

In addition to the fractures sustained concomitantly, patients may experience head injury, with intracranial bleeds, further exacerbated by their medications, of which DOACS are common. While data suggest that the use of DOACS did not demonstrate increased mortality as compared to patients without anticoagulation, the risk of surgical intervention and resulting morbidity remains unclear. Limiting the use of these medications when appropriate may assist in improved outcomes after falls.

Motor Vehicle Crashes

In the older population, minor car crashes are associated with significant injury. Further, several studies have shown increasing age to be a risk factor for pedestrian versus vehicle.

Contributing factors range from the gait of the older individual to the decrease in hearing and vision. Interventions that address the physiological progression as well as balance exercises like Tai Chi can aid in injury prevention. Public health initiatives that focus on changing the timing of stop lights and increasing the lighting at specific locations all work towards decreasing the incidence of elderly patients being struck by vehicles.

Older patients are more likely to wear seatbelts while driving. Despite this, they are at an increased risk of death and significant morbidity if involved in a crash, as compared to the younger population. Factors described previously such as vision and hearing loss can impact the ability to drive safely, but an important concern is the how the individual "fits into the car."

National educational programs like "Car Fit" teaches the aging how to determine how well they fit their vehicle; are they too close to the steering wheel, do seats need to be raised, or do they even need a differently sized vehicle. Other focus is on teaching driver safety and increasing awareness while maintaining independence.

Summary

The demographic of the trauma patients is rapidly changing, consistent with the changing face of the country. Older patients have physiological changes and underlying medical conditions that make them prone to traumatic injuries and their mechanism of injury varies from that of the younger patient. There is an urgent need to focus on the specific issues facing that population with a concerted effort to support the physiologic changes that occur. Vision and hearing impairment, limited gait and mobility, environmental challenges, decreased cognition, substance use, inappropriate polypharmacy, increased comorbidities, and orthostatic hypotension are some of the main risk factors for traumatic injuries. Falls and motor vehicle crashes with pedestrian versus vehicle as a significant cause of injury, means that injury prevention should also involve public health initiatives to decrease the incidence of injury. Recognizing risk factors, screening for them in the hospital and at primary care visits and implementing interventions specific for the elderly population can help to prevent injuries. Optimal injury prevention should involve optimization of the limitations in this population, as well as legislature.

References

1. Llompart-Pou JA, Pérez-Bárcena J, Chico-Fernández M, Sánchez-Casado M, Raurich JM. Severe trauma in the geriatric population. World J Crit Care Med. 2017;6(2):99–106. https://doi.org/10.5492/wjccm.v6.i2.99.
2. US Preventive Services Taskforce. Hearing loss in older adults: screening|United States Preventive Services Taskforce. 2021. November 20, 2022. https://www.uspreventiveservicestaskforce.org/uspstf/recommendation/hearing-loss-in-older-adults-screening#citation18
3. Steinman BA, Nguyen AQD, Pynoos J, Leland NE. Falls-prevention interventions for persons who are blind or visually impaired. Insight (Lawrence). 2011;4(2):83–91.
4. Pynoos J, Steinman BA, Nguyen AQ. Environmental assessment and modification as fall-prevention strategies for older adults. Clin Geriatr Med. 2010;26(4):633–44. https://doi.org/10.1016/j.cger.2010.07.001.
5. Pega F, Kvizhinadze G, Blakely T, Atkinson J, Wilson N. Home safety assessment and modification to reduce injurious falls in community-dwelling older adults: cost-utility and equity analysis. Inj Prev. 2016;22:420–6. https://doi.org/10.1136/injuryprev-2016-041999.
6. Duim E, Lebrão ML, Ferreira Antunes JL. Walking speed of older people and pedestrian crossing time. J Transport Health. 2017;5:70–6. https://doi.org/10.1016/j.jth.2017.02.001.
7. Rimland JM, Abraha I, Dell' Aquila G, Cruz-Jentoft A, Soiza R, Gudmusson A, et al. Effectiveness of non-pharmacological interventions to prevent falls in older people: a systematic overview. The SENATOR project ONTOP series. PLoS One. 2016;11(8):e0161579. https://doi.org/10.1371/journal.pone.0161579.
8. Guirguis-Blake JM, Michael YL, Perdue LA, Coppola EL, Beil TL, Thompson JH. Interventions to prevent falls in community-dwelling older adults: a systematic review for the U.S. Preventive Services Task Force. Rockville (MD): Agency for Healthcare Research and Quality (US). 2018. Report No.: 17–05232-EF-1.
9. van Schoor NM, Smit JH, Pluijm SMF, Jonker C, Lips P. Different cognitive functions in relation to falls among older persons: immediate memory as an independent risk factor for falls. J Clin Epidemiol. 2002;55(9):855–62. https://doi.org/10.1016/s0895-4356(02)00438-9.
10. Chan WC, Yeung JWF, Wong CSM, Lam LCW, Chung KF, Luk JKH, et al. Efficacy of physical exercise in preventing falls in older adults with cognitive impairment: a systematic review and meta-analysis. J Am Med Dir Assoc. 2015;16(2):149–54. https://doi.org/10.1016/j.jamda.2014.08.007.
11. Hammond T, Wilson A. Polypharmacy and falls in the elderly: a literature review. Nurs Midwifery Stud. 2013;2(2):171–5. https://doi.org/10.5812/nms.10709.
12. Machado-Duque ME, Castaño-Montoya JP, Medina-Morales DA, Castro-Rodríguez A, González-Montoya A, Machado-Alba JE. Association between the use of benzodiazepines and opioids with the risk of falls and hip fractures in older adults. Int Psychogeriatr. 2018;30(7):941–6. https://doi.org/10.1017/S1041610217002745.
13. Anam AK, Insogna K. Update on osteoporosis screening and management. Med Clin North Am. 2021;105(6):1117–34. https://doi.org/10.1016/j.mcna.2021.05.016.
14. Immonen M, Haapea M, Similä H, Enwald H, Keränen N, Kangas M, et al. Association between chronic diseases and falls among a sample of older people in Finland. BMC Geriatr. 2020;20:225. https://doi.org/10.1186/s12877-020-01621-9.
15. Dani M, Dirksen A, Taraborrelli P, Panagopolous D, Torocastro M, Sutton R, Lim PB. Orthostatic hypotension in older people: considerations, diagnosis and management. Clin Med (Lond). 2021;21(3):e275–82. https://doi.org/10.7861/clinmed.2020-1044.

Neurobehavioral Aspects of Acute Care Surgery in Geriatric Patients

11

Aaron Pinkhasov and Anna Jaysing

The Prevalence of Neurocognitive Impairment and Psychiatric Illness Among Geriatric Patients

During normal aging, the brain undergoes morphological changes with gradual loss of synapse number, decline in major neurotransmitters availability and reduction in neuroplasticity. This makes the geriatric population particularly vulnerable to the cognitive and emotional burdens of surgery. Neurocognitive impairment and psychiatric illness are highly prevalent among geriatric patients. At an average age of 70 year, about two thirds of Americans experience some level of cognitive impairment. Among adults over 60 years of age undergoing elective non-cardiac surgery, an estimated 18% have diagnosed cognitive impairment and 37% have unrecognized cognitive impairment. Among the community dwelling geriatric population, the prevalence of depression is estimated to be between 5 and 10%. Around 11.4% of geriatrics patients have an anxiety disorder, with 2.8% having generalized anxiety disorder and 3.5% having post-traumatic stress disorder (PTSD). Moreover, amid the COVID-19 pandemic, 25% of the geriatric population reported anxiety or depression.

A. Pinkhasov (✉)
Department of Psychiatry, NYU Long Island School of Medicine, Mineola, NY, USA

Department of Medicine, NYU Long Island School of Medicine, Mineola, NY, USA

Deparment of Psychiatry, NYU Langone Hospital—Long Island, NYU Long Island School of Medicine, Mineola, NY, USA
e-mail: Aron.Pinkhasov@nyulangone.org

A. Jaysing
Department of Psychiatry, NYU Long Island School of Medicine, Mineola, NY, USA
e-mail: Anna.Jaysing@nyulangone.org

The Interplay Between Injury and the Baseline Neuropsychiatric Health of Geriatric Patients

The presence of neurocognitive impairment in geriatric patients correlates with the surgical acuity, type, and outcome. Geriatric patients with dementia, who undergo a major surgical procedure as part of an inpatient admission, are more likely to undergo an emergent operation as compared to geriatric patients without dementia. Moreover, geriatric patients with dementia most frequently undergo treatment for a dislocated or fracture hip and femur, while geriatric patients without dementia most frequently undergo knee arthroplasty, a finding likely mediated in part by the increased risk for falls among patients with dementia. Furthermore, geriatric patients with underlying dementia who undergo surgery for bone fracture, hip replacement, lower extremity amputation, percutaneous transluminal coronary angioplasty, and urinary tract pathology are more

P. Petrone, C. E.M. Brathwaite (eds.), *Acute Care Surgery in Geriatric Patients*,
https://doi.org/10.1007/978-3-031-30651-8_11

likely to suffer in-hospital mortality, are less likely to be discharge home, and are more likely to experience a longer length of stay as compared to patients without dementia.

Fall risk factors in the geriatric population include age-related neurosensory decline, loss of agility, impaired balance, medical and psychiatric comorbidities, and risk associated with pharmacologic treatment. In turn, falls are a risk factor for exacerbation of cognitive impairment and psychiatric illness among geriatric patients. Elderly patients with dementia are at particular risk for delirium post hip fracture. However, falls may also be associated with cognitive decline in patients cognitively intact at baseline. The mechanism by which this bidirectional impact occurs is thought to be via decreased physical performance and depressive mood. A decline in physical performance combined with a fear of falling can have a compound effect on patients' social activities. The resultant social isolation can lead to the development of a depressed mood, which can in turn further affect physical function, laying the foundation for a vicious cycle.

A similar bidirectional relationship is described between traumatic brain injury (TBI) and neuropsychiatric illness. Both dementia and depression are associated with late life TBI risk. The prevalence of depression in the elderly following TBI is up to 37%. Though the mechanism remains to be fully understood, the chronic neuroinflammation caused by TBIs is a likely mediator. TBI is associated with a 50% increased risk of new-onset PTSD among geriatric patients and 37% of patients report clinically significant levels of anxiety post TBI. Both PTSD and anxiety have been shown to impede TBI recovery. Moreover, TBI can impede a patient's ability to recover from PTSD. Of particular consequence to the geriatric population, moderate to severe TBIs increase the risk of dementia up to four-fold.

The Interplay Between Stroke and the Baseline Neuropsychiatric Health of Geriatric Patients

Both pre-existing cognitive dysfunction and psychiatric illness can impact post-stroke cognition among geriatric patients. Similarly, stroke can impact geriatric neurocognitive function and mental health. It is estimated that 20–50% of stroke patients develop mood symptoms, with depression being the most frequent psychiatric consequence of brain ischemia. Though the exact mechanism of post-stroke depression has yet to be elucidated, synaptic alterations in the prefrontal cortex and hippocampus, stroke elicited neuroinflammatory changes, and the disruption of neural circuits connecting areas of the prefrontal cortex, basal ganglia, and the limbic system have all been hypothesized to be etiologically implicated. In addition to the challenges that come with the depressive symptoms themselves, post-stroke depression is associated with reduced functional recovery, cognition, and social reintegration. Regarding post-stroke mania, lesions in paleocortical areas of the right hemisphere, head of the caudate, and dorsomedial thalamus are thought to be risk factors. Post-stroke anxiety has been associated with right hemisphere lesions and anterior circulation territory lesions. Screening tools that can be used to identify post-stroke neuropsychiatric disorders are outlined in Table 11.1.

Table 11.1 Post-stroke neuropsychiatric disorder prevalence, screening, and management (adapted from Zhang et al., 2020)

	Prevalence	Screening tools
Post-stroke depressive disorder	5–84%	– Geriatric Depression Scale (GDS)
		– Hospital Anxiety and Depression Scale (HADS)
		– Patient Health Questionnaire–9 (PHQ-9)
		– Beck Depression Inventory (BDI-II)
		– Center for Epidemiological Studies Depression Scale (CES-D)
		– Stroke Aphasic Depression Questionnaire–10 (SADQ-10)
Post-stroke anxiety disorders	20–24%	– Hamilton Anxiety Scale
		– Hospital Anxiety and Depression Scale (HADS)–Anxiety Sub-Scale
Post-stroke PTSD (PAS)	8.3–29.6%	– Post-traumatic Adjustment Scale
Post-stroke psychosis and psychotic disorders	4.67–5.05%	

Postoperative Delirium

Delirium is a common and potentially devastating complication of geriatric comorbidities. It is defined as an acute or subacute change in mental status with associated cognitive and behavioral disturbances. The incidence of postoperative delirium varies by surgical procedure and anesthesia type. The awareness about postoperative delirium increased considerably between 1995 and 2020. However, it remains severely undiagnosed and is missed in up to two-thirds of patients. The incidence of postoperative delirium by surgery time is outlined in Table 11.2.

Table 11.2 Incidence of postoperative delirium by surgery type (adapted From Rudolph et al., 2011)

Surgery	Incidence
Abdominal aortic aneurysm (Infrarenal)	33–54%
Abdominal	5–51%
Coronary artery bypass graft	37–52%
Elective orthopedic	9–15%
Head and neck cancer (major surgery)	17%
Hip fracture	35–65%
Peripheral vascular	30–48%
Urologic	4–7%

The Risk Factors for Postoperative Delirium

The risk of postoperative delirium among geriatric patients is influenced by both pre-existing and precipitating factors as shown in Table 11.3. As some pre-existing risk factors can be modified prior to surgery, they are important to be aware of. It is equally important to identify and address intraoperative and postoperative delirium risk factors, whenever possible. Taking care to appropriately manage patient pain, limit disturbances during sleep and avoid psychotropic medications can protect patients from the harmful effects of postoperative delirium.

Intraoperative Hypotension

While intraoperative hypotension is theorized to be a risk factor for neurocognitive decline, as mediated by the impact on blood flow and tissue perfusion, clinical evidence linking the phenomenon to the development of postoperative delirium is mixed. This is largely due to the presence of various confounding factors as well as a heterogenous definition of hypotension. Nevertheless, available evidence does suggest a tailored approach to arterial pressure management based on advanced hemodynamic monitoring is preferable to using existing cut-off points.

Hyponatremia

Both preoperative and postoperative hyponatremia have been shown to be risk factors for postoperative delirium among patients undergoing

Table 11.3 Pre-existing and precipitating risk factors for postoperative delirium (adapted from Schenning et al., 2015)

Pre-existing risk factors	Precipitating risk factors
Pre-surgical	*Intraoperative*
• Age >65 years	– Blood loss
– Neuropsychiatric conditions	– Blood transfusion
– Pre-existing cognitive dysfunction	– Prolonged surgery
– Prior history of delirium	– Surgical urgency
– Depression	– Surgical complexity
– History of stroke	
– Substance use and withdrawal	
(EtOH, tobacco, illicit drugs, narcotics)	*Postoperative*
• Use of psychotropic medications	– Intensive care unit admission
• Poor physical status	– Increased hospital course length
• Loss of hearing and vision	– Increased mechanical ventilation duration
• Medical comorbidities	– Use of physical restraints
– Heart failure	– Sleep disruption
– Renal failure	– Pain
– Diabetes mellitus	– Use of CNS active medications
– Atrial fibrillation	
– Anemia	
– Atherosclerosis	

orthopedic, spinal, and thoracic surgery. Moreover, the use of postoperative hypotonic maintenance fluid can be associated with a higher risk of postoperative delirium as compared to the use of isotonic maintenance fluid.

Identifying Postoperative Delirium and Postoperative Cognitive Decline

The presentation of delirium falls into five overarching domains: global disturbance of cognition, psychomotor disturbance, emotional dysregulation, sleep-wake cycle disturbance, and impaired consciousness and attention. Global disturbance of cognition includes perceptual distortions, impaired abstract thinking and comprehension, and/or disorientation. Emotional dysregulation can manifest as irritability, anger, fear, anxiety, and/or perplexity. Impaired consciousness and attention presents as a reduced ability to direct, focus, sustain, and sift attention.

The symptoms of delirium can progress in a variety of ways. Hyperactive delirium, which is seen in 77% of delirium cases, is characterized by agitation, restlessness, and combative, uncooperative behavior. Hypoactive delirium, seen in 23% of delirium cases, is accompanied by withdrawn and depressed affect, psychomotor retardation, apathy, and lethargy. A mixed-type characterized by an overlapping presentation may also be seen. While agitated delirium patients draw attention and response of health care providers, patients with hypoactive delirium frequently go unnoticed and undertreated making their prognosis worse compared to hyperactive or mixed types of delirium.

Diagnosing Delirium

According to DSM-5 criteria, delirium is a disturbance in attention and awareness that is a change from baseline, develops over a short period of time (usually hours to days) and tends to fluctuate in severity during the course of a day. There are additional disturbances in cognition such as memory deficits, disorientation, language disturbances, impaired visuospatial ability, and/or altered perception. All aforementioned disturbance are not explained by another pre-existing, established, or evolving neurocognitive disorder and do not occur in the context of a severely reduced state of arousal (i.e., coma). Finally, there must be evidence from history, physical exam, or laboratory tests that the disturbance is a direct physiological consequence of another or multiple other etiologies (i.e., medical condition, substance intoxication or withdrawal, toxin exposure).

The differential diagnosis of postoperative delirium is broad and includes emergence delir-

Table 11.4 Validated delirium screening tools (Adapted from Schenning et al., 2015)

	Sensitivity	Specificity
Confusion assessment method (CAM)	94–100%	90–95%
Confusion assessment method for the intensive care unit (CAM-ICU)	95–100%	89–93%
Delirium symptom interview (DSI)	90%	80%
Nursing delirium screening scale (NuDESC)	85.7%	86.8%
Intensive care delirium screening checklist (ICDSC)	99%	64%
NEECHAM confusion scale	95%	78%

ium (defined as an acute confusion state during recovery from anesthesia), postoperative cognitive dysfunction (defined as an acute to subacute, quantifiable decline in cognition), cerebrovascular accident, transient ischemic attack, dementia, and depression. As a diagnosis of exclusion, other etiologies must be ruled out before the diagnosis of postoperative delirium can be made.

Screening for delirium before each shift is essential to capturing changes in mental status. (APSS 2022) There are many validated screening tools for assessing delirium which include the Confusion Assessment Method, the Confusion Assessment Method for the Intensive Care Unit, the Delirium Symptom Interview, the Nursing Delirium Screening Scale, the Intensive Care Delirium Screening Checklist, and the NEECHAM Confusion Scale. Their sensitivity and specificity are outlined in Table 11.4. For older adults in a general hospital setting, the Confusion Assessment Method is preferred, whereas for older adults in an intensive care unit, the Intensive Care Delirium Screening Checklist and the Confusion Assessment Method for the Intensive Care Unit are preferred.

The benefits of the CAM screening tool is that it is available in over 20 languages. There is a short, 4 item version that is commonly used for screening, and a longer, 10 item version that provides information on every subtypes.

Preventing and Managing Neurocognitive and Psychiatric Sequelae of Surgery and Anesthesia

Given the high prevalence of cognitive impairment among geriatric patients, an understanding of baseline cognitive function is instrumental to the assessment of mental status changes in the postoperative period. As baseline cognitive impairment is too often unrecognized, preoperative cognitive evaluation is recommended for patients without a known history of cognitive impairment or dementia. Moreover, major risk factors for delirium such as age greater than 65 years, pre-existing cognitive decline or dementia, current hip fracture, and the presence of severe illness should also be routinely assessed.

When assessing for preoperative delirium, patient risk can be stratified into low (2%), medium (13%), and high (50%) delirium risk using the Marcantonio clinical prediction tools, which is based on six preoperative risk factors (age ≥70, alcohol abuse, cognitive impairment, low activity level, abnormal electrolytes, and invasive surgery).

The management of postoperative delirium includes preventative measures and identification of the underlying cause. Preventative measures include patient-specific habilitation programs that target predisposing risk factors, frequent patient orientation, increasing patient mobility, promoting patient sleep hygiene, appropriated medication management (i.e., adequate pain control, limited use of medications with psychoactive properties, avoidance of polypharmacy), and ensuring access to glasses, hearing aids, and dentures. Hearing aids are of particular importance as severe hearing loss is associated with a greater number of neuropsychiatric symptoms and progression of dementia.

Postoperative delirium management begins with non-pharmacologic interventions aimed at addressing patient activity, comfort, and environment. Activity can be promoted through early involvement of PMNR department and focus on ambulation and cognitive stimulation.

Moving patients out of bed into chairs and proactively removing lines such as Foley catheters, NG tubes, and leads helps patients ambulate sooner. Orienting patients to person, place, time, and situation, as well as engaging them with puzzles, and mindfulness coloring activities support cognitive stimulation.

To promote patient comfort, ensuring patients have sensory correction and communication devices is essential. Make sure patients have access to hearing aids, glasses, and interpreter services if necessary. Additionally, promote adequate feeding and elimination by ensuring dental comfort, reassessing dietary restrictions daily, assisting in feeding during mealtimes, encouraging fluid intake, toileting every 2 h during the day, and bladder scanning patients if no urine has been passed in an 8-h period.

Despite the challenges of the hospital environment, it is important to promote proper sleep hygiene and provide familiar stimuli. To facilitate proper sleep hygiene, expose patients to natural daylight and avoid caffeinated beverages after 2 pm. At night, turn off all lights and screens, offer eye masks, minimize noise, and avoid non-urgent test and medicines. To promote a familiar environment, ensure there is a visible clock in the room, play personalized music, and encourage family to visit and bring personal items from home, such as favorite blankets or family photographs to improve patients' comfort.

Should delirium persist despite these non-pharmacologic interventions, pharmacologic interventions aimed at managing pain and supporting sleep can be considered. When feasible use acetaminophen for pain and melatonin for sleep phase regulation. Limit the use of benzodiazepines, anticholinergics, and opiates and consult psychiatry before using antipsychotics for agitation or psychosis.

Most importantly, continue to address underlying causes of delirium, such as infection and polypharmacy. When considering which medications to use in geriatric patients, Beers Criteria can be used as safety guidelines as outlined in Table 11.5.

Table 11.5 Medications to avoid in geriatric patients (Adapted from Fixen, 2019)

Anticholinergic	First-generation antihistamines
	Anti-parkinsonian agents (benztropine, trihexyphenidyl)
	Antispasmodics
Antithrombotics	Dipyridamole
Cardiovascular	Peripheral alpha-1 blockers
	Centrally acting alpha-2 agonists (clonidine, guanabenz, guanfacine, methyldopa, reserpine)
	Disopyramide
	Dronedarone
	Digoxin
	Nifedipine (immediate release)
	Amiodarone
CNS	Tricyclic antidepressants
	Antipsychotics (except in schizophrenia or bipolar disorder)
	Barbiturates
	Benzodiazepines
	Meprobamate
	Nonbenzodiazepine (benzodiazepine receptor agonist hypnotics)
	Ergoloid mesylates
Endocrine	Desiccated thyroid
	Long-acting sulfonylureas
	Sliding-scale insulin
Genitourinary	Desmopressin
Pain	Nonselective NSAIDs
	Skeletal muscle relaxants

Pathophysiology of Postoperative Delirium and Postoperative Cognitive Dysfunction

While the etiology of postoperative delirium is multifactorial, greater cognitive reserve is associated with lower delirium incidence post-surgery. Therefore, postoperative delirium is postulated to arise when the physiologic stresses of surgery and anesthesia are greater than a patient's cognitive reserve.

Cognitive reserve is the brain's capacity to overcome injury. Low educational attainment, limited participation in cognitive leisure activities, and low levels of physical activity have been shown to be associated with an increased risk of dementia or cognitive decline. However, increased participation in cognitive activities (i.e., doing puzzles, knitting, writing, card games), in particular, has been found to decrease delirium incidence and severity in older surgical patients.

The mechanism by which surgery and anesthesia cause physiology stress to the brain has yet to be clearly defined. However, the processes of neuroinflammation, neurochemical changes, and hyponatremia are likely to be implicated.

Neuroinflammation

Neuroinflammation is the peripheral neuroendocrine response to the physiologic stress of surgery and anesthesia. Associated physiological and behavioral changes such as depression, cognitive deficits, and social withdrawal are thought to be an adaptive response to injury. Using this framework, altered mental status, also termed delirium, is considered an exaggerated version of this response. This impact of surgery and anesthesia on neuroinflammation is laid out in Fig. 11.1.

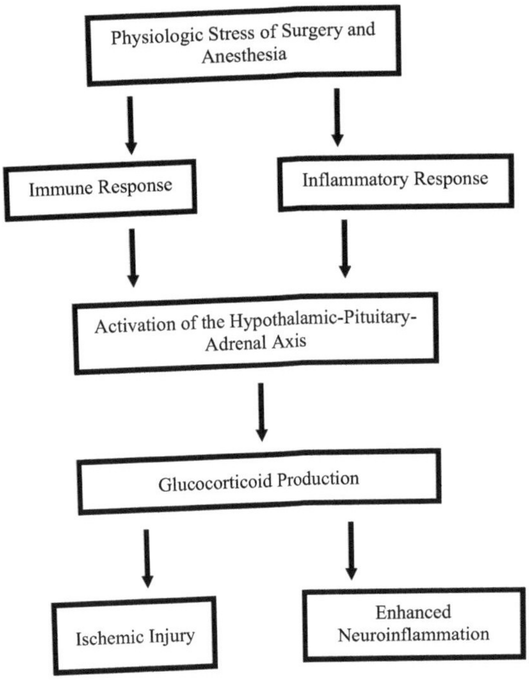

Fig. 11.1 Impact of surgery and anesthesia on neuroinflammation

Neurochemical Changes

Another theory regarding the mechanism of postoperative delirium emphasizes the role the impact of neurochemical imbalances on neurotransmission. It highlights in particular the effect of the changes seen in the acetylcholine, dopamine, gamma-aminobutyric acid, glutamate, and serotonin systems. By using functional magnetic resonance imaging to examine the strength of resting-state functional connectivity between regions producing or utilizing acetylcholine and dopamine during and after an episode of delirium, patients with delirium have been shown to have disruption in reciprocity of the dorsolateral prefrontal cortex with the posterior cingulate cortex, reversible reduction of subcortical functional connectivity, and dysregulation of the suprachiasmatic nucleus of the hypothalamus.

Oxidative Stress

The theory of oxidative stress is that brain hypoperfusion induces local ischemia that triggers increased production of reactive oxygen species, which lead to excitotoxicity, apoptosis, and local inflammation. However, there is little clinical evidence to suggest that global cerebral desaturation is a common cause of delirium and the administration of drugs that increase free radical scavengers have not reduced the incidence or duration of delirium.

When Neurologic Burden Overwhelms Cognitive Reserve

When the neurologic stresses of anesthesia and surgery overcome a patient's cognitive reserve, postoperative delirium may emerge. It is imperative to address postoperative delirium as it creates a toxic environment that can increase length of hospital stay, further erode cognitive reserve via increased risk of long-term cognitive impairment and increase mortality risk. Postoperative delirium has also been found to be associated with an increased incidence of new onset disability and increased risk for discharge to a nursing home.

Postoperative delirium is a risk factor for posttraumatic stress disorder among geriatric patients, with the prevalence being particularly high 3 months after surgery. It is important to note that traumatic stress can be associated with lasting changes in the amygdala, hippocampus, and prefrontal cortex, which are areas of the brain implicated in the stress response. Not only can subsequent stressors result in increased cortisol and norepinephrine responses, but patients with post-traumatic stress disorder (PTSD) may demonstrate smaller hippocampal and anterior cingulate volumes, increased amygdala function, and decreased medial prefrontal/anterior cingulate function. However, treatments for PTSD have shown to improve memory and increased hippocampal volume.

Given the protective effects of increased cognitive reserve, pre-surgical optimization aimed at bolstering brain function and capacity should be considered, especially in particularly at-risk patients.

Conclusion

The geriatric population is especially vulnerable to the burdens of surgery and injury due to the high prevalence of pre-existing illness and overall decreased neuroplasticity. Understanding the interplay between these burdens and the baseline neuropsychiatric health of geriatric patients can help clinicians identify which patients may be particularly at risk for poor outcomes. Presurgical neurocognitive screening serves to not only establish this population's baseline function, which is essential when evaluating for postoperative delirium, but also to capture their overall risk for post-surgical cognitive impairment and psychiatric illness.

With an appreciation for the preoperative and postoperative interventions that may alter the geriatric population's risk for delirium and psychiatric illness, clinicians can better safeguard their neuropsychiatric health. Optimizing patients before surgery, avoiding medications known to be high risk for the geriatric population, and facilitating patient comfort and cognitive stimulation can all help prevent against delirium. When, despite the employment of preventive interventions, delirium arises, it can be promptly diagnosed through routine screenings for changes in a patient's mental status at the beginning of each shift. Screening and management of highly prevalent comorbid psychiatric conditions, such as anxiety, depression, and psychosis of paramount importance. Once diagnosed, establishing and addressing the underlying etiology is crucial for preserving functional status and improving healthcare outcomes in this vulnerable population.

References

1. American Psychiatric Association. American Psychiatric Association DSM-5 Task Force. In: American Psychiatric Association, editor. Diagnostic and statistical manual of mental disorders: DSM-5, vol. xliv. 5th ed; 2013. p. 947.
2. Bremner JD. Traumatic stress: effects on the brain. Dialogues Clin Neurosci. 2006;8(4):445–61.
3. Choi SH, Lee H, Chung TS, et al. Neural network functional connectivity during and after an episode of delirium. Am J Psychiatry. 2012;169(5):498–507. https://doi.org/10.1176/appi.ajp.2012.11060976.
4. Chow WB, Rosenthal RA, Merkow RP, et al. Optimal preoperative assessment of the geriatric surgical patient: a best practices guideline from the American College of Surgeons National Surgical Quality Improvement Program and the American Geriatrics Society. J Am Coll Surg. 2012;215(4):453–66. https://doi.org/10.1016/j.jamcollsurg.2012.06.017.
5. Deiner S, Liu X, Lin HM, et al. Does postoperative cognitive decline result in new disability after surgery? Ann Surg. 2021;274(6):e1108–14. https://doi.org/10.1097/SLA.0000000000003764.
6. Fixen DR. 2019 AGS beers criteria for older adults. Pharmacy Today. 2019;25(11):42–54.
7. Jones RN, Fong TG, Metzger E, et al. Aging, brain disease, and reserve: implications for delirium. Am J Geriatr Psychiatry. 2010;18(2):117–27. https://doi.org/10.1097/JGP.0b013e3181b972e8.
8. Marcantonio ER, Goldman L, Mangione CM, et al. A clinical prediction rule for delirium after elective noncardiac surgery. JAMA. 1994;271(2):134–9.
9. Masutani R, Pawar A, Lee H, Weissman JS, Kim DH. Outcomes of common major surgical procedures in older adults with and without dementia. JAMA Netw Open. 2020;3(7):e2010395. https://doi.org/10.1001/jamanetworkopen.2020.10395.
10. Mohanty S, Rosenthal RA, Russell MM, Neuman MD, Ko CY, Esnaola NF. Optimal

perioperative Management of the Geriatric Patient: a best practices guideline from the American College of Surgeons NSQIP and the American Geriatrics Society. J Am Coll Surg. 2016;222(5):930–47. https://doi.org/10.1016/j.jamcollsurg.2015.12.026.
11. Reynolds K, Pietrzak RH, El-Gabalawy R, Mackenzie CS, Sareen J. Prevalence of psychiatric disorders in U.S. older adults: findings from a nationally representative survey. World Psychiatry. 2015;14(1):74–81. https://doi.org/10.1002/wps.20193.
12. Rudolph JL, Marcantonio ER. Review articles: postoperative delirium: acute change with long-term implications. Anesth Analg. 2011;112(5):1202–11. https://doi.org/10.1213/ANE.0b013e3182147f6d.
13. Schenning KJ, Deiner SG. Postoperative delirium in the geriatric patient. Anesthesiol Clin. 2015;33(3):505–16. https://doi.org/10.1016/j.anclin.2015.05.007.
14. Wilson JE, Mart MF, Cunningham C, et al. Delirium. Nat Rev Dis Primers. 2020;6(1):90. https://doi.org/10.1038/s41572-020-00223-4.
15. Zhang S, Xu M, Liu ZJ, Feng J, Ma Y. Neuropsychiatric issues after stroke: clinical significance and therapeutic implications. World J Psychiatry. 2020;10(6):125–38. https://doi.org/10.5498/wjp.v10.i6.125.

12 Initial Evaluation of the Geriatric Injured Patient

Ricardo Jacquez

General Evaluation

Airway

Assessment of the elderly airway begins by asking the patient to speak. While it is wrong to assume that your patient is hard of hearing and raise you voice at the outset, one should remain open to the need to step closer and speak more loudly and clearly. If the patient is speaking, then a patent airway is present. The speech need not be fluent, only present. Slurred speech following a stroke in years past remains a reliable sign of a patent airway.

If the patient does not have a protected airway, *then you must give them one.* Table 12.1 lists common airway problems specific to the elderly patient. The jaw thrust maneuver should be used to open the trauma patient's airway because it assumes a cervical spine injury may be present and causes little to no neck movement. An oral airway can be inserted to temporarily displace the tongue anteriorly. The airway is likely to require suctioning of emesis, and/or secretions. Dependent on the level of consciousness, the patient may require that you remove their dentures either by hand or with forceps. In facial trauma, the dentures may have become dislodged and displaced into the oropharynx. A comatose patient (GCS 8 or less) requires a definitive airway which by definition is an airway preventing aspiration below the level of the vocal cords. The gold standard definitive airway is an endotracheal tube placed trans orally with its cuff balloon placed just below the vocal cords. Approach the airway with an expectation of limited neck movement either from arthritic changes limiting atlanto-occipital joint movement or cervical hardware placed in years passed.

Table 12.1 Common airway problems specific to the elderly patient

• Emesis occluding the airway	• Tongue occluding the airway.
• Dentures occluding the airway	• Tracheal crush injury
• Neck bleeding obstructing the trachea	• Angioedema related to medications

If orotracheal intubation is not possible, then prepare for a cricothyrotomy surgical airway. An ETT 6.0 can be inserted into your cricothyrotomy. In the event, the patient presents with an open tracheal wound, *one attempt* at insertion of an ETT 6.0 can be made. Avoid more than one attempt as insertion is difficult and unlikely to succeed. Attempts at orotracheal intubation should immediately follow.

R. Jacquez (✉)
Division of Trauma and Acute Care Surgery, Department of Surgery, NYU Long Island School of Medicine, NYU Langone Hospital—Long Island, Mineola, NY, USA
e-mail: ricardo.jacquez@nyulangone.org

P. Petrone, C. E.M. Brathwaite (eds.), *Acute Care Surgery in Geriatric Patients*,
https://doi.org/10.1007/978-3-031-30651-8_12

Breathing

Breath sounds should be heard clearly in the right and left lung. Note that a respiratory rate greater than 35 breaths per minute is not effective breathing and immediately requires that ventilation be supported.

If the patient is not breathing, your assessment must discover why—and fix the problem. Table 12.2 lists common breathing problems specific to the elderly patient. It is important also to maintain awareness of the respiratory changes, which come with age. Table 12.3 lists physiologic respiratory changes specific to the elderly patient.

If the patient is not breathing effectively, then you must breathe for them. Breathing for the patient is quickly achieved with bag valve mask (BVM) ventilation. Connect the BVM to oxygen 15 lpm as soon as possible, but do not wait—ventilation without supplemental oxygen is better than no ventilation at all. Approach BVM ventilation with the expectation that mandibular resorption, loss of dentition, and alveolar retraction will lead to a poor face mask fit. Releasing some air from the face mask ring seal can help obtain a better seal.

If you suspect a pneumothorax is present based on lack of breath sounds, tracheal deviation, distended neck veins, or subcutaneous emphysema you must immediately decompress the chest. A scalpel thoracostomy ensures creation of a finger-sized thoracostomy—thus allowing trapped air to escape. Another option for decompression is lateral chest wall needle decompression into the fifth intercostal space. Insertion of more than one needle or catheter into the fifth intercostal space will increase the speed of decompression. *Note* that chest tube placement is not specifically mentioned. The thoracostomy and egress of pneumothorax is *much more important* than the chest tube itself. Any delay for water chamber set up or chest tube obtainment is an unconscionable delay in life-saving treatment.

If you are presented with a sucking chest wound, then the thoracostomy has been created for you. Apply an occlusive dressing taped on *only three sides*. One side of the dressing must be allowed to open, and vent should a tension pneumothorax develop.

If breath sounds remain absent after thoracostomy, then consider other causes as mentioned above in Table 12.2. If asthmatic bronchospasm is suspected, administer Albuterol via nebulizer until wheezing is heard. A wheezing asthmatic is much better than a silent asthmatic. Also take into consideration redundant pharyngeal tissue which will benefit from placement of a nasal or oral airway.

Table 12.2 Common breathing problems specific to the elderly

• Hemothorax (think rib fractures and anticoagulation)	• Foreign body occluding the bronchus (think unchewed food)
• Asthmatic bronchospasm	• Sucking chest wound causing pneumothorax
• Pneumothorax (check for tracheal deviation, distended neck veins, subcutaneous emphysema)	

Table 12.3 Physiologic respiratory changes specific to the elderly patient

• Decreased tidal volume	• Blunted response to hypoxemia
• Decreased vital capacity	• Blunted response to hypercarbia
• Alveolar wall thickening	• Decreased pulmonary elasticity
• Reduced oxygen delivery	• Possible COPD / bronchiectasis

Circulation

Circulation evaluation also begins by listening to the patient. If they are talking, then they have enough blood pressure to perfuse the brain. Always remember that your patient may have bled a lot before the ambulance arrived, especially if a fall resulted in a significant scalp laceration. The use of anticoagulation may have significantly increased the amount of on-scene blood loss. Do not underestimate the volume of scalp bleeding which occurred on scene. Many

Table 12.4 Common hypotensive causes to look out for in the elderly trauma patient

• Bleeding into the chest	• Bleeding from the spleen
• Bleeding from a long bone	• Bleeding into the pelvis
• Bleeding onto the floor • Preinjury dehydration • Bleeding from the liver	• Bleeding from the scalp • Bleeding into a gluteal or thigh hematoma • Bleeding into the retroperitoneum

elderly patients with scalp lacerations will compensate until arrival to the trauma bay at which point they will demonstrate profound hypotension. Table 12.4 lists common hypotensive causes specific to the elderly trauma patient.

Beta blockade may mask the true level of hypovolemic shock in the elderly trauma patient through all but the most severe phases of shock. Anticoagulants are another class of medication which complicates the initial assessment. Elderly bleeding may be exaggerated and may require anticoagulation reversal before hemostasis can be ultimately achieved. The elderly patient may also provide a more fragile hemodynamic picture with a decreased maximal heart rate and decreased cardiac output present before the time of injury and blood loss. I propose that fear of sudden hemodynamic compensation is not strictly limited to the pediatric trauma patient but also the elderly trauma patient. The elderly trauma patient will provide limited compensation for a limited period of time with limited reserve—an abrupt crash will follow unless the physician is prepared to act aggressively and preemptively.

If the patient does not have enough volume, then you must give them volume. Table 12.5 lists physiologic circulatory changes specific to the elderly patient. Assume that you are already behind on resuscitation of the elderly trauma patient and consider early activation of massive transfusion protocol. Replace the patients lost blood by ensuring transfused products maintain a 1:1:1 ratio. Avoid excessive transfusion of packed red blood cells at the expense of hemostatic components such as platelets or plasma. The elderly

Table 12.5 Physiologic circulatory changes specific to the elderly patient

• Use of betablockers	• Decreased arterial compliance
• Use of anticoagulation/antiplatelet	• Decreased maximal heart rate
• Increased dysrhythmias	• Possible baseline hypovolemia
• Decreased cardiac output	• Possible congestive heart failure

patient on daily diuretics may suffer injury in a relative hypovolemic state prior to the development of pelvic fracture bleeding. Liberal use of CT with IV contrast may allow for demonstration of an arterial blush and thus expedite embolization by interventional radiology.

If the patient is hemorrhaging, then you must stop the bleeding. The steps to stop bleeding are sequential. The first step involves a hemostatic tool every physician, nurse, or EMT is born with—the human hand. Direct pressure to stop bleeding is always step 1.

If bleeding cannot be controlled with direct pressure, then we move up the ladder-packing the wound directly with hemostatic gauze. The next move up the ladder is applications of a tourniquet to stop bleeding. If two tourniquets are required to stop extremity bleeding, then two tourniquets are required. Application of a second tourniquet should immediately follow failure of the first tourniquet to provide hemorrhage control. A second tourniquet is simply an additional life-saving tool and is not deserving of any hesitancy. At the top of the ladder to control bleeding are exploratory laparotomy and/or exploratory thoracotomy.

Disability

Disability evaluation begins by listening to the patient. If they are talking, then they can protect their own airway. Confirm both pupils are reactive to light and the same size.

Calculate the Glasgow Coma Score

The score is the sum of the scores for these individual elements: Eye + Verbal + Motor.

Eye response	Verbal response	Motor response
1. Eyes open spontaneously	1. Orientated	1. Obeys commands
2. Eye opening to sound	2. Confused	2. Localizing pain
3. Eye opening to pain	3. Inappropriate words	3. Withdrawal from pain
4. No eye opening	4. Incomprehensible sounds	4. Abnormal flexion to pain
	5. No verbal response	5. Abnormal extension to pain
		6. No motor response

Table 12.6 Neurologic changes in the elderly brain

• Generalized brain atrophy • Loss of neurons • Accumulation of amyloid and pathologic proteins • Anticholinergic medications	• Decreased body temperature regulation • Bridging veins under increased tension • Dementia

Minor brain injury = GCS 13–15/**Moderate** brain injury = GCS 9–12/**Severe** brain injury = GCS 3–8.

Calculate GCS based on the *best* score obtained (i.e., Localizing pain with the left hand is *more prognostic* than no motor response with the right hand).

The neurologic exam of the elderly trauma patient must quickly determine the degree of traumatic brain injury present. Examine eyes for reactivity and asymmetry. A large, dilated pupil is the hallmark of impending brain herniation and requires immediate actions to decrease intracranial pressure such as hyperventilation and or hypertonic saline. It is important also maintain awareness of the neurologic changes which come with age. Table 12.6 lists neurologic changes specific to the elderly trauma patient.

Intubate for GCS less than 8 as this patient is unable to protect their airway. Unfortunately, in moderate and severe brain injury the damage is already done. However, by avoidance of worsening secondary brain injury—we can provide the patient with the best possible neurologic recovery. The main drivers of secondary brain injury are hypoxia and hypotension; therefore, we must make certain to avoid hypoxia and avoid hypotension. Care should also be taken to avoid hypoglycemia.

The elderly brain due to generalized atrophy may be more prone to tearing of bridging veins which find themselves under more and more tension as brain atrophy increases. There is no reason to assume that only a head strike is required to create intracranial bleeding. Minimal trauma such as a cough may tear bridging veins. An aneurysm may only require one additional hypertensive emergency before rupturing. Maintain a high index of suspicion for elderly traumatic brain injury.

Many elderly traumatic brain injuries will overlap with symptoms concerning for transient ischemic event or stroke. When in doubt, the patient can only benefit from a dual trauma and stroke code activation. Often the stroke workup can be initiated with trauma imagining with the addition of CT angiography of the head and neck as well as CT perfusion scans. While minutes will be added to the trauma workup—the benefits far outweigh the additional time required for imaging.

Exposure

Exposure evaluation begins by examining the body from head to toe for contusions, lacerations, punctures, and open fractures. Exposure requires that you log roll the patient to examine the spine for injuries and the back for contusions, lacerations, and punctures. Remember that due to age-related hypothalamic changes, temperature regulation is more difficult. The exposed elderly patient may become hypothermic quickly, thus warm blankets should be provided soon after exposure.

Standardize your own head to toe examination and perform the same exam on every patient every time. Diligence will be required on your part as every trauma provider encounters an injury that distracts you. The most difficult way to learn this difficult lesson is to miss a second or third injury in a patient which remains unaddressed and thus hampers patient survival. Do not allow the bleeding scalp wound to monopolize your attention away from the unstable pelvic fracture which is also bleeding into the pelvis.

Place the cervical collar *after the endotracheal tube has been secured*. Remember, there is no collar, airway, breath, and circulation algorithm—the collar will never be more important than the airway, breathing, and circulation. As you examine the patient from head to toe vocalize your findings confidently to the room so that situational awareness of the various injuries is carried by all members of the trauma team. Following examination of the anterior patient body, log roll the patient with no fewer than three persons: one person for cervical stabilization and two persons to roll the trunk, pelvis, and thigh.

Document your physical exam so that continuity of care can be provided. This is especially true should your patient require transfer to another hospital for higher level of care. Do not forget to maintain temperature control of the patient. Warm the cold patient. Cool the hot patient.

The next step is the Secondary Survey. The first step of the Secondary Survey is to **repeat the Primary Survey and ensure that you missed no life-threatening injuries**.

References

1. Luchette FA, Yelon J. Geriatric trauma and critical care. 2nd ed. New York: Springer; 2017.
2. Wijdicks E. The practice of emergency and critical care neurology. Oxford: Oxford University Press; 2010.
3. Committee on Trauma. ATLS Advanced Trauma Life Support. 10th ed. Chicago: American College of Surgeons; 2018.
4. Kahn M, McMonagle M. Trauma: code red. London: Taylor & Francis; 2019.

Emergency Medical Services and the Elderly Patient: Prehospital Management

13

Jonathan Berkowitz, Adrian Cotarelo, Jonathan Washko, and Brian Levinsky

Introduction

Emergency Medical Services (EMS) play a critical role in the healthcare system. Well-functioning prehospital care systems have been shown to improve outcomes in important emergencies such as cardiac arrest, myocardial infarction, stroke, and many others. Although the inception of EMS in the US focused on trauma care, EMS has evolved to deliver care for many different populations.

There are many challenges to providing care for geriatric patients, regardless of the patient is in a hospital bed, operating room, or the back of an ambulance. EMS continues to adapt to demographic changes and medical innovation. The backbone of prehospital care is provided by the different types of prehospital providers, ranging from first responders to paramedics. The training and skillsets vary significantly between these categories and the overlay of different abilities is fundamental to how many prehospital systems function. Expansion of prehospital care into critical care and community paramedicine is a relatively recent advance that is in response of the increasing complexity of care and the focus on the Institute for Healthcare Improvement (IHI) triple aim: improving patient satisfaction, outcomes, and cost-effectiveness. The future of EMS and the greying of America are interwoven together.

The Evolving Importance of Geriatrics to EMS

Older adults have always been an important special population for EMS, but the coming decades will see older adults become one of the most common populations that EMS responds to. By 2030, all baby boomers will be 65 and older and approximately 1/5 of the US population will be over age 65. The year 2034 is projected to be the first year that there are more people older than 65 than less than 18. Given that, the elderly already makes up 40% of all transports and a third of all emergency/911 responses. These changes suggest that in the future the majority of EMS

J. Berkowitz (✉) · J. Washko
Division of Prehospital and Disaster Medicine, Department of Emergency Medicine, Zucker School of Medicine, Hempstead, NY, USA

Northwell Center for EMS, Northwell Health, New Hyde Park, NY, USA
e-mail: jberkowitz3@northwell.edu

A. Cotarelo
Office of Medical Affairs, FDNY, New York, NY, USA

Long Island Jewish Medical Center, Northwell Health, New Hyde Park, NY, USA

B. Levinsky
Northwell Center for EMS, Northwell Health, New Hyde Park, NY, USA

P. Petrone, C. E.M. Brathwaite (eds.), *Acute Care Surgery in Geriatric Patients*, https://doi.org/10.1007/978-3-031-30651-8_13

responses will be to care for an elderly patient. Some models suggest that by 2030 more than half of EMS responses will be for the elderly.

EMS History in US

The history of EMS sheds significant light on the current state of prehospital care. The seminal publication from the National Academy of Sciences (NAS) in 1966 *Accidental Death and Disability: The Neglected Disease of Modern Society* shepherded the modern age of EMS. This document focused on gaps in the response to trauma generally and specifically to motor vehicle accidents. Although it clearly was instrumental in the formation of EMS, it also was very important in the creation of trauma systems as it clearly described the need for specialized facilities to manage critical patients. The NAS report led to the Highway Safety Act, which established the Department of Transportation (DOT). The DOT was in turn responsible for developing standards and programs for the implementation of prehospital care systems.

Professional organizations such as the American College of Surgeons, American Association of Orthopedic Surgeons, American Heart Association and American Society of Anesthesiologists were directly involved in providing medical input into the newly formed prehospital care systems. In addition, new organizations were founded with a focus on EMS and significant efforts were made to improve prehospital care. In 1972, the NAS published a follow-up report titled *Roles & Resources of Federal Agencies in Support of Comprehensive Emergency Medical Services*. This new publication endorsed further federal involvement with EMS and spurred the EMS systems act in 1973. This law promoted EMS grants to develop research and comprehensive prehospital care systems. The law established 15 key components of EMS.

From the mid 1970s forward EMS continued its evolution. However, it has always maintained close ties to transportation. EMS made significant progress to self-sufficiency, but there were still significant gaps. There were major variations in financing across the country. This was partially resolved with Medicare national ambulance fee schedule that was enacted in 2002. The fee schedule established seven categories: BLS, ALS 1 (simple), ALS 2 (advanced), ALS intercept, Specialty Care, Rotary Wing, and Fixed Wing. To this day, EMS financing is predicated on transport rather than care—in most cases, EMS is not reimbursed unless a patient is transported to a hospital. While the financial model continued to view EMS as a transportation benefit, the clinical model has matured. The backbone of the EMS system is the tiered layering of EMS providers and how they are trained. This was formalized in 2007, with the release of the National EMS Scope of Practice Model which propelled further standardization in training and care delivery.

EMS Training and the National Model

EMS clinicians of different training levels comprise a wide range of education and skills. Familiarity with the training models within EMS can provide a framework for understanding the skill sets and knowledge bases of various providers. While EMS certifications are conducted at the state level, with variation between state-specific protocols and policies, the National EMS Education Standards were developed to outline the core competencies for entry-level EMS providers. In order to further standardize the care delivered by EMS providers, the National Association of State EMS Officials (NASEMSO) developed the National Model EMS Guidelines. These guidelines provide an evidence-based resource for EMS practice and are meant to be used as a framework for the development of state and local practice. However, protocol variation still exists between regions, at both the local and state levels.

The National EMS Education Standards recognize four levels of EMS provider: the Emergency Medical Responder (EMR), Emergency Medical Technician (EMT),

Advanced Emergency Medical Technician (AEMT), and Paramedic. Each level is briefly summarized below.

Emergency Medical Responder (EMR)

The training of an EMR is focused on basic, immediate lifesaving interventions often as a part of a greater prehospital team. An EMR is often the entry level EMS position. They are trained to recognize signs of immediate threats to life and provide basic first aid interventions while awaiting additional resources. While they are often on scene first, they are not typically the EMS provider transporting a patient to the hospital without additional support. An EMR is trained in the use of a BVM, but is not trained in intubation, supraglottic airway placement, or advanced airway management. Further, while an EMR is trained in basic CPR and the use of an AED, they do not receive training in EKG interpretation or the use of an automatic CPR device. An EMR is not trained in the placement of peripheral IV access. EMR certification consists of a minimum of approximately 48 h of training.

Emergency Medical Technician (EMT)

An EMT is able to provide basic evaluation and transportation for patients requiring emergency care. In addition to the skills of an EMR, an EMT receives additional training in providing blood glucose monitoring, oxygen therapy, pulse oximetry, traction splinting, the use of mechanical CPR devices, cardiac monitoring including obtaining and transmitting a 12 lead EKG. They are not trained in the interpretation of an EKG. They also receive training in the administration of a limited number of medications, including oral aspirin, oral glucose, acetaminophen, inhaled bronchodilators, and assisted administration of a patient's prescribed nitroglycerin. They are not trained in peripheral IV access. EMT certification requires a minimum of approximately 150 h of training, including both classroom and field time, with both skills stations and written exams required for state certification.

Advanced Emergency Medical Technician (AEMT)

The AEMT is able to provide a limited amount of Advanced Life Support beyond the scope of an EMT, but significantly more limited than that of a Paramedic. In addition to the skills of an EMT, the AEMT is trained in supraglottic airway insertion, end-tidal CO_2 monitoring and interpretation, peripheral IV and IO access and medication administration, venous blood draws, and initiation of non-medicated IV fluids. AEMT certification is often pursued after initial EMT certification, requiring an average of 200 additional hours of training beyond those required to certify as an EMT.

Paramedic

The Paramedic is the most advanced EMS provider in the National EMS Model and is able to provide advanced emergency care in the field. Paramedics are trained to interpret and apply diagnostic findings to provide targeted treatment of medically complex patients. Paramedics are certified in ACLS and carry and administer a wide variety of medications including narcotics, vasopressors, sedatives, antiarrhythmics, antiemetics, and more. Paramedics may work in ground or air transport, hospital, or community settings. In addition to the skills of the AEMT, Paramedics are trained in needle chest decompression, cricothyrotomy, NG and OG tube placement, endotracheal intubation, 12-lead EKG interpretation, transcutaneous cardiac pacing, and blood product infusion. Paramedic training hours vary significantly by program and region, but involve over 1600 h split between didactic sessions and simulation training, field time on an ambulance, and clinical time between the Emergency Department and other hospital settings.

State Variation in EMS Practice

While the National EMS Education Standard outlines the foundation of knowledge expected of an entry-level EMS practitioner, there is significant variation in EMS practice by state. State protocols vary in specific protocols, including which level of EMS provider may administer different medications. Local protocols may vary further still. The National Registry of Emergency Medical Technicians (NREMT) administers national-level certification for each of the four primary training levels—NREMR, NREMT, NRAEMT, and NRP. Certification with the National Registry involves written and skills-based exams and is sometimes required for state-level certification. National Registry certification alone does not allow an EMS provider to practice in a given state unless otherwise specified by the state licensing board. Familiarity with specific local protocols is crucial to understanding the scope of practice of responders of different levels in a given region.

Geriatric Training in EMS

As the number of older adults in the general population continues to increase, EMS providers are responding to a rising number of geriatric patients. While some degree of geriatric considerations has long since been integrated into the scope of EMS education, EMS providers may have limited training directly related to the needs of older adults. The National EMS Education Standards recommends integrating geriatric care into other sections of the curricula without a dedicated section, as a longitudinal approach to the considerations of elderly populations. However, this makes it difficult to estimate the number of hours of coursework dedicated to geriatric care.

There are few standardized approaches for gauging EMS provider training with regard to geriatric populations. The National Model EMS Guidelines detail specific considerations for geriatric patients, interwoven throughout the practice recommendations. All EMS providers, from EMR to Paramedic, are trained to recognize and report signs of elder abuse and mistreatment. Beyond this, as geriatric considerations are integrated throughout other sections of the EMS curricula, one should expect increasing familiarity with geriatric care with increasing levels of certification.

The National Model EMS Guidelines outline several specific considerations for the care of geriatric patients. These include medication dosing variations in the elderly, including risk of polypharmacy, susceptibility to dehydration, shock, atypical presentation of pathology, and susceptibility to heat and cold-related illness. Further recommendations are made regarding changes to the trauma assessment, including additional padding for patients with significant kyphosis if spinal immobilization is indicated, and consideration for traumatic injury in seemingly lower risk mechanisms including falls from standing. Abuse and maltreatment are highlighted as key considerations for vulnerable populations, including the elderly, with dementia limiting the ability to report mechanisms of injury. While the National Model EMS Guidelines can serve as a framework for regional protocols, they may not reflect specific regional training models.

The National EMS Education Standards detail several core competencies for the EMS clinician, many of which direct responders of all levels to consider age-related variations in geriatric patients. These include the approach to patient assessment, Public Health considerations, airway management, psychosocial considerations, age-related considerations by organ system, treatment modifications and precautions in the elderly, and geriatric considerations in the trauma assessment and management. The Paramedic instructional guidelines further outline age-related considerations, including physiologic and sensory changes in the elderly, pharmacokinetic changes including increased drug sensitivity and increased risk of adverse drug reactions, complex medical histories due to multiple chronic illnesses, the risk of polypharmacy and accidental overdose, and further considerations for functional assessment in those with limited mobility in their activities of daily living.

Those seeking further education on geriatric care may pursue dedicated coursework, such as certification via the Geriatric Education for Emergency Medical Services (GEMS) course. GEMS offers two, 8-h long courses each providing a 4-year-long accreditation as a GEMS provider. The Core Provider course offers further dedicated education on age-related changes and considerations, including approaches to the assessment of geriatric patients, identification of psychosocial challenges, end-of-life care, and specific systems-based pathologies. The Advanced Provider course offers further in-depth content and clinical scenarios.

The Impact of Geriatrics to EMS

The change in demographics to more elderly EMS responses is significant not just in magnitude but because geriatric responses tend to have very different needs than non-geriatric responses (Table 13.1).

The prehospital management of geriatric trauma is also significantly more complex. Historically considered low risk mechanisms, such as ground level falls, pose a more significant risk to the elderly population. What may be considered a minor motor vehicle accident can be much more significant. In addition, given that prehospital providers have minimal diagnostic capabilities and rely on vital sign abnormalities, the fact that geriatric patients may not exhibit tachycardia or that a systolic blood pressure <110 mmHg might be indicative of shock means that these patients are at increased risk of under triage. The *2021 National Guideline for Field Triage of Injured Patients*, published by the American College of Surgeons include specific vital signs criteria for patients 65 and older as well as provide for EMS judgment patients in this age group.

Table 13.1 Summary of geriatric responses across several dimensions

Dimension	Difference
Field operations	The duration that EMS spends treating the patient on scene prior to transport is longer. Geriatric patients are more likely to be transported (rather than refuse care). There is a higher incidence of termination of resuscitation on scene. Geriatric patients more frequently reside in nursing, assisted living or other specialized facilities
Communication	Communication barriers are more likely to be present and they may impede accurate information gathering from both a medical dispatch and field operations perspective
Clinical conditions	Geriatric EMS responses are significantly more likely to be cardiovascular or respiratory in nature
Interventions	Almost all EMS interventions are more common in geriatric EMS responses. This includes IV placement, EKGs, monitoring, defibrillation, pacing, CPR, bag-valve-mask ventilation, intubation, and supraglottic airway use. Bi-pap and CPAP are significantly more common in the elderly population
Medications	Medications used for symptomatic relief, such as intravenous analgesics and antiemetics, are used less frequently. Cardiac and respiratory medications are used with greater frequency. Geriatric patients have more complicated medication regimens

Community Paramedicine

For the past two decades, a new model for healthcare delivery utilizing EMS has been showing promise in improving care for elderly patients. Community paramedicine (CP) is the use of paramedics not to treat and transport but to evaluate and treat patients and when appropriate, avoid transport. Several populations have been a focus of community paramedicine efforts and outcomes; The geriatric population is one of the most common.

CP has been shown to both reduce ER visits and hospitalizations amongst the elderly, with no increase in mortality. In-depth assessments have found a very low rate of ER presentation after a community paramedic visit and high patient and provider satisfaction. In addition, numerous studies have demonstrated the value of CP to geriatric patients for specific illness that commonly affect the elderly. Community paramedics have been shown to reduce repeat ED visits for dementia patients when utilized as part of an organized transitions of care plan. Heart failure patients were found to be less likely to present and require admission when those patients had access to CP.

The utility of CP for geriatrics is focused on the ability of a trained paramedic to provide an ad hoc visit with a geriatric patient at risk. Several programs have also explored standing visits as well. Specific skills relate to specific disease conditions, such as IV furosemide for heart failure and IV fluids and ondansetron for vomiting and dehydration. Paramedics are able to draw blood work, and in some systems, they are exploring point-of-care testing and point-of-care ultrasound. The telehealth and remote patient monitoring revolution have further advanced the ability of paramedics to take care of sicker patients at home and the ability of CPs to function as remote physician extenders continues to be significantly advanced through technology.

Aside from specific disease conditions specific sub-population of geriatric patients have had great success with Community Paramedicine. Hospice programs integrating community paramedics have been found to have significantly reduced unnecessary transports and improved end-of-life care. Numerous advanced illness management programs utilize community paramedics to ensure that patients with goals of care to avoid unnecessary hospitalization are able to meet their personal wishes.

These programs are usually focused around at-risk programs where the CP is an important tool for cost reduction. As mentioned above, the cost structure for EMS does not readily include payment for the clinical care given by the EMS provider; payment is strictly for transport to an emergency room. However, recently a new demonstration project, ET3 (Emergency Triage Treat and Transport) is in some regions offering a new model that may ultimately lead to additional utilization of EMS providers as a way to reduce unnecessary healthcare utilization. The literature around the impact of community paramedicine in achieving the IHI triple aim is clear, and it is very likely that there will be continued growth in this new area.

Conclusion

Many geriatric emergencies start with an EMS response, and the emergency medical system provides many critical services to the elderly. From the numerous simple "lift assists" when EMS is called to assist a patient who has fallen and needs help getting up, to cardiac, neurologic, and traumatic emergencies, EMS is the primary method of delivering emergency care to the elderly in the out-of-hospital environment. It should be expected that EMS be comfortable caring for these emergencies. Advances in healthcare delivery that directly impact geriatric patients are heavily reliant on EMS. Continued investment in the EMS system will directly benefit elderly patients.

References

1. Krohmer JR. History of emergency medical services. In: Cone DC, Brice JH, Delbridge TR, Myers JB, editors. Emergency Medical Services; 2021. https://doi.org/10.1002/9781119756279.ch1.
2. Duong HV, Herrera LN, Moore JX, Donnelly J, Jacobson KE, Carlson JN, et al. National characteristics of emergency medical services responses for older adults in the United States. Prehosp Emerg Care. 2018;22(1):7–14. https://doi.org/10.1080/10903127.2017.1347223.
3. Platts-Mills TF, Leacock B, Cabanas JG, Shofer FS, McLean SA. Emergency medical services use by the elderly: analysis of a statewide database. Prehosp Emerg Care. 2010;14(3):329–33. https://doi.org/10.3109/10903127.2010.481759.

4. Tohira H, Masters S, Ngo H, Bailey P, Ball S, Finn J, Arendts G. Descriptive study of ambulance attendances for older adults with and without dementia in Western Australia. Prehosp Emerg Care. 2022:1–8. https://doi.org/10.1080/10903127.2022.2096947.
5. Newgard CD, Lin A, Caughey AB, McConnell KJ, Bulger E, Malveau S, et al. Falls in older adults requiring emergency services: mortality, use of healthcare resources, and prognostication to one year. West J Emerg Med. 2022;23(3):375–85. https://doi.org/10.5811/westjem.2021.11.54327.
6. Peterson LK, Fairbanks RJ, Hettinger AZ, Shah MN. Emergency medical service attitudes toward geriatric prehospital care and continuing medical education in geriatrics. J Am Geriatr Soc. 2009;57(3):530–5. https://doi.org/10.1111/j.1532-5415.2008.02108.x.
7. Adams BL, McKenna KD. EMS practitioner education. In: Cone DC, Brice JH, Delbridge TR, Myers JB, editors. Emergency Medical Services; 2021. https://doi.org/10.1002/9781119756279.ch82.
8. Abrashkin KA, Washko J, Zhang J, Poku A, Kim H, Smith KL. Providing acute care at home: community paramedics enhance an advanced illness management program—preliminary data. J Am Geriatr Soc. 2016;64(12):2572–6. https://doi.org/10.1111/jgs.14484.
9. Saario EL, Mäkinen MT, Jämsen ER, Nikander P, Castrén MK. Screening of community-dwelling older patients by the emergency medical services: an observational retrospective registry study. Int Emerg Nurs. 2021;59:101078. https://doi.org/10.1016/j.ienj.2021.101078.
10. Forsgärde ES, Elmqvist C, Fridlund B, Svensson A, Andersson R, Rööst M. Patients' aged ≥65 years dispositions during ambulance assignments, including factors associated with non-conveyance to hospital: a longitudinal and comparative study. BMJ Open. 2020;10(11):e038885. https://doi.org/10.1136/bmjopen-2020-038885.
11. van Vuuren J, Thomas B, Agarwal G, MacDermott S, Kinsman L, O'Meara P, Spelten E. Reshaping healthcare delivery for elderly patients: the role of community paramedicine; a systematic review. BMC Health Serv Res. 2021;21(1):29. https://doi.org/10.1186/s12913-020-06037-0.

Discussing Goals of Care in the Geriatric Acute Care Surgery Patient

14

Sheila Rugnao and Anastasia Kunac

Vignette

Emergent surgical consultation is requested for a 91-year-old female presenting with depressed GCS, large frontal head contusion, and externally rotated and shortened left leg. She was brought to the emergency department by EMS after being found down by her home health aide. Further imaging reveals a subdural hematoma and femoral neck fracture. Her health aide discloses that she is on warfarin for atrial fibrillation but is otherwise healthy. She is ADL-independent and ambulates with a rolling walker. On exam, her thin, frail frame lays listless in the stretcher and her white hair appears matted with blood. Chart review yields a phone number to the patient's daughter who first expresses how upset her mother would be if she knew she was in the hospital. She comments on her mother's headstrong

S. Rugnao
Rutgers New Jersey Medical School, Newark, NJ, USA
e-mail: Sheila.Rugnao@rutgers.edu

A. Kunac (✉)
East Orange Veterans Affairs Medical Center, East Orange, NJ, USA
e-mail: kunacan@njms.rutgers.edu

P. Petrone, C. E.M. Brathwaite (eds.), *Acute Care Surgery in Geriatric Patients*, https://doi.org/10.1007/978-3-031-30651-8_14

and ornery character and further comments: "if she wasn't so insistent on living alone, this wouldn't have happened!" How do you approach the conversation about her injuries? How does knowing the patient's desire to live independently and preference to not be in the hospital inform the discussion? Knowing her injuries will cause significant functional decline and she will be unable resume living alone, what does her immediate and future care look like? While there are orthopedic, neurosurgical, and palliative therapies available, what is the most appropriate recommendation to make?

Introduction

Most surgeons have been engaged in the care of a severely ill patient with multiple medical comorbidities who has a diagnosis that would, in most circumstances, be treated with surgery. Every surgeon also knows despite recent medical advances the combination of high-risk surgery and multiple medical comorbidities equate to increased perioperative morbidity and mortality. This is exacerbated in geriatric populations, where frailty independently increases perioperative complications. In these challenging clinical scenarios, the best treatment may not be clear. How does one decide what treatment to recommend? While treatments can be disease focused and curative or symptom based and palliative, the aim is to provide care that aligns with the patient's goals. The goal may be obvious in certain scenarios: uncomplicated acute appendicitis in a healthy and athletic 70-year-old patient with no comorbid conditions can be easily remedied by surgery with a reasonable expectation that within a few weeks the patient should return to their baseline functional status. However, in geriatric patients who suffer from multiple significant comorbid conditions, serious acute illness, or significant traumatic injury, the goals of the patient and risks and benefits of surgical intervention may be nuanced and require a more in-depth conversation.

Patient-centered care is the foundation of modern clinical practice. Over time medical dogma has shifted from paternalistic to collaborative, requiring that physicians develop new communication skills and tools. Traditional medical education highlights medical acumen, diagnostic prowess, physical exam skills and interviewing, while training on how to talk about death and dying or discussing palliative and end-of-life care are absent or insufficient. Here we outline the importance of and approach to goals of care conversations in an acute setting.

Determination of Decision-Making Capacity

With an expanding geriatric population in the USA, more frequently surgeons will be called upon to treat patients with cognitive deficits and advanced dementia, making it increasingly more critical for clinicians to understand decision-making capacity. The principle of autonomy and foundation of shared decision-making is built on the assumption that the patient understands the risks and benefits of treatment or no treatment and can make decisions regarding their own care. However, at times, and especially in the setting of acute care surgery, patients may be sedated, obtunded or simply too sick to participate in these conversations.

If1 a patient is not able to communicate an understanding of their illness, acknowledge in their own words the risk and benefits of pursing or declining the proposed treatments, and use this

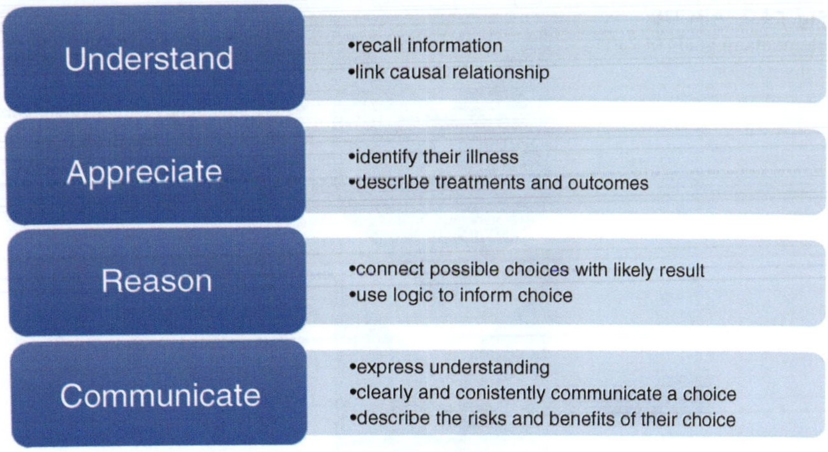

Fig. 14.1 Principles of decision-making capacity

information logically, a surrogate decision-maker should be involved (Fig. 14.1). Typically, surrogate decisions-makers will be identified in a living will or advanced directive; however, often these documents do not address specific clinical scenarios or circumstances. As mentioned before, it is the duty of the surgeon to review advanced directives and living wills with both the patient and surrogate pre-operatively. Multiple studies have shown that the earlier these conversations happen the less conflict there is in future discussions regarding end-of-life care, withdrawal of care, and do not resuscitate orders. Early and ongoing conversations also aid in management of family grief and bereavement.

If the patient is determined to not have decision-making capacity, and has not previously designated a health care proxy, the legal next-of-kin is called upon to assist with medical decisions. In the setting where a patient is deemed to not have capacity and there is no legal next of kin, literature suggests either a physician approach, ethics committee approach or legal guardianship be pursued. Additionally, there will be times when a patient does have capacity but does not wish to participate in medical decisions for various reasons; in this circumstance, it is within their right to designate another party to do so.

Setting the Stage

Ideally, the goals of care conversation will take place in a room large enough to allow all parties to sit and face each other. It is important to sit while having these discussions so as not to unintentionally communicate hastiness, impatience, or dismissiveness. Full attention is required with active effort to minimize interruptions from phones and pagers. Gathering all appropriate services and consultants who can lend additional perspectives can also be helpful in clarifying expectations. If a palliative specialist is desired and available, they should be involved as early as possible.

Once the stage has been set, there are multiple ways to approach the conversation. Previously published blueprints for sharing bad news (SPIKES, ABCDE), goals of care conversations (REMAP), and communication in the setting of trauma (ABCDE), were adapted here for the Acute Care Surgeon to create a simple ABCDE format that addresses the critical aspects of goals of care conversations (Fig. 14.2).

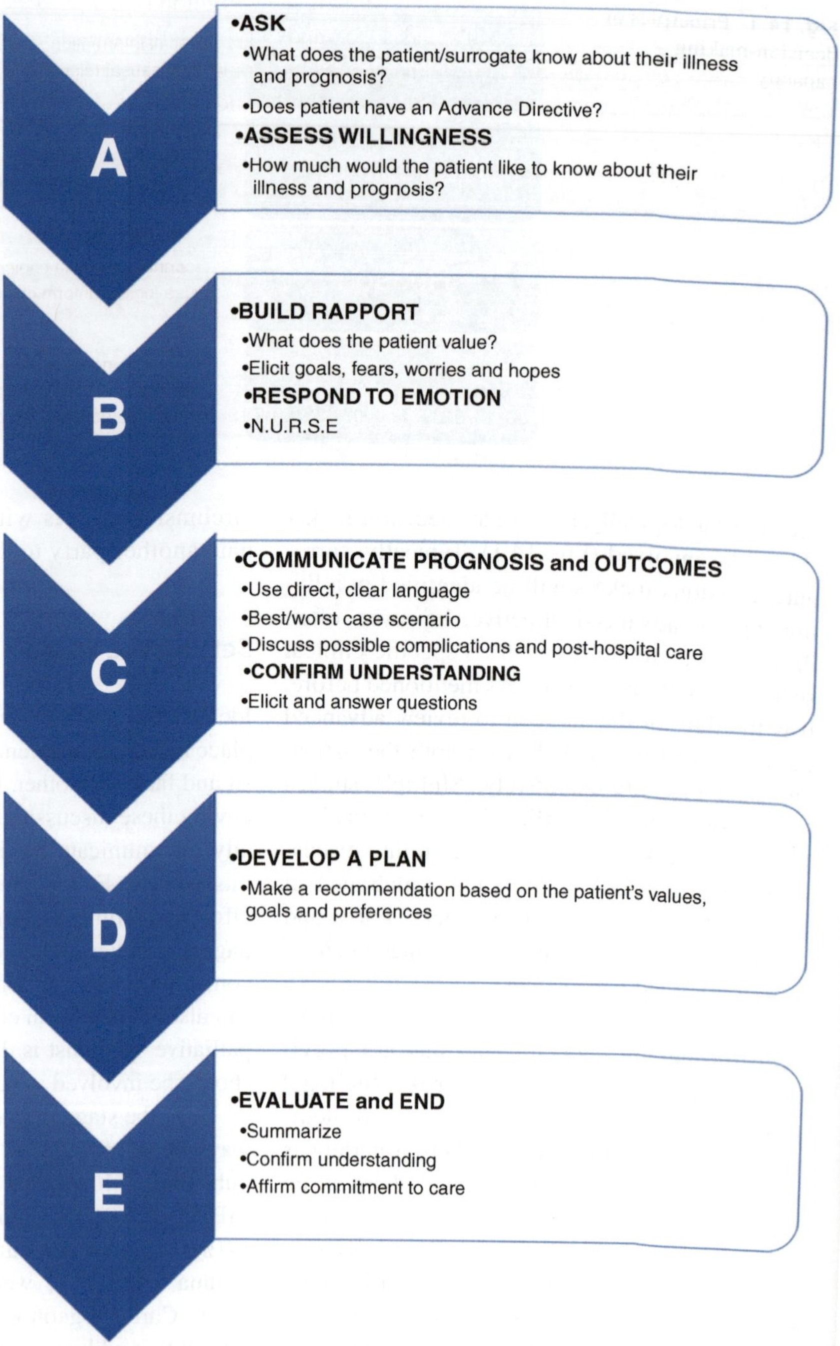

Fig. 14.2 ABCDE: elements in goals of care conversation

Goals of Care

Goals of care conversations aim to clarify the patients understanding of their illness and treatment options, illuminate their values, preferences and wishes and enable the patient and physician to collaboratively develop a plan that aligns with these goals. These conversations can sometimes be truncated to a decision on CPR or intubation leading to interactions regarding code-status that come off transactional, pressured, or even adversarial in nature. Goal-directed conversations should be exploratory, conversational, comprehensive, and frequently revisited. They should not be limited to discussion around medical treatments but should incorporate how the patient desires to live.

As surgeons, we must remind ourselves that much of the patient's experience happens after surgery. At times, a patient's personal goals may take priority over medical goals influencing a choice of non-operative treatment, or no treatment at all. It may be uncommon or uncomfortable for the surgeon to recommend against surgery; however, it is important to remind ourselves that the best treatment plan is one that is aligned with the patient's goals, not our own. In 2007, UCSF's Tracy Minichiello in an article on breaking bad news, emphasized how providers' thoughts and negative emotions around the subject can translate into perceived disengagement or disinterest by patients; she proposes that familiarity with helpful phrases and using a conversation guide can help to alleviate some stress and ameliorate these unwanted outcomes.

Despite having morbid illness, majority of moribund patients have often not had end-of-life discussions with their physicians. Though it is not ideal to have such discussions in an acute setting, especially when a patient has longstanding illness, it is appropriate and necessary to do so. It should first be determined if goals of care discussion has previously been had or if an advanced directive (AD) exists. If the topic is familiar with the patient or surrogate, the ensuring discussion may be easier to have. If an AD exists, it is important to review it in detail with the patient and/or surrogate. This allows for clarification and gives the provider an opportunity to better understand the patient's wishes and values regarding certain treatments. Studies have shown that having advanced care-planning conversations with patients improves end-of-life care and patient satisfaction, while reducing both patient and families' stress and anxiety.

Table 14.1 Ask and assess: phrases to initiate goals of care conversations

"A lot has happened recently. What is your understanding of your illness and the treatments being offered?"
"What have you been told about your condition/illness/injury so far?
"Have you spoken with anyone about the treatments you would want if you were seriously ill?"

Ask and Assess Understanding

A good way to begin the conversation is to ask an open-ended question, such as, "A lot has happened recently. What is your understanding of your illness or injury and the treatments being offered?" Allowing the patient to describe in their own words, their understanding will culminate a foundation for ongoing discussion (Table 14.1). This is an opportunity for the provider to mainly listen. Understanding the patient's preferences for information and for involvement in decision-making helps the patient retain control and allows the physician to provide the desired information. As mentioned above, it is also important at this "Ask" stage to ascertain if the patient has an existing Advance Directive. If meeting with a surrogate decision-maker, in cases where the patient lacks decision-making capacity, it may be prudent to ask if the patient has otherwise communicated their wishes even without a paper Advance Directive or Living Will.

Build Rapport

A critical step to having an effective goal-directed conversation is rapport building. An Australian study which randomized severely ill patients to receive advanced care planning or nothing, found that without structured conversations around Goals of Care (GOC) and End-of-Life (EOL) patients felt unheard, unimportant, uninformed, and simply in the way during their hospitalization. Asking patients their perspectives and eliciting their hopes, worries, and fears communicates empathy and support while also empowering patients to feel they have a role in their care. Even if the patient lacks the ability to make complex decisions, involving them in the GOC meeting is important to solicit their values and priorities.

The provider should seek to understand what outcome would be acceptable to the patient. This is pinnacle in the goals of care conversation. Statements such as, "What sort of quality of life would be unacceptable to you?" and "Which types of conditions would you say make life not worth living?" or "Is there any situation that you see being worse than death?" can help illuminate a patient's goals and values (Table 14.2). Rather than focusing on risks and benefits of treatment, the physician's intention should be to further their own understanding of the patient's goal and values.

Table 14.2 Build rapport: phrases to elicit understanding of patient values

"What sort of quality of life would be unacceptable to you?"
"What conditions would you say make life not worth living?"
"Is there any situation that you see being worse than death?"
"When considering end of life, what is most important to you?"

Inevitably, these topics will provoke a wide range of emotions. Go to statements like, "We've discussed many sensitive subjects, would you share with me how that makes you feel?", help to facilitate discussion and communicate empathy. Patients may or may not be ready to communicate how they feel. Remember that providing space for emotion to be felt by lending silence also communicates empathy. This can be prefaced with a statement such as, "It's natural that talking about these things can be upsetting—it's okay to take some time." If the patient/surrogate is too emotional to continue, it may be best to take a short break, allow space and revisit the conversation. While it is often perceived that decisions need to be made in an immediate fashion, outside of a hemodynamically unstable patient, most surgical intervention can be safely delayed with close observation for a short period. When revisiting a delicate conversation, various communication tools may come in handy. The mnemonic NURSE is a commonly used framework for addressing emotions (Fig. 14.3) For example, "As I listen, it sounds like you are worried/scared/anxious about x/y/z. Would you mind sharing more about that?" By acknowledging the patient's emotions, the provider creates an open and supportive atmosphere, which communicates an alliance.

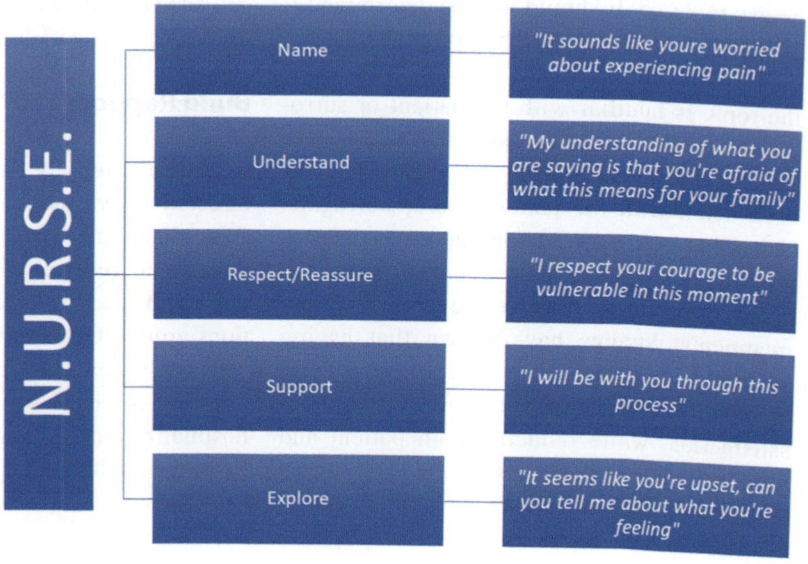

Fig. 14.3 Nurse mnemonic for responding to emotions

Communicate Prognosis and Outcomes

This is when the provider transitions the conversation from evocative to explanatory. Using statements such as, "Is it okay if we now discuss your prognosis?", or, "Now I'd like to share with you what I know about your disease/injury/illness and what some possible outcomes are." This readies the listener to receive the information. Always, fire a warning shot first to allow them to prepare psychologically for the bad news. When communicating bad news direct language is best. Avoid using medical jargon or complicated terminology. Physicians tend to be overly optimistic or paint information more favorably when communicating bad news and poor outcomes. Attempts to soften the message may result in inadvertent miscommunication, which can translate into mistrust between patient and provider. Once you have communicated the news, pause for 10–15 s, this allow them to process what was just said and react.

Easy-to-use prognostication tools like surgical risk calculators such as The American College of Surgeons National Surgical Quality Improvement Program (ACS NSQIP) risk calculator, frailty scales, and the Palliative Performance Scale are readily available, easy to use, and provide immediate information that can be used to create a common ground and established expected outcomes. One previously suggested and widely adopted approach for presenting possible outcomes when navigating high-risk procedures is to present best case and worst-case scenarios. Dr. Margaret "Gretchen" Schwartze has published and spoken widely about a tool surgeons can use for contrasting best case/worst case with surgery versus best case/worst case with palliative care (or any alternate treatment option). During this exchange, the spectrum of possible interventions, range of outcomes, and most likely outcomes of each of the proposed treatment option can be presented and discussed.

Of critical importance at this step is to confirm understanding of not only the diagnosis, but also the prognosis. If the patient or surrogate had previously been advised of their diagnosis/injuries and volunteered a comprehensive understanding, the surgeon may still have to confirm that they have integrated this information in the context of age, comorbidities, and frailty and clearly understand their likely outcomes. Eliciting and answering questions is an effective way to confirm understanding before moving forward to decide on a therapeutic strategy.

Develop a Treatment Plan

The intention of having comprehensive goals of care discussion is so that the provider is equipped to develop a patient-centered plan with the stated goals and values in mind. The surgeon's expertise, experience, and education allow them to create a plan of action that integrates the patient's goals with available medical therapy. It may be uncomfortable for a surgeon to recommend against surgery and propose conservative treatment or even palliative care; however, these options may be best if the operative mortality risk is too great or there is a probable outcome that is incongruent with the patient's desires. A provider's underlying core values—to sustain and prolong life—may be incongruent with the patient's values and desire for quality rather than quantity of life. We must always remind ourselves that the best choice is the one that respects the *patient's goals* and honors *their* autonomy. While mortality is commonly thought of as an unwanted outcome, most hospitalized older patients imagine living with conditions such as incontinence, gastrostomy or tracheostomy, and debilitating conditions that necessitate continuous care, an outcome worse than death.

As previously suggested, it is good practice to reframe and summarize the patient's values and goals as they pertain to treatment options before recommending a plan. This allows for clarification and patient-provider alignment prior to moving forward. Once any discrepancies have been resolved, establishing a recommendation is about to be made with a statement such as "is it okay if I propose a plan now?" can help to reorient and focus the conversation.

The plan should incorporate specifics around code-status, vasopressors/ionotropic medications, mechanical ventilation, IV fluids, nutritional support, blood products, and dialysis. Each of these interventions should be framed with the patient's goals in mind, and there must be agreement on the plan. It is worth noting that once a code-status is determined, it is simply designated in a patient's chart as "DNR." As one can imagine, this does not convey much to caregivers about the patient's values and preferences. A patient may accept cardiopulmonary resuscitation if the inciting event is something easily reversible and the physician anticipates full or meaningful recovery; though concurrently the patient may have stated that living with anoxic brain injury is a fate worse than death. Similarly, a patient may be okay with a trial of mechanical ventilation but not okay with long-term ventilator dependence. Likewise, a person may find that obtaining nutrition via gastrostomy is acceptable only if necessary for a limited time but believes never being able to eat again is an unacceptable way of life. It is imperative that the surgeon understand these nuances and consider them when making the decision to progress or withdraw care. As the patient's clinical status changes and their prognosis with it, these conversations should be revisited.

Evaluate and End

We recommend closing the loop with a summary statement such as, "What I've heard you say is important to you is [summary]. Have I understood you correctly?". Follow up by restating the plan as it pertains to and aligns with the patient's goals. For example, "Given that being around family and avoiding painful procedures is most important to you we will proceed with arranging home hospice." Always confirm agreement and understanding. End with an affirmation that you plan to support them and be there with them through the process.

Conclusion

As the paradigm in medicine has shifted, collaborative rather than directive approaches have become paramount in delivering high-quality care with respect to patient autonomy. When geriatric and moribund patients are faced with surgical disease, having comprehensive goals of care discussions has been shown to improve patient satisfaction and reduce suffering. By using a shared decision-making strategy and the proposed ABCDE framework, surgeons can increase their understanding of the patient's values; provide an opportunity for the patient to gain clarification of their illness, treatment, and prognosis; build rapport; facilitate a therapeutic alliance; and develop a treatment plan that is aligned with the patient's goals.

References

1. Makary MA, Segev DL, Pronovost PJ, Syin D, Bandeen-Roche K, Patel P, et al. Frailty as a predictor of surgical outcomes in older patients. J Am Coll Surg. 2010;210(6):901–8. https://doi.org/10.1016/j.jamcollsurg.2010.01.028.
2. Detering KM, Hancock AD, Reade MC, Silvester W. The impact of advance care planning on end of life care in elderly patients: randomised controlled trial. BMJ. 2010;340:c1345–5. https://doi.org/10.1136/bmj.c1345.
3. Minichiello TA, Ling D, Ucci DK. Breaking bad news: a practical approach for the hospitalist. J Hosp Med. 2007;2(6):415–21. https://doi.org/10.1002/jhm.271.
4. Back AL, Arnold RM, Baile WF, Tulsky JA, Fryer-Edwards K. Approaching difficult communication tasks in oncology. CA Cancer J Clin. 2005;55(3):164–77. https://doi.org/10.3322/canjclin.55.3.164.
5. Bernacki RE, Block SD. Communication about serious illness care goals. JAMA Intern Med. 2014;174(12):1994. https://doi.org/10.1001/jamainternmed.2014.5271.
6. Tyrie L, Mosenthal A, Bryczkowski S, Laboy C, Lamba S. Difficult conversations after resuscitation in trauma: video education E-module. MedEd PORTAL. 2015; https://doi.org/10.15766/mep_2374-8265.10092.

7. Krumholz HM, Phillips RS, Hamel MB, Teno JM, Bellamy P, Broste SK, et al. Resuscitation preferences among patients with severe congestive heart failure. Circulation. 1998;98(7):648–55. https://doi.org/10.1161/01.cir.98.7.648.
8. Dunlay SM, Strand JJ. How to discuss goals of care with patients. Trends Cardiovasc Med. 2016;26(1):36–43. https://doi.org/10.1016/j.tcm.2015.03.018.
9. Advance Care Planning (ACP) Decisions. (2021). The goals-of-care conversation: a best-practice, Step-By-Step Approach. https://acpdecisions.org/goals-of-care-conversations-a-best-practice-step-by-step-approach/.
10. Childers JW, Back AL, Tulsky JA, Arnold RM. REMAP: a framework for goals of care conversations. J Oncol Pract. 2017;13(10):e844–50. https://doi.org/10.1200/JOP.2016.018796.
11. Havens JM, Peetz AB, Do WS, Cooper Z, Kelly E, Askari R, et al. The excess morbidity and mortality of emergency general surgery. J Trauma Acute Care Surg. 2015;78(2):306–11. https://doi.org/10.1097/TA.0000000000000517.
12. Lynn J. Death foretold: prophecy and prognosis in medical care. BMJ. 2001;322(7283):437. https://www.ncbi.nlm.nih.gov/pmc/articles/PMC1119657/. Accessed 14 Jul 2022
13. Schwarze ML, Kehler JM, Campbell TC. Navigating high risk procedures with more than just a street map. J Palliat Med. 2013;16(10):1169–71. https://doi.org/10.1089/jpm.2013.0221.
14. Rubin EB, Buehler AE, Halpern SD. States worse than death among hospitalized patients with serious illnesses. JAMA Intern Med. 2016;176(10):1557–9. https://doi.org/10.1001/jamainternmed.2016.4362.
15. Shapiro ME, Singer EA. Perioperative advance directives: do not resuscitate in the operating room. Surg Clin North Am. 2019;99(5):859–65. https://doi.org/10.1016/j.suc.2019.06.006.

Traumatic Brain Injury

15

Lee Tessler and David Chen

Traumatic Brain Injury

Traumatic brain injury (TBI) can be devastating at any age though the geriatric population is uniquely susceptible to both immediate disability and long-term effects as compared with other age groups. This can be due to both confounding medical comorbidities that increase as patients age, as well as the increased likelihood of pre-existing neuro-degenerative disease in the elderly. Prior to discussing the impact and treatment of traumatic brain injury in this population, we must define exactly what it is we are trying to study. In this chapter, TBI will represent any alteration in brain function, or other evidence of brain pathology, caused by an external force. As we will see, this definition will allow us to include diagnoses such as concussion, which by its own definition presents with an altered state of brain function. In addition, this definition will also encompass entities such as traumatic subarachnoid hemorrhage and subdural hematoma, which at times may only exhibit radiographic evidence of head trauma, but can nonetheless have equally, or worse, long-term neurological consequences.

The global incidence of traumatic brain injury is estimated to be between 27 and 69 million annually. In the United States alone, this number is thought to be approximately 1.6 million, with those in the geriatric population comprising almost 200,000 of those injuries, representing the age group with the highest incidence. Just under half that number was hospitalized for their injury, and of those patients, almost 15,000 resulted in death. As we will see, though, death is not the only potential adverse outcome after TBI in the elderly.

Concussion

As stated by the definition of traumatic brain injury in the previous section, we will define concussion as an alteration in brain function caused by an external force. For the purposes of our discussion, this can be accompanied by transient

L. Tessler (✉)
Neurosurgery, NYU Langone Hospital–Long Island, East Meadow, NY, USA

Neurosurgery, NYU Grossman School of Medicine, New York, NY, USA

New York State Fraternal Order of Police, Hicksville, NY, USA

New York State Neurosurgical Society, New York, NY, USA
e-mail: lee.tessler@nyulangone.org

D. Chen
Neurosurgery, NYU Langone Hospital–Long Island, East Meadow, NY, USA

Neurosurgery, NYU Grossman School of Medicine, New York, NY, USA

Trauma Neurosurgery, NYU Langone Hospital–Long Island, Mineola, NY, USA
e-mail: david.chen2@nyulangone.org

P. Petrone, C. E.M. Brathwaite (eds.), *Acute Care Surgery in Geriatric Patients*,
https://doi.org/10.1007/978-3-031-30651-8_15

neurological symptoms, or a temporary loss of consciousness, but will exclude those TBIs accompanied by abnormal radiographic studies. While the number of patients presenting to medical attention for TBI and concussion can be calculated at approximately 1.6 million per year, it is estimated that at least half, if not more, of all concussions go unreported.

Falls are the leading cause of TBI in all age groups and remain a significant cause of concussion in the elderly population. Geriatric patients are more prone to falls due to confounding medical conditions such as gait difficulty from neurological or orthopedic etiologies, declining vision, and degenerative conditions such as dementia. Similar to other age groups, motor vehicle crashes make up the second largest cause of concussion. Other etiologies, though, are more common in this population as compared to younger patients, such as what we consider minor head trauma like bumping one's head on a cabinet door, or when exiting a car. In addition, treating medical professionals must also consider elder abuse in the right clinical setting.

The pathophysiology of concussion is thought to be represented by two major forces: impact loading and inertial loading. Impact loading occurs at the site of the applied external force by directly conveying mechanical energy to the underlying tissue. Inertial loading occurs from the movement of the brain inside the skull. This can occur in the absence of a direct force, such as when the brain of a passenger in a car that stops short continues to move within the skull. Both linear and rotational acceleration can result, which can lead to shear injury of the neurons within the brain. This type of mechanical insult can then result in alterations at the neurotransmitter/receptor level, causing neuronal dysfunction and leading to the symptomatology seen with concussion.

Concussion can but does not necessarily have to be accompanied by a transient loss of consciousness. Symptoms often include headache, altered mental status, and confusion. These initial symptoms can last from several minutes to several hours. In the elderly, it can often times be difficult to diagnose concussion if the inciting trauma was not witnessed by others. Patients who present with symptoms of altered mental status can be dismissed as having progressive dementia, urinary tract infections, or other etiology. Especially in geriatric patients who are on antiplatelet agents or anticoagulants, if concussive symptoms or traumatic mechanism is suspected, additional studies should be performed to rule out more significant pathology, such as intracranial hemorrhage.

In addition to obtaining advanced imaging if warranted, initial management of concussion includes observation to assess for ongoing neurological deficit. Patients should also be discouraged from strenuous physical and mental exertion, even more so if symptoms are worsened during such activities. This includes limiting driving, which can be uniquely compromised in this patient population with respect to reaction time and cognitive processing. After this initial period, which can last 7–10 days, many patients experience Post-Concussive Syndrome (PCS). This is characterized by symptoms which may include persistent headache, difficulty concentrating, loss of appetite, insomnia, balance difficulty, and especially in the geriatric population, mood disturbances, and depression. PCS symptoms typically last for 6 weeks on average. Patients and their families should be counseled of this likelihood, not to upset them that symptoms will last, but to reassure them that if they still have symptoms several weeks after the initial event, they should not be discouraged, as PCS is self-limiting and resolves in the majority of cases. With that said, patients and families should also be counseled that the expectation is that although symptoms can persist, they should improve over time, and that if they worsen, they should seek medical attention immediately.

If long-term symptoms persist, patients can be referred for neuropsychological testing or vestibular therapy, depending on exact complaints. Patients should also be counseled of the dangers of Second Impact Syndrome (SIS), which can result in cerebral edema if the patient suffers a second concussion prior to resolution of symptoms from the primary trauma. Geriatric patients specifically should be supervised, if possible, during this initial time period, given their increased incidence of imbalance and falls.

Traumatic Subarachnoid Hemorrhage

The primary protection for the brain is the skull, which essentially represents a "fixed box." Although it is responsible for displacement and absorption of a significant amount of mechanical energy from external trauma, it is not the only barrier of brain protection. The covering of the brain, or meninges, is made up of three distinct layers. The dura mater, literally meaning "tough mother" in Latin, is the leathery outer layer, and is responsible for protection from traumatic pathology such as skull fracture fragments and epidural hematomas. The inner layer of the meninges is known as the pia, and is a very thin, delicate membrane that is densely adherent to the parenchymal convolutions and allows blood vessels to traverse to and from the brain. The middle layer is composed of a spider-web like membrane known as the arachnoid (think arachnid/spider web). Cerebrospinal fluid (CSF), which is produced by the choroid plexus of the ventricular system, flows in between the arachnoid and pial layers, in a compartment known as the subarachnoid space. The CSF is then absorbed along the midline convexity of the brain by what are known as arachnoid villi, a fact which will become important as we further discuss head trauma and its long-term consequences.

Subarachnoid hemorrhage refers to extra vascular blood found in the subarachnoid space between the arachnoid and pial layers (Fig. 15.1). Due to the fact that many blood vessels traverse this space en route to and from the brain, this is a common location of bleeding from ruptured intracranial aneurysms. However, the most common cause of subarachnoid hemorrhage by far is head trauma (tSAH). While the incidence of tSAH can be difficult to assess, it is reported as being anywhere from 2.9 to 61%, depending on whether the patient is admitted to an ICU or if there were other associated intracranial injuries. Similar to other forms of traumatic brain injury,

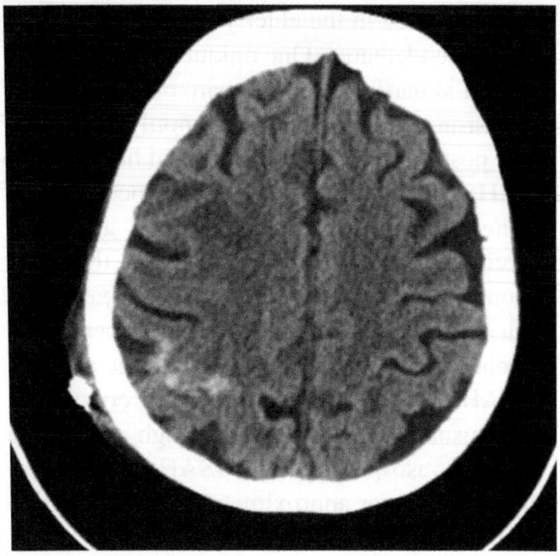

Fig. 15.1 Right parietal subarachnoid hemorrhage with overlying scalp laceration

the leading causes of isolated tSAH in the elderly are falls, minor head trauma, and motor vehicle crashes. Typical presentation of patients with subarachnoid hemorrhage is similar to that of concussion, with some patients being asymptomatic at the time of diagnosis. When present on initial scans, tSAH it is associated with a two-fold increase in mortality from head trauma.

The initial management of patients with isolated tSAH requires a slightly increased vigilance when compared to that of concussion alone. Patients are typically observed in a monitored unit with frequent neuro checks, and often obtain at least one follow-up CT scan to assess for progression of hemorrhage or the development of associated hemorrhages such as extra-axial bleeds or evolution of intraparenchymal contusions that were not seen on the presenting film. In addition, especially of concern in the geriatric population, is the presence of anti-platelet or anticoagulation medication, which is typically temporarily held, though can be reversed in the setting of extensive hemorrhage and based on the initial indication for the medication. Patients are also placed on 1 week of an anti-seizure medication given the data to support decreased incidence of early seizure, though not late seizure activity, with the understanding that lower doses may have to be used in the elderly due to side effects of increased lethargy. One unique short-term risk of tSAH in particular to be aware of is the risk of vasospasm. Though more commonly described in the post-aneurysmal subarachnoid hemorrhage (aSAH) population, vasospasm can occur in the setting of traumatic brain injury of all types, especially with associated tSAH. With that said, although the development of aSAH appears to be related to clot burden, the fact that vasospasm is associated with head trauma, even in the absence of tSAH, hints towards a separate or concurrent mechanism. Additionally, although the time course of vasospasm seen in tSAH is similar to aSAH, lasting for approximately 10 days, it can occur earlier after the initial insult than its atraumatic counterpart. Vasospasm can be detected in head trauma anywhere from 2 to 41% of cases through angiography and should be considered if there are acute changes in mental status without concurrent imaging findings, as the development of radiographic evidence of infarct may be too late to intervene. If vasospasm is being considered, treatment options include the use of "Triple-H" therapy of hemodilution, hypertension, and hypervolemia, along with use of calcium channel blockers or angiographic intervention in severe cases.

Earlier in this chapter, when discussing the physiologic flow of cerebral spinal fluid, it was discussed that in general, the CSF is produced by the choroid plexus, travels in the subarachnoid layer of the meninges, and is then reabsorbed along the cerebral convexity by the arachnoid villi. This can lead to another late risk, especially in elderly patients who are put back on antiplatelet and anticoagulants shortly after the initial trauma—the development of hygromas. Since the CSF is generally produced at the same rate it is absorbed, approximately 20 cc per hour, if there is something that decreases the absorption of CSF but does not alter the production, CSF can build up. If subarachnoid blood is present, which is more commonly along the convexity, especially when compared to aSAH, it can essentially clog the arachnoid vili, which in turn, can result in the development of hygromas, or fluid along the convexity (Fig. 15.2). Although this is often

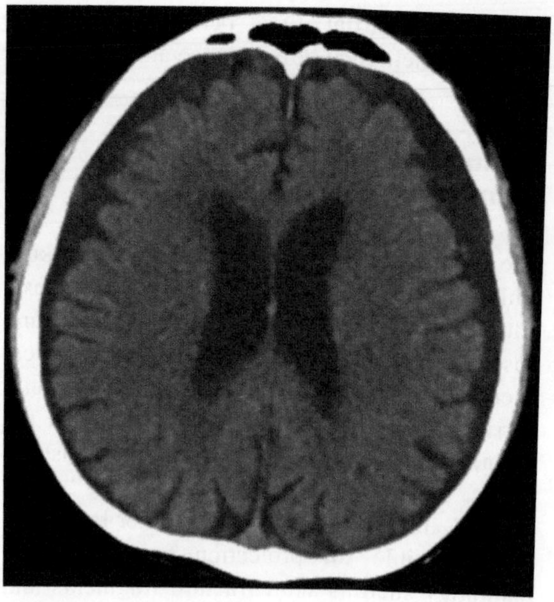

Fig. 15.2 Bilateral subdural hygromas

self-limiting, hygroma development can put bridging veins on stretch, and even with minor repeat trauma, can more frequently result in acute or subacute subdural hematoma. Because of this, it is recommended that a short-term follow-up scan be obtained within the first month to assess for hygroma development prior to restarting antiplatelet or anticoagulants, if possible from a medical standpoint. This is especially true in the geriatric population, as one study found that patients with isolated tSAH and age greater than 76 were more likely to have a worse outcome when combined with other factors.

Subdural Hematoma

As stated in the previous section, although traumatic subarachnoid hemorrhage can lead to development of subdural hygromas and ultimately subdural hematoma (SDH), the majority of traumatic subdural hematomas occur at the time of the initial injury. As we have for our other sections, we will start with a brief working definition. Whereas traumatic subarachnoid hemorrhage described blood between the arachnoid and pial layers of the meninges, the term subdural hematoma will be used to describe blood between

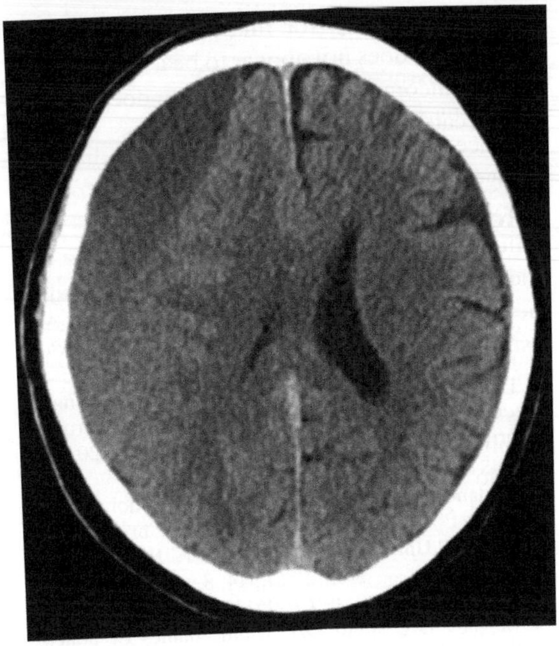

Fig. 15.3 Right frontoparietal mixed density subdural hematoma

the dura mater and the arachnoid layers, and for our purposes, that which is caused by a traumatic event (Fig. 15.3). Subdural hematomas can be characterized by the age of the blood seen on imaging. Within the first few days, they are referred to as acute, and are represented by extra-axial hyperdensity seen on CT. After about 2 weeks, they are described as subacute, and are seen as isodense to the brain on CT. After a month or so, they are categorized as chronic, and appear hypodense to the brain on CT. All three phases have their own distinct consistency, which will be used to determine prospective treatment. The incidence of acute subdural hematoma in the setting of severe traumatic brain injury is in the range of 21%, and approximately 11% when mild and moderate TBI is considered as well. Somewhat expectedly in the younger population, the mechanism of injury tends to be motor vehicle crash, whereas in geriatric patients the mechanism is more commonly falls, especially when combined with anti-platelet and anticoagulant use. The mechanism is generally accepted to be tearing of bridging veins that traverse the subdural space between the brain and dura. Elderly patients are in a unique position to develop SDH with even minor trauma due to the fact that the brain tends to lose volume during the aging process with expansion of the subarachnoid CSF space, therefore resulting in more "stretch" on existing bridging veins. Presentation of patients with SDH tend to be more severe and focal than other types of injuries. Concussion and subarachnoid hemorrhage is a more diffuse process. With epidural hematoma, the brain has the benefit of the tough dura mater layer protection until there is enough volume to cause a rise in intracranial pressure. Subdural hematoma, on the other hand, is beneath the dura, and therefore applies direct pressure to the brain parenchyma itself, which is at that point only protected by the very thin arachnoid and pial meningeal layers. This can result in focal deficits such as hemiparesis and aphasia, depending on laterality, or more global effects due to a rise in intracranial pressure, such as depressed mental status if there is concomitant midline shift, loss of basal cisterns, or herniation syndromes.

Initial management of acute subdural hematoma in the geriatric population follows the same algorithm as in other age groups. Surgical decisions are generally made based on clinical information, such as Glasgow Coma Scale (GCS) and the presence of neurological deficits, radiographic data, such as clot thickness, degree of midline shift, and visibility of basal cisterns, as well as patient and family discussions surrounding salvageability and expectations of postoperative care, such as likelihood of ventilator dependence or the need of feeding tube placement. It is in this last category that there may be some differences in the decision of whether to surgically treat a patient with an acute subdural hematoma based on age. Studies have shown a significant increase in both mortality (50% age >70; 26% age <70) and poor outcome as defined by Glasgow Outcome Score (74.1% age >70; 48% between 40 and 70; 30% > 40), which may lead to decisions to treat the geriatric population with nonsurgical intervention. If surgical intervention is ultimately warranted, the choice of surgical techniques is somewhat dependent on the acuity of the blood, and more specifically the consistency. Acute subdural hematomas tend to consist of thicker, clot-ted blood, and therefore necessitate a formal craniotomy to adequately evacuate, with or without craniectomy depending on the degree of underlying cerebral edema. Subacute subdural hematomas are more liquid, but still thick in consistency. In certain cases, burr holes may be used, however, if the blood is too thick, or there is the presence of membranes, a craniotomy may need to be performed as well. Once a subdural hematoma reaches the chronic phase, it typically has a very thin, liquid consistency. At this point, burr holes can often successfully drain the collection, though once again, if there are significant membranes, a craniotomy may still be required. It is for this reason, specifically in the geriatric population, that if there is no neurological deficit, there is a benefit to waiting until a subdural is "liquified" in order to perform a less invasive surgical procedure, such as burr holes, if one is needed. Non-operative management of subdurals of all ages are accompanied by serial imaging and neuro exams. Imaging is typically continued until complete resolution of the subdural, which can often take months. For patients on anti-platelet or anticoagulation medications, which is more common as the age of patients increase, a risk/benefit analysis must be performed by the neurosurgeon and the involved medical doctor or cardiologist to determine when to resume, as the incidence of recurrence or worsening of hematoma can increase with the use of these agents prior to complete resolution. Outcome data for geriatric patients undergoing treatment for subdural hematomas tend to show improvements in neurological status though this may not be accompanied by improvements in functional status.

Conclusion

To summarize, although there are some unique challenges and characteristics regarding the care of geriatric patients with head trauma, similar treatment algorithms are used as compared to younger patients. Medical comorbidities, use of anti-platelet and anticoagulant medications, and patient and family expectations must all be considered specifically for this population. Age in and of itself, does not appear to be a sole determinant of outcome, and advanced age does not preclude treatment in appropriate patients.

References

1. Menon DK, Schwab K, Wright DW, et al. Position statement: definition of traumatic brain injury. Arch Phys Med Rehabil. 2010;91:1637–40. https://doi.org/10.1016/j.apmr.2010.05.017.
2. Dewan MC, Rattani A, Gupta S, et al. Estimating the global incidence of traumatic brain injury. J Neurosurg. 2018;130:1–18. https://doi.org/10.3171/2017.10.JNS17352.
3. Rutland-Brown W, Langlois JA, Thomas KE, Xi YL. Incidence of traumatic brain injury in the United States, 2003. J Head Trauma Rehabil. 2006;21(6):544–8. https://doi.org/10.1097/00001199-200611000-00009.
4. Meaney DF, Smith DH. Biomechanics of concussion. Clin Sports Med. 2011;30(1):19–31. https://doi.org/10.1016/j.csm.2010.08.009.
5. Modi NJ, Agrawal M, Sinha VD. Post-traumatic subarachnoid hemorrhage: a review. Neurol India. 2016;64(Suppl):S8–S13. https://doi.org/10.4103/0028-3886.178030.
6. Eisenberg HM, Gary HE Jr, Aldrich EF, Saydjari C, Turner B, Foulkes MA, et al. Initial CT findings in 753 patients with severe head injury. A report from the NIH traumatic coma data bank. J Neurosurg. 1990;73:688–98. https://doi.org/10.3171/jns.1990.73.5.0688.
7. Armin SS, Colohan AR, Zhang JH. Vasospasm in traumatic brain injury. Acta Neurochir Suppl. 2008;104(13):421–5. https://doi.org/10.1007/978-3-211-75718-5.
8. Rau CS, Wu SC, Chien PC, Kuo PJ, Chen YC, Hsieh HY, Hsieh CH. Prediction of mortality in patients with isolated traumatic subarachnoid hemorrhage using a decision tree classifier: a retrospective analysis based on a trauma registry system. Int J Environ Res Public Health. 2017;14(11):1420. https://doi.org/10.3390/ijerph14111420.
9. Bullock MR, Chesnut R, Ghajar J, Gordon D, Hartl R, Newell DW, et al. Surgical management of acute subdural hematomas. Neurosurgery. 2006;58(3 Suppl):S16–24.
10. Hanif S, Abodunde O, Ali Z, Pidgeon C. Age related outcome in acute subdural haematoma following traumatic head injury. Ir Med J. 2009;102(8):255–7.
11. Mulligan P, Raore B, Liu S, Olson JJ. Neurological and functional outcomes of subdural hematoma evacuation in patients over 70 years of age. J Neurosci Rural Pract. 2013;4(3):250–6. https://doi.org/10.4103/0976-3147.118760.

16 Neurocritical Care in the Elderly

Rajanandini Muralidharan and Sok Lee

Traumatic Brain Injury

Epidemiology

Traumatic brain injury (TBI) is one of the leading causes of disability in the elderly. The incidence of TBI is highest among older patients. Furthermore, TBI-related hospital visits, hospital admissions, and death have increased the most among adults older than 75 years old age. In 2013, adults older than 75 years old accounted for 26.5% of all TBI-related deaths and 31.4% of all TBI-related hospitalizations. Unlike children and younger adults where the most common mechanism of TBI is related to motor vehicle collision, older adults suffer TBIs most commonly due to low energy impacts such as ground-level falls. This is likely due to diminished baseline function, pre-existing comorbidities including cognitive and visual impairment, coordination, and gait abnormalities, as well as medication side effects.

R. Muralidharan (✉) · S. Lee
Department of Neurology, NYU Long Island School of Medicine, NYU Langone Hospital—Long Island, Mineola, NY, USA
e-mail: Rajanandini.Muralidharan@nyulangone.org; Sok.Lee@nyulangone.org

Clinical Assessments

Several different modalities are used for the initial assessment of traumatic brain injury including clinical examination, Glasgow Coma Scale (GCS), and neuroimaging which is mainly computed tomography (CT) of head. In older adults, the early stage of clinical exams and GCS may overestimate the true severity of the brain injury due to pre-existing neurological diseases such as dementia, prior ischemic stroke and intracranial hemorrhage (ICH), or degenerative spine diseases. In addition, adverse effects of baseline medication and pre-existing medical comorbidities can make the initial assessment even more challenging. On the other hand, ICH may present even in the absence of any significant neurological deficits on presentation due to a variety of reasons including physiological changes and atrophy of the brain from aging. As shown in a Swedish study, 57% of adults greater than 60 years of age with ICH on CT head presented with normal GCS. Therefore, it is important to raise high suspicion for ICH in elderly with TBI even with a normal neurological exam, anticipate possible early clinical deterioration, and have a lower threshold to obtain CT head. The American College of Emergency Physicians recommends obtaining CT head in all patients greater than 65 years of age even in mild TBI without loss of

P. Petrone, C. E.M. Brathwaite (eds.), *Acute Care Surgery in Geriatric Patients*,
https://doi.org/10.1007/978-3-031-30651-8_16

consciousness and in all patients greater than 60 years old with TBI and loss of consciousness.

Intracranial Pressure Monitoring

Intracranial hypertension (IHT) is often encountered in severe TBI, and it has been associated with worse outcomes. Despite this, monitoring of intracranial pressure in patients with severe TBI remains to be a contentious issue due to conflicting results on the benefits of ICP monitoring on functional outcome and mortality. Moreover, the benefit of ICP monitoring in older patients with severe TBI remains unclear. As a result, there is considerable variation in the indications and the use of ICP monitoring across hospitals and intensive care units. The rate of ICP monitor placement decreases with older age across hospitals. The National Trauma Data Bank from 2010 to 2014 showed that patients 65 years of age or older were significantly less likely to have ICP monitoring than those younger than 65 years old. Due to the mixed results of ICP monitoring on the outcome of severe TBI, the most recent Brain Trauma Foundation (BTF) guidelines downgraded its level of evidence and although it is still recommended, the indication is less clear and largely depends on the experience of its use in hospitals and local policies.

Intracranial Pressure and Cerebral Perfusion Pressure Goal

The most recent BTF guideline recommends treating ICP greater than 22 mmHg while maintaining cerebral perfusion pressure (CPP) between 60 and 70 mmHg. In addition, it recommends maintaining systolic blood pressure at or greater than 110 mmHg for patients older than 70 years old. Studies have shown that older patients with TBI have lower ICP than younger patients due to cerebral atrophy and increased cerebrospinal fluid (CSF) space. Hence, CPP is generally higher in elderly patients. In addition, older patients with TBI are more likely to have impaired cerebrovascular autoregulation and pressure reactivity. These differences along with medical comorbidities such as hypertension and baseline medications such as antihypertensives make it difficult to predict whether current CPP and ICP treatment guidelines can be applied to elderly patients.

Medical Management of Intracranial Hypertension

Intracranial components are composed of brain parenchyma, arterial and venous blood, and cerebrospinal fluids which are all stored in a rigid skull. Therefore, an increase of an intracranial component comes at the expense of another component until the compensatory mechanism reaches its limit and results in decreased intracranial compliance with an exponential rise in intracranial pressure. Although the treatments of IHT can be generally effective in lowering ICP at least temporarily, they have potential adverse effects and thus the measures should be approached in a stepwise fashion. In addition, it is crucial to determine the etiology of IHT to implement the most effective treatment strategy early on, such as the placement of external ventricular drainage in obstructive hydrocephalus or evacuation of mass lesions in ICH with mass effects. General measures should include neutral head positioning, head of bed elevation to 30°, and ensuring jugular veins are free of compression from any lines or cervical collars. In addition, seizures, pain, agitation, fever, and shivering should be treated appropriately with antiepileptics, sedation, and analgesia to minimize metabolic demands and cerebral hyperemia. Also, intubation and mechanical ventilation should be considered to administer sedation and avoid hypoxemia while maintaining normocapnia. Neuromuscular blockers can be effective in lowering ICP; however, due to their adverse effects including masking the neurological examination, they are not routinely used unless in specific situations such as in shivering or difficulty with ventilation.

The next tier of ICP management includes hyperosmolar therapy, namely mannitol and hypertonic saline (HTS) solution which are the two most commonly used agents. Hyperosmolar therapy works by creating an osmotic gradient and shifting fluid from the interstitial to intravascular space, as well as by decreasing blood viscosity and increasing cerebral blood flow, which in turn leads to vasoconstriction and lowering of ICP. A meta-analysis that compared the efficacy of mannitol and HTS in TBI showed that HTS was more effective in lowering ICP; however, there were no differences in functional outcome or mortality. In the elderly TBI population, therapy should be selected based on the patient's medical comorbidities while considering the adverse effects of each therapy (mainly volume depletion and kidney failure with mannitol and volume overload with HTS) and closely monitor volume status, serum osmolarity and osmolarity gap. Hyperventilation which exerts its effects via hypocapnia and vasoconstriction can be used as a temporizing measure in emergent situations. However, due to its short-lasting effects and concern for cerebral ischemia and rebound IHT, it should not be used prophylactically or for a prolonged period. In cases of refractory IHT, third-tier treatment should be considered which includes barbiturates, hypothermia, and decompressive craniectomy.

Surgical Management of Intracranial Hypertension

ICP elevation refractory to medical management should be evaluated for decompressive craniectomy (DC). In DC, opening the skull increases intracranial compartment size which reduces ICP. The first major randomized trial to evaluate the efficacy of DC in traumatic brain injury was the Decompressive Craniectomy in Diffuse Traumatic Brain Injury (DECRA) study. The multi-centered trial included 155 patients aged 15 to 59 with diffuse TBI, GCS 3 to 8, and ICP ≥20 mmHg for more than 15 min despite first-tier interventions of IHT. A group undergoing bifrontal craniectomy was compared to a group receiving continued medical interventions. The results showed that the surgical group had lower ICP and less ventilatory support and ICU days but had worse functional outcomes at 6 months with similar mortality rates. However, the study had several important limiting factors including baseline patient characteristics where a higher rate of patients with unreactive pupils was enrolled in the surgical group, early surgical interventions were done with lower ICP thresholds than the current standard, and the use of extensive bilateral craniectomy. In the RESCUEicp trial, 408 TBI patients aged 10 to 65 with ICP ≥25 mmHg for 1–12 h despite first and second-tier medical therapy were randomized into the decompressive craniectomy (bifrontal or hemicraniectomy) group and medical treatment group. At 6 months, the DC group had lower mortality but higher rates of vegetative state and severe disability, and similar rates of moderate disability or good functional recovery. However, further prespecified analysis showed that, at 12 months, surgical patients had higher rates of favorable outcome defined by "upper severe disability" or better. Current BTF guideline recommends DC for severe TBI with sustained ICP refractory to medical intervention. However, given these trials excluded older TBI patients, data on the efficacy of DC in the elderly is not clearly established. Putting things together, in severe TBI with sustained and refractory IHT, bifrontal or hemicraniectomy reduces mortality but with increased both upper and lower severe disability (i.e., functionally independent within the home or better). Given the limited data on the elderly, discussion with surrogates should be done while considering the current data on DC, predicted risk of unfavorable outcomes, patient's age, and medical comorbidities.

Other Complications of Traumatic Brain Injury to Consider in the Elderly

Delirium in the Elderly

Delirium is a common complication of TBI, but it is even more common in elderly patients. One study showed that 75% of elderly with TBI in ICU suffer from delirium. The underlying pathophysiology of delirium in TBI is complex and along with primary brain injury, likely involves secondary brain injury with subsequent inflammation and molecular, biochemical, and cellular changes that lead to neuronal damage and apoptosis. Risk factors of delirium in TBI include older age, seizures, drugs (benzodiazepines, opiates, propofol, neurotransmitter receptor modulators), hyperosmolar therapy, organ failure, sepsis, sleep deprivation, sensory deprivation/overstimulation, and pre-existing pathology. To minimize the risk of delirium, the Society of Critical Care Medicine recommends minimizing sedation, adequately assessing and addressing pain, and encouraging early mobilization. In addition, certain drugs that may exacerbate delirium such as benzodiazepines and antipsychotics should be avoided, and beta blockers or antiepileptics such as valproic acid or carbamazepine which have shown potential benefits in post-traumatic delirium should be considered.

Post-Traumatic Seizures

Early post-traumatic seizures are common in the first 7 days post-TBI and have been shown to occur in 10.8% of patients. Furthermore, electrographic seizures defined as seizures seen on electroencephalogram (EEG) without clinical activities, occur in up to 25% of TBI patients. Early post-traumatic seizures are associated with worse functional outcomes and mortality. Compared to younger adults, older adults are at higher risk of post-traumatic epilepsy likely due to pre-existing neurological diseases such as dementia and prior strokes. Therefore, subclinical seizures should be investigated when older patients with moderate to severe TBI remain in a coma, have neurological exams not explained by imaging, or have fluctuating mental status. The most recent BTF guidelines provide level IIA recommendation for the use of phenytoin in the first 7 days post-injury to decrease the incidence of early post-traumatic seizure. However, it remains uncertain whether early use of antiepileptic drugs (AED) provides any benefit to the older population with severe TBI given the adverse effects of AED. A recent retrospective study showed that, in older patients with TBI, early use of antiseizure medication reduced both short- and long-term mortality across all severity of TBI without reducing the incidence of early seizure, a finding likely explained by subclinical seizures. Yet, the optimal AED type and duration in the elderly population with TBI are not well established. Although phenytoin is recommended by BTF guidelines, it is likely not the optimal AED in the elderly due to nonlinear pharmacokinetics, propensity for drug–drug interaction, and cognitive side effects. A recent meta-analysis that compared the efficacy of levetiracetam and phenytoin in early post-traumatic seizure revealed a similar efficacy in seizure prevention, but fewer adverse effects were seen in the levetiracetam group. In summary, there is no clear evidence to support the use of any one type of AED above the others, and so it should be chosen based on the adverse effect profile. In addition, prolonged prophylactic use should be discouraged to avoid adverse effects.

When to Restart Antithrombotic Agents After Traumatic Brain Injury

Many elderly patients are on antithrombotic therapy due to a variety of conditions, but with the increasing incidence of TBI in the elderly, there is a higher incidence of antithrombotic-related ICH in TBI cases. Antithrombotic use in the elderly is associated with higher rates of traumatic brain injury as well as higher risk of suffering ICH and higher mortality. Preinjury warfarin use has been associated with higher rates of hematoma expansion on follow-up CT head. Preinjury use of anticoagulation or dual antiplatelet therapy with aspirin and clopidogrel was associated with higher mortality in patients with TBI. Hence, the timing of antithrombotic therapy resumption as well as thromboprophylaxis initiation can be challenging. The majority of recent literature supports starting prophylactic anticoagulation within 24–72 h post-injury with a stable CT head. BTF and the American Association for the Surgery of Trauma Critical Care Committee consensus both support either unfractionated heparin (UH) or low molecular weight heparin (LMWH) for prophylactic anticoagulation. Data supports the use of LMWH over UH based on lower venous thromboembolism (VTE) and higher survival rates seen in TBI patients on LMWH. As for therapeutic anticoagulation, patients at high risk of thrombotic complications, such as those with a mechanical heart valve, should be considered for restarting therapeutic anticoagulation at 7–12 days post-injury while carefully weighing the risks and benefits. For patients with high thrombotic risk requiring antiplatelet therapy, starting antiplatelet monotherapy can be considered as early as 24 h following a stable repeat CT head.

Prognosis of Traumatic Brain Injury in the Elderly

Several studies have shown older patients with severe TBI are more likely to have worse functional outcomes, higher mortality, medical complications, longer hospital stays, and continued medical care post-discharge when compared to younger patients. The findings are due to several factors including the mechanism of TBI in elderly patients which includes a higher incidence of ground-level falls with subsequent SDH which is associated with worse outcomes. In addition, pre-injury comorbidities as well as higher use of anti-thrombotic agents are known to be associated with increased expansion of intracranial hemorrhage and worse outcomes. Also, diminished brain reserve in older patients limits the potential for plasticity and neural repair, and cognitive impairments limit the success of rehabilitation. Finally, elderly patients with severe TBI receive less aggressive treatment likely due to the perception that such patients have unfavorable prognosis. Although older adults with severe TBI have worse outcomes, a substantial number of these patients recover well and warrant continued aggressive management. Currently, there are two prognostic models (CRASH-CT and IMPACT) that incorporate age to predict functional outcomes and mortality. However, their performance on outcome prediction in the older TBI population have not been very accurate largely due to the failure to incorporate pre-existing comorbidities into the model. Therefore, when determining the prognosis of the elderly with TBI, one should consider the severity of brain injury along with the age of the patient as well as pre-existing comorbidities while being aware of the limitations of different predictive models.

Ischemic and Hemorrhagic Stroke

Background

Acute ischemic stroke (AIS) is a leading global cause of death and chronic disability. Perioperative stroke is a potentially devastating complication for patients and surgeons alike. Age is the most important non-modifiable risk factor for stroke. The cumulative effects of cardiovascular risk factors and aging-related changes on cerebral macro- and microcirculations, make the elderly particularly prone to both ischemic and hemorrhagic forms of stroke. Despite the reduction in the incidence of stroke due to advances in acute stroke care, aggressive primary prevention and improved management of stroke-related complications, its prevalence is projected to rise due to the aging population. There is also an increased number of elderly patients with significant cardiovascular risk factors undergoing surgery leading to an increase in the incidence of perioperative stroke despite advances in perioperative care and surgical technique.

Perioperative stroke is an ischemic or hemorrhagic brain infarction which occurs during surgery, during emergence from anesthesia, and/or up to 30 days after surgery. More strokes occur after urgent surgery than after elective surgery. Most perioperative strokes are ischemic rather than hemorrhagic (<5% of strokes) and their incidence varies based on the type of surgical procedure. General surgery poses the lowest risk of perioperative stroke with an incidence of between 0.1% and 1.0% according to retrospective studies. However, it may occur in up to 10% of patients undergoing high-risk cardiac, vascular or neurological surgery. In patients undergoing non-cardiac or nonvascular surgery, more than half of strokes occur within the first 24 h and up to 93% occur within the first 72 h of the perioperative setting. These strokes may be symptomatic as manifested by motor, sensory, or cognitive dysfunction, or may be silent, otherwise known as covert infarctions. The incidence of covert infarctions is variably reported in the literature, but is highest in patients undergoing high-risk cardiac, vascular, or neurological surgery. Procedures such as carotid artery stenting, open surgical valve replacements involving the mitral valve, and transcatheter aortic valve replacements carry highest risk of covert infarctions, which are often uncovered by magnetic resonance imaging (MRI). MRI here often demonstrates scattered ischemic lesions across multiple vascular territories given that many of these strokes are embolic in nature. To refer to these infarcts as silent is a misnomer as they have been associated with cognitive impairment and dementia, particularly in patients undergoing cardiac surgery, increased risk of subsequent stroke, and increased length of stay and mortality.

Pathophysiology and Causal Mechanisms

Ischemic thromboembolic complications are not uncommon in the perioperative period. Surgical trauma creates endothelial injury with tissue factor release that promotes hypercoagulability in part through activation of the coagulation cascade and reduction in fibrinolysis. The perioperative period is also characterized by a pro-inflammatory state with increased platelet production, aggregation, and reactivity that facilitate thrombosis. Furthermore, rebound hypercoagulability may occur in patients who have discontinued their anticoagulant or antiplatelet medications in preparation for surgery. Hemorrhagic stroke may be precipitated by antiplatelet and/or anticoagulant therapy, and uncontrolled hypertension caused by postoperative pain, sympathetic nervous system upregulation, or missing antihypertensive medications in the perioperative period. In the elderly, cerebral amyloid angiopathy is a major cause of lobar hemorrhagic stroke. Combined with other physiological stressors such as anemia from acute blood loss, dehydration, hypoxia, hypothermia, and fasting, the perioperative period is a perfect storm for the development of stroke.

Both ischemic and hemorrhagic perioperative stroke have different causal mechanisms and distinct pathophysiology. Ischemic strokes can be further subdivided into thromboembolic and hypoperfusion-related strokes. Thrombotic large vessel stroke may occur after embolization of thrombi formed over atherosclerotic plaques in patients with intracranial or extracranial large artery stenosis. In patients undergoing cardiac surgery, nearly two-thirds are the result of proximal embolism related to the procedure itself or embolic complications of myocardial infarction and/or atrial fibrillation. Intraoperative embolism may originate from aortic manipulation and subsequent dislodgement of atherosclerotic plaques as encountered in cardiac surgeries such as cardiopulmonary bypass, proximal aorta replacement surgery and valvular surgery, and from direct cardiac manipulation. Atrial fibrillation is a major cause of embolic stroke in the elderly and occurs in 15–42% of patients after cardiac surgery and roughly 10% in noncardiac surgery. Thrombus formation in the left atrial appendage and subsequent systemic embolization leads to cerebral infarction. In a recent meta-analysis, new-onset postoperative/perioperative atrial fibrillation (POAF) had 62% higher odds of early stroke compared with those without POAF. Hypoperfusion strokes occur as a result of hypotension or low-flow states with or without the presence of high-grade large vessel stenosis, and lead to watershed distribution strokes. Hypoperfusion may be induced by anesthesia-related decrease in systemic vascular resistance and vasodilatation, anesthesia-related myocardial depression, other causes of low cardiac output, acute blood loss, or shock states. Other types of rare ischemic infarctions include spinal cord infarctions after thoraco-abdominal aortic aneurysm surgery, and fat embolism after orthopedic surgery or traumatic bone injuries.

Hemorrhagic perioperative stroke is rare and has a few causes including uncontrolled hypertension, use of anticoagulant and antiplatelet agents, and cerebral hyperperfusion syndrome (CHS) observed after carotid endarterectomy and stenting. CHS results from the central nervous system (CNS) autoregulatory failure in the setting of flow limiting vascular lesions such as severe carotid artery stenosis. These patients typically have maximally dilated cerebral blood arteries with limited cerebrovascular reserve and elevated blood pressure to maintain constant cerebral blood flow in light of this flow limitation. However, after vessel revascularization, blood pressure remains elevated and autoregulatory impairment prevents reflex vasoconstriction of cerebral arteries leading to hyperprefusion. If postoperative hypertension is left untreated, the resultant increased cerebral blood flow creates a hyperperfusion state that may lead to the development of intracranial hemorrhage, subarachnoid hemorrhage, and cerebral edema formation.

Prevention

Prevention of perioperative stroke begins with the identification of high-risk patients such as those with a history of stroke and symptomatic carotid artery stenosis. A history of stroke is directly linked to the risk of perioperative stroke, and the timing of surgery from the most recent stroke further affects this risk. It is currently recommended that elective surgery, excluding cardiac and neurologic procedures, be deferred at least 6–9 months after a prior stroke to reduce the risk of perioperative stroke. The decision to delay surgery must take a patient-centered approach with a discussion of the risks and benefits of delaying surgical treatment. High-grade carotid artery stenosis (>70%) with symptoms of ischemic stroke or transient ischemic attack ipsilateral to the stenosis should be strongly considered for revascularization by Carotid Endarterectomy (CEA) or Carotid Artery Stent (CAS) within 6 months. Recommendations on medical and/or surgical management of patients with asymptomatic high-grade carotid stenosis undergoing noncardiac and non-neurological surgery is currently unknown. This is because intensive medical management with drug therapy and lifestyle modification in recent years has delivered promising results with markedly lower stroke rates compared with traditional medically treated cohorts. In patients with symptomatic and asymptomatic high-grade carotid artery stenosis who require emergency cardiac surgery such as coronary artery bypass grafting (CABG), the timing of CEA is unclear. Options include performing carotid revascularization concomitantly with CABG or after CABG, with the former carrying a higher risk of morbidity and perioperative stroke and death in certain studies.

The use of certain medications also modulates perioperative stroke risk. Though statin medications do not decrease perioperative stroke, their anti-inflammatory effects in particular confer cardiovascular protection. Antiplatelet therapy with aspirin should be held preoperatively, unless patients have had prior percutaneous coronary intervention, given higher perioperative bleeding risk without a reduction in nonfatal MI or mortality. There is also evidence that initiation of antiplatelet therapy such as aspirin after carotid and cardiac surgeries reduces perioperative stroke without increasing hemorrhagic complications. Lastly, perioperative beta blocker has been shown to reduce adverse cardiac events and the 2014 American College of Cardiology/American Heart Association Guideline on Perioperative Cardiovascular Evaluation and Management strongly supports continuing β-blockers in patients who are on β-blockers long term. Though β-blockers reduce risk of arrhythmias such as atrial fibrillation, sympathetic activity, and MI, they have not been shown to reduce perioperative stroke risk. In fact, β-blockers such as metoprolol have been associated with perioperative hypotension and associated with higher overall mortality rates and perioperative stroke.

Risk Factors

In addition to the type and nature of the surgical procedure, other intraoperative risk factors can affect perioperative stroke risk. Though anesthetic technique (regional, general, or neuraxial) has been examined in the literature as a risk factor, there is insufficient evidence to make clear suggestions on the use of general anesthesia vs regional anesthesia. Intraoperative hypotension, most commonly defined as systolic blood pressure <80 mmHg or 20% below baseline, seems to be associated with perioperative stroke. CNS autoregulatory failure can occur below a mean arterial pressure (MAP) of 50, and the resultant decrease in the cerebral perfusion pressure and cerebral blood flow can lead to cerebral infarctions. Autoregulatory thresholds may even be higher for elderly patients, especially those with recent ischemic stroke and chronic hypertension. Strong associations regarding hypotension have not been found in the literature but may be due to low incidence of clinical evident strokes, undetected covert strokes, and the lack of standardized definitions for intraoperative hypotension. The 2021 American Heart Association/American Stroke Association perioperative guidelines on noncardiac and nonneurological surgery suggest that MAP goals be maintained above 70 mmHg to reduce the risk of perioperative stroke.

Presentation

Identifying stroke in the elderly may be very challenging in the perioperative period. Prolonged intubation after surgery and pre-existing cognitive impairment may preclude accurate neurologic assessments. Nonspecific findings such as difficulty awakening from anesthesia may itself be a sign of stroke and can also mask focal deficits on the exam. Focal deficits such as aphasia may be mistaken for delirium and confusion, particularly in the setting of opioid and psychoactive medication use. This makes it difficult to establish a time of symptom onset, which is essential to determine appropriate stroke treatment. Neuromonitoring such as somatosensory evoked potentials and continuous electroencephalography deployed during certain high-risk neurosurgical procedures such as CEA can help detect early ischemia and can help overcome some of these challenges.

Treatment

Activation of a stroke response team should take place immediately after recognition of an acute stroke in the perioperative setting in order to obtain pretreatment neurologic examination and National Institutes of Health Stroke Scale (NIHSS) score, establish a last known well time which may be the time of anesthetic induction, and facilitate appropriate imaging studies to determine the appropriate treatment. A noncontrast head CT scan should be obtained first to rule out intracranial hemorrhage, with additional CT angiography and perfusion studies in patients suspected of having a large artery vessel occlusion (LVO). LVO is suspected when NIHSS >6 and/or cortical deficits such as aphasia or visual field defects are present on examination. The incidence of LVO is 10.9% in patients with perioperative ischemic strokes after cardiac surgery. LVO portends poor neurologic outcomes if left untreated.

Treatment of ischemic stroke in the perioperative setting has its limitations as patients are often ineligible for intravenous alteplase because of the risk of bleeding from the surgical site. However, patients may be eligible for mechanical thrombectomy in the presence of LVO up to 24 h after the onset of stroke symptoms with appropriate clinical and imaging characteristics as outlined by the inclusion and exclusion criteria of recent stroke trials. Though these trials boast promising benefit of mechanical thrombectomy in reducing disability in select patients with LVO, disparities in treatment and stroke guideline adherence are not uncommon for the very elderly. The very elderly have been traditionally excluded from randomized clinical trials and the results from the trials may not be generalizable to this group. Furthermore, frailty and poor baseline functionality, multiple medical comorbidities, and polypharmacy may impact the response to acute and chronic stroke therapies and recovery. Therefore, the decision to pursue mechanical thrombectomy in elderly perioperative patients with stroke needs an individualized risk/benefit assessment taking into account these complexities.

References

1. Gardner RC, Dams-O'Connor K, Morrissey MR, Manley GT. Geriatric traumatic brain injury: epidemiology, outcomes, knowledge gaps, and future directions. J Neurotrauma. 2018;35:889–906. https://doi.org/10.1089/neu.2017.5371.
2. Stocchetti N, Paternò R, Citerio G, Beretta L, Colombo A. Traumatic brain injury in an aging population. J Neurotrauma. 2012;29:1119–25. https://doi.org/10.1089/neu.2011.1995.
3. Schupper AJ, Berndtson AE, Smith A, Godat L, Costantini TW. Respect your elders: effects of ageing on intracranial pressure monitor use in traumatic brain injury. Trauma Surg Acute Care Open. 2019;4(1):e000306. https://doi.org/10.1136/tsaco-2019-000306.
4. San Martino P, Graziano F, Rebora P, Elli F, Giussani C, Oddo M, et al. Intracranial pressure monitoring in patients with acute brain injury in the intensive care unit (SYNAPSE-ICU): an international, prospective observational cohort study. Lancet Neurol. 2021;20(7):548–58. https://doi.org/10.1016/S1474-4422(21)00138-1.
5. Godoy DA, Lubillo S, Rabinstein AA. Pathophysiology and management of intracranial hypertension and tissular brain hypoxia after severe traumatic brain injury: an integrative approach. Neurosurg Clin N Am. 2018;29:195–212. https://doi.org/10.1016/j.nec.2017.12.001.
6. Gu J, Huang H, Huang Y, Sun H, Xu H. Hypertonic saline or mannitol for treating elevated intracranial pressure in traumatic brain injury: a meta-analysis of randomized controlled trials. Neurosurg Rev. 2019;42:499–509. https://doi.org/10.1007/s10143-018-0991-8.
7. Stocchetti N, Carbonara M, Citerio G, Ercole A, Skrifvars MB, Smielewski P, et al. Severe traumatic brain injury: targeted management in the intensive care unit. Lancet Neurol. 2017;16(6):452–64. https://doi.org/10.1016/S1474-4422(17)30118-7.
8. De Bonis P, Pompucci A, Mangiola A, D'Alessandris QG, Rigante L, Anile C. Decompressive craniectomy for the treatment of traumatic brain injury: does an age limit exist? A review. J Neurosurg. 2013;112:1150–3. https://doi.org/10.3171/2009.7.JNS09505.
9. Roberson SW, Patel MB, Dabrowski W, Ely EW, Pakulski C, Kotfis K. Challenges of delirium management in patients with traumatic brain injury: from pathophysiology to clinical practice. Curr Neuropharmacol. 2021;19:1519–44. https://doi.org/10.2174/1570159X19666210119153839.
10. Glaser AC, Kanter JH, Martinez-Camblor P, Taenzer A, Anderson MV, Buhl L, et al. The effect of antiseizure medication administration on mortality and early posttraumatic seizures in critically ill older adults with traumatic brain injury. Neurocrit Care. 2022;37(2):538–46. https://doi.org/10.1007/s12028-022-01531-1.
11. Xu JC, Shen J, Shao WZ, Tang LJ, Sun YZ, Zhai XF, et al. The safety and efficacy of levetiracetam versus phenytoin for seizure prophylaxis after traumatic brain injury: a systematic review and meta-analysis. Brain Inj. 2016;30:1054–61. https://doi.org/10.3109/02699052.2016.1170882.
12. Scotti P, Séguin C, Lo BWY, de Guise E, Troquet JM, Marcoux J. Antithrombotic agents and traumatic brain injury in the elderly population: hemorrhage patterns and outcomes. J Neurosurg. 2019:1–10. https://doi.org/10.3171/2019.4.JNS19252.
13. Ng IC, Barnes C, Biswas S, Wright D, Dagal A. When is it safe to resume anticoagulation in traumatic brain injury? Curr Opin Anaesthesiol. 2022;35:166–71. https://doi.org/10.1097/ACO.0000000000001117.
14. Meschia JF, Bushnell C, Boden-Albala B, Braun LT, Bravata DM, Chaturvedi S, et al. Guidelines for the primary prevention of stroke: a statement for healthcare professionals from the American Heart Association/American Stroke Association. Stroke. 2014;45(12):3754–832. https://doi.org/10.1161/STR.0000000000000046.
15. Benesch C, Glance LG, Derdeyn CP, Fleisher LA, Holloway RG, Messé SR, et al. Perioperative neurological evaluation and management to lower the risk of acute stroke in patients undergoing noncardiac, nonneurological surgery: a scientific statement from the American Heart Association/American Stroke Association. Circulation. 2021;143(19):e923–46. https://doi.org/10.1161/CIR.0000000000000968.

Cervical and Thoracic Spine Trauma in the Elderly

17

Carlos Yáñez Benítez, Alejandra Utrilla, Luca Ponchietti, and Patrizio Petrone

Elderly Population Worldwide

The conventional indicator for "old age" is based on the chronological age, or years since birth, considering "old age" for those 65 or over. Those from 65 to 74 years old are referred to as "early elderly" and those older than 75 as "late elderly." Worldwide the population is aging; this is due to the decline in fertility and the advances in sophisticated medical care, all leading to increased longevity and life expectancy. In 2019 there were over 703 million older persons worldwide; over the next three decades, this number is projected to double, reaching 1.5 billion by 2050. The elderly population is more vulnerable to falls and low-energy trauma than the young; the sum of extrinsic (environment) and intrinsic (cognitive impairment, physical comorbidities, loss of visual acuity) factors increase the risk of falling during daily activities. These falls are commonly produced from a standing height, sitting height, from a bed, or down a flight of stairs.

C. Yáñez Benítez (✉) · A. Utrilla · L. Ponchietti
San Jorge University Hospital, Huesca, Spain

P. Petrone
NYU Langone Hospital—Long Island, Mineola, New York, USA
e-mail: Patrizio.Petrone@nyulangone.org

Any fall in this frail population can potentially lead to severe injuries or fractures, even those deemed to be low-energy trauma or low-level falls. Cervical spine fractures account for over 55% of all spinal injuries and can be potentially life-threatening in the elderly. The neck mobility and the exposure of the cervical spine make it highly vulnerable to injuries during falls. In addition, the upper cervical spine, with a particular interest in the atlantoaxial complex and odontoid process, is fragile in degenerative spinal disease, this explains why odontoid fractures are the most prevalent type of cervical spine injury in elderly patients (Fig. 17.1).

Loss of bone density and advanced osteoporosis, most prevalent in women over 85, can lead to thoracic vertebral compression fractures with very low-energy trauma. These fractures are among the most frequent types of injuries in the dorsal spine, commonly seen in women over 60, and are associated with significant morbidity. With this background, it is essential to understand the importance of fall prevention in the elderly and attending trauma teams must maintain a high index of suspicion for cervical and dorsal spine injuries during any fall or trauma in the elderly.

P. Petrone, C. E.M. Brathwaite (eds.), *Acute Care Surgery in Geriatric Patients*,
https://doi.org/10.1007/978-3-031-30651-8_17

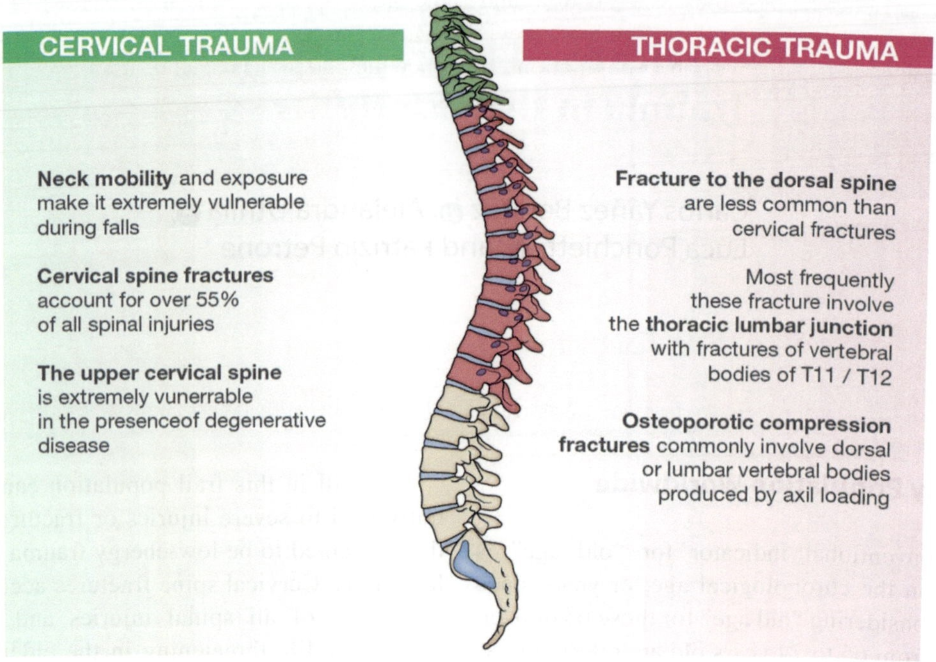

Fig. 17.1 Characteristics of cervical and thoracic spine trauma in the elderly (Illustration by Ilaria Bondi)

Basic Cervical and Thoracic Spine Anatomy

The human spine comprises 7 cervical, 12 thoracic, and 5 lumbar vertebrae, followed by the sacrum and the coccyx, formed by the fusion of 5 and 4 vertebrae, respectively. Each vertebra has a cylindrical vertebral body that bears the most weight; these are separated by the intervertebral disks held together by five longitudinal ligaments. These ligaments are present throughout the entire spine (anterior and posterior longitudinal ligaments, the ligamentum flavum, the interspinous ligament, and the supraspinous ligament) (Fig. 17.2).

The bony structures connect each vertebra's anterior and posterior portions to the termed posterior elements, including the pedicles, lamina, spinous, and transverse processes. The facet joints, interspinous ligaments, and paraspinal muscles are all responsible for providing spine stability and normal range of motion during the daily activities (Fig. 17.3).

The cervical spine has a curvature with posterior concavity termed cervical lordosis, which is typical among adults (Fig. 17.4). Of all the spine segments, the cervical spine is the most vulnerable to injuries due to its significant mobility and greater exposure than the dorsal or lumbar spine, protected by the ribcage and lumbar muscles. The upper cervical spine has some distinctive features: the first vertebrae, termed atlas or C1, has no vertebral body and creates the occipital-atlantal joint with the skull's base. The second cervical vertebrae termed axis or C2 forms the atlantoaxial

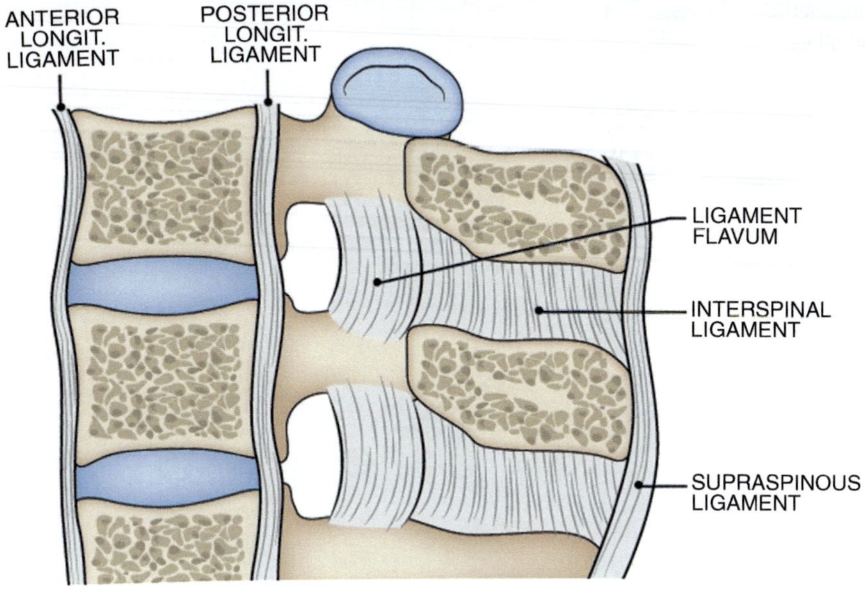

Fig. 17.2 Longitudinal ligaments of the spine (Illustration by Ilaria Bondi)

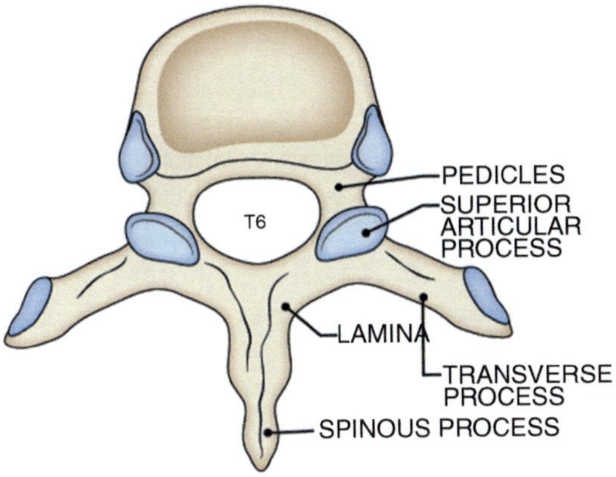

Fig. 17.3 Basic morphology and elements of a vertebra (Illustration by Ilaria Bondi)

joint. The cervical canal is also different in the upper cervical spine; it is broader from the foramen magnum to the inferior portion of C2, so surviving patients with injuries in C1 or C2 may arrive at the hospital without neurological deficits. However, significant trauma in the upper cervical spine above C3 is a high risk of death on the scene type of injury due to apnea and loss of innervation of the phrenic nerves. Below this level, from C3 to C7, the spinal canal is smaller, so vertebral injuries associated with spinal cord injuries are more common (Fig. 17.4).

The dorsal spine runs from the base of the neck to the bottom of the ribcage (Fig. 17.5). It is the most extended section of the spine. The normal dorsal spine has a curvature with anterior concavity termed normal dorsal kyphosis that contributes to maintaining balance when standing up and walking. This natural kyphosis is from 20–45°. Curvatures outside this range are abnormal and termed hyperkyphosis. In addition, the dorsal spine has unique articulations with the ribs; these are two for each rib, the costovertebral joint and the costotransverse joint (Fig. 17.5).

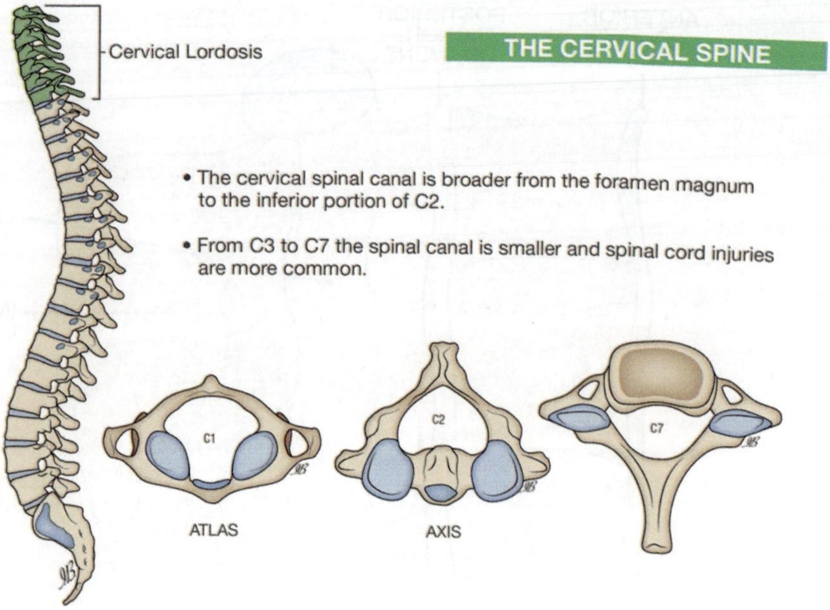

Fig. 17.4 Characteristics of the cervical spine (Illustration by Ilaria Bondi)

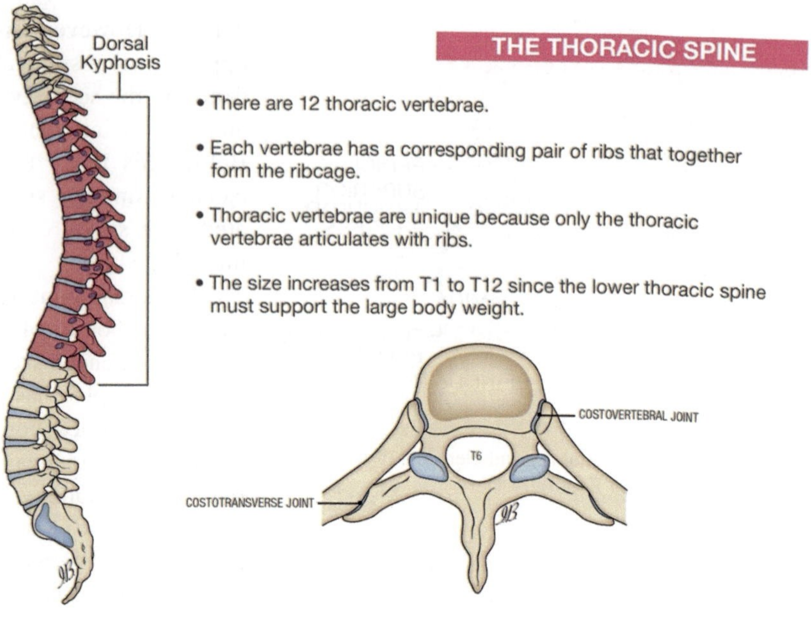

Fig. 17.5 Characteristics of the thoracic spine (Illustration by Ilaria Bondi)

Spinal Cord Anatomy

The spinal cord is an extension of the central nervous system that runs from the foramen magnum and ends in adults close to L1–L2. It is formed by a central area of gray matter corresponding to the neuronal cell bodies comprising the ventral, lateral, and dorsal horns, organized into segments forming the motor and sensory nerves. There are 31 pairs of spinal nerves. However, not all arise from the spinal cord at the level of the vertebrae exit, mainly in the lumbar and sacral regions.

In contrast to the brain, the spinal cord's white matter is on the outside (myelin-containing regions composed of axons) surrounding the gray matter (cell bodies and dendrites), forming the spinal cord's longitudinal ascending or descending tracts. These are the pathways that communicate the brain with the body. In general, the ascending tracts carry sensory information from the body to the brain, and the descending tracts deliver motor information from the brain to body muscles. There are three main spinal cord tracts: the lateral corticospinal tract (controls motor functions on the same side of the body), the spinothalamic tract or anterolateral system (transmits pain and temperature sensation from the opposite side of the body), and the dorsal columns (proprioception, vibration, and light-touch sensation from the same side of the body).

These paired tracts that can be injured on one or both sides of the spinal cord. To adequately explore the patient, we must assess all dermatomes (area of the skin innervated by the sensory axons of a segmental nerve or root) and the myotomes (muscle groups innervated by the motor axons from a spinal nerve or root). The cervical section of the spine has 8 nerve roots (C1–C8), and each is named according to the vertebrae immediately above. The thoracic spine has 12 nerve roots and the lumbar spine 5; however, below L1–L2, we find the most distal part of the spinal cord; from here on, it adopts the form of a cone termed "conus medullaris." Below this level, we find the cauda equina formed by paired lumbosacral nerves less susceptible to injuries and the filum terminale.

Spinal Cord Assessment

For adequate assessment of spinal cord integrity, the American Spinal Cord Injury Association (ASIA) has developed a worksheet that provides detailed information on the patient's spinal function integrity in a simple-to-use format. The International Standards for Neurological Classification of Spinal Cord Injury (ISNCSCI) allows the motor and sensory response registration on both the right and left sides of the body and has a classification score for a motor response from 0 to 5, where 0 is complete paralysis and 5 is an active movement against total resistance. The superficial sensation is graded from 0 to 2, being 0 absence of sense and 2 normal sensation. The utility of using this system is that it allows systematization of the neurological assessment among different teams and gives clear indication of when to test non-key muscles to assess the different root levels. Finally, the ISNCSCI assessment tool also provides an impairment assessment scale (IAS), a step-by-step approach to the neurological level of injury, and a guideline to determine if the spinal cord injury is complete or incomplete (Fig. 17.6).

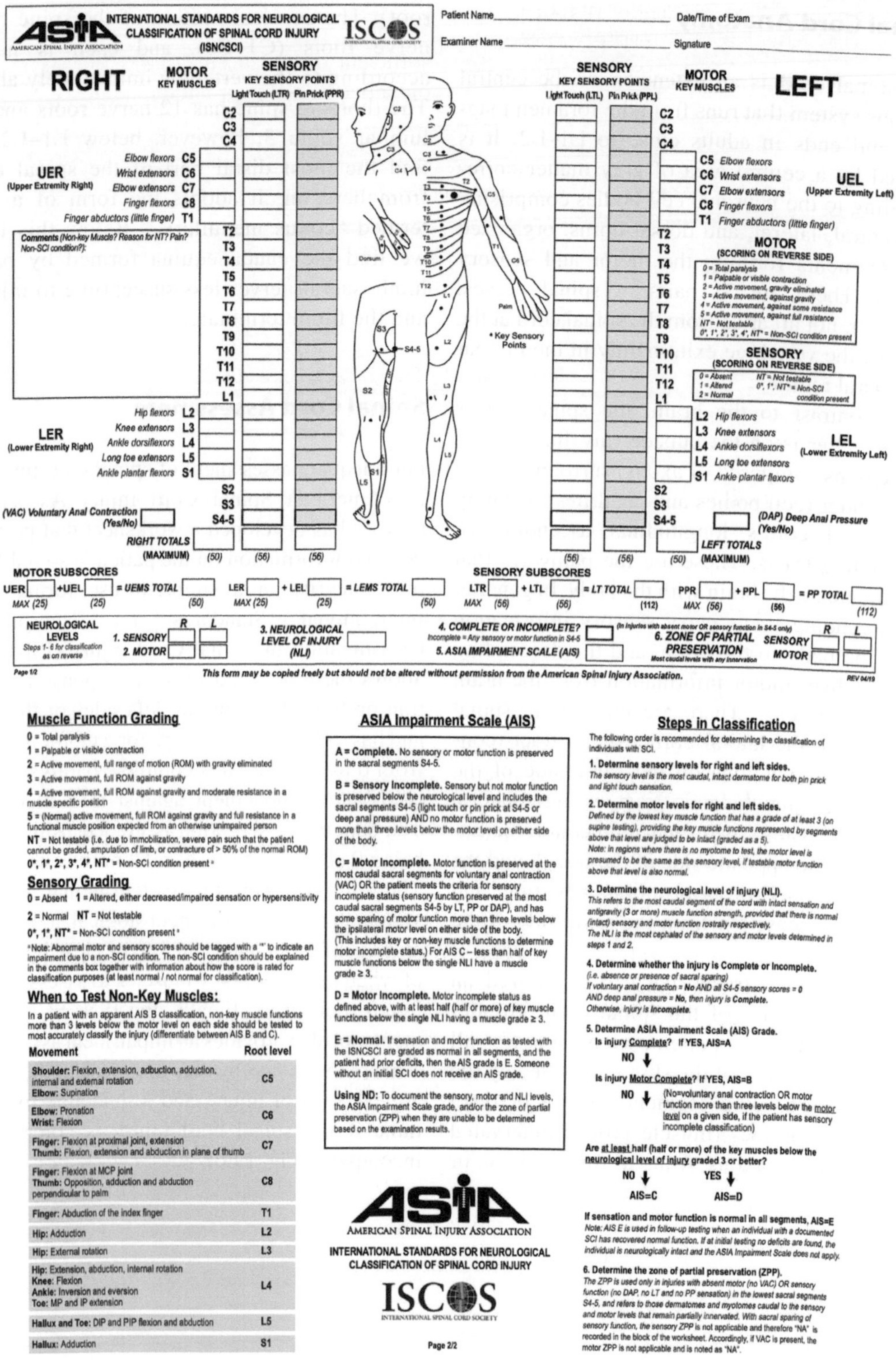

INTERNATIONAL STANDARDS FOR NEUROLOGICAL CLASSIFICATION OF SPINAL CORD INJURY (ISNCSCI)

AMERICAN SPINAL INJURY ASSOCIATION — ISCOS

Patient Name________ Date/Time of Exam________

Examiner Name________ Signature________

RIGHT — MOTOR KEY MUSCLES — SENSORY KEY SENSORY POINTS Light Touch (LTR) Pin Prick (PPR)

SENSORY KEY SENSORY POINTS Light Touch (LTL) Pin Prick (PPL) — MOTOR KEY MUSCLES — LEFT

C2, C3, C4

UER (Upper Extremity Right): Elbow flexors C5; Wrist extensors C6; Elbow extensors C7; Finger flexors C8; Finger abductors (little finger) T1

UEL (Upper Extremity Left): C5 Elbow flexors; C6 Wrist extensors; C7 Elbow extensors; C8 Finger flexors; T1 Finger abductors (little finger)

Comments (Non-key Muscle? Reason for NT? Pain? Non-SCI condition?):

T2, T3, T4, T5, T6, T7, T8, T9, T10, T11, T12, L1

LER (Lower Extremity Right): Hip flexors L2; Knee extensors L3; Ankle dorsiflexors L4; Long toe extensors L5; Ankle plantar flexors S1

LEL (Lower Extremity Left): L2 Hip flexors; L3 Knee extensors; L4 Ankle dorsiflexors; L5 Long toe extensors; S1 Ankle plantar flexors

S2, S3, S4-5

(VAC) Voluntary Anal Contraction (Yes/No)

(DAP) Deep Anal Pressure (Yes/No)

Dorsum · Palm · • Key Sensory Points

MOTOR (SCORING ON REVERSE SIDE)
0 = Total paralysis
1 = Palpable or visible contraction
2 = Active movement, gravity eliminated
3 = Active movement, against gravity
4 = Active movement, against some resistance
5 = Active movement, against full resistance
NT = Not testable
0*, 1*, 2*, 3*, 4*, NT* = Non-SCI condition present

SENSORY (SCORING ON REVERSE SIDE)
0 = Absent NT = Not testable
1 = Altered 0*, 1*, NT* = Non-SCI condition present
2 = Normal

RIGHT TOTALS (MAXIMUM) (50) (56) (56)

LEFT TOTALS (MAXIMUM) (56) (56) (50)

MOTOR SUBSCORES

UER [ ] + UEL [ ] = UEMS TOTAL [ ] — MAX (25) (25) (50)

LER [ ] + LEL [ ] = LEMS TOTAL [ ] — MAX (25) (25) (50)

SENSORY SUBSCORES

LTR [ ] + LTL [ ] = LT TOTAL [ ] — MAX (56) (56) (112)

PPR [ ] + PPL [ ] = PP TOTAL [ ] — MAX (56) (56) (112)

NEUROLOGICAL LEVELS (Steps 1-6 for classification as on reverse) R L
1. SENSORY
2. MOTOR

3. NEUROLOGICAL LEVEL OF INJURY (NLI)

4. COMPLETE OR INCOMPLETE? Incomplete = Any sensory or motor function in S4-5

5. ASIA IMPAIRMENT SCALE (AIS)

6. ZONE OF PARTIAL PRESERVATION (In injuries with absent motor OR sensory function in S4-5 only) Most caudal levels with any innervation — SENSORY R L — MOTOR

Page 1/2 This form may be copied freely but should not be altered without permission from the American Spinal Injury Association. REV 04/19

Muscle Function Grading

0 = Total paralysis

1 = Palpable or visible contraction

2 = Active movement, full range of motion (ROM) with gravity eliminated

3 = Active movement, full ROM against gravity

4 = Active movement, full ROM against gravity and moderate resistance in a muscle specific position

5 = (Normal) active movement, full ROM against gravity and full resistance in a functional muscle position expected from an otherwise unimpaired person

NT = Not testable (i.e. due to immobilization, severe pain such that the patient cannot be graded, amputation of limb, or contracture of > 50% of the normal ROM)

0*, 1*, 2*, 3*, 4*, NT* = Non-SCI condition present *

Sensory Grading

0 = Absent **1** = Altered, either decreased/impaired sensation or hypersensitivity

2 = Normal **NT** = Not testable

0*, 1*, NT* = Non-SCI condition present *

Note: Abnormal motor and sensory scores should be tagged with a "" to indicate an impairment due to a non-SCI condition. The non-SCI condition should be explained in the comments box together with information about how the score is rated for classification purposes (at least normal / not normal for classification).

When to Test Non-Key Muscles:

In a patient with an apparent AIS B classification, non-key muscle functions more than 3 levels below the motor level on each side should be tested to most accurately classify the injury (differentiate between AIS B and C).

Movement	Root level
Shoulder: Flexion, extension, adbuction, adduction, internal and external rotation **Elbow:** Supination	C5
Elbow: Pronation **Wrist:** Flexion	C6
Finger: Flexion at proximal joint, extension **Thumb:** Flexion, extension and abduction in plane of thumb	C7
Finger: Flexion at MCP joint **Thumb:** Opposition, adduction and abduction perpendicular to palm	C8
Finger: Abduction of the index finger	T1
Hip: Adduction	L2
Hip: External rotation	L3
Hip: Extension, abduction, internal rotation **Knee:** Flexion **Ankle:** Inversion and eversion **Toe:** MP and IP extension	L4
Hallux and Toe: DIP and PIP flexion and abduction	L5
Hallux: Adduction	S1

ASIA Impairment Scale (AIS)

A = Complete. No sensory or motor function is preserved in the sacral segments S4-5.

B = Sensory Incomplete. Sensory but not motor function is preserved below the neurological level and includes the sacral segments S4-5 (light touch or pin prick at S4-5 or deep anal pressure) AND no motor function is preserved more than three levels below the motor level on either side of the body.

C = Motor Incomplete. Motor function is preserved at the most caudal sacral segments for voluntary anal contraction (VAC) OR the patient meets the criteria for sensory incomplete status (sensory function preserved at the most caudal sacral segments S4-5 by LT, PP or DAP), and has some sparing of motor function more than three levels below the ipsilateral motor level on either side of the body. (This includes key or non-key muscle functions to determine motor incomplete status.) For AIS C – less than half of key muscle functions below the single NLI have a muscle grade ≥ 3.

D = Motor Incomplete. Motor incomplete status as defined above, with at least half (half or more) of key muscle functions below the single NLI having a muscle grade ≥ 3.

E = Normal. If sensation and motor function as tested with the ISNCSCI are graded as normal in all segments, and the patient had prior deficits, then the AIS grade is E. Someone without an initial SCI does not receive an AIS grade.

Using ND: To document the sensory, motor and NLI levels, the ASIA Impairment Scale grade, and/or the zone of partial preservation (ZPP) when they are unable to be determined based on the examination results.

AMERICAN SPINAL INJURY ASSOCIATION

INTERNATIONAL STANDARDS FOR NEUROLOGICAL CLASSIFICATION OF SPINAL CORD INJURY

ISCOS — INTERNATIONAL SPINAL CORD SOCIETY

Steps in Classification

The following order is recommended for determining the classification of individuals with SCI.

1. Determine sensory levels for right and left sides.
The sensory level is the most caudal, intact dermatome for both pin prick and light touch sensation.

2. Determine motor levels for right and left sides.
Defined by the lowest key muscle function that has a grade of at least 3 (on supine testing), providing the key muscle functions represented by segments above that level are judged to be intact (graded as a 5).
Note: in regions where there is no myotome to test, the motor level is presumed to be the same as the sensory level, if testable motor function above that level is also normal.

3. Determine the neurological level of injury (NLI).
This refers to the most caudal segment of the cord with intact sensation and antigravity (3 or more) muscle function strength, provided that there is normal (intact) sensory and motor function rostrally respectively.
The NLI is the most cephalad of the sensory and motor levels determined in steps 1 and 2.

4. Determine whether the injury is Complete or Incomplete.
(i.e. absence or presence of sacral sparing)
*If voluntary anal contraction = **No** AND all S4-5 sensory scores = 0 AND deep anal pressure = **No**, then injury is **Complete**.*
*Otherwise, injury is **Incomplete**.*

5. Determine ASIA Impairment Scale (AIS) Grade.
Is injury Complete? If YES, AIS=A
NO ↓
Is injury Motor Complete? If YES, AIS=B
NO ↓ (No=voluntary anal contraction OR motor function more than three levels below the motor level on a given side, if the patient has sensory incomplete classification)

Are at least half (half or more) of the key muscles below the neurological level of injury graded 3 or better?
NO ↓ **AIS=C** **YES** ↓ **AIS=D**

If sensation and motor function is normal in all segments, AIS=E
Note: AIS E is used in follow-up testing when an individual with a documented SCI has recovered normal function. If at initial testing no deficits are found, the individual is neurologically intact and the ASIA Impairment Scale does not apply.

6. Determine the zone of partial preservation (ZPP).
The ZPP is used only in injuries with absent motor (no VAC) OR sensory function (no DAP, no LT and no PP sensation) in the lowest sacral segments S4-5, and refers to those dermatomes and myotomes caudal to the sensory and motor levels that remain partially innervated. With sacral sparing of sensory function, the sensory ZPP is not applicable and therefore "NA" is recorded in the block of the worksheet. Accordingly, if VAC is present, the motor ZPP is not applicable and is noted as "NA".

Page 2/2

Fig. 17.6 American spinal injury association: International standards for neurological classification of spinal cord injury, revised 2019; Richmond, VA (With permission)

Patterns of Incomplete Injuries

Spinal cord injuries (SCI) can compromise both sensory and motor signals bilaterally at the level of injury. However, there are situations in which the patient can suffer incomplete injury patterns, known as incomplete injury syndromes, which should be recognized.

Central cord syndrome: This is the most common incomplete injury pattern encountered after falls with or without fractures or dislocations. It is frequently found in patients with cervical spondylosis that suffer hyperextension injuries and is characterized by incomplete injury with greater weakness in the upper extremities than in the lower extremities.

Brown-Séquard syndrome: This rare syndrome is characterized by a spinal cord hemisection that causes ipsilateral loss of proprioception, vibration, and motor response at the level of the injury and below and contralateral loss of pain and temperature.

Anterior cord syndrome: A rare syndrome caused by a decreased blood supply to the anterior two-thirds of the spinal cord that compromises the corticospinal and spinothalamic tracts while sparing the dorsal columns. It is characterized by loss of motor function, pain, and temperature sensation at the level of the injury and below while preserving light touch sensation and position sense of the joint.

Cervical and Thoracic Spine in the Elderly

Muscle strength, mobility, bone mineral density, and soft tissue elasticity are lost as the body ages. As a result, the spine reduces its range of motion and elasticity. Injury severity caused by a compressive load on the spine depends on gender, age, the mineral density of the vertebral body, and the magnitude of the loading force during blunt trauma. While younger patients can resist heavier loads and suffer injuries only with high energy transfer or heavy loading, elderly patients may suffer injuries with low energy or light loading. In addition, the decreased mineral density of the vertebral body makes the elderly spine more susceptible to axial loading injuries with low-impact falls.

Additionally, the spine suffers from spondylosis deformans and degenerative changes, causing increased thoracic kyphosis and loss of cervical lordosis (Fig. 17.8). These can be found in both the supporting connective tissue as well as in the ligaments. Spondylosis deformans is a common condition in the elderly population associated with degeneration of the intervertebral disks and the presence of osteophytes in the vertebral bodies. Patients with spondylosis deformans have an increased risk of spinal injuries caused by reduced spine flexibility. Another common finding among elderly patients is paravertebral ligamentous ossification; these can be in the form of diffuse idiopathic skeletal hyperostosis (DISH), ossification of the posterior longitudinal ligament (OPLL), or ossification of the ligamentum flavum (OLF). These conditions can have a partial or complete fusion of spinal segments with the narrowed spinal canal. These degenerative conditions may increase the risk of spinal cord injuries even after minor trauma, such as falling from a standing position or bed (Fig. 17.7).

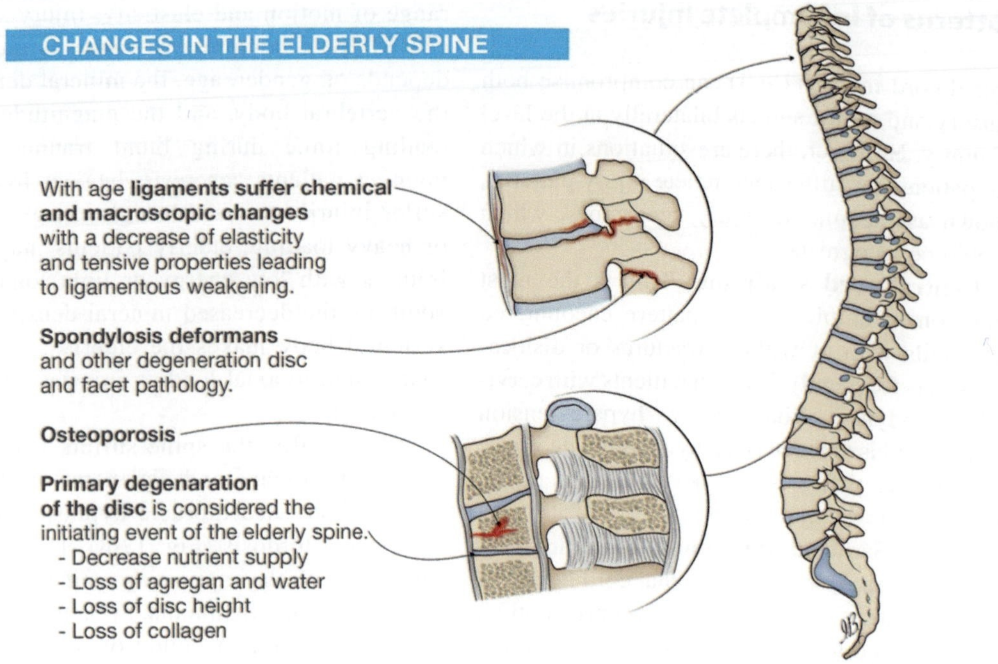

Fig. 17.7 Characteristics of the changes commonly identified in the elderly spine. (Illustration by Ilaria Bondi)

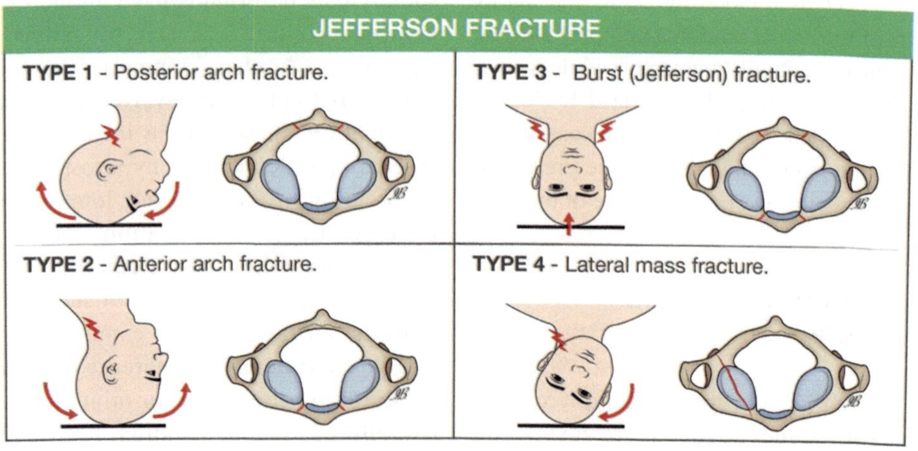

Fig. 17.8 Jefferson classification of C1 fractures (Illustration by Ilaria Bondi)

Cinematics of injuries

Energy transfer to the spine can cause injuries by several mechanisms: compression or axial loading, tension, torsion or rotation, bending, and distraction. Compression injuries of the spine are commonly reproduced by the kinetic energy transmitted from the moving torso to the neck or thoracic spine or by pressure caused by loading forces. Tension injuries are produced by deacceleration forces commonly generated by automotive restrain systems or airbag deployments. Finally, torsion of the spine can cause unilateral facet or atlantoaxial dislocation injuries commonly seen on lateral impacts.

Mechanism of Injury

Traffic accidents and falls are the most common mechanisms of injury in the elderly. Motor vehicle accidents are the most crucial cause of injury-related deaths among the elderly worldwide, followed by falls. Elderly patients are not commonly exposed to injuries during sports; however, many elderly patients have an active lifestyle, travel, and perform outdoor recreational activities. Even though anybody can have a potential fall with a spine injury, elderly patients often have physical, perceptual, and even cognitive deterioration, making them more susceptible to falls indoors and outdoors. Reports from the World Health Organization (WHO) suggest an increase in fall risk for those over 65 and an increase for those over 70. Falls can be responsible for up to 30% of severe injuries in this population.

The injuries encountered in elderly patients after falls will also depend on the pattern of the fall; the patient can fall from a standing height, from a height, or, most commonly, down a staircase. Low-level falls are those produced from a height of 2 m or lower and are the leading cause of trauma in some European countries. Also, the elderly will have more direct anterior craniofacial trauma compared with younger patients. The typical injury will be a fall forward from a standing height and hitting the forehead of the face against a wall or the floor.

Specific Types of Cervical Vertebral Fractures

Cervical fractures have a bimodal distribution, with the first peak affecting young male adults, primarily due to road accidents related to motor vehicle injuries, sports injuries, and assaults. The second peak, however, is seen in patients over 55 and elderly who suffer accidental falls. Recent studies suggest a reduction in cervical injuries in the young with most lesions affecting the lower cervical spine (LCS) and an increase in cervical injuries in the elderly, mostly affecting the upper cervical spine (UCS). In this elderly population, degenerative spinal disease increases the risk of upper cervical spine fractures. The most common fractures in elderly patients involve C1 and C2, particularly those of the atlanto-axial complex and the odontoid.

Atlas fractures represent near to 25% of all cranio-cervical injuries, close to 11% of all cervical fractures, and between 1 and 3% of all the spinal fractures. Over 80% of them are caused by motor vehicle accidents due to axial loading. When the atlas fracture is associated with a transverse atlantal ligament (TAL) tear the UCS is usually unstable and may require surgical treatment. The use of Magnetic Resonance Imaging (MRI) can help confirm the diagnosis by means of the Rule of Spence that determines the level of lateral mass displacement: when is >than 6.9 mm is associated with TAL tear. There are two main classifications systems for C1 fractures: the Landell and Van Peteghem classification and the Jefferson classification. The Jefferson classification (Fig. 17.8) considers the location of the fracture with regard to the anterior ring only (Type I), posterior ring (Type II), both anterior and posterior (Type III or classical burst fracture of C1 with disruption on the anterior and posterior rings) caused by axial loading by either large objects falling directly to the head or when the patient falls and lands headfirst, and fracture to the lateral masses of C1 (Type IV) (Fig. 17.8).

C1 and C2 are classically explored with the open mouth plain X-ray film that provides antero-posterior cervical spine view. Though not frequently associated with neurologic deficits, several UCS injuries are considered unstable and should be treated with a hard C-collar until evaluated by a neurosurgeon or orthopedic surgical team. The two most common classification systems for odontoid fractures are the Roy-Camille and the Anderson-D'Alonzo classification systems (Fig. 17.9). These consider the fracture's location and the fracture line's direction to create the scoring system. In the elderly, the fractures of the odontoid process of the axis are the most common type of UCS injury, being the D'Alonzo type II the most common of all. Most of these patients' neurological status will be unaffected and will have very few if any, clinical signs.

The traumatic spondylolisthesis of the axis is a fracture of the posterior elements of C2

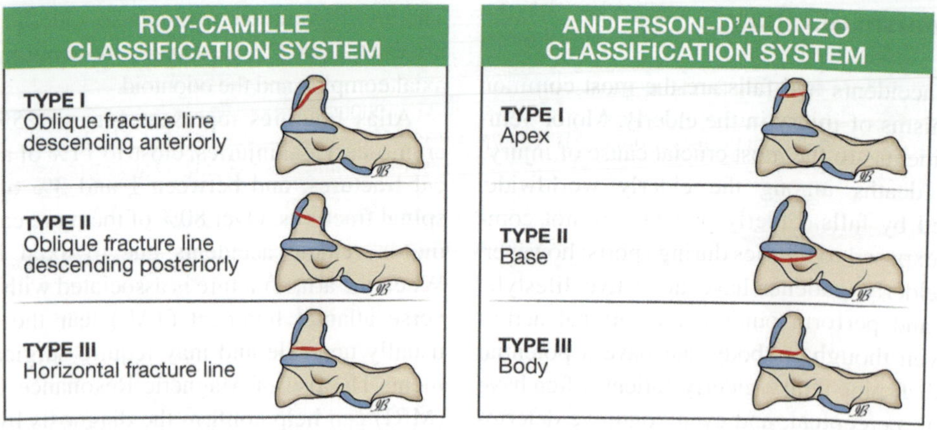

Fig. 17.9 Roy-Camille and Anderson-D'Alonzo classification systems of C2 fractures (Illustration by Ilaria Bondi)

caused by extension of the cervical spine; they account for 4–7% of all cervical spine fracture. Described as the Hangman's fracture by Schneider in 1965; however, it is present in only 10% of injuries related to hangings. There are several classifications systems for these types of injuries but the most commonly used is the Levine and Edwards classification system that classifies the injuries based on the mechanism of injury.

Fractures to the Thoracic Spine

Fractures to the thoracic spine are less common than cervical fractures; however, they can be present in elderly osteopenic patients due to several mechanisms of injury. Most post-traumatic fractures affect the thoracolumbar junction with fractures of vertebral bodies at T11/T12 or L1/L2. The German AO Foundation (Arbeitsgemeinschaft Osteosynthese) has developed a classification that differentiates compression fractures (Type A) from flexion-distraction (Type B) and highly unstable fractures (Type C). Anterior wedge compression Type A fractures are produced with axial loading with flexion of the torso. Due to the strength of the rib cage, surrounding muscles are most commonly stable. If the trauma has severe axial compression, burst injuries of the spinal body can be seen, especially in the elderly with a reduced mineral density of the vertebral bodies. Type B transverse fractures through the vertebral body, termed Chance fractures, are caused by severe flexion and may be seen in patients with inadequately placed lap belts or other forms of automotive retrain systems. These are commonly associated with both retroperitoneal and abdominal visceral injuries. Fracture dislocations in the thoracic spine are rare; however, due to the narrowness of the spinal canal in relation to the spinal cord, any fracture subluxation may potentially result in a neurological deficit. The indications for conservative vs. surgical management will depend on the patient's comorbidity and the grade of fracture instability. Except for the compression fractures, all the rest of the dorsal vertebral fractures usually will need specialized consultation and, most commonly, internal fixation.

Initial Assessment

One crucial element in patients suspected of suffering traumatic spine injuries is to avoid additional neurological damage during transport or manipulation, so it is essential to prevent further spinal movement. Conventionally, the use of primary cervical immobilization with stiff collars (C-collar) and a spinal board for the dorsal-lumbar spine is considered appropriate during rescue and transport. However, these devices, when applied to elderly patients with degenerative deformity, rigidity, and loss of elasticity, are not only poorly tolerated but may also cause additional injury by worsening fractures and even causing neurologic damage. Recent recommendations suggest the convenience of individual patient assessment, opting for soft padding and tape as a valid alternative to rigid hard C-collars in elderly patients with severe deformities. These simple measures will facilitate transfer while reducing the risk of additional neurologic injury or stiff collar-induced injury in an elderly deformed spine.

Spine Clearance

Cervical spine injury (CSI) clearance in elderly noncooperative patients is exceptionally challenging. The use of validated criteria to decide which patients do not require cervical spine imaging, such as the National Emergency X-Radiography Utilization Study or NEXUS (alert and stable, no neurological deficit, no altered level of consciousness, not intoxicated, no midline spinal tenderness, no distracting injuries) or the Canadian C-spine rule (CCR) are unreliable for patients over 65. Most authors advocate for maintaining a high index of suspicion, systematic examination to rule out midline tenderness, detailed focal neurological examination, and search for any sign of head-facial trauma. However, despite the lack of findings, most authors agree that cervical spine imaging is recommended in elderly trauma patients 65 years and older.

Imaging and Workup

The radiological diagnosis of cervical and thoracic spine injuries in the elderly is challenging due to degenerative arthritis that may affect both the vertebrae's anterior and posterior segments and the fixed deformities. These changes can frequently render the search for radiological landmarks in conventional plain X-ray imaging useless. However, a standard cervical radiographic series should include an anterior-posterior view, open mouth, and complete lateral projections. A swimmer's view should be included if the lateral view does not show the cervicothoracic junction. The dorsal spine series should consist of a complete anterior-posterior and lateral projection of the dorsal spine, including the dorsal-lumbar junction.

Additionally, conventional X-ray studies can provide some clues that suggest significant osteopenia. The typical finding in the osteoporotic spine is the "picture framing sign" produced by a highly demarcated vertebral body outline produced by radiolucency of the vertebral body. Other characteristics are the augmented biconcavity of the vertebral endplates and a protrusion of the intervertebral disk into the vertebral body.

Despite having a complete conventional X-ray series, it is not uncommon to miss cervical spine injuries in the geriatric population during routine radiographic imaging. The best approach for assessing this population's cervical and dorsal spine injuries is unknown. Computed tomography (CT) and MRI protocols are essential to rule out vertebral or spinal cord injuries in elderly patients with cranial, facial, or cervical trauma. Conventional indications for cervical CT scans in non-elderly patients include high-speed motor vehicle accidents, falls from heights, significant head trauma, neurological deficits, and multiple associated injuries. However, since in the elderly, even low-energy trauma can lead to severe injury, most consider good practice to perform CT scans routinely.

Indication for cervical MRI is suspected spinal cord injuries, SCIWORA, Central Cord Syndrome, or abnormal findings on CT scans. MRI is the most crucial imaging assessment tool for elderly patients with spine trauma and suspected spinal cord injury since it differentiates acute injury from degenerative changes. Findings of spinal cord edema, spinal cord hematomas, prevertebral hematomas, intervertebral disk blood collections, or disruption of spine ligaments are all possible using MRI. The use of midsagittal T1- and T2-weighted images is considered by many experts as one of the best methods to rule out spinal cord injury. In addition, MRI is highly effective in assessing hyperextension injuries with damage to the anterior longitudinal ligament and endplate fractures. It is also helpful in evaluating central cord hemorrhagic necrosis not detected by other imaging methods. However, one of the limitations of MRI is its lack of availability compared to CT scans more readily available, and its inability to distinguish between acute traumatic cord edema and spondylosis chronic cord compression.

Therapeutic Options

Therapeutic option for upper spine injuries in the elderly is different from the young and active population, the optimal treatment option remains controversial until today. There are three methods to treat these types of injuries: rigid cervical collar immobilization without fracture reduction, Halo-vest (HV) with progressive fracture reduction and surgical treatment. There is a lack of consensus when treating these types of injuries in the elderly, and an in-depth analysis of the patients' comorbidities, American Society of Anesthesiologist (ASA) grade, level of autonomy prior to the injury and life expectancy should be balanced when discussing treatment options. Controversies on different treatments option are common due to the elevated risk of surgical procedures in the elderly population versus the complications associated to prolonged cervical immobilization.

For those patients with relatively stable injuries and significant comorbidity or loss of autonomy the use of hard cervical collar is a non-rigid external immobilization method associated with low risk. This noninvasive method is usually well tolerated; however, it does have a high rate of non-union with the risk of fracture displacement. Despite the risk of non-union some authors consider that in the elderly population bony union is not always the objective, instead achieving a stable fibrous union could be suffice.

The Halo-vest is a rigid external immobilization device for non-operative management developed by Perry and Nickel for poliomyelitis patients and through the years it has suffered modifications in design and materials; today, it is used on several types of cervical fractures. It provides better immobilization than the rigid collar by means of a cranial pin halo ring and a thoracic jacket. It is considered by many experts as inadequate for upper cervical spine fractures in the elderly due to the high rate of morbidity and mortality.

Finally, surgical fixation could be the best option for a selected group of elderly patients with active lifestyles and few comorbidities, especially for D'Alonzo type II odontoid fractures and other unstable UCS fractures. Currently, there are several techniques for surgical stabilization of the fractured spine in the elderly. The surgical fixation can be accomplished by either an anterior or posterior approach. The first provides immediate spinal stability while preserving normal rotation range. Posterior approach arthrodesis is another method used in UCS injuries that consists of wiring, transarticular screws, and even C1 lateral mass and C2 pars interarticularis screws. However, posterior approach can drastically reduce cervical rotation and range of movement of the cervical spine. Since it has the lowest rate of non-union. However, when compared with cervical collar immobilization it has a higher rate of complications and mortality.

For thoracic spine fractures without neurologic injury with a reduction in the height of the anterior column < than 50% and a reduction of the spinal canal < than 30%, non-operative treatment can be considered a suitable option. When surgical fixation is required, there are several open treatment options. One of the most recent advances for spine surgical fixation, particularly for thoracolumbar fractures is the development of minimally invasive fixation techniques that offer a faster rehabilitation, lower amount of blood loss and less pain when compared with open techniques. The introduction of systems like the NForce allow percutaneous reduction and instrumentation by a posterior approach of thoracolumbar fractures.

References

1. Delcourt T, Bégué T, Saintyves G, Mebtouche N, Cottin P. Management of upper cervical spine fractures in elderly patients: current trends and outcomes. Injury. 2015;46(Suppl 1):S24–7. https://doi.org/10.1016/S0020-1383(15)70007-0.

2. Engelbart J, Zhou P, Johnson J, Lilienthal M, Zhou Y, Ten-Eyck P, et al. Geriatric clinical screening tool for cervical spine injury after ground-level falls. Emerg Med J. 2022;39(4):301–7. https://doi.org/10.1136/emermed-2020-210693.
3. Hoffman JR, Wolfson AB, Todd K, Mower WR. Selective cervical spine radiography in blunt trauma: methodology of the National Emergency X-radiography utilization study (NEXUS). Ann Emerg Med. 1998;32(4):461–9. https://doi.org/10.1016/s0196-0644(98)70176-3.
4. Cushing CH, Holmes JF, Tyler KR. Cervical spine injuries in older patients with falls found on magnetic resonance imaging after computed tomography. West J Emerg Med. 2021;22(5):1190–5. https://doi.org/10.5811/westjem.2021.5.51844.
5. Pagliei V, Bruno F, Battista G, Iacopino A, Riva C, Arrigoni F, et al. Cervical spine trauma: impact of different imaging classification systems in the clinical decision-making. Acta Biomed. 2021;92(S5):e2021404. https://doi.org/10.23750/abm.v92iS5.11877.
6. Roy-Camille R, Saillant G, Judet T, de Botton G, Michel G. Factors of severity in the fractures of the odontoid process (author's transl). Rev Chir Orthop Reparatrice Appar Mot. 1980;66:183–6.
7. Hadley MN, Browner CM, Liu SS, Sonntag VK. New sub-type of acute odontoid fractures (type IIA). Neurosurgery. 1988;22:67–71.
8. Jubert P, Lonjon G, Garreau de Loubresse C, Bone and Joint Trauma Study Group GETRAUM. Complications of upper cervical spine trauma in elderly subjects. A systematic review of the literature. Orthop Traumatol Surg Res. 2013;99(6 Suppl):S301–12. https://doi.org/10.1016/j.otsr.2013.07.007.
9. Anderson LD, D'Alonso RT. Fracture of the odontoid process of the atlas. J Bone Joint Surg Am. 1974;56:1663–74.
10. Macki M, Hamilton T, Pawloski J, Chang V. Occipital fixation techniques and complications. J Spine Surg. 2020;6(1):145–55. https://doi.org/10.21037/jss.2019.12.01.
11. Pal D, Sell P, Grevitt M. Type II odontoid fractures in the elderly: an evidence-based narrative review of management. Eur Spine J. 2011;20(2):195–204. https://doi.org/10.1007/s00586-010-1507-6.
12. Linhart C, Becker CA, Befrui N, Suero EM, Kussmaul AC, Böcker W, et al. A novel device for closed reduction and percutaneous fixation of thoracolumbar fractures. In Vivo. 2022;36(1):384–90. https://doi.org/10.21873/invivo.12715.
13. Stadhouder A, Buskens E, Vergroesen DA, Fidler MW, de Nies F, Oner FC. Nonoperative treatment of thoracic and lumbar spine fractures: a prospective randomized study of different treatment options. J Orthop Trauma. 2009;23(8):588–94. https://doi.org/10.1097/BOT.0b013e3181a18728.

Hollow Viscus Injury

18

Soledad Montón, Felipe Pareja, José Manuel Aranda, Ignacio Monzón, and José María Jover

Injury to the Stomach

Introduction

It is necessary to reinforce the idea that although trauma remains a leading cause of morbidity and mortality across all ages, geriatric patients differ significantly from their younger counterparts in their greater number of comorbidities, and higher risk of severe disability and death. After this little clarification, let us focus directly on the topic of concern.

Gastrointestinal system injuries that can affect the stomach, small intestine, colon, and rectum, like the rest of the organs of our anatomy, can be caused by two types of mechanism: blunt or penetrating trauma.

S. Montón
Hospital García Orcoyen, Estella, Navarra, Spain

F. Pareja
Hospital Universitario Virgen del Rocío, Sevilla, Spain

J. M. Aranda
Hospital Regional Universitario de Málaga, Málaga, Spain

I. Monzón
School of Medicine, University of Pretoria, Pretoria, South Africa

J. M. Jover (✉)
Hospital Universitario de Getafe, Madrid, Spain
e-mail: josemjover@aecirujanos.es

Injuries range from small ecchymosis in the organ wall, to complete necrosis from devascularization for blunt trauma, to perforation in penetrating trauma. Association with solid visceral injuries is frequent, which makes it more difficult at the time of diagnosis.

In this part of the chapter, we will review injuries that specifically affect the stomach.

Incidence

Most gastric injuries are caused by penetrating mechanism, of which 20% are by firearm and 10% by knife. Blunt trauma injuries are rarer. The East Coast American Association for the Surgery of Trauma (EAST) in its multicenter study, reports that the prevalence of gastric injury in blunt abdominal trauma was 0.06% and 2.1% of patients who presented hollow viscus injuries.

Degrees of Injury

The classification of the grades of injury of the different organs of the American Association for the Surgery of Trauma (Table 18.1) is the most widely used classification of traumatic injuries, including gastric injuries. Although injury management does not exactly correlate with grade, this classification provides a practical means of describing injury severity and can guide treat-

P. Petrone, C. E.M. Brathwaite (eds.), *Acute Care Surgery in Geriatric Patients*,
https://doi.org/10.1007/978-3-031-30651-8_18

Table 18.1 American Association for the Surgery of Trauma (AAST) for stomach injuries

Grade	Injury	Description
I	Hematoma	Intramural hematoma <3 cm Partial wall thickness laceration
II	Laceration	Laceration: <2 cm in gastroesophageal junction/pylorus <5 cm in proximal (one-third) <10 cm in distal (two-third)
III	Laceration	Laceration: >2 cm at gastroesophageal junction/pylorus >5 cm in proximal (one-third) >10 cm distal (two thirds)
IV	Vascular	Tissue loss/devascularization of < two-thirds of the stomach
V	Vascular	Tissue loss/devascularization of > two-thirds of the stomach

ment decisions regarding primary repair and/or the need for resection a part of the hollow viscera in particular.

Diagnosis

Like any traumatic patient, the initial evaluation, resuscitation, diagnosis, and treatment are carried out following the protocols of the Advanced Trauma Life Support (ATLS).

A patient with suspected hypotensive abdominal trauma or signs of peritonitis, or both, should be transferred immediately to the operating room. On the other hand, if the clinical situation allows it, a Focused Abdominal Sonography for Trauma (FAST) should be performed during the initial evaluation.

Although FAST is a good tool, in fact, it is the test of choice for the detection of free intra-abdominal fluid in a hemodynamically compromised trauma patient. The presence of free fluid is highly suggestive of blood, most of the time, and is an indication for urgent laparotomy. FAST is not sensitive enough to detect the presence of gastrointestinal injury unless there is a significant amount of fluid within the abdomen from damaged hollow viscus or blood from injury to the mesentery or solid viscus. Although, to tell the truth, the objective of FAST is only the detection of free fluid in the abdomen, without discerning whether it is blood or another fluid and its mission does not consist of the specific detection of lesions, neither hollow nor solid viscera.

Regarding penetrating trauma, FAST has a limited role in its initial evaluation, although it could be useful in decision-making in a trauma patient with more than one injured cavity.

On the other hand and more specifically related to the issue that concerns us, the great dilemma in cases of gastric injuries is the difficulty in making a preoperative diagnosis, which causes a delay in surgical treatment, which entails morbidity and mortality. Abdominal pain and signs of peritoneal irritation are the most frequent clinical findings. Other signs that we could also find on examination are abdominal wall ecchymosis and abdominal distention. However, these findings are not specific for gastrointestinal injury. It is important to reinforce that the absence of these signs considerably decreases the possibility of the presence of these gastrointestinal lesions. In addition, physical examination may be masked in a patient with a low level of consciousness for different reasons or due to the presence of other associated lesions in other nearby compartments such as the head, spine, chest or extremities, among others.

Although abdominal injury patterns are similar in older and younger adult trauma patients, diminished pain sensation and increased laxity of abdominal wall musculature make the abdominal examination less reliable in geriatric patients. Thus, early evaluation to detect intraperitoneal hemorrhage using ultrasound is important.

Within the diagnosis, there are no specific laboratory parameters for gastric lesions. An initial elevation of leukocytosis is relatively common in trauma patients due to the stress produced by the injury itself. In the mentioned EAST study, no statistically significant differences were found in the elevation of leukocytes between those patients who presented hollow viscus perforation versus those who did not. However, the progressive increase and persistence in the number of white blood cells in a patient with suspected abdominal trauma may be indicative of the development of an intra-abdominal injury.

One of the diagnostic challenges is to distinguish whether the injury is hollow or solid viscus, since it compromises the decision to perform a laparotomy or not, especially in patients without hemodynamic compromise.

For this reason, Computerized Tomography (CT) is the test of choice for the specific diagnosis of gastric lesions, like the rest of gastrointestinal lesions, in a situation of hemodynamic stability.

After closed abdominal trauma, CT has been shown to be very specific in ruling out injuries, especially in asymptomatic patients. The role of CT in penetrating trauma is less well defined. In addition, CT can be useful in differentiating patients who will require surgical exploration versus those who will be managed conservatively.

The signs that we could objectify find in the CT suggestive of gastric injury and could be extrapolated to any hollow viscus injury would be:

- Pneumoperitoneum (free or retroperitoneal)
- Mesenteric air
- Discontinuity in the gastric wall
- Extravasation of intravenous contrast
- Free intra-abdominal fluid in the absence of solid visceral injury
- Edema or bowel wall thickening
- Mesenteric hematoma or expansion of it

Observational studies report different results on the efficacy of CT scanning in the diagnosis of gastrointestinal injuries due to blunt trauma. Some said 100% accuracy in diagnosis compared to others who report that 20% of blunt gastrointestinal injuries can be missed by CT. Several authors have sought to identify.

The risk of contrast-induced nephropathy is higher in older adult patients, particularly in the presence of hypovolemia, chronic renal disease, or diabetes, and measurements should be taken to avoid this complication.

Contrary to blunt trauma, the accuracy of CT in penetrating trauma in the context of a hemodynamically stable situation without a clear indication for urgent surgical exploration has been studied less.

Another diagnostic tool that is essential to talk about is laparoscopy. The number of indications for the use of laparoscopy has been continuously expanding in recent years. At the same time, however, the diagnostic and therapeutic role of laparoscopy in the treatment of penetrating and blunt abdominal trauma remains controversial.

There is no doubt that laparoscopy has screening, diagnostic, and therapeutic functions above all, particularly when a diaphragmatic injury is suspected. It is extremely sensitive in determining the need for laparotomy, reducing the percentage of unnecessary laparotomies. In addition, it helps in the diagnosis of solid viscera injuries. However, the sensitivity in detecting hollow viscus injuries is low and less reliable.

Although there is still a debate about the optimal role of laparoscopy in the trauma setting, it may offer advantages over traditional exploratory laparotomy. Laparoscopy can play a very advantageous role in the diagnosis, especially of penetrating abdominal trauma in a group of selected patients, where the experience of the surgeon is a very important and essential factor. The development of specific guidelines and protocols may increase the value of laparoscopy in trauma, but this would require higher quality evidence.

Treatment

The absolute indications for emergency surgery in gastrointestinal injuries are:

Hemodynamic instability, diffuse abdominal pain and/or peritonitis on physical examination, or radiological findings of gastrointestinal perforation such as pneumoperitoneum, contrast leak, or organ wall ischemia.

It is important to take into account that older patients have reduced vital capacity with less profound tachycardic response to hemorrhage or pain, for example. The absence of an absolute tachycardia due to this blunted response may create a false sense of security. Systemic vascular resistance is increased, often contributing to baseline hypertension, which can lead to the misinterpretation of blood pressure readings following trauma when expected declines may not manifest despite the onset of shock. The effect of medications the patient takes regularly can further obscure the reading of vital sign measurements.

For that reason, it is essential to obtain early surgical consultation for known or suspected intra-abdominal injury because operative management of these gastrointestinal injuries may be preferable to non-operative management.

Patients with hemodynamic stability and abdominal trauma without peritonitis or clear radiological signs of gastric injury, non-operative conservative management can be performed. As an example, the presence of a gastric wall hematoma without contrast extravasation on CT can be treated conservatively as long as the presence of other associated injuries that require surgical treatment are ruled out.

Although still controversial, in recent years there has been an increase in the level of evidence supporting the non-operative management of penetrating abdominal injuries. A retrospective study of 792 patients without hemodynamic compromise and with gunshot wounds without signs of peritonism were managed conservatively by means of serial physical examinations plus repeated blood tests. Of all of them, 10% developed late symptoms that required laparotomy. The percentage of blank laparotomies was 14%. Complications attributed to delay in surgical indication were 0.3% with no increase in mortality. Although the duration of observation was individually tailored, the minimum observation time was 12 h for stab injuries and 24 h for firearm injuries.

Treatment with non-operative selective observation consists of serial physical examinations of the abdomen every 1 or 2 h by the same medical team, accompanied by analytical determinations (monitoring of leukocytes) and repeat CT if necessary. Any change in the examination such as abdominal pain, peritoneal irritation, or hemodynamic compromise will require a change in therapeutic approach.

Patients with associated traumatic brain injury or spinal cord injury who have an impaired level of consciousness are not candidates for conservative management.

Surgical treatment of gastric injuries is largely conditioned by the degree of injury, which defines the type of injury (hematoma or laceration), their extent and location, as well as the presence of associated injuries. Aboobakar et al. suggest a practical algorithm depending on the type of injury (Fig. 18.1). Depending on the grade of injury:

Grade I to III: They are the majority of gastric injuries and can be repaired with primary suture in a single line of suture or two; that second line of suture is recommended to reinforce hemostasis if necessary since the stomach is a widely vascularized organ.

Grade IV: (tissue loss or devascularization of less than 50% of the stomach) to **V** (tissue loss or devascularization of more than 50% of the stomach): these are much less frequent injuries, they are usually associated with other abdominal injuries, in addition to a high mortality. Due to the extent of the damage in grades IV and V, primary repair of them is not feasible. Depending on the location of the affected tissue, proximal or distal, and the extent of the devascularized tissue, a partial or total gastrectomy will be necessary.

When considering the reconstruction of intestinal transit after gastric resection, the type of reconstruction (gastroduodenostomy, gastrojejunostomy, or Roux-en-Y) will be conditioned by the type of associated injury (duodenum, bile duct, and pancreas).

Once inside the abdomen, it is important to be systematic in the examination of each abdominal organ, hence when we face the stomach, we must explore its anterior and posterior sides, looking for hematomas or lacerations. To access the posterior surface, it is necessary to open the lesser sac. Ligating a few of the short vessels allows a better exposure, especially of the gastric fundus and the gastroesophageal junction on its posterior face. Small perforations can be identified by injecting air or methylene blue through a nasogastric tube. A wound near or over the pylorus should be repaired transversally, in the same way as when a pyloroplasty is performed, to maintain a wide gastric outlet.

Regarding the placement of drains, the data in the literature are limited when referring to

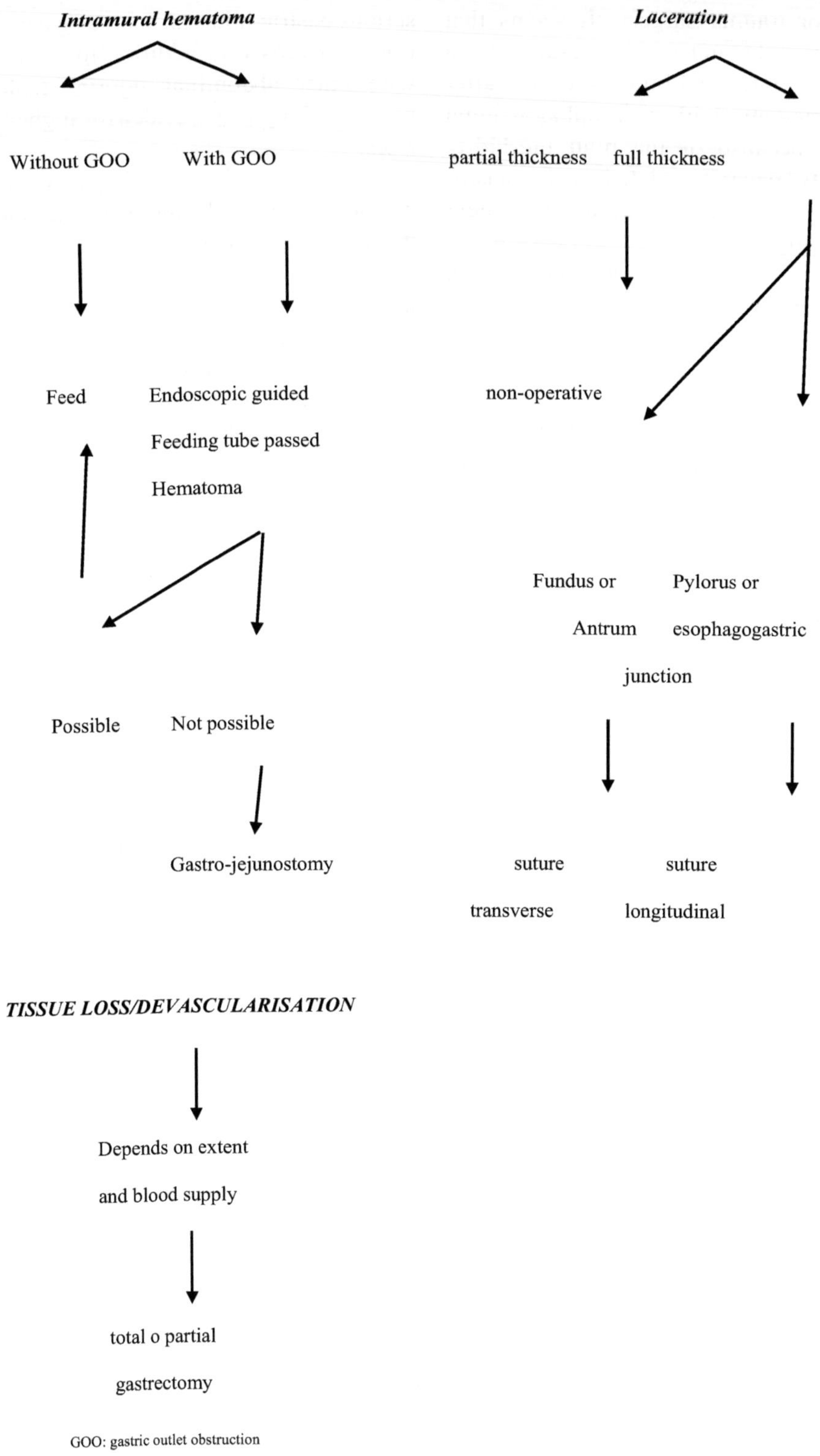

Fig. 18.1 Algorithm for gastric injuries based on the degree of injury

emergency or trauma surgery. It seems that most authors prefer not to leave drains when repairing gastrointestinal injuries, except after a total gastrectomy, with an esophagojejunal anastomosis because of the high morbidity and mortality rates associated with anastomotic leak. They recommend its placement prophylactically.

An injury at the gastroesophageal junction should be repaired in one or two layers over a nasogastric tube with closed-suction drainage and consideration of a fundoplication to buttress the repair.

Again, the role of laparoscopy in the treatment of gastrointestinal injuries is controversial. Although laparoscopy is an effective and safe diagnostic and therapeutic tool in elective surgery, it is less used in trauma surgery. An important role in the evaluation in hemodynamically stable patients with penetrating injuries to evaluate peritoneal penetration, but at the same time it has also been used to evaluate gastrointestinal injuries by blunt mechanism. Once the laparoscopic procedure has begun, the ability to also repair the injuries will depend on the experience of the surgeon and his or her ability to perform the same exhaustive exploration of the abdominal cavity as would be done in open procedures. This maneuvers in laparoscopic surgery requires much more experience and skill.

Complications

After repair of gastrointestinal injuries, in general, the incidence of complications ranges between 22 and 29%. Among the frequent systemic complications would be pneumonia, sepsis, renal dysfunction, and thromboembolism. Among the specific complications of the repair, infections dominate and would be surgical wound infection, intra-abdominal abscess (24%), suture dehiscence, among others.

Mortality rates of patients who have suffered a gastric rupture ranges from 28 to 66%. The highest mortality is related to very severe injury mechanisms that have been necessary to cause serious gastric injuries, such as gastric perforation or necrosis, in addition to the association with other abdominal injuries (spleen, diaphragm, lung), or evidence higher severity rates.

The challenge in gastric injuries is its prompt diagnosis and timely intervention, conditioning the prognosis of these patients and greatly limiting mortality and morbidity associated to these injuries.

According to trauma patient management protocols, gastrointestinal injuries should be evaluated and repaired following a systematic method, where bleeding control should be the first priority to minimize fluid requirements and the need for transfusion, followed by the control of contamination produced by gastrointestinal lesions.

Injury to the Small Bowel and Mesentery

Introduction

The management of these injuries is a clinical challenge mainly due to their relative infrequency, uncertain diagnosis and deleterious consequences when not promptly treated. The care of elderly patients with trauma represents a unique set of challenges. In geriatric patients, the combination of comorbid health conditions, prescribed medications, and frailty makes them more vulnerable to trauma and subsequent complications, including infections, pneumonia, venous thromboembolism, and multisystem organ failure. Patients 65 year-old and older are twice as likely to die compared with younger patients with similar injury severity score (ISS). Studies suggest that mortality increases 6.8% for every year beyond age 65 years. Elderly patients are undertriaged a significant portion of the time and are more likely to go to a non-trauma center than younger patients. It is recommended that any patient older than 70 years with trauma should be transported to a trauma center regardless of their ISS.

Table 18.2 American Association for the Surgery of Trauma (AAST) for small bowel injuries

Grade	Injury	Description
I	Hematoma	Contusion or hematoma without revascularization
	Laceration	Partial, without perforation
II	Laceration	Laceración <50% of the circumference
III	Laceration	Laceración >50% of the circumference without transect
IV	Laceration	Small intestine transection
V	Laceration	Small intestine transection with tissue loss
	Vascular	Devascularized segment

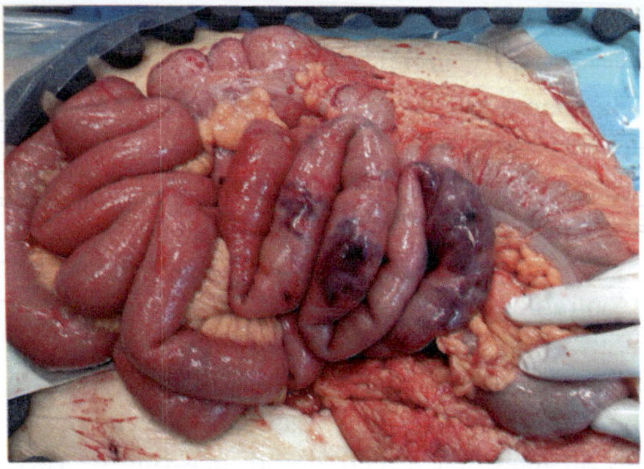

Fig. 18.2 Grade I hematoma (Photo courtesy of Felipe Pareja)

Incidence

Small bowel and mesenteric traumatic injuries are uncommon, with a prevalence of approximately 1% in blunt trauma and 17% in penetrating trauma.

Degrees of Injury

The most used classification to evaluate these injuries is that of the AAST that establishes 5° of injury that will help us with decision-making (Table 18.2). The key is to differentiate the most destructive injuries from the non-destructive ones (Fig. 18.2), in order to decide on a primary repair, primary anastomosis, damage control with delayed anastomosis or jejunostomy/ileostomy.

Diagnosis

The initial evaluation of elderly patients following major trauma should be based on ATLS protocols and the priorities of treatment are the same irrespective of the age of the patient. Immediate recognition and management of life-threatening injuries is essential. History and physical examination should be obtained, focusing on mechanism of injury, presence of (uncontrolled) comorbidities, and the chronic use of drugs that may influence the normal response to trauma (beta blockers, anticoagulation, etc.).

In hemodynamically compensated patients with no peritonitis or abdominal tenderness with a tangential injury and clear CT evidence of no intra-abdominal injury is possible a non-operatory management (NOM), but CT is inferior to clinical examination to detect the need for surgical intervention. The specificity and sensitivity for bowel injury through clinical examination is 99% and 100%, respectively, as compared to 84% and 31% with CT.

In the setting of abdominal trauma with or without solid organ injury, intestinal injuries are often omitted, so a high index of suspicion is required since the delay in the diagnosis of intestinal injury is related to increased morbidity and mortality. A lower limit should be used for surgical exploration in the elderly in both penetrating and blunt trauma, and occasionally in hemodynamically stable patients the use of laparoscopy may be useful, but with low conversion threshold. Management of small bowel injuries should aim to restore intestinal transit and prevent intestinal failure. Small bowel continuity is preferable to diversion; however, the occurrence of an anastomotic leak in trauma patients is associated with a sharp increase in mortality (46% versus 1%) in patients with or without an anastomotic leak, respectively.

Treatment

The management of these injuries does not differ in the elderly patient, except for needing a higher degree of suspicion and not delaying the definitive treatment of them. Bowel injuries should be managed by primary repair, when feasible. Contraindications include destructive injuries with >50% disruption of the bowel circumference, and mesenteric devascularization with bowel ischemia. In these cases, it is necessary to do an intestinal resection and anastomosis (primary or delayed after damage control surgery). It is very important to avoid massive resections and preserve as much of the well-vascularized intestine as possible, and if a jejunostomy or ileostomy is necessary, a distal mucosal fistula should be performed to allow distal feeding for future reconstruction. In patients undergoing damage control, if restoration of transit within 48 h is not possible, it is preferable to perform a jejunostomy/ileostomy instead of delaying it for a longer time.

Regarding to the performance of anastomosis, it is necessary to take into account that not only local factors but also others such as the presence of significant peritonitis, intestinal edema, use of vasopressors, need for massive transfusion, significant comorbidity, and associated injuries. There is no evidence showing the superiority of any anastomotic technique after bowel resection in trauma, so the use of mechanical sutures or manual sutures must be individualized based on local conditions and surgeon experience.

In the context of trauma, both primary repair and small bowel anastomosis (primary and after damage control) have a better prognosis in the general population, and in the elderly, than colon anastomosis. Anastomotic leak rate is around 3%, so the patient's prognosis will be more influenced by the severity of the trauma and the comorbidity than the anastomotic failure. Although reliable data are not yet available, the use of indocyanine green in the trauma setting could be useful in evaluating intestinal vascularization, especially in patients with severe injuries, as it may improve the prognosis of the anastomosis and limit the length of the intestinal resections.

Injuries to the Large Intestine

Introduction

Colon trauma in elderly patients (65 years and older) is particularly important. Older patients have reduced physiological reserves affecting all organ systems and comorbidities that makes them more susceptible to complications and increased mortality. The physiological decline of age and the use of chronic medication significantly influence the response to injury and the outcome of these patients.

Blunt trauma mechanisms are the most common causes of injury in the elderly (falls and motor vehicle crashes), however reports have shown that penetrating injuries cause up to 50% of deaths in older victims of assault. Abuse and neglect are also responsible for repeated trauma in the elderly.

The management of colonic trauma has evolved over the past 150 years. Colonic trauma has transformed from a near-absolute death sentence to a commonly survivable injury due to advances in surgical technique, antimicrobial therapy, and critical care. Much has been learned from military and civilian practice that is applicable to the management of colonic trauma today. However, discrepancy still exists concerning the best modality of treatment when managing colonic injuries. Major concerns are the potential for anastomosis failure, the development of intestinal fistulae and intra-abdominal abscesses following trauma, with the associated risks of high mortality and long hospital stay. There are no age-specific protocols for the management of colonic trauma.

Incidence

Elderly patients have a preponderance for blunt mechanisms of injury. The incidence of hollow viscera injury in this population group is small compared to younger patients, but the risk of mortality is increased.

Colonic trauma can be secondary to penetrating or blunt trauma. Penetrating injuries are by far the most common, comprising over 98% of cases, affecting any part of the colon. Blunt colonic injuries, occurring in about 5% of cases, are secondary to rapid decelerating injuries; these can affect any area but are more common in the transverse and sigmoid colon due to their relative mobility. Irrespective of mechanism, large intestine injuries combined rupture and perforation of the organ wall with significant mesenteric lacerations resulting in ischemic segments and spillage of colonic content. Severe associated intra- and extra-abdominal injuries are present in many of these patients, in many cases determining the outcome following trauma.

In older patients, the diminished ability to mount a response following trauma and the potential for altered level of consciousness makes the physical examination of the abdomen difficult. Low Glasgow Coma Score and hypotension on admission are markers of poor outcome in this population group.

Degrees of Injury

A commonly used classification of colonic injuries is the one proposed by the AAST-OIS. This classification comprises five incremental grades of severity of injury that help in the decision-making regarding treatment. However, a better distinction should be established between non-destructive and destructive colonic injuries, in the authors' opinion this allows a more accurate way of deciding whether to perform a primary anastomotic repair or exteriorize a colostomy following resection of the affected segment. Destructive colonic injuries are more commonly associated with gunshot wounds.

Destructive colonic injuries are described as:

- Laceration affecting more than 50% of the colonic wall circumference (AAST Grade III)
- Injuries with complete colonic transection (AAST Grade IV)
- Injuries with associated mesenteric laceration causing devascularized segments

Diagnosis

The initial evaluation of elderly patients following major trauma should be based on ATLS protocols. The priorities of treatment are the same irrespective of the age of the patient. Immediate recognition and management of life-threatening injuries is essential. History and physical examination should be obtained, focusing on mechanism of injury, presence of (uncontrolled) comorbidities, and the chronic use of drugs that may influence the normal response to trauma (beta blockers, anticoagulation, etc.). Rapid identification of life-threatening bleeding and/or need for immediate surgical intervention using risk stratification parameters based on mechanism of injury, presenting physiology, signs and symptoms and the anatomical location of the injury should be the main priority.

Most colonic injuries are easily diagnosed during laparotomy performed for hemodynamic instability or peritonitis. A diagnostic problem arises in patients with a significant mechanism of injury, hemodynamic stability and no signs of peritonitis in whom non-operative management is being considered but have suspicious CT findings.

There are no investigations that are sensitive and specific enough to diagnose a colonic trauma. Penetrating injuries in the vicinity of the colon with normal hemodynamic status and no indication for emergency surgery should be managed using a combination of repeated physical examination, imaging with contrast-enhanced CT scanning. Surgery, including laparoscopic evaluation, should be the default position when diagnostic doubt exists. The same should apply to those patients with blunt trauma.

CT evaluation in hemodynamically normal ("stable") patients with blunt or penetrating abdominal trauma may find indirect signs of a potential bowel or colonic injury; a CT scoring proposed by Faget and colleagues for blunt trauma is recommended by the World Society of Emergency Surgery (WSES) to be used in these patients, the score indicates the need for surgical exploration if 5 or more points are present (Table 18.3).

Table 18.3 CT scoring system recommended by WSES

CT sign	Score
Hemoperitoneum, small	1
Hemoperitoneum, abundant	3
Mesenteric pneumo-peritoneum	5
Bowell wall thickness	2
Arterial mesenteric vessel (contrast) extravasation	3
Mesenteric (fatty) stranding	2
Reduced bowel wall enhancement	1
Bowel wall discontinuity	5
Splenic injury	1
Abdominal wall injury (i.e., seat belt sign)	2

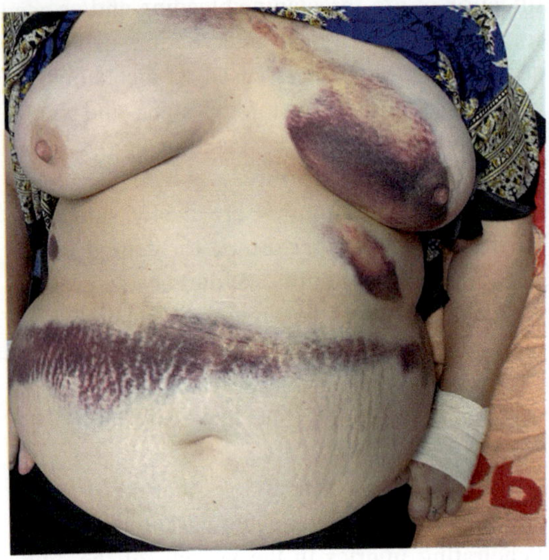

Fig. 18.3 Seat belt sign (Photo courtesy of Ignacio Monzón)

Often, penetrating trauma victims will require an emergency laparotomy, making the diagnosis of colonic trauma relatively easy. In general, patients with a seat belt sign (Fig. 18.3) and those with free peritoneal fluid seen on CT without a "solid" organ injury, raising suspicion of mesenteric or colonic trauma, as well as small intestine and urinary bladder, should be considered for immediate abdominal exploration (laparotomy or laparoscopy), instead of a passive attitude involving clinical observation and further investigations that may lead to delayed institution of treatment with the development of significant complications and mortality.

Recommendations such as performing diagnostic peritoneal lavage, serial abdominal examination, measurement of serum amylase and inflammatory markers as indicators of bowel injury remain nonspecific for the diagnosis of hollow viscera injury and could potentially delay appropriate surgical treatment.

Treatment

The definitive treatment for colonic trauma is surgery. However, there is no agreement as to what constitute the best modality of treatment for civilian colonic trauma; multiple reports have stressed the fact that civilian practice encounter less significant colonic injuries, thus a less aggressive approach using primary repair should be considered, this approach is believed to prevent the complications and risk of a colostomy. The choice of surgical intervention should aim at preventing anastomotic failure, enteric fistula formation, and development of intra-abdominal abscesses.

Historically, the surgical treatment of colonic trauma has been performed using three distinct techniques: primary repair, which may include direct repair of minor injuries or resection and primary anastomosis; exteriorization of a repaired segment without colostomy; and fecal diversion, such as loop colostomy, Hartmann's colostomy, or end colostomy with mucous fistula with delayed reconstruction.

Exteriorizing repaired segments was popular during the 1970s and 1980s but was abandoned as it offered very little in terms of prevention of suture line leakage and fistula formation. Nowadays, the management consists of either primary repair or diversion; the choice between one or the other is based in several important predictors of complications.

The most important predictors for diversion are the hemodynamic and physiological status on arrival and the presence of a destructive colonic injury. Patients presenting in shock with acidosis, hypothermia, and ongoing coagulopathy and those with a destructive injury should be managed using damage control surgery principles. During the abbreviated surgery, these patients should be offered immediate bleeding and fecal contamination control; the latter is usually accomplished by resecting the affected colonic segment and performing a delayed primary repair or a diversion once physiology and coagulopathy are restored ("clip and drop" principle). Attempting a primary anastomosis in these conditions is simply doomed to failure. In patients who have been shot, irrespective of the choice of colonic repair, the missile tract should be laid open, debrided, profusely washed, and drained to prevent necrotizing soft-tissue sepsis.

Other factors to be considered when choosing between primary repair and diversion are:

- Delayed presentation of injury (>6 h) with significant fecal contamination or established sepsis.
- Presence of bowel edema.
- Ongoing use of vasopressor therapy.
- Need for massive transfusion.
- Presence of uncontrolled comorbidities, especially cardiac, renal, or hepatic.
- High Injury Severity Score (ISS).
- Presence of severe associated injuries (solid organ injury, Traumatic Brain Injury).
- Location of colonic injury (left sided are considered at higher risk).
- Injuries secondary to gunshot wounds.

An effort should be made to develop and institute local protocols and management algorithms with clear recommendations for intervention. Recent reports have found that primary repair of colon offers similar results when compared to diversion for colonic trauma.

Complications

Management using designated algorithms seem to reduce the rate of complications and mortality, but most trauma centers do not have a defined protocol for the management of colonic trauma.

Following colonic trauma, the overall incidence of intra-abdominal complications can be as high as 30%; abscess formation occurs in nearly 15% of cases, and enteric fistula in about 8%, anastomotic failure occurs in about 40% of cases in whom a massive transfusion is administered and uncontrolled comorbidities are present and nearly always if a patient had a primary repair in the presence of shock and a destructive colonic trauma.

Intra-abdominal abscess is common in patients with significant fecal contamination and those in whom a single antimicrobial agent is used as prophylaxis; however, several reports have failed to find an association between abscess formation and anastomotic failure. Superficial surgical site infection (wound sepsis) is the most common complication following surgery for colonic injury, occurring in up to 50% of patients. Stoma complications including necrosis, obstruction and para-stomal hernia are seen in 14% of cases, nearly all require surgical correction. A commonly missed source of complication is the missile or blade tract, debris form colonic injuries contaminating the wound tract could lead to severe necrotizing soft-tissue infections.

Early mortality is related to exsanguination from associated injuries; late colon-related mortality ranges from 1 to 4% resulting from severe sepsis and organ failure. Mortality is more common in patients with diversion, possibly reflecting the severity of the injury rather than the colostomy itself.

Colonic trauma in the elderly is not frequent, the evaluation to exclude these injuries and the management should follow the same principles used in a younger patient. Special attention should be paid to those patients who are "stable" but have free abdominal fluid seen on CT that cannot be explained. The default approach in these cases should be based in a high index of suspicion of mesenteric and hollow organ injury and aggressive abdominal exploration using laparoscopy or laparotomy to identify and repair a possible colonic injury. Choosing between primary repair and diversion will depend on the hemodynamic status, degree of physiological deterioration, and the type of colonic injury present.

Rectal Trauma

Introduction

After a prohibitive high mortality rate was communicated from the US Civil War with expectant management of rectal injuries, in later military conflicts surgery was the rule and several techniques were described for the treatment of rectal trauma: fecal diversion in World Wars I and II, presacral drainage in Korea and distal rectal washout in Vietnam. This is how the dogma of the "four Ds" (debridement, diversion, drainage, and distal washout) was defined for the treatment of rectal injuries, which became the standard of surgical care. However, even when important key concepts may be extracted from military knowledge of trauma injuries, clear differences may be established between military and civilian environments, and modern literature has shown that not all the pillars from the four Ds have to be always indicated and performed. Modern wartimes have also introduced the damage control surgery philosophy that may be of course applied for rectal injuries.

Incidence

Fortunately, incidence of rectal trauma is low, 1–3% in civilian field, and 5% has been established for military environment from modern wartime data. However, mortality and morbidity remain between 3–10% and 18–21%, respectively. Most of them are derived from gunshot wounds, and frequency of rectal injuries from stab wounds or blunt trauma are only up to 15%. Due to the proximity of pelvic organs and a prolific blood supply, isolated rectal trauma is rarely seen.

Degrees of Injury

Flint et al. published the Colon Injury Score, defining three groups with increasing severity based on the type of injury, grade of contamination, the presence or absence of associated injuries, the hemodynamic status, and the interval to definitive treatment. Later on, Moore et al. defined the Organ Injury Scale for visceral and hollow viscus trauma, including the rectum (Table 18.4). Based on these two classifications, several authors have tried to define different criteria to classify rectal injuries into two different groups with different surgical approaches: destructive and non-destructive. Even when these criteria are not universal and a definitive consensus has not been reached, these variables must be considered when deciding for a conservative or a more aggressive surgical approach for the management of a rectal injury. Location is another important aspect to decide surgical approach for rectal trauma. Extraperitoneal rectum includes lower one-third and posterior upper two-thirds,

Table 18.4 Classification of rectal trauma

CIS					
Grade	Injury	Contamination	Associated injuries	Hemodynamic status	Interval
I	Contusion, partial laceration	Minimal	No	Stable	<6 h
II	Full-thickness perforation	Moderate	Yes	Unstable	6–12 h
III	Tissular loss	Severe	Yes	Shock	>12 h

AAST-OIS		
Grade	Injury	Description
I	Hematoma	Contusion or hematoma without devascularization
	Laceration	Partial-thickness laceration
II	Laceration	Laceration <50% circumference
III	Laceration	Laceration ≥50% circumference
IV	Laceration	Full-thickness laceration with extension into the perineum
V	Vascular	Devascularized segment

CIS colon injury score, *AAST* American Association for the Surgery of Trauma, *OIS* organ injury scale meanwhile only anterior and lateral upper two-thirds are intraperitoneal.

Diagnosis

Due to the deep location within the pelvis, surgeon's level of suspicion must be high for rectal trauma concerning certain mechanisms of injury, especially high-velocity pelvic trauma, transpelvic gunshot wounds or impaled patients. Digital rectal examination must be the initial exploration, and it must be performed after an exhaustive initial assessment of the trauma patient. The presence of gross blood, a clear defect in the rectal wall and the presence of bony fragments may be detected, and the anal sphincter tone may be evaluated. After this, while hemodynamic instability indicates that a suspected rectal injury must be evaluated in the operating room, stable trauma patients must undergo a CT scan and a proctoscopy. A pararectal wound tract, extravasation of contrast, a rectal wall defect, extraluminal free air, rectal wall thickening or perirectal fat stranding are radiological signs of rectal injury. Rectal contrast may be used to improve CT accuracy but it must be taken into account that there is no clear evidence for a definitive recommendation and may not evaluate adequately distal third of the rectum due to occlusion of the device's balloon. Sensitivity of proctoscopy determining size and extent of the rectal injury is high especially for extraperitoneal area though it may be decreased by the lack of bowel preparation or the presence of associated injuries, more frequently when performed at the trauma bay. If doubts concerning intraperitoneal injury exist, exploratory and even therapeutic laparoscopy may be indicated.

Treatment

These general principles must be followed when considering surgical management of rectal trauma:

- Isolated rectal trauma is rare, so patients with a suspected injury must be correctly evaluated with an initial general assessment according to the ATLS principles.
- Unstable patients must be evaluated in the operating room, and damage control surgery principles must be accomplished with bleeding and contamination control to differ definitive surgical treatment until the physiological status of the trauma patient has been improved.
- Even when principles of the four Ds continue being adequate for military environment, in the civilian setting is not always necessary to use all of them. Several criteria have to be included as part of the algorithm for the treatment of the rectal injury, as patient characteristics, mechanism, interval, type of the lesion, grade of contamination, location, and associated injuries.
- Generally, it may be considered that intraperitoneal rectal injuries may be treated as if they were colonic. Non-destructive injuries may be securely sutured while destructive ones must be resected. Anastomosis may be performed most of the times, immediately in stable patients or in definitive surgery if damage control was applied because of hemodynamic instability. Diversion, terminal or proximal, must be only indicated in the presence of gross contamination or high transfusion requirements.
- For extraperitoneal rectal injuries, several studies have shown that systematic use of diversion, presacral drainage and distal rectal washout confers no benefit. Far from this, morbidity of ostomies by themselves or during surgical reversal and associated potential dissemination of pelvic contamination by opening presacral space or by performing a washout may worsen results of a more conservative surgical approach of extraperitoneal rectal trauma. So, these techniques must be only recommended in severe and destructive rectal injuries with large soft-tissue defects and/or involving the bony pelvis given the concern for open fractures and pelvic sepsis. Primary repair of extraperitoneal injuries constitutes a choice only if accessible transanally and possible to perform without mobilizing additional surgical planes; otherwise, it must be left open as spontaneous healing is going to

be the rule. Transanal minimally invasive surgery (TAMIS) and endoscopic clips has been successfully used for closing rectal defects.

– Sphincter repair of anal injuries must be only faced if an adequate knowledge of these particular surgical techniques is warranted. Otherwise, definitive repair must be delayed until an experienced surgeon is available. Proximal diversion must be considered only if dealing with a severely destructive anal injury.

The United States National Trauma Data Bank published data related with rectal trauma injuries over a 2-year period, concerning injuries, surgical management, and outcomes. On a multivariate regression analysis, older age was associated with a higher rate of mortality together with other factors, while stoma formation was associated with a lower mortality rate when considering especially intraperitoneal or combined injuries. Conclusion from this must be that a low threshold must be defined to perform a diversion when considering rectal trauma in the elderly, as there is only a very narrow margin with this special population, and associated trauma morbidity must be minimized to ensure satisfactory clinical response.

References

1. Bruscagin V, Coimbra R, Rasslan S, Abrantes WL, Souza H, Neto G, Dalcin RR, Drumond RJR. Blunt gastric injury. A multicentre experience. Injury. 2001;32:761.
2. Hefny AF, Kunhivalappil FT, Matev N, Ávila N, Bashir MO, Abu-Zidan FM. Usefulness of free intraperitoneal air detected by CT in diagnosing bowel perforation in blunt trauma: experience from a community-based hospital. Injury. 2015;46:100.
3. Beltzer C, Bachmann R, Strohaker J, Axt S, Schmidt R, Kuper M, Königsrainer A. Value of laparoscopy in blunt trauma and penetrating abdominal trauma a systematic review. Chirurg. 2020;91(7):567–75.
4. Aboobakar MR, Singh JP, Maharaj K, Mewa KS. Gastric perforation following blunt abdominal trauma. Trauma Case Rep. 2017;10:12–5.
5. Velmahos G, Vasiliu P, Demetriades D, Chan L, Murray J, Salim A, Sava J, Katkhouda N, Berne T. Wound management after colon injury: open or closed? A prospective randomized trial. Am Surg. 2002;68:795.
6. Lin HF, Chen YD, Lin KL, Wu MC, Wu CY, Chen SC. Laparoscopy decreases the laparotomy rate form hemodynamically stable patients with blunt hollow viscus and mesenteric injuries. Am J Surg. 2015;210:326.
7. Bonomi AM, Granieri S, Gupta S, Altomare M, Cioffi SP, Sammartano F, Cimbanassi S, Chiara O. Traumatic hollow viscus and mesenteric injury: role of CT and potential diagnostic–therapeutic algorithm. Updat Surg. 2021;73(2):703–10.
8. Zafar SN, Shah AA, Zogg CK, et al. Morbidity or mortality? Variations in trauma centres in the rescue of older injured patients. Injury. 2016;47(5):1091–7.
9. Smyth L, Bendinelli C, Lee N, et al. WSES guidelines on blunt and penetrating bowel injury: diagnosis, investigations, and treatment. World J Emerg Surg. 2022;17(1):13.
10. Sharpe JP, Magnotti LJ, Fabian TC, Croce MA. Evolution of the operative management of colon trauma. Trauma Acute Care Surg Open. 2017;2:1–7. https://doi.org/10.1136/tsaco-2017-000092.
11. Zheng YX, Chen L, Tao SF, Song P, Xu SM. Diagnosis and management of colonic injuries following blunt trauma. World J Gastroenterol. 2007;13(4):633–6. https://doi.org/10.3748/wjg.v13.i4.633.
12. Cullinane DC, Jawa RS, Como LL, et al. Management of penetrating colonic injuries: a meta-analysis and practice management guideline from the Eastern Association for the Surgery of trauma. J Trauma Acute Care. 2019;86(3):505–15. https://doi.org/10.1097/TA.0000000000002146.
13. Gash KJ, Suradkar K, Kiran RP. Rectal trauma injuries: outcomes from the US national trauma data Bank. Tech Coloproctol. 2018;22:847–55. https://doi.org/10.1007/s10151-018-1856-4.
14. Biffl WL, Moore EE, Feliciano DV, Albrecht RM, Croce MA, Karmy-Jones R, et al. Management of colorectal injuries: a Western trauma association critical decisions algorithm. J Trauma Acute Care Surg. 2018;85(5):1016–20. https://doi.org/10.1097/TA.0000000000001929.
15. Clemens MS, Peace KM, Yi F. Rectal trauma: evidence-based practices. Clin Colon Rectal Surg. 2018;31:17–23. https://doi.org/10.1055/s-0037-1602182.

Management of Pancreatic Trauma

19

Kemp Anderson, Areg Grigorian, and Kenji Inaba

Introduction

The pancreas is a complicated organ with its anatomic structure, location, and function presenting unique challenges to the trauma care provider. Given the old surgical adage that strongly warns against interfering with the pancreas, this view has likely been held by surgeons for generations, and much of that apprehension remains today. This can be particularly true in the trauma setting where pancreatic injuries are infrequently encountered with most historical studies suggesting that pancreatic injuries occur less than 5% of trauma patients with a recent NTDB study suggesting that pancreatic injuries are present in less than 1% of trauma admissions. Furthermore, most of these studies reflect the incidence of this injury at large Level 1 trauma centers. At smaller, lower volume centers obtaining and maintaining sufficient experience in the management of these injuries becomes increasingly difficult. When broken down between penetrating and blunt trauma, each category likely accounts for between 39–44% and 56–61%, respectively. Reported mortality for penetrating and blunt injuries varies from 8–27% to 5–18%, respectively. Patients 65 years and older account for about 7% of pancreatic injuries with the majority of those being from blunt mechanisms.

From an overall outcome standpoint, it is difficult to accurately parse out the contribution of pancreatic injury as these are almost always accompanied by injuries to other organ systems. Common mechanisms of blunt pancreatic injury are motor-vehicle and motorcycle collisions, falls from height, assaults with abdominal impact, and bicycle crashes.

Anatomy

Anatomically, the pancreas lies deep within the retroperitoneum, buttressed on all sides. The pancreas is encapsulated by mesothelium and has a smooth, lobulated surface. It is most commonly divided into four anatomical sections: head, neck, body, and tail. The superior mesenteric artery (SMA) and superior mesenteric vein (SMV) run posterior to the neck of the pancreas, and much of what is described in the surgical management of trauma patients references the anatomical location of injury relative to these vessels.

The pancreas provides a combination of both exocrine and endocrine function. By mass, exocrine tissue makes up the majority of pancreatic parenchyma. The exocrine component secretes between 500 and 800 mL/day of iso-osmotic pancreatic fluid. This fluid contains amylases,

K. Anderson · A. Grigorian · K. Inaba (✉)
Division of Trauma and Surgical Critical Care, Department of Surgery, LAC+USC Medical Center, University of Southern California, Los Angeles, CA, USA
e-mail: Kenji.Inaba@med.usc.edu

P. Petrone, C. E.M. Brathwaite (eds.), *Acute Care Surgery in Geriatric Patients*,
https://doi.org/10.1007/978-3-031-30651-8_19

proteases, and lipases. While amylases are secreted in their active form, proteases and lipases are secreted as inactive precursors, relying upon contact with duodenal secreted enterokinase for activation of trypsinogen to trypsin. In turn, trypsin auto-activates the precursor enzymes for all pancreatic proteases and lipases. With pancreatic injury, these enzymes can become auto-activated within the pancreas, which in turn yields the destructive feed-forward loop of auto-digestion. The endocrine component is contained within islets of Langerhans, and several distinct cellular sub-types are responsible for secretion of glucagon, insulin, somatostatin, ghrelin, and pancreatic polypeptide. Damage to pancreatic endocrine function can lead to dysregulation of hormones, and particular attention must be paid to blood sugar.

The main pancreatic duct, also called the duct of Wirsung, lies centrally within the parenchyma, usually equi-distant from the superior and inferior borders of the gland. The main pancreatic duct joins with the common bile duct (CBD) and empties into the duodenum via the major papilla called the ampulla of Vater. The accessory duct of Santorini has some variability in location of drainage and function based upon its embryologic movement. Most commonly, the accessory duct drains a small portion of the pancreatic outflow and also empties into the duodenum. When present, the lesser papilla is found in close proximity to the ampulla of Vater.

The pancreatic blood supply is derived from both the celiac axis and the SMA, yielding significant collateral flow that is protective against ischemic damage to the organ. The splenic artery comes off the celiac axis and perfuses the body and tail via a number of branches, most prominently the dorsal pancreatic artery. The dorsal pancreatic artery has a left branch that feeds the tail and a right branch that feeds the body, eventually anastomosing with the blood supply to the head. The head is perfused by the anterior and posterior superior pancreaticoduodenal arteries, both arising from the gastroduodenal artery. These join with their inferior counterparts coming off the SMA. There is a rich shared blood supply through these arcades that also contributes to perfusing the duodenum. The body and tail are drained through direct branches by the splenic vein. The inferior mesenteric vein feeds into the splenic vein approximately midway through the body. The head and neck are also drained by direct branches into the SMV.

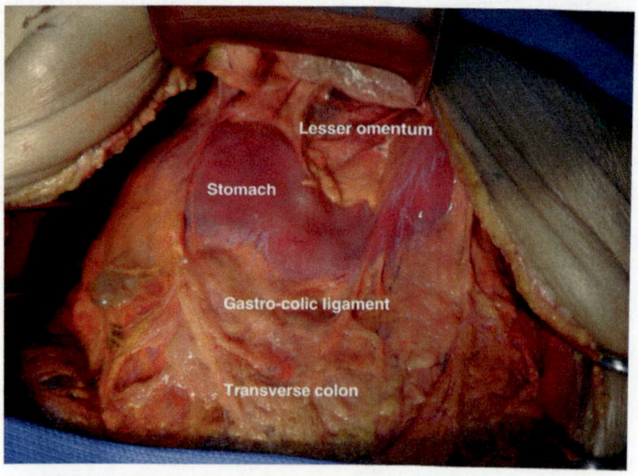

Fig. 19.1 Initial view on laparotomy

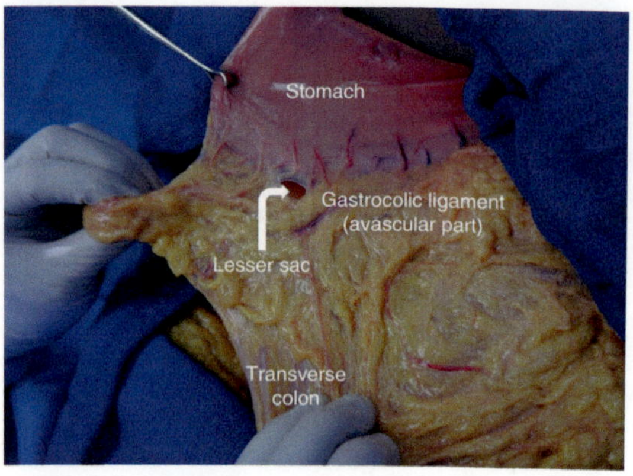

Fig. 19.2 Approach toward pancreas

The surrounding structures account for the rarity of finding a pancreatic injury in isolation. The pancreas lies deep to portions of the stomach, greater omentum, and the transverse colon (Fig. 19.1). The pancreatic body and neck lie inferior and adjacent to the gastric antrum and pylorus (Fig. 19.2). The head becomes contiguous with the c-loop of the duodenum, over which lies the transverse colon and small bowel. As the mesenteric veins converge, the portal vein originates deep and superior to the pancreas. The aorta lies deep to the junction of the neck and body.

These key relationships, as well as the close proximity of the IVC, liver, biliary tree, and right renal vein account for the poly-organ injury pattern often observed when managing pancreatic trauma.

Diagnosis

The diagnostic approach to pancreatic injuries has changed substantially over the last several decades with the ever-improving quality of cross-sectional imaging.

After blunt trauma, it is rare for a pancreatic injury to be symptomatic and trigger abdominal exploration. Consequently, the diagnosis of a blunt pancreatic injury is most commonly made on CT scan, which is the gold standard screening modality for this injury.

For penetrating injuries, if the patient is hemodynamically unstable, unevaluable, or has diffuse peritonitis, they should proceed directly to the OR, where the pancreas can be visually inspected. If not, however, the patient should undergo a CT scan, which, as in blunt injuries, is the standard diagnostic screening modality.

While CT image resolution has greatly improved, caution must be taken as it is not perfect. A recent study from a high-volume trauma center suggested that the CT sensitivity and specificity for pancreatic injury were 36.4% and 68.2%, respectively. This group found that CT alone missed 78.8% of pancreatic injuries, using a combination of 64 and 40 slice dedicated trauma scanners. A recent systematic review found that reported sensitivities for CT identification of pancreatic injuries range from 33 to 100% and specificities from 62 to 97%. This variance can likely be attributed to differences in technology between centers and to variations of interpretations. The sensitivity and specificity for clinically significant injury is likely better. Additionally, in one study, 92% of the missed injuries would have been considered low grade. While these limitations must be recognized, without question, CT scan should be the primary diagnostic modality used to evaluate the pancreas. If there is a need for further evaluation of the duct, Magnetic Resonance Cholangiopancreatography (MRCP) should be considered.

For diagnostic confirmation, Endoscopic Retrograde Cholangiopancreatography (ERCP) may also be considered. Historically, the role of intraoperative duct imaging was often discussed; however, contemporary management approaches have made these relatively obsolete.

The American Association for the Surgery of Trauma Organ Injury Scale (AAST-OIS) has been used as a uniform way to classify the severity of pancreatic injuries. This scale has been used heavily in research to delineate severity and describe outcomes; however, for practical use in the clinical setting, this scale has limited utility. Indeed, experts within the field have recently proposed a newer scale that may provide a more useful framework for classification and decision-making. At the time of writing, these changes have not been widely adopted but are likely to become more common in the future.

Management

Blunt

As previously discussed, blunt trauma rarely results in pancreatic injury that requires operative intervention. Moreover, about 83% of pancreatic injuries resulting from blunt trauma are defined as low grade in the AAST-OIS scoring system. For minor blunt pancreatic trauma, non-operative management is sufficient; however, for severe blunt pancreatic trauma definitive operative management has been associated with lower mortality and shorter length of stay. Thus, delineating those who do and do not need an operation is critical.

In general, most blunt pancreatic injuries will not require operative intervention. For those that require laparotomy for some other indication, operative inspection of the pancreas is often sufficient to delineate whether or not intervention is required. The two major factors that will drive operative decision-making are the presence of a destructive pancreatic injury and the pattern of damage relative to the SMA and SMV. Non-destructive parenchymal and branch duct injuries can be managed with closed suction drainage alone.

Destructive injuries to the pancreas will require operative intervention. For injuries to the left of the vessels, a distal pancreatectomy is indicated. For the distal pancreatectomy, splenic preservation may be considered in stable patients. While splenic preservation is generally advocated, the actual risk of Overwhelming Post-Splenectomy Infection in adults is unclear. In the geriatric population, increased operative time and increased risk of short-term morbidity may push the surgeon to choose splenectomy over preservation. Likewise, if there is a concurrent splenic injury, the architecture of the older spleen and lack of physiologic reserve should be taken into consideration, when considering splenic preservation.

Whenever possible, injuries to the right of the superior mesenteric vessels are best managed with closed suction drainage, even if a ductal injury is suspected (Fig. 19.3). Both isolated pancreatic head resection and pancreaticoduodenectomy, or colloquially the Whipple procedure, have high associated rates of morbidity and mortality. In the geriatric population, the complicated reconstruction presents even further risk to the patient and is more likely to fail. In the setting of pancreatic head trauma where there is associated destruction of the duodenum that cannot be repaired, a Whipple procedure may be considered. In this case, it is important to remember that none of these injuries must be addressed in the index operation. In an unstable patient, particularly in the geriatric population, damage control principles should be followed.

Penetrating

The majority of operative injuries to the pancreas result from penetrating mechanisms. Gunshot wounds are the most frequent mechanism, as stab wounds and other penetrating injuries often fail to reach the pancreas. Isolated injuries to the pancreas from a penetrating mechanism are exceedingly rare, and most penetrating injuries to the pancreas will be associated with multiple other

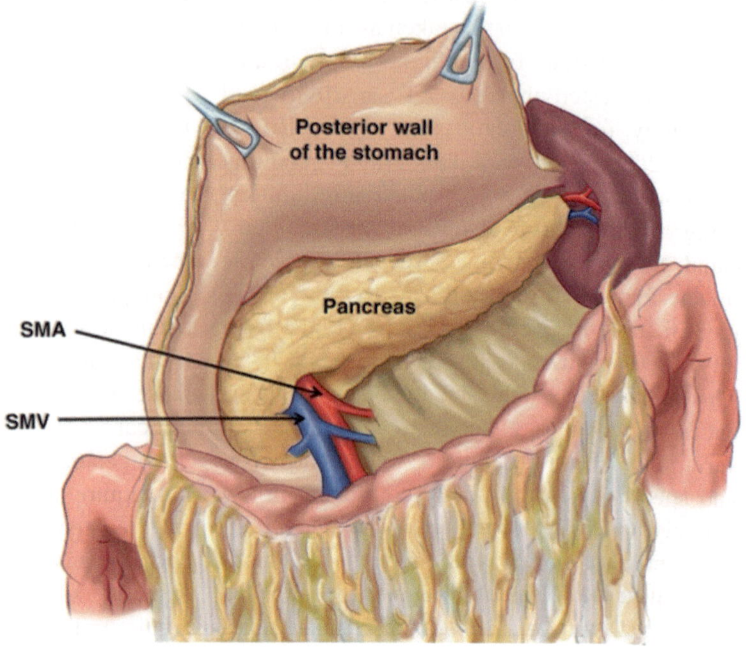

Fig. 19.3 View of pancreas on opening the lesser sac

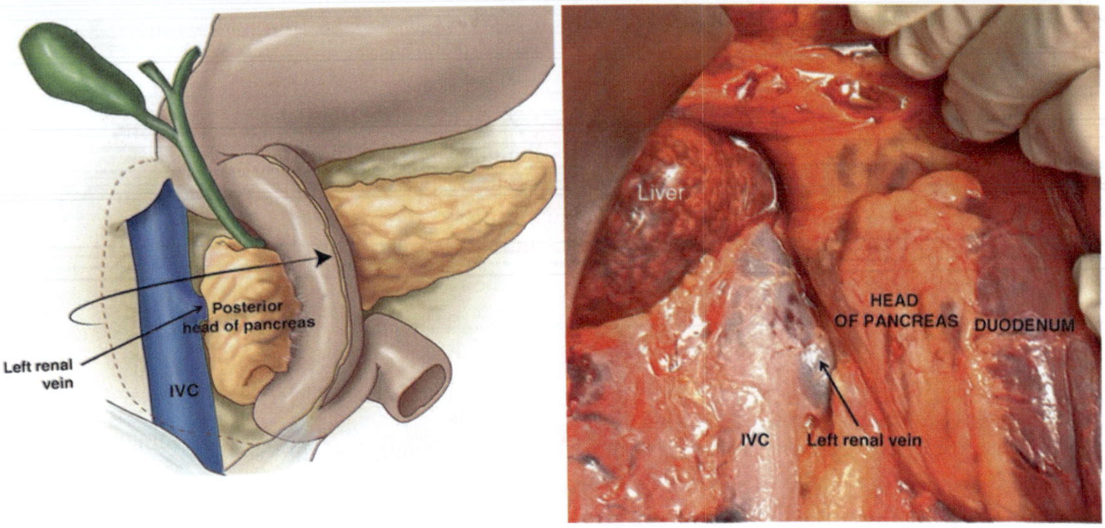

Fig. 19.4 Mobilization of the duodenum

injuries. At laparotomy, the pancreas should always be carefully examined. As mentioned previously, visual inspection of the pancreas is sufficient to identify the majority of injuries. For anterior injuries, the stomach, small bowel, and transverse colon may also be in the path of injury. Attention must also be paid to possible injuries to the surrounding structures, such as the liver, duodenum, portal vein, IVC, Aorta, CBD, SMA, SMV, and any other structures within the path of injury (Fig. 19.4).

As with blunt trauma, the two major factors that will drive operative decision-making are the extent of destruction to the parenchyma and the pattern of damage relative to the SMA and SMV. Isolated small parenchymal and branch duct injuries can be managed with closed suction drainage alone. Destructive injuries to the left of the vessels can be managed with a distal pancreatectomy with or without splenectomy, depending upon individual patient factors, including age (Figs. 19.5 and 19.6). Injuries to the head of the pancreas are best managed with closed-suction drainage whenever possible, as resection and reconstruction are technically difficult as previously discussed, in the geriatric population. If

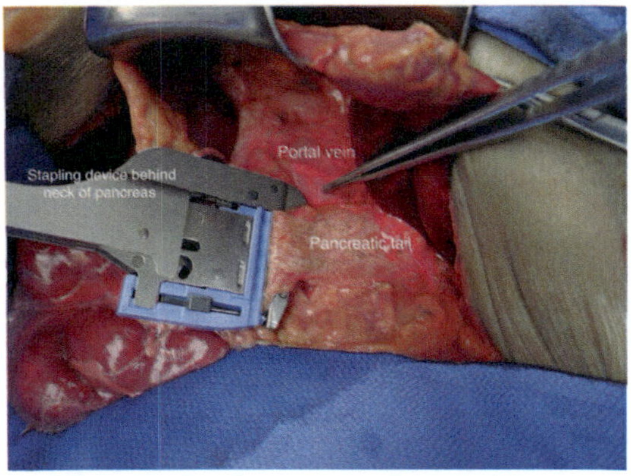

Fig. 19.5 Landmarks for distal pancreatectomy

there is concurrent destruction of the duodenum, a Whipple procedure may be considered. Given that ballistic injuries can be severe and highly destructive, many of these patients will have a more significant total injury burden and may be more hemodynamically deranged. As such, it is important to re-emphasize that none of these pancreatic injuries require definitive repair during the index operation, and in the setting of damage control surgery, they are likely better addressed once the patient has been resuscitated.

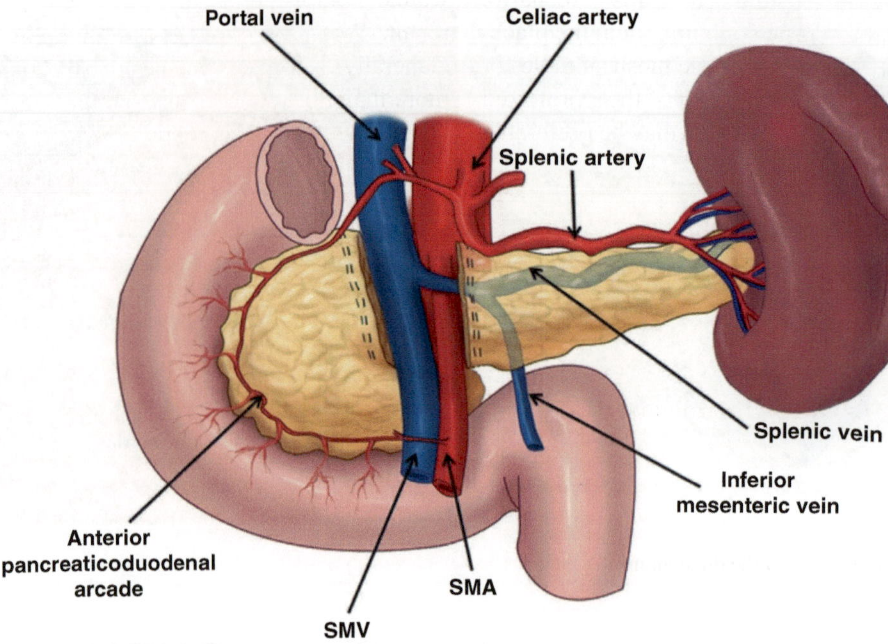

Fig. 19.6 Stapled distal pancreatectomy

Conclusions

While the overall treatment approach to pancreatic trauma is the same in the geriatric and broader adult population, the general trend toward more conservative management is of even greater importance within the geriatric population. The physiologic demands of a polytraumatic event especially in the face of decreased physiologic reserve must be weighed when considering treatment for this population. Thankfully, these injuries are quite rare among this population.

References

1. Kuza CM, Hirji SA, Englum BR, Ganapathi AM, Speicher PJ, Scarborough JE. Pancreatic injuries in abdominal trauma in US adults: analysis of the National Trauma Data Bank on management, outcomes, and predictors of mortality. Scand J Surg. 2020;109(3):193–204.
2. Biffl WL, Ball CG, Moore EE, West M, Russo RM, Balogh Z, Kornblith L, Callcut R, Schaffer KB, Castelo M. A comparison of management and outcomes following blunt versus penetrating pancreatic trauma: a secondary analysis from the WTA multicenter trials group on pancreatic injuries. J Trauma Acute Care Surg. 2022;93:620. https://doi.org/10.1097/TA.0000000000003651.
3. Buitendag JJP, Kong VY, Laing GL, Bruce JL, Manchev V, Clarke DL. A comparison of blunt and penetrating pancreatic trauma. S Afr J Surg. 2020;58(4):218.
4. Colney L, Tandon N, Garg PK, Gupta N, Sagar S, Gupta A, Kumar A, Kumar S. Exocrine and endocrine functions and pancreatic volume in patients with pancreatic trauma. Eur J Trauma Emerg Surg. 2022;48(1):97–105.
5. Vasquez M, Cardarelli C, Glaser J, Murthi S, Stein D, Scalea T. The ABC's of pancreatic trauma: airway, breathing, and computerized tomography scan? Mil Med. 2017;182(S1):66–71.
6. Odedra D, Mellnick VM, Patlas MN. Imaging of blunt pancreatic trauma: a systematic review. Can Assoc Radiol J. 2020;71(3):344–51.
7. Ball CG, Biffl WL, Moore EE. Time to update the American Association for the Surgery of Trauma pancreas injury grading lexicon? J Trauma Acute Care Surg. 2022;92(3):e38–40.
8. Siboni S, Kwon E, Benjamin E, Inaba K, Demetriades D. Isolated blunt pancreatic trauma: a benign injury? J Trauma Acute Care Surg. 2016;81(5):855–9.
9. Byrge N, Heilbrun M, Winkler N, Sommers D, Evans H, Cattin LM, Scalea T, Stein DM, Neideen T, Walsh P, Sims CA, Brahmbhatt TS, Galante JM, Phan HH, Malhotra A, Stovall RT, Jurkovich GJ, Coimbra

R, Berndtson AE, O'Callaghan TA, Gaspard SF, Schreiber MA, Cook MR, Demetriades D, Rivera O, Velmahos GC, Zhao T, Park PK, Machado-Aranda D, Ahmad S, Lewis J, Hoff WS, Suleiman G, Sperry J, Zolin S, Carrick MM, Mallory GR, Nunez J, Colonna A, Enniss T, Nirula R. An AAST-MITC analysis of pancreatic trauma: staple or sew? Resect or drain? J Trauma Acute Care Surg. 2018;85(3):435–43.

10. Schellenberg M, Inaba K, Cheng V, Bardes JM, Lam L, Benjamin E, Matsushima K, Demetriades D. Spleen-preserving distal pancreatectomy in trauma. J Trauma Acute Care Surg. 2018;84(1):118–22.
11. Schellenberg M, Inaba K, Bardes JM, Cheng V, Matsushima K, Lam L, Benjamin E, Demetriades D. Detection of traumatic pancreatic duct disruption in the modern era. Am J Surg. 2018;216(2):299–303.

Injury to the Spleen

20

Johannes Wiik Larsen and Kjetil Søreide

Introduction

Abdominal trauma remains a frequent cause of morbidity and mortality worldwide. While the liver is the most frequently reported solid organ injury in abdominal trauma, abdominal injury often results in injury to the spleen—either in isolation or combined with other injuries—and, as such, places splenic injury as one of the most frequently encountered solid organ injuries globally. Historically, the epidemiology of such solid organ injuries has been dominated by young male patients and children. The elderly population is less frequently represented and hence fewer reports specifically aimed to this population. Indeed, in cohorts of abdominal trauma, one Australian study reported only a quarter of all patients being over 51 years of age. Less than 12% of admitted patients were >65 years of age in a Norwegian cohort study. A large historic cohort from the 1990s in the United States also reported the geriatric population (≥65 years) to account for less than 7% of all splenic injuries. Hence, most data available on splenic injury stem from the younger patient population (children and young adults) and adapting this experience to the elderly population should be done with some reservations as results are partly extrapolated from cohorts with different comorbidity, medication, and physiological reserve profile than normally displayed in the elderly.

With the worldwide aging of the population, an increasing proportion of geriatric patients will also be reflected in this injury category. Additionally, increased mobility and active lifestyles at a more advanced age will inevitably increase the number of elderly suffering from traumatic injuries, including injury to the spleen. In this chapter, we will specifically cover management issues of splenic trauma when seen in the geriatric population.

Injury Mechanisms with Risks of Splenic Injury

The elderly population is at risk for any type of injuries associated with low energy impacts and associated bleeding risk from medications. Blunt trauma is by far the most predominant mechanism of splenic injury—reported between 75 and 90%—and is similar across age groups including the geriatric population. In frail patients, any blunt trauma to the left flank, even in the assumption of low energy impact as ground-level falls, should lead to a suspicion of splenic injury and sufficient diagnostic measures. Elderly patients on anticoagulation or antithrombotic therapy are

J. Wiik Larsen · K. Søreide (✉)
Department of Gastrointestinal Surgery, HPB Unit, Stavanger University Hospital, Stavanger, Norway

Department of Clinical Medicine, University of Bergen, Bergen, Norway

P. Petrone, C. E.M. Brathwaite (eds.), *Acute Care Surgery in Geriatric Patients*,
https://doi.org/10.1007/978-3-031-30651-8_20

prone to suffer bleeding complications even from relatively minor insults.

Motor vehicle crashes are still contesting falls as the most frequent cause of abdominal solid organ injury in geriatric patients. Even if older people are said to drive shorter distances at lower speeds than younger drivers, both reduced physical/mental reserves (limited mobility, slower reaction times, decreased vision/hearing, and cognitive impairment), and more often medical conditions that can precipitate a collision, make them more vulnerable to such event. Any impact to the left side of the body with or within a vehicle in motion has the potential energy to cause damage to the splenic tissue in elderly patients.

Although penetrating injuries are significantly less common than blunt injuries in geriatric abdominal trauma, stab injuries and gunshot wounds to the spleen can be seen both following acts of violence and as a result of intentional self-harm or suicide. Regardless of the type of injury mechanism, the team providing treatment should remain vigilant to elder maltreatment and abuse, as this is often unrecognized and underreported.

Injury Work-Up

General principle of trauma care applies and includes primary survey in adherence to ATLS principles, as covered in detail elsewhere in this book. Patients in extremis are immediately treated according to damage control resuscitation protocols. In case of patients not responding to transfusion therapy and showing persistent hemodynamic instability they are taken to theater for resuscitative emergency surgery, if not deemed futile in the emergency room.

For all other patients, the clinical work-up, establishment of diagnosis and severity assessment involves cross-sectional imaging, with computed tomography with intravenous contrast as the gold standard. Modern CT scanners will be able to diagnose splenic and any associated injuries and score the anatomical severity grade, according to AAST-OIS definitions.

Severity Scores and Classification

The most utilized classification of splenic injury is the American Association for the Surgery of Trauma (AAST)—Organ Injury Scale (OIS) (Table 20.1). With the seminal paper published by Moore et al. in 1989, an initial classification system was in place which standardized splenic injury severity scoring from grade I to V. OIS is based purely on spleen lesion anatomy. This classification has been updated several times, including the latest revision in 2018.

Notably, the purely anatomically based injury scale has some limitations, including inconsistent reliability across score values and that it does not include physiological parameters. Consequently, an additional scoring tool that includes the patients physiological state by incorporating hemodynamic status has been proposed by the World Society of Emergency Surgery (WSES) in

Table 20.1 AAST-OIS for splenic injuries

Grade	Injury description	
I	Hematoma	Subcapsular, <10% surface area
	Laceration	Capsular tear, <1 cm parenchymal depth
II	Hematoma	Subcapsular, 10–50% surface area
		Intraparenchymal, <5 cm diameter
	Laceration	1–3 cm parenchymal depth not involving a parenchymal vessel
III	Hematoma	Subcapsular, >50% surface area or expanding
		Ruptured subcapsular or parenchymal hematoma
		Intraparenchymal hematoma >5 cm
	Laceration	>3 cm parenchymal depth or involving trabecular vessels
IV	Laceration	Laceration of segmental or hilar vessels producing major devascularization (>25% of spleen)
V	Laceration	Completely shatters spleen
	Vascular	Hilar vascular injury which devascularized spleen

Table 20.2 WSES spleen trauma classification for adults (modified table to report recommendations for adults only (with pediatric population excluded))

	WSES class	Mechanism of injury	AAST	Hemodynamic status[a]	CT scan	First-line treatment in adults
Minor	WSES I	Blunt/penetrating	I–II	Stable	Yes + local exploration in SW[c]	NOM[b] + serial clinical/laboratory/radiological evaluation Consider angiography/angioembolization
Moderate	WSES II	Blunt/penetrating	III	Stable		
	WSES III	Blunt/penetrating	IV–V	Stable		NOM[b] All angiography/angioembolization + serial clinical/laboratory/radiological evaluation
Severe	WSES IV	Blunt/penetrating	I–V	Unstable	No	OM

SW stab wound, *GSW* gunshot wound [a, b, c] refer to @, *, and # in Fig. 20.1.

their guidelines and includes three classes (Table 20.2):

- Minor (WSES Class I)
- Moderate (WSES Class II-III)
- Severe (WSES Class IV)

Of note, the WSES severity scoring system is not without discrepancy nor debate, yet may provide a better understanding of variation in care when considering both anatomy and physiology. Common to all classification systems for splenic injuries is that they describe the injury in pediatric and adult patient cohorts without special consideration for geriatric patients.

Management of Splenic Injury in the Elderly

The management of splenic injury follows essentially two pathways, either non-operative management (NOM) or operative management (OM). In historic cohorts, an emphasis on "splenic salvage" procedures were emphasized, including splenoraphy and use of mesh wrappings to cover the shattered spleen. In current practice, this has largely been replaced by either a non-operative strategy supported by splenic angioembolization by interventional radiology; or an operative strategy. An operation is indicated in the hemodynamic unstable patient for which open splenectomy is the preferred treatment. Failed NOM is also an indication for splenectomy, for example, when splenic artery embolization fails to cease ongoing bleeding or contrast-blush on CT, or multiple injuries with the subsequent need for laparotomy to ensure control of potential bleeding sources. Consensus is hardly an exact science in this regard, as reflected in nuances and opinions across guidelines and expert opinions. However, systematic assessment of available data suggests that splenic angioembolization should be strongly considered as an adjunct to non-operative management in patients with AAST Grade IV and Grade V blunt splenic injury but should not be routinely recommended in patients with AAST Grade I to Grade III injuries. In Fig. 20.1, the algorithm suggested for non-operative or operative management of splenic injuries in the adult population is presented. This algorithm is conditional on the use of the WSES severity classes but can be incorporated with use of AAST-OIS anatomical grading systems, assessment of patient physiology and radiological findings on initial or repeated scans.

For patients treated non-operatively (with or without splenic angioembolization), the duration of bedrest and start of mobilization is controversial, extrapolated from predominantly younger cohorts and hence should be individualized according to the estimated physical reserve, associated other injuries and severity of the splenic injury. Suffice to say is that early involvement by physical therapist to facilitate early mobilization should be prioritized, as duration of immobiliza-

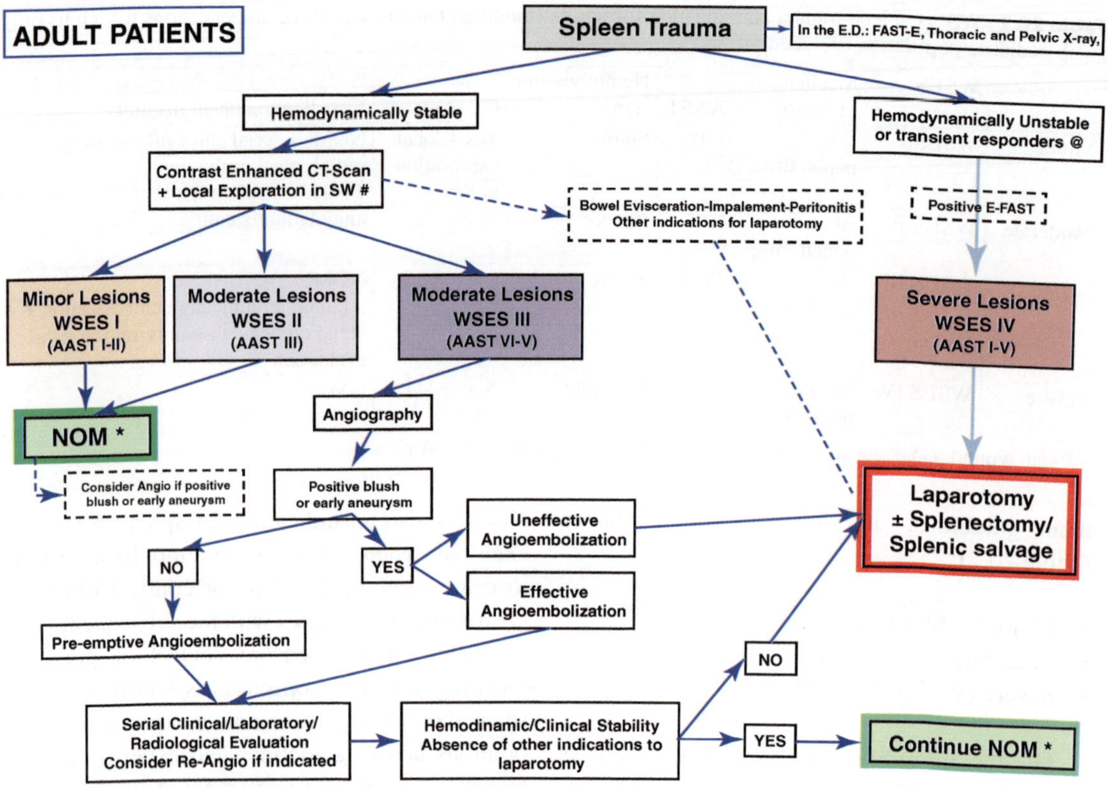

Fig. 20.1 Spleen trauma management algorithm for Adult Patients. Copyright© The Author(s) 2017, reproduced with permission from Coccolini et al. World J Emerg Surg. 2017; 12: 40 under the terms of the Creative Commons Attribution 4.0 International License (http://creativecommons.org/licenses/by/4.0/), which permits unrestricted use, distribution, and reproduction in any medium, provided you give appropriate credit to the original author(s) and the source, provide a link to the Creative Commons license, and indicate if changes were made. *SW* stab wound; *GSW* gunshot wound. (*) NOM should only be attempted in centers capable of a precise diagnosis of the severity of spleen injuries and capable of intensive management including close clinical observation and hemodynamic monitoring in a high dependency/intensive care environment, including serial clinical examination and laboratory assay, with immediate access to diagnostics, interventional radiology, and surgery and immediately available access to blood and blood products or alternatively in the presence of a rapid centralization system in those patients amenable to be transferred. (@) Hemodynamic instability is considered the condition in which the patient has an admission systolic blood pressure <90 mmHg with evidence of skin vasoconstriction (cool, clammy, decreased capillary refill), altered level of consciousness and/or shortness of breath, or >90 mmHg but requiring bolus infusions/transfusions and/or vasopressor drugs and/or admission base excess (BE) >−5 mmol/L and/or shock index >1 and/or transfusion requirement of at least 4–6 units of packed red blood cells within the first 24 h; moreover, transient responder patients (those showing an initial response to adequate fluid resuscitation, and then signs of ongoing loss and perfusion deficits), and more in general those responding to therapy but not amenable of sufficient stabilization to be undergone to interventional radiology treatments. (#) Wound exploration near the inferior costal margin should be avoided if not strictly necessary because of the high risk to damage the intercostal vessels)

tion increases time to recovery and time to return to the pre-injury state.

Thromboprophylaxis should be started at time when bleeding control is ensured, and preferably within 48 h. Patients that are on oral anticoagulation drugs should restart the medication as soon as food is tolerated and per indication for their anticoagulation.

Much controversy and debate concern such issues of care, and it should be noted that data are scarce and extrapolated from the general population of trauma patients.

Outcomes

Data from the geriatric population is scarce, yet one study found that failure of NOM in splenic injury was associated with increasing age as well as higher injury severity grade. Another study also found a higher failure rate of NOM in the geriatric population. Failed NOM in elderly patients was not associated with increased mortality, as mortality was associated to injury severity and other injuries. In one study, mortality in splenic injury was associated to other associated injuries (specifically severe head injuries) rather than the splenic injury per se. An increased mortality in failed NOM in the elderly population is associated with higher injury burden and associated injuries (e.g., neurotrauma), but based on observational data it is hard to propose that operative management may have altered the outcome. Notably, higher age per se is a risk factor for prolonged ICU stay, longer hospital stay and increased mortality even for isolated splenic injuries.

Vaccination After Splenectomy or Angioembolization

Routine vaccination after splenectomy for trauma is recommended across most national guidelines with variation in the suggested use of routine life-long use of antibiotics, but recommendations are less clear for patients who undergo angioembolization. Current data suggests that the immune function is maintained and, vaccination is not necessary after splenic angioembolization.

References

1. Han J, Dudi-Venkata NN, Jolly S, Ting YY, Lu H, Thomas M, et al. Splenic artery embolization improves outcomes and decreases the length of stay in hemodynamically stable blunt splenic injuries–a level 1 Australian trauma Centre experience. Injury. 2022;53(5):1620–6. https://doi.org/10.1016/j.injury.2021.12.043.
2. Wiik Larsen J, Søreide K, Søreide JA, Tjosevik K, Kvaløy JT, Thorsen K. Epidemiology of abdominal trauma: an age- and sex-adjusted incidence analysis with mortality patterns. Injury. 2022;53:3130. https://doi.org/10.1016/j.injury.2022.06.020.
3. Clancy TV, Ramshaw DG, Maxwell JG, Covington DL, Churchill MP, Rutledge R, et al. Management outcomes in splenic injury: a statewide trauma center review. Ann Surg. 1997;226(1):17–24. https://doi.org/10.1097/00000658-199707000-00003.
4. Moore EE, Shackford SR, Pachter HL, McAninch JW, Browner BD, Champion HR, et al. Organ injury scaling: spleen, liver, and kidney. J Trauma. 1989;29(12):1664–6.
5. Coccolini F, Montori G, Catena F, Kluger Y, Biffl W, Moore EE, et al. Splenic trauma: WSES classification and guidelines for adult and pediatric patients. World J Emerg Surg. 2017;12:40. https://doi.org/10.1186/s13017-017-0151-4.
6. Søndenaa K, Tasdemir I, Andersen E, Skadberg JE, Søreide JA. Treatment of blunt injury of the spleen: is there a place for mesh wrapping? Eur J Surg. 1994;160(12):669–73.
7. Watson GA, Hoffman MK, Peitzman AB. Nonoperative management of blunt splenic injury: what is new? Eur J Trauma Emerg Surg. 2015;41(3):219–28. https://doi.org/10.1007/s00068-015-0520-1.
8. Amico F, Anning R, Bendinelli C, Balogh ZJ. Grade III blunt splenic injury without contrast extravasation–world Society of Emergency Surgery Nijmegen consensus practice. World J Emerg Surg. 2020;15(1):46. https://doi.org/10.1186/s13017-020-00319-y.
9. Stassen NA, Bhullar I, Cheng JD, Crandall ML, Friese RS, Guillamondegui OD, et al. Selective nonoperative management of blunt splenic injury: an eastern Association for the Surgery of trauma practice management guideline. J Trauma Acute Care Surg. 2012;73(5 Suppl 4):S294–300. https://doi.org/10.1097/TA.0b013e3182702afc.
10. Crichton JCI, Naidoo K, Yet B, Brundage SI, Perkins Z. The role of splenic angioembolization as an adjunct to nonoperative management of blunt splenic injuries: a systematic review and meta-analysis. J Trauma Acute Care Surg. 2017;83(5):934–43. https://doi.org/10.1097/ta.0000000000001649.
11. Ong AW, Eilertson KE, Reilly EF, Geng TA, Madbak F, McNicholas A, et al. Nonoperative management of splenic injuries: significance of age. J Surg Res. 2016;201(1):134–40. https://doi.org/10.1016/j.jss.2015.10.014.
12. Trust MD, Teixeira PG, Brown LH, Ali S, Coopwood B, Aydelotte JD, et al. Is it safe? Nonoperative management of blunt splenic injuries in geriatric trauma patients. J Trauma Acute Care Surg. 2018;84(1):123–7. https://doi.org/10.1097/ta.0000000000001731.
13. Bashir R, Grigorian A, Lekawa M, Joe V, Schubl SD, Chin TL, et al. Octogenarians with blunt

splenic injury: not all geriatrics are the same. Updat Surg. 2021;73(4):1533–9. https://doi.org/10.1007/s13304-020-00765-y.
14. Warnack E, Bukur M, Frangos S, DiMaggio C, Kozar R, Klein M, et al. Age is a predictor for mortality after blunt splenic injury. Am J Surg. 2020;220(3):778–82. https://doi.org/10.1016/j.amjsurg.2020.01.053.
15. Freeman JJ, Yorkgitis BK, Haines K, Koganti D, Patel N, Maine R, et al. Vaccination after spleen embolization: a practice management guideline from the eastern Association for the Surgery of trauma. Injury. 2022;53:3569. https://doi.org/10.1016/j.injury.2022.08.006.

Geriatric Liver Trauma

21

Erik J. Teicher, Paula A. Ferrada, and David V. Feliciano

Introduction

As the population ages, geriatric trauma has become an increasing problem. Trauma patients aged >65 years have a higher risk of severe disability and death even with similar injury severity scores (ISS) when compared with younger trauma patients. Reasons for these poorer outcomes among geriatric trauma patients include a diminished response to physiologic stress, higher incidence of medical comorbidities, and polypharmacy. Elderly patients generally do not tolerate alterations of normal physiologic parameters when challenged with trauma or major surgery. Medical comorbidities have been found to be an independent predictor of mortality for trauma patients, with the strongest being hepatic disease, renal disease, and cancer. These result in a blunted response to injury, increased risk of bleeding, and others. Elderly patients are more likely to experience blunt rather than penetrating trauma which accounts for less than 5% of cases and, unfortunately, with most being self-inflicted. The most common blunt mechanisms are falls, followed by motor vehicle collisions.

The liver is the largest solid abdominal organ and the most frequently injured in blunt abdominal trauma, abdominal stab wounds, and third most commonly injured in abdominal gunshot wounds. The liver accounts for 22% of all abdominal injuries. It has been reported that hepatic injury occurs in 20%, 30%, and 40% of those operated on for blunt, gunshot, and stab wounds to the abdomen, respectively. Injury to the liver is rarely in isolation with an associated injury rate of 83%, including injury to the chest in over half the cases. The most commonly associated abdominal injuries include those to the spleen and small bowel in blunt trauma and stomach, colon, and small bowel in penetrating trauma. The overall mortality attributed to hepatic injury is about 8.6–11.7%. This usually results from a combination of associated injuries, uncontrolled hemorrhage, and subsequent development of septic complications. Mortality rates associated with hepatic injuries have steadily declined in the past decades due to advances in selective non-operative management (SNOM) and surgical critical care.

The liver is organized anatomically into two lobes and eight segments around the hepatic veins and receives blood from the hepatic artery and portal vein. The hepatic artery supplies about 25% of the total hepatic blood flow and 50% of its oxygen requirements, while the portal vein provides about 75% of the total hepatic blood flow and 50% of its oxygen requirements. The

E. J. Teicher (✉) · P. A. Ferrada
Trauma and Acute Care Surgery, Inova Health System, Falls Church, VA, USA
e-mail: Erik.Teicher@inova.org

D. V. Feliciano
Department of Surgery, University of Maryland, Baltimore, MD, USA

P. Petrone, C. E.M. Brathwaite (eds.), *Acute Care Surgery in Geriatric Patients*,
https://doi.org/10.1007/978-3-031-30651-8_21

parenchyma is covered by a fibrous Glisson's capsule and is attached to the abdominal wall by the falciform, triangular, and coronary ligaments. High energy blunt mechanisms, such as motor vehicle collisions or falls from heights, cause hepatic injuries on impact when the liver continues to move and produces an injury to Glisson's capsule and to the parenchyma at sites of ligamentous attachment to the abdominal wall. The liver usually fractures between the lateral segments VI and VII and the medial segments V and VIII of the right lobe. Lower energy blunt mechanisms, such as a direct blow to the abdomen, usually cause damage to the central segments IV, V, VIII, or even segment I (caudate lobe). Low-energy penetrating mechanisms, such as stab wounds, produce injury that is dependent on the depth of penetration and whether an intraparenchymal vessel is involved. High-energy penetrating mechanisms, such as rifle wounds, create extensive hepatic injuries due to the cavitary effect of the missile as it traverses the liver.

Patient Assessment and Initial Diagnostic Studies

All trauma patients should be fully evaluated using the guidelines in the Advanced Trauma Life Support course established by the American College of Surgeons Committee on Trauma. Patients with blunt or penetrating abdominal trauma who are hemodynamically unstable or have peritonitis need operative exploration. Those that are hemodynamically normal and without peritonitis, however, should undergo further radiological imaging of the abdomen (Fig. 21.1). It has been estimated that about 85%

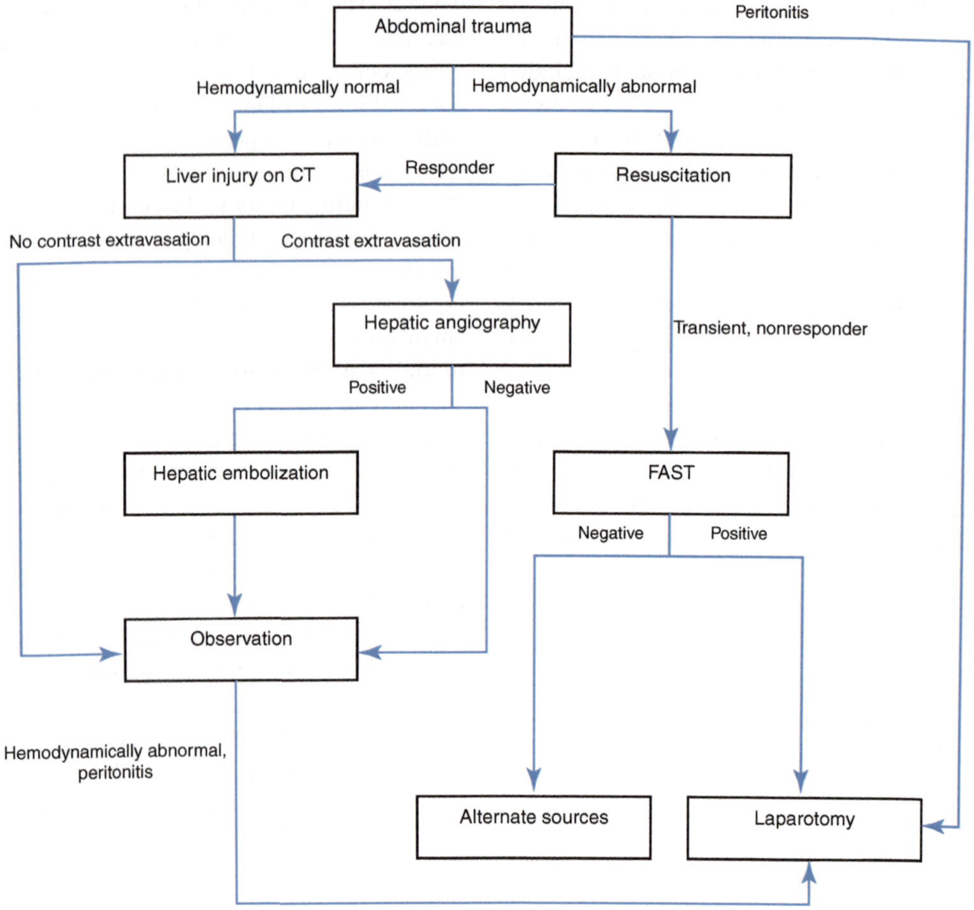

Fig. 21.1 Initial management approach to hepatic trauma

of patients with blunt hepatic injuries are hemodynamically stable upon presentation. It has been well established that patients with low-energy penetrating abdominal trauma and who are hemodynamically stable and without peritonitis, even with peritoneal violation, may undergo SNOM with or without further radiological imaging. This is particularly true for those with right thoracoabdominal wounds. Those with high-energy penetrating abdominal trauma, regardless of patient hemodynamics or physical examination, have historically undergone laparotomy; however, this mandate has changed in the last few decades. Management of patients who are hemodynamically stable and without peritonitis and who have had additional radiological imaging involves observation with serial physical examinations. Therefore, patients with altered sensorium or intoxication must be observed with particular care based on changes in vital signs or signs of sepsis.

Computed tomography (CT) has become the most important tool in assessing the hemodynamically stable patient following abdominal trauma. CT is able to define the severity of injury to the liver and to quantify the amount of hemoperitoneum. Intravenous contrast is mandatory as ongoing hemorrhage can be seen as active extravasation on CT and is predictive of failure with SNOM. CT has been shown to have a 65–100% sensitivity and 76–85% specificity for detection of a hepatic vascular injury while also having the benefit of finding associated injuries in the abdomen. It is important to remember that CT involves exposure to high levels of ionizing radiation and that the use of intravenous contrast may compromise renal function. In the majority of institutions the use of CT involves transport of the patient away from the resuscitation area to the radiology department. Hence, such patients should be hemodynamically stable, even if methods for bleeding control have been used to attain this. The use of the Resuscitative Endovascular Balloon Occlusion of the Aorta (REBOA) has been described to help stabilize hemorrhaging patients until the final control of bleeding is achieved.

Table 21.1 AAST liver injury scale (2018 Revision)

Grade		Injury description
I	Hematoma	Subcapsular, non-expanding, <10% surface area
	Laceration	Capsular tear, non-bleeding, <1 cm parenchymal depth
II	Hematoma	Subcapsular, non-expanding, 10–50% surface area; intraparenchymal <10 cm in diameter
	Laceration	Capsular tear, active bleeding; 1–3 cm parenchymal depth, <10 cm in length
III	Hematoma	Subcapsular, >50% surface area or expanding; ruptured subcapsular hematoma with active bleeding; intraparenchymal hematoma >10 cm depth or expanding
	Laceration	>3 cm parenchymal depth
IV	Hematoma	Ruptured intraparenchymal hematoma with active bleeding
	Laceration	Parenchymal disruption involving 25–75% of hepatic lobe or 1–3 Couinaud's segments within a single lobe
V	Laceration	Parenchymal disruption involving >75% of hepatic lobe or >3 Couinaud's segments within a single lobe
	Vascular	Juxtahepatic venous injury (retrohepatic vena cava/central major hepatic veins)

The severity of hepatic trauma is a spectrum from a minor capsular tear to extensive lobar disruption. The Organ Injury Scaling Committee of the American Association for the Surgery of Trauma developed a Liver Injury Scale that was most recently updated in 2018 (Table 21.1). Grades I and II are regarded as minor injuries, and grades III, IV, and V represent severe injuries as seen on imaging (Fig. 21.2a–e). or during laparotomy The success of SNOM is less likely as the grade of injury increases.

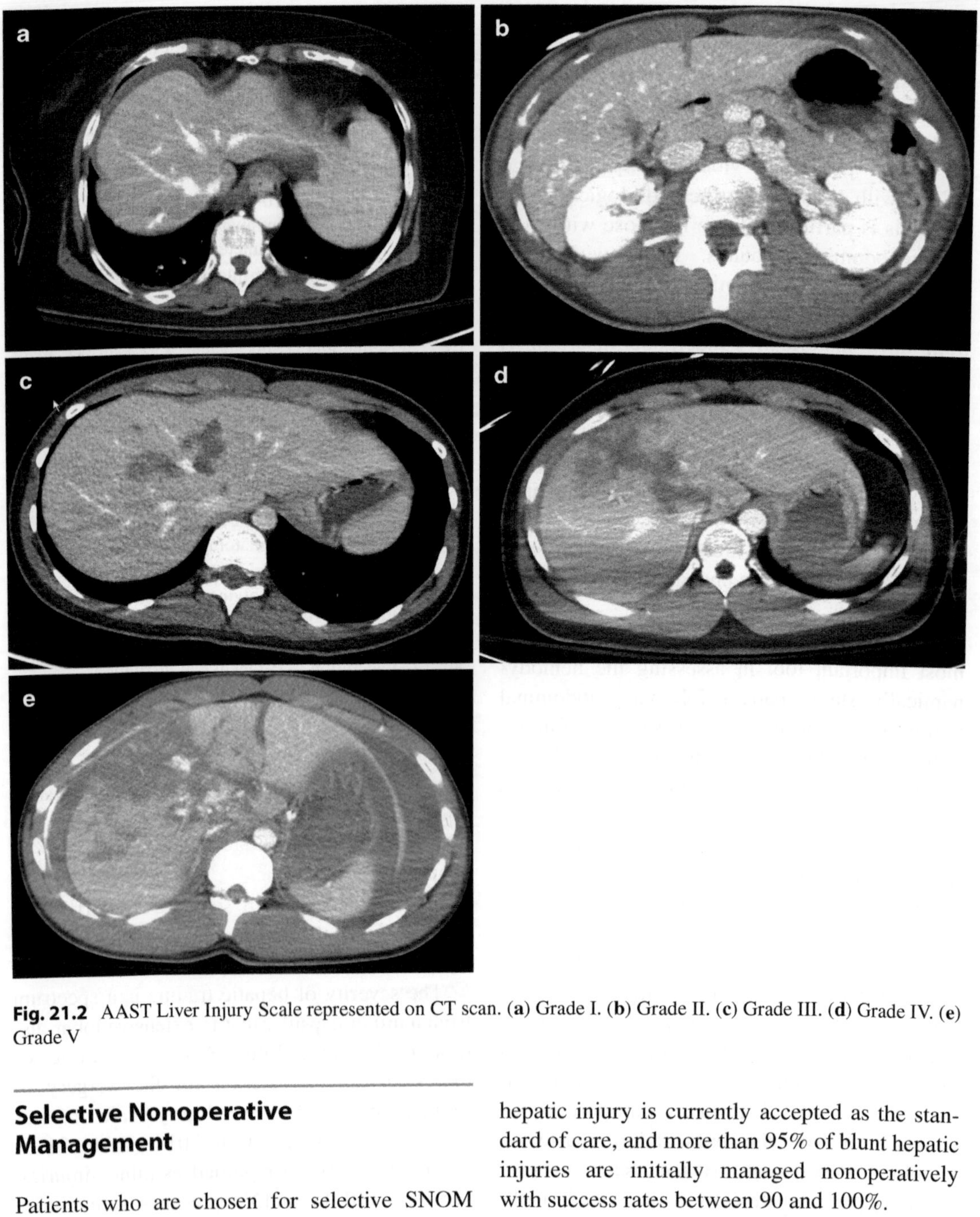

Fig. 21.2 AAST Liver Injury Scale represented on CT scan. (**a**) Grade I. (**b**) Grade II. (**c**) Grade III. (**d**) Grade IV. (**e**) Grade V

Selective Nonoperative Management

Patients who are chosen for selective SNOM must be hemodynamically stable, without peritonitis, and able to undergo serial abdominal examinations. The hepatic injury grade should not determine candidacy for SNOM as 50–80% of bleeding from the liver injury stops without intervention. While controversial, age should not be a contraindication for SNOM. SNOM of a blunt hepatic injury is currently accepted as the standard of care, and more than 95% of blunt hepatic injuries are initially managed nonoperatively with success rates between 90 and 100%.

Interventional radiological techniques are commonly used in the management of patients with abdominal trauma, and hepatic angioembolization has emerged as an important adjunct in hemorrhage control. It has been shown that patients with active extravasation of contrast on CT are 20 times more likely to undergo hepatic angioembolization than those without. Patients who are hemodynamically stable with active extravasation of contrast from the injured liver and who undergo hepatic angioembolization have their site of bleeding controlled 68–87% of the time.

Failure rates of SNOM are about 3–7.5% for all grades and about 65% for grades IV and V. This failure of SNOM appears to be associated with the overall burden of injury rather than the liver injury grade as only 47% of patients who fail initial SNOM have ongoing hepatic bleeding. The rest have associated injuries often missed on the original abdominal CT. Other factors identified as predictors of failure of SNOM include age, hemoglobin, blood pressure, need for transfusion, and active extravasation of contrast on CT. Failure of SNOM due to delayed hepatic bleeding is rare and occurs less than 3.5% of the time. It has been shown, however, that SNOM in the elderly is associated with increased transfusion requirements.

Operative Management

When SNOM is not possible, fails, and hepatic angioembolization is contraindicated, the patient needs an exploratory laparotomy. Mortality of hepatic operations for trauma can be significant and approaches 66% in grade IV and V injuries with 59% as a result of uncontrolled hemorrhage. The standard approach is through a midline incision, which can be extended to a median sternotomy, or on rare occasions, to a right thoracoabdominal incision. The liver should immediately be manually compressed, and tamponade can then be maintained by perihepatic packing, which will control hemorrhage in up to 80% of patients and allow for continued resuscitation. The method of perihepatic packing varies, but generally involves insertion of laparotomy packs over the diaphragmatic surface of the liver to produce a tamponade effect between the liver, abdominal wall, and thoracic cage.

If bleeding remains uncontrolled, then compression of the portal triad (Pringle maneuver) should be applied digitally or by using an atraumatic clamp. This can be therapeutic and diagnostic. If a Pringle maneuver controls bleeding, then there is likely an intraparenchymal hepatic arterial or portal venous injury. If a Pringle maneuver does not control bleeding, then an injury to a hepatic vein or the retrohepatic vena cava is likely. These measures for rapid hemorrhage control should be maintained to allow effective resuscitation. Any attempt to identify and repair a hepatic vascular injury before hemodynamic stabilization should be avoided as further bleeding will lead to hypotension, acidosis, and a coagulopathy. While controversial, it has been generally accepted that up to 1 h of compression of the portal trial can be tolerated in the non-cirrhotic patient.

If the bleeding has stopped after the removal of packing then nothing further is required. If bleeding continues, then it becomes necessary to decide on whether to continue with exploration or perform definitive perihepatic packing and damage control. This decision is based on the patient's hemodynamics and measures of resuscitation. The use of packs directly over the inferior vena cava should be avoided in a damage control situation because of an increased risk of compression of the right renal vein and inferior vena cava leading to an acute kidney injury. Following this damage control procedure, resuscitation is continued with correction of metabolic parameters, and packs are removed at a reoperation within 36–48 h. Some advocate for insertion of a plastic sheet such as a bowel bag, or omentum between the liver and packing to help reduce the risk of additional bleeding during the subsequent removal of packing.

If the liver continues to bleed, but damage control is not thought to be necessary, there are additional operative techniques available. Release of the Pringle maneuver may allow for identification of bleeding sites that can be selectively ligated. Appropriate mobilization of the liver is important to obtain a thorough examination of the injured liver unless the injured area is easily accessible. The liver is mobilized by dividing the falciform, triangular, and anterior coronary ligaments. Additional exposure can also be achieved with extension of the initial incision into a median sternotomy in obese patients. Hepatotomy and vascular ligation may be utilized for continued bleeding from a deep laceration or a missile tract. This should be performed while using the Pringle maneuver and involves blunt finger fracture, electrocautery, or stapling for extension of the hepatic wound. This now allows for either direct suture or clip ligation of bleeding vessels. It is important to realize that hepatotomy may result in additional bleeding arising from normal hepatic parenchyma, but there is a low risk of rebleeding, necrosis, or sepsis when performed properly. Hepatorrhaphy involves wide placement of large sutures through hepatic parenchyma for compression and tamponade of bleeding and may result in extensive necrosis of the liver but can be used if a coagulopathy is present or if damage control is necessary.

If viable pieces of the liver are still attached to the hilum, or in patients with loss of Glisson's capsule, mesh wrapping has been employed for tamponade of the fractured liver. Synthetic absorbable mesh is used to wrap either the right or left lobe of the liver under tension and secured with suture. A cholecystectomy is recommended when the right lobe is wrapped to avoid necrosis of the gallbladder. Another option is to use a viable omental pedicle that can be mobilized and placed within a hepatic laceration or hepatotomy site to slow additional hepatic venous and portal bleeding. The omentum is then secured within the wound with absorbable sutures that cross the wound edges. Penetrating liver injuries can result in well-defined tracks and techniques have been described to control bleeding within these tracks without the need for an extensive hepatotomy. Several Penrose drains can be passed through the track under tension and when the tension is released the drains shorten and tamponade the track. Balloon tamponade is performed by passing a red rubber catheter through a Penrose drain and then tying the proximal and distal ends of the Penrose drain around the red rubber catheter. This 2-drain system is then passed through the track, and saline infusion through the red rubber drain inflates the Penrose drain to tamponade a bleeder in the track.

Non-anatomical resection refers to removal of injured hepatic parenchyma using the border of injury as the extent of resection rather than a standard surgical plane. This may be performed with blunt finger fracture, a Kelly clamp, or stapling. The rationale is to limit the extent of parenchymal dissection so that additional bleeding is not encountered and that the time required is less than an anatomic resection. Anatomic resection can be performed by experienced surgeons without control of inflow and outflow vessels. Historically, this procedure has been associated with a mortality of 25–50%, is now rarely performed, and reserved for those circumstances when other methods to control bleeding have failed. Total vascular exclusion involves control of the portal triad and suprahepatic and intrahepatic vena cava after complete mobilization of the liver. It is important to note that clamping of the inferior vena cava results in decreased venous return and worsening hemodynamics. This may be avoided by the atriocaval (Schrock) shunt that is placed through the right atrial appendage and advanced through the inferior vena cava below the renal veins and secured above and below the liver. The insertion of the atriocaval shunt, combined with occlusion of the portal triad, allows total vascular exclusion of the liver while preserving venous return to the heart. Unfortunately, the use of the atriocaval shunt for retrohepatic venous injuries is associated with a mortality rate of 50–90% often because insertion is delayed until irreversible shock is present. Instead of inserting an atriocaval shunt, a commercially available bridge balloon can be passed via a femoral vein to tamponade the hole in the cava until the surgical team decides on the best operating approach.

Drainage after repair of a hepatic injury has no influence on mortality, development of a liver abscess, or formation of a biliary fistula. Closed suction drains, however, should be placed when there is a large dead space after extensive resection or debridement, when there is continued oozing after the hepatic repair, or when sutures are likely to cause liver necrosis. Routine postoperative angioembolization is indicated after definitive perihepatic packing and damage control laparotomy when there is continued bleeding from closed suction drains or the need for continued transfusion.

Complications

Complications following SNOM of a hepatic injury may occur in 12–14% of patients and increase with the grade of injury. The complication rates after laparotomy are 1%, 21%, and 63% for grade III, IV, and V injuries, respectively. Elderly patients have an increased risk of general complications including pneumonia, subphrenic abscess, and urinary tract infections with sepsis related to bedrest and the presence of a urinary catheter. Repeat CT scans are indicated if the patient develops increasing abdominal pain, fever, jaundice, or a decrease in hemoglobin. Surveillance CT scan following management of a hepatic injury is not indicated in patients with an uneventful hospital course.

Recurrent bleeding, abdominal compartment syndrome, a subphrenic abscess, bile leak, hemobilia, bilhemia, bile peritonitis, and necrosis of the parenchyma are the most frequent complications after management of a major hepatic injury. Recurrent bleeding is the most dreaded complication with a rate of about 2–7% and is usually caused by extension of a subcapsular hematoma or rupture of a pseudoaneurysm and can usually be treated with angioembolization.

Bile leaks can present in about 3–10% of patients and result in bilomas or bile peritonitis. Most bilomas regress spontaneously but those that enlarge or become infected can be successfully managed with percutaneous drainage that may be combined with an endoscopic sphincterotomy. Bile peritonitis after SNOM is treated with laparoscopy, placement of closed suction drains, and possible sphincterotomy. In patients with post-observation or postoperative melena or hematemesis with bleeding from the ampulla of Vater diagnosed on upper gastrointestinal endoscopy, angioembolization should be used to control the hemobilia resulting from an arteriobilious fistula. With increasing jaundice, endoscopic retrograde cholangiography can be used to treat the bilhemia resulting from a biliovenous fistula, which is quite rare. Perihepatic abscesses can occur in 5–10% of patients with percutaneous drainage as the treatment. When hemorrhage control has resulted in hepatic necrosis that affects the condition of the patient, surgical management is indicated. This is usually done with a non-anatomic resection of the necrotic liver, but an anatomic resection may be indicated if much of a lobe is necrotic. Unplanned interventions such as laparotomy, angioembolization, percutaneous drainage, and endoscopic procedures for complications resulting from hepatic trauma are more commonly observed in patients with higher grades of injury as previously noted.

Geriatric patients managed either with SNOM or with an operation have a longer hospital length of stay than younger patients. Mortality after any operative intervention increases with age with an operative mortality of 42.8% in geriatric patients and 20.4% in younger patients with the most severe injuries. Mortality following SNOM of hepatic injury was 1.3% in geriatric patients and 0.3% in younger patients in one review. It should also be noted that failed SNOM is an independent predictor of mortality.

Acute care surgeons must understand the inferior outcomes in the geriatric patient with hepatic trauma when deciding on management options. The increased morbidity and mortality observed in this patient population should allow for early goals of care discussions following initial resuscitation and intervention. Specific validated scoring systems, such as the Trauma-Specific Frailty Index (TSFI), have been developed to identify elderly trauma patients at risk for poor outcomes following injury and help the acute care surgeon with discussions and disposition. This index has been validated and is expressed as a ratio of points/15 with frailty defined as TSFI >0.25 (Table 21.2). In literature reviews, frail patients were older, had a higher incidence of comorbidities, and were more likely to sustain falls resulting in a higher ISS. Also, frail patients had an increase in hospital complications, transfer to a skilled nursing facility, mortality, and 30-day readmission. An unfavorable discharge disposition is seen more frequently when the TSFI >0.27.

Table 21.2 15 Variable trauma-specific frailty index

Comorbidities	Points
Cancer history	
Yes	1
No	0
Coronary heart disease	
Myocardial infarction	1
Coronary artery bypass grafting	0.75
Percutaneous coronary intervention	0.5
Medication	0.25
No medication	0
Dementia	
Severe	1
Moderate	0.5
Mild	0.25
None	0
Daily activities	
Help with grooming	
Yes	1
No	0
Help with managing money	
Yes	1
No	0
Help doing household work	
Yes	1
No	0
Help toileting	
Yes	1
No	0
Help walking	
Wheelchair	1
Walker	0.75
Cane	0.25
None	0
Health attitude	
Feel less useful	
Most time	1
Sometimes	0.5
Never	0
Feel sad	
Most time	1
Sometimes	0.5
Never	0
Feel effort to do everything	
Most time	1
Sometimes	0.5
Never	0
Falls	
Most time	1
Sometimes	0.5
Never	0
Feel lonely	
Most time	1
Sometimes	0.5
Never	0
Sexually active	
Yes	1
No	0
Albumin	
<3	1
>3	0

References

1. Llompart-Pou JA, Perex-Barcena J, Chico-Fernandez M, et al. Severe trauma in the geriatric population. World J Crit Care Med. 2017;6:99–106.
2. Parks RW, Chrysos R, Diamond T. Management of liver trauma. Br J Surg. 1999;86:1121–35.
3. Badger SA, Barclay R, Campbell R, et al. Management of liver trauma. World J Surg. 2009;33:2522–37.
4. Kozar RA, Crandall M, Shanmuganathan K, et al. Organ injury scaling 2018 update: spleen, liver, and kidney. Trauma Acute Care Surg. 2018;85:1119–22.
5. Poletti PA, Mirvis SE, Shanmuganathan K, et al. CT criteria for management of blunt liver trauma: correlation with angiographic and surgical findings. Radiology. 2000;216:418–27.
6. Sharma OP, Oswanski MF, Singer D, et al. Assessment of nonoperative management of blunt spleen and liver trauma. Am Surg. 2005;71:379–86.
7. Piper GL, Peitzman AB. Current management of hepatic trauma. Surg Clin North Am. 2010;90:775–85.
8. Misselbeck TS, Teicher EJ, Cipolle MD, et al. Hepatic angioembolization in trauma patients: indications and complications. J Trauma. 2009;67:769–73.
9. Carrillo EH, Spain DA, Wohltmann CD, et al. Interventional techniques are useful adjuncts in nonoperative management of hepatic injuries. J Trauma. 2000;46:619–24.
10. Hurtuk M, Reed RL, Esposito TJ, et al. Trauma surgeons practice what they preach: the NTSB

story on solid organ injury management. J Trauma. 2006;61:243–54.
11. Pacher HL, Knudson MM, Esrig N, et al. Status of nonoperative management of blunt hepatic injuries in 1995: a multicenter experience in 404 patients. J Trauma. 1996;40:31–8.
12. Bruns B, Kozar R. Liver and biliary tract. In: Feliciano DV, Mattox KL, Moore EE, editors. Trauma. 9th ed. New York: McGraw Hill; 2020.
13. Gorman E, Bukur M, Frangos S, et al. Increasing age is associated with worse outcomes in elderly patients with severe liver injury. Am J Surg. 2020;220:1308–11.
14. Edalatpour A, Young BT, Brown LR, et al. Grade of injury, not initial management is associated with unplanned interventions in liver injury. Injury. 2020;51:1301–5.
15. Hamidi M, Haddadin Z, Zeeshan M, et al. Prospective evaluation and comparison of the predictive ability of different frailty scores to predict outcomes in geriatric trauma patients. Trauma Acute Care Surg. 2019;87:1172–80.

Injury to Kidney

22

Nezih Akkapulu and Aytekin Ünlü

Introduction

The world's current population is aging, and the geriatric (65 years old and older) population is rapidly growing. Furthermore, it is predicted that about 70 and 90 million US citizens will be older than 65 by 2030 and 2050, respectively. Parallel to this growth, the number of elderly trauma patients is expected to increase.

According to population-based studies, the renal injury rate of hospitalized trauma patients is about 1.5%, and less than 25% are older than 65 years old. Although geriatric renal trauma patients' proportion is a small percentage, it is crucial in terms of patients' outcomes. Regardless of injury mechanisms, management choice, and surgical intervention, geriatric trauma patients have a longer length of hospital stay, higher complication and mortality risks than younger counterparts.

N. Akkapulu (✉)
Faculty of Medicine, Department of General Surgery, Hacettepe University, Ankara, Turkey
e-mail: akkapulu@hacettepe.edu.tr

A. Ünlü
Division of War Surgery, Department of General Surgery, Gulhane Training and Research Hospital, Ankara, Turkey
e-mail: aytekin.unlu@sbu.edu.tr

Physiologic Changes of Kidney in Elderly

Fibrous tissue replaces normal glomerular tissue gradually with aging; this phenomenon is known as glomerulosclerosis and results from an approximate loss of 50% of normal glomerular tissue by 70 years of age. Another aging change is the intimal thickening of renal arterioles due to smooth muscle atrophy and atherosclerosis. These changes in geriatric patients lead to diminishing average capacity for maintaining renal functions and may result in acute kidney injury even in a slight deviation of hemostasis like a trauma.

Besides these alterations, other age-related changes such as frailty, limited physiologic capacity, multiple comorbidities, and multimedications lead to demanding challenges in the medical and surgical management of geriatric trauma patients with renal injury.

Trauma Mechanisms and Diagnosis

Renal trauma incidence is 10% of all abdominal trauma, and the kidney is the most affected organ in the genitourinary system in the geriatric population as in other age groups. The rate of renal injury is lower than other solid organ traumas, independent of the mechanism. However, these injuries can be associated with higher mortality

P. Petrone, C. E.M. Brathwaite (eds.), *Acute Care Surgery in Geriatric Patients*,
https://doi.org/10.1007/978-3-031-30651-8_22

when renal hemorrhage is the most acute and dramatic.

Labib et al. reveal that falls are the most common trauma mechanism in the elderly, with a 72% rate, followed by motor vehicle accidents (25%). Penetrating and other trauma mechanisms comprise nearly 3% of the severely injured geriatric population. Blunt trauma is the primary mechanism for renal injury in geriatric trauma patients. In addition to this rate, penetrating injuries predominate in some level I urban trauma centers. As a result, the overwhelming majority of renal trauma, 90%, occurs from blunt mechanisms also in geriatric trauma patients.

Symptomatology and physical exam findings of renal injury include a broad spectrum. Gross or microscopic hematuria, clues of significant flank trauma such as ecchymosis, rib fractures, or penetrating trauma of the abdomen, flank, or lower chest can herald renal injury.

Comorbid states and medication usage can becloud clinic diagnosis of the geriatric patient. Pre-existing conditions like hypertension and beta-blocker medications can disguise vital signs in significant hemorrhage of a geriatric patient with renal trauma.

The Focused Assessment for Sonography in Trauma (FAST) is the first-line modality to assess for free intra-abdominal fluid and the specification of an injury to solid organs, especially kidneys. Doppler technique for evaluating vascular anatomy and renal perfusion can be used in renal trauma. However, a negative FAST does not exclude renal injury.

The threshold for using computed tomography (CT) should be kept low, as management of the geriatric patient with only clinical or FAST evaluation will not be appropriate. Grading of renal trauma is based on the American Association for the Surgery of Trauma (AAST) Organ Injury Scale for Kidney Injuries (Table 22.1). Although the scale has not been validated in the elderly cohort, it has many modifications, and it was validated in a national cohort that includes 742,774 trauma patients. It predicts morbidity and mortality in blunt trauma and for morbidity in penetrating trauma.

Table 22.1 AAST organ injury scale for kidney injuries

Grade[a]	Type of injury	Description of injury
I	Contusion	Microscopic or gross hematuria, urologic studies normal
	Hematoma	Subcapsular, non-expanding without parenchymal laceration
II	Hematoma	Non-expanding perirenal hematoma confirmed to renal retroperitoneum
	Laceration	<1.0 cm parenchymal depth of renal cortex without urinary extravasation
III	Laceration	>1.0 cm parenchymal depth of renal cortex without collecting system rupture or urinary extravasation
IV	Laceration	Parenchymal laceration extending through renal cortex, medulla, and collecting system
	Vascular	Main renal artery or vein injury with contained hemorrhage
V	Laceration	Completely shattered kidney
	Vascular	Avulsion of the renal hilum, which devascularizes the kidney

[a]Advance one grade for bilateral injuries up to grade III

Recent guidelines offer intravenous contrast-enhanced abdominal and pelvic CT with early and delayed (10–20 min) phases should be performed in suspicion of renal trauma to evaluate renal laceration and collecting system injury. Intravenous administration of contrast agents does not increase the risk of acute kidney injury in a geriatric trauma patient.

Management

Experience and knowledge related to the management of geriatric trauma patients are growing in the literature; however, there are no guideline statements regarding the recommended evaluation and management of geriatric patients with renal injuries.

The first step of evaluating and managing the geriatric patient with renal trauma is hemodynamic stability regardless of trauma mechanism. Transient responder to IV fluid resuscitation or hemodynamically unstable patient with renal trauma should be performed through an intervention like surgery or angioembolization according to the form of trauma, logistics, and experience of the institution.

The surgery's aim should consist of damage control principles; first, uncontrolled bleeding should be stopped, avoid nephrectomy if possible and obtain the perinephric drainage. The presence of concomitant abdominal trauma, Grade V injuries, life-threatening hemorrhage from the renovascular bundle, ureteropelvic junction avulsion, and persistent urinoma despite perinephric drainage or ureteral stenting are the main indications of surgery.

Endovascular approaches, especially selective embolization (Figs. 22.1 and 22.2), are an excellent option for controlling renovascular bleeding in selected patients with penetrating and blunt trauma. Patient selection for embolization is based on criteria such as contrast extravasation, perinephric hematoma greater than 3.5 cm, and complex vascular injury (including pseudoaneurysm and fistula). The success rate can reach 80% in high-volume centers. Fails of intervention rates are three times higher in penetrating injuries. Besides, geriatric patients are at higher risk of failure due to age-related vascular discrepancies, and needing additional intervention like surgery can increase the risk of morbidity and mortality in elderly patients.

Non-operative management is also the mainstay option for hemodynamically stable geriatric patients with renal trauma. Patients with regular CT scans and AAST Grade I–II injuries did not need observation longer than 24 h and hospitalization regardless of trauma mechanism. Patients with AAST Grade III renal injuries are a candidate for bed rest, supportive care, and observation. AAST Grade I to III traumas have a low risk of early and late complications. Therefore, follow-up CT scan is recommended if the patient becomes clinically deteriorated. AAST Grade IV and V geriatric patients with renal trauma can be managed conservatively, but the threshold of the intervention should be kept lower in the geriatric population. A follow-up CT scan after 24 or 48 h is cautious in patients with AAST Grade IV and V because of the risk of developing complications such as urinoma and hemorrhage.

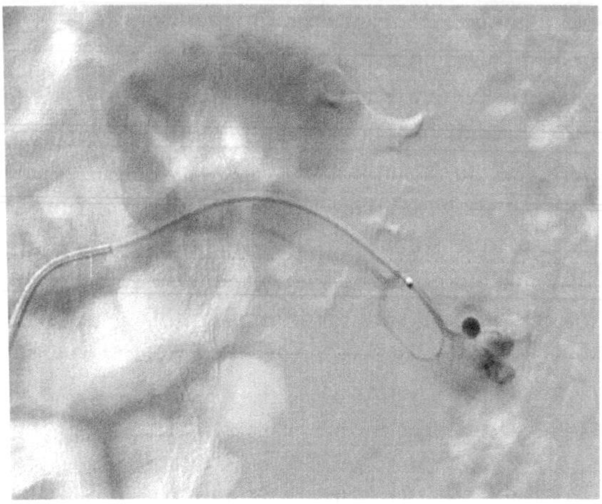

Fig. 22.1 Selective angiography of a geriatric patient with blunt trauma: a complex lobulated pseudoaneurysm is visualized on the left lower pole interlobar artery (courtesy of Gonca Eldem, MD)

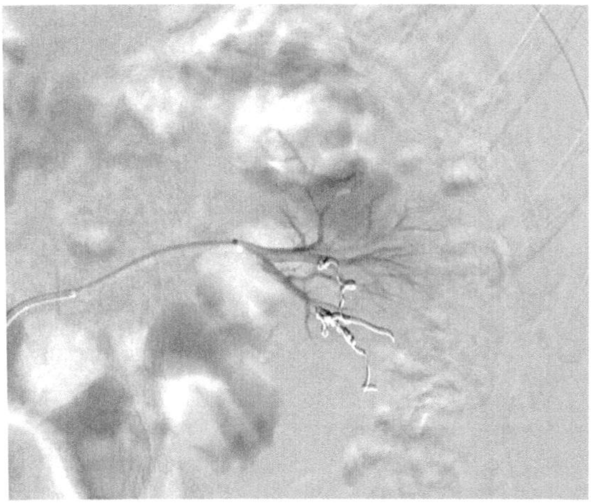

Fig. 22.2 Post-embolization angiography image of the same patient: the interlobar arteries of the pseudoaneurysms are embolized with detachable coils (courtesy of Gonca Eldem, MD)

Conclusions

The geriatric population and as well as the number of geriatric trauma patients are increasing. Physiologic changes in the elderly become a unique and challenging population in trauma management. Falls are the most common mechanism in the geriatric trauma and renal trauma of geriatric patients. Hemodynamic stability is the most crucial decision-making factor in geriatric patients with renal trauma. CT scans and conservative management are the cornerstones in hemodynamically stable patients. Age-related grading systems and guidelines are necessary for managing geriatric patients with renal injury.

References

1. Clare D, Zink KL. Geriatric Trauma. Emerg Med Clin North Am. 2021;39(2):257–71.
2. Wessells H, et al. Renal injury and operative management in the United States: results of a population-based study. J Trauma. 2003;54(3):423–30.
3. Nakao S, et al. Trends and outcomes of blunt renal trauma management: a nationwide cohort study in Japan. World J Emerg Surg. 2020;15(1):50.
4. Bonne S, Schuerer DJ. Trauma in the older adult: epidemiology and evolving geriatric trauma principles. Clin Geriatr Med. 2013;29(1):137–50.
5. Metcalf M, Broghammer JA. Genitourinary trauma in geriatric patients. Curr Opin Urol. 2016;26(2):165–70.
6. Brooks SE, Peetz AB. Evidence-based care of geriatric trauma patients. Surg Clin North Am. 2017;97(5):1157–74.
7. Myers JB, Brant WO, Broghammer JA. High-grade renal injuries: radiographic findings correlated with intervention for renal hemorrhage. Urol Clin North Am. 2013;40(3):335–41.
8. Labib N, et al. Severely injured geriatric population: morbidity, mortality, and risk factors. J Trauma. 2011;71(6):1908–14.
9. Buckley JC, McAninch JW. Selective management of isolated and nonisolated grade IV renal injuries. J Urol. 2006;176(6 Pt 1):2498–502.
10. Morey AF, et al. Urotrauma: AUA guideline. J Urol. 2014;192(2):327–35.
11. Sadro CT, et al. Geriatric trauma: a Radiologist's guide to imaging trauma patients aged 65 years and older. Radiographics. 2015;35(4):1263–85.
12. Serafetinides E, et al. Review of the current management of upper urinary tract injuries by the EAU trauma guidelines panel. Eur Urol. 2015;67(5):930–6.
13. Moore EE, et al. Organ injury scaling: spleen, liver, and kidney. J Trauma. 1989;29(12):1664–6.
14. Kuan JK, et al. American Association for the Surgery of Trauma organ injury scale for kidney injuries predicts nephrectomy, dialysis, and death in patients with blunt injury and nephrectomy for penetrating injuries. J Trauma. 2006;60(2):351–6.
15. Johnsen NV, et al. Surgical Management of Solid Organ Injuries. Surg Clin North Am. 2017;97(5):1077–105.

23 Emergency Hernia Repair in the Elderly

David K. Halpern

Introduction

Urgent hernia repair is one of the most common general surgery emergencies. The risk of ventral incisional hernia after midline laparotomy incision is at least 20% and is predicted to be twice as high in patients with associated comorbidities. The obesity crisis in America has further challenged the general surgeon and herniologist. Increasing abdominal circumference is associated with a corresponding increasing risk of hernia recurrence. Studies have shown that BMI >50 may be associated with hernia recurrence of close to 100%. With each recurrence, hernias become more complex. Fibrosis from previous repairs, altered anatomy and mesh prosthesis make subsequent repairs more difficult.

On a similar note, the percentage of the US population over 65 is increasing dramatically. Current models predict the population of geriatric patients in the USA to double in the next 30 years, with a potential for almost 70 million patients by the year 2030. Geriatric patients are more likely to develop hernia due to issues such as constipation, prostatism, chronic cough, and malnutrition. Age has been shown to be an independent risk factor for morbidity and mortality in patients undergoing emergency hernia repair. Polypharmacy, comorbidities, frailty, and delirium in this population further complicate surgical recovery. Knowing when and how to operate is paramount to having good outcomes.

General surgeons and internists often recommend watchful waiting for geriatric patients with asymptomatic hernias. Fear of surgical complications or decompensation in frail elderly patients with comorbidities is generally the rationale for this recommendation. Multiple studies have supported the role for watchful waiting in this scenario, with the 4-year risk of acute emergency likely less than 5%. While the risk of acute incarceration and strangulation is not high, the outcomes of intervention in the acute scenario are often poor in the geriatric population. Wound morbidity rates, hospital length of stay, need for bowel resection, hernia recurrence rates, and mortality rates are significant in geriatric patients undergoing emergent repair. The anesthetic choice may also be suboptimal as almost all patients undergoing emergent repair will require general anesthesia. Those who undergo elective repair may be candidates for local anesthesia and sedation. Because of the above factors, all patients who are acceptable candidates for surgery should strongly be considered for elective repair. Symptomatic patients, on the other hand, have a higher incidence to progress to incarceration and strangulation. Patients with symptomatic hernias should be encouraged to undergo elective repair.

D. K. Halpern (✉)
Department of Surgery, NYU Langone Hospital—Long Island, Mineola, NY, USA
e-mail: david.halpern@nyulangone.org

P. Petrone, C. E.M. Brathwaite (eds.), *Acute Care Surgery in Geriatric Patients*,
https://doi.org/10.1007/978-3-031-30651-8_23

Basic Principles of Emergency Hernia Repair in the Geriatric Patient

When faced with an acutely incarcerated hernia in an elderly patient, the algorithm towards surgery shifts. Despite associated comorbidities, a surgical emergency cannot be ignored. Delaying intervention beyond 24 h of onset of symptoms has a significant effect on surgical outcomes. All patients with painful, irreducible hernias require urgent surgical evaluation. Findings such as skin erythema, bowel obstruction at the neck of an irreducible hernia, or signs of systemic sepsis often prompt urgent surgical intervention. If there are no signs of bowel compromise, an attempt at manual reduction of the hernia with or without sedation should be made.

There are instances, however, when the need for surgical intervention may not be so clear. Patients with wide neck ventral hernias or voluminous hernia sacs may present with abdominal pain and distention. If radiographic evaluation demonstrates a bowel obstruction, it is important to discern whether the hernia is the culprit, or whether an adhesive obstruction exists that is unrelated to the hernia anatomy. The former will require urgent surgical exploration, while the latter may benefit from a conservative trial.

The general surgeon must use sound judgment and practical thinking in the acute care setting. The surgeon should be encouraged to operate within their ability and must have the knowledge to discern which techniques are feasible in the emergency setting. The goal of surgery must be clearly defined. In an elderly decompensated patient, one should strive to fix the problem at hand with the least intervention. A suboptimal repair in an alive patient is preferable to a surgical mortality. Damage control laparotomy with resection of necrotic bowel, temporary abdominal closure device with second look and definitive closure is a sound option in the appropriate clinical setting.

Patients with complex or recurrent hernias present unique challenges in the emergency setting. The management of these patients will be discussed at length later in the chapter. Simply put, the idea is not to get fancy. Formal abdominal wall reconstruction with myofascial advancement should be discouraged. Mesh explantation should be avoided if possible. Sac closure, bridging mesh, incorporation of previous mesh and simple closure are all feasible options. The use of permanent suture and prosthesis should be balanced with the degree of surgical contamination and wound morbidity. The concept of accepting a higher risk of hernia recurrence and utilization of damage control techniques should be a recurring theme in the acute management of hernia in the geriatric population.

Lastly, hubris has no place in the operating room. Some of us practice in rural settings or with limited resources. In that situation, we operate to the best of our ability and use what is at hand to remedy the situation. Some of us work in academic medical centers where there are experts in the delivery of tertiary care. For those of us so fortunate, when we encounter difficult problem, call for help. Two sets of eyes are better than one, and discussion often brings clarity as to the best approach to achieve a favorable outcome.

Preoperative Workup

In evaluating the geriatric patient in the acute care setting, one should have a unique toolbox to assess the challenges associated with treating this population. All geriatric patients should undergo some form of functional assessment, including dementia screening, fall risk assessment, delirium screening and frailty score. Risk assessment tools serve as prognostic indicators of surgical outcome. While not absolute, they are useful in guiding patients, family members and caretakers as to expected convalescence. Quality of life after emergency surgery in the elderly is often significantly impacted. In the rare instance that a patient with acute hernia presents in severe extremis or is deemed unsalvageable, comfort measures may be appropriate rather than an attempt at heroic intervention.

Mortality rates after emergency hernia repair in the elderly are reported in the literature to be 2.8%. Almost all patients can be expected to undergo emergent repair. A complete history and physical evaluation should be obtained on all patients. Tobacco usage, presence of diabetes, pulmonary disease, and use of immunomodulators should be noted. Patients should be queried as to the number of previous hernia repairs, presence of mesh or prior wound complications. Directed physical examination with attention to the integrity of overlying skin, presence or absence of draining sinuses, previous scars, abdominal obesity, and body contour. HbA1c testing should be conducted on all patients with history of diabetes, glucose intolerance, or risk factors for diabetes. Body mass index should be calculated, and a nutritional assessment should be performed. Patients with nausea and vomiting may present with dehydration and electrolyte abnormalities. Fluid resuscitation and any metabolic derangements should be corrected.

Approximately 20% of elderly patients requiring acute hernia surgery will be on some form of anticoagulation. Coumadin-induced coagulopathy can be rapidly reversed with prothrombin complex concentrate, Vitamin K or fresh frozen plasma. Direct acting oral anticoagulants can be reversed with their respective reversal agents: idarucizumab for dabigatran and andexanet alfa for apixaban and rivaroxaban. Prothrombin complex concentrate can also be used in this scenario. The effects of antiplatelet therapy from clopidogrel, prasugrel, and ticagrelor can be controlled with DDAVP and perioperative platelet transfusions as needed.

Radiographic imaging is helpful in the workup of hernia in the acute setting. Although the diagnosis of incarcerated hernia in a patient presenting with sudden onset of a painful irreducible groin mass in the face of a clinical bowel obstruction may be obvious, the information obtained from cross sectional radiographic imaging is useful. The availability of rapid CT scanning in the emergency department has increased in recent years. CT scan is useful in delineating hernia anatomy and complexity. A fat containing hernia with acute incarceration becomes less of an emergency than that of a similar hernia containing compromised bowel. Such findings may allow more time for fluid resuscitation, correction of electrolyte abnormalities or reversal of anticoagulants if needed. CT may also help define whether there is a hernia-specific emergency, or whether there is some other emergency that may be amenable to nonoperative management. The size and number of hernia defects, the presence of previous mesh and the proximity of the hernia orifice to bony structures can all be readily assessed with CT scan. This information is useful in planning the approach and technique of hernia repair in the emergency setting.

Ventral Hernia Repair

Emergent ventral hernia repair in the elderly population remains a costly burden on the health care system. Advanced age has been shown to be a negative independent prognostic indicator upon both morbidity and mortality of urgent hernia repair. Prompt recognition and appropriate planning are important to achieve favorable outcomes.

When evaluating a patient with abdominal pain and ventral hernia, it is important to discern whether the acute pathology is related to the hernia, or some other abdominal pathology. A patient with a tender, irreducible hernia with overlying skin changes or peritonitis will need urgent surgical exploration. As hernia size and complexity increase, the ability to discern whether there is a hernia-specific emergency may become more confounded. CT imaging can be very useful in this regard. Stable patients with imaging findings suggestive of an adhesive obstruction unrelated to the hernia anatomy may be managed conservatively if there are no signs of bowel compromise. NPO status and iv hydration should be commenced with the addition of nasogastric decompression at the discretion of the surgeon. Delayed imaging looking for progression of oral contrast beyond the area of obstruction may be useful to evaluate resolution of the obstruction. Gastrografin challenge has been advocated to assist in the paradigm as to whether surgical intervention is necessary. Gastrografin should be used with caution in the elderly population. This is particularly important if there are risk factors for aspiration such as altered mental status, dysphagia, or gastric distention. Pneumonitis caused by aspiration of gastrografin can be quite potent and cause a rapid decline in patients respiratory status resulting in the need for endotracheal intubation, and sometimes causing the patient's demise.

If initial CT imaging demonstrated obstruction at the hernia neck, signs of a closed loop obstruction, or evidence of vascular compromise, a conservative trial is inappropriate. These patients should be taken urgently to the operating room. Additionally, when there is uncertainty, it is better to err on the side of a more aggressive approach. Delay to surgery beyond 24 h and need for bowel resection have been found to be risk factors for morbidity and mortality in this patient population.

Once a decision for surgery is made, the surgeon must now decide whether a definitive repair will be performed or whether a staged approach will be used. Ventral hernia represents a broad array of pathology. In the acute setting, a simple umbilical hernia can be repaired with suture technique or mesh technique with favorable results. The approach to repair will vary based on the complexity of the hernia, wound-specific factors, and patient characteristics. The principles of modern definitive hernia repair are based upon the concept of defect closure and restoring the native anatomy of the abdominal wall as best possible. This is usually followed by reinforcement of the repair with a mesh prosthesis. Placement of a permanent mesh prosthesis has been shown to have superior results in terms of hernia recurrence.

Wound morbidity is a significant risk factor for hernia recurrence. There is a preponderance of evidence supporting the concept of preoptimization of specific patient factors prior elective hernia repair to improve hernia recurrence rates and decrease wound morbidity. The same principle should be applied to hernia repair in the emergent setting. The surgeon should be aware that a patient with a BMI >35, HbA1c >7.2, tobacco usage, use of immunosuppressive medications, chronic pulmonary disease or malnutrition will be more likely to experience postoperative wound complications and have a higher incidence of hernia recurrence. For such patients in the acute setting, it may be wiser to perform a tissue repair or use a bioabsorbable mesh. These approaches have a higher incidence of hernia recurrence but are associated with decreased wound morbidity. Definitive repair of a recurrent hernia can be delayed to the elective setting when the patient is properly optimized.

Wound classification will also influence the decision as to whether a definitive or staged approach is used. In clean or clean contaminated wounds (class 1 and 2), a permanent mesh prosthesis can be utilized with favorable results. As the degree of wound contamination increases, the risk of wound complications and mesh infection increases. With contaminated or dirty wounds (class 3 and 4), the use of a permanent mesh prosthesis should be avoided. The surgeon may elect to perform primary fascial repair with or without the use of a bioabsorbable mesh. In severely contaminated wounds temporary abdominal closure with a wound vac or similar dressing may be appropriate. The patient may be returned to the OR for primary closure with or without reinforcement with a bioabsorbable mesh.

Elderly patients with large complex or recurrent incisional hernias present formidable challenges. Proper repair of these defects often requires techniques of abdominal wall reconstruction (AWR). AWR involves the development of myofascial advancement flaps to repair the hernia(s). The goal is restoration of the midline fascia or central tendon of the abdomen, followed by reinforcement with a mesh prosthesis. Many geriatric patients with complex hernias defer elective repair because of comorbidities or deconditioning. When these patients present acutely, the proper approach becomes even more challenging. In most instances, formal abdominal wall reconstruction with component separation techniques should be avoided in the acute setting. Patients may not be adequately optimized for definitive repair, and the catabolic state associated with acute surgical emergencies hinders wound healing. There is an increased risk of perioperative wound morbidity, and the opportunity for future definitive repair is compromised.

Additionally, the postoperative physiology associated with complex abdominal wall reconstruction and midline repair such as increased intra-abdominal pressure may cause decreased cardiac output and respiratory compromise.

In almost all instances of acute hernia incarceration with complex hernia or need for bowel resection, the abdominal wall can be safely temporized. If previous mesh is present, one should make an assessment as to the integrity and condition of the existing mesh. If the mesh is well incorporated, explantation should be avoided in the emergency setting. It is acceptable to incorporate old mesh into the repair in this situation. One must realize that mesh will not heal to mesh. If a permanent suture is not used, the hernia will recur as the suture resorbs. One must balance the risk of wound complications and suture granuloma formation with hernia recurrence. The approach will vary based on the complexity of the hernia. With large defects, it is acceptable to place a bridging mesh to achieve abdominal closure. The prosthesis should be appropriate for the degree of wound contamination. If a permanent or synthetic bioabsorbable prosthesis is selected, one with an adhesion barrier should be used. Alternatively, hernia sac or omentum can be harvested for use as an adhesion barrier. On occasion, skin only closure may be appropriate. One must be aware that this technique places the patient at risk for postoperative wound dehiscence and evisceration, The consequences of such may be catastrophic with the development of enterocutaneous or enteroatmospheric fistula if not properly managed. Additionally, leaving the midline fascia separated without any support or bridge allows for unopposed lateral pull of the oblique muscles. Over time, this will often lead to the development of giant abdominal wall defects with loss of domain.

One must employ common sense and be cognizant of what techniques will work and which will fail in temporizing complex hernia in the acute setting. For instance, sac only closure of complex hernia with a large thin sac extending into an abdominal pannus on an obese patient will likely not work. This patient may be better served with a bridge repair. On the other hand, a patient with a thick, fibrotic sac of a complex recurrent hernia with retracted musculature may do fine with sac and skin only closure as a temporizing repair.

Traditional approaches to emergent ventral repair have been described using open techniques. There is increasing evidence to the safety and efficacy of minimally invasive (MIS) repair. MIS repair offers the advantage of decreased wound complication and may allow definitive repair in a patient who may otherwise have not been properly optimized. Defect closure can be performed with a suture passer, or with laparoscopic suturing. The robotic platform has facilitated the ability to close fascial defects. Immunofluorescence angiography may also be used to assess the viability of the viscera if there is concern for vascular compromise. If an MIS approach is used and the viscera cannot be reduced, a hybrid approach may be used. One can explore the hernia sac through a limited incision, reduce the contents of the hernia, drop the mesh into the abdomen through the hernia defect, and complete the defect closure through the limited incision. One can then return to laparoscopy for final mesh positioning and fixation. This technique may offer advantages particularly on morbidly obese patients with complex hernias.

Mesh Selection

There is plethora on hernia mesh available. An in-depth review of hernia mesh is beyond the scope of this chapter. Mesh placement during hernia repair is associated with decreased risk of hernia recurrence. A basic knowledge of types of hernia mesh available in today's market, their characteristics and indications for usage is a minimal requirement for the general or acute care surgeon dealing with hernia in the emergent situation. A review will be provided below.

Polypropylene (PPP) mesh has been the mainstay of hernia repair. Introduced in 1958 by Usher, it is probably the most used and best studied mesh on the market. PPP is a permanent monofilament. The mesh is available in both microporous (heavyweight) or macroporous (midweight/lightweight) weave. Macroporous mesh allows for increased tissue ingrowth and less foreign body reaction, whereas microporous mesh has a higher tensile strength and may be more suited for bridging repairs. Microporous heavyweight PPP mesh may cause intense foreign body reaction like fibrosis in some patients.

Polyester mesh is also available as a permanent prosthesis. The mesh is more hydrophilic than polypropylene and which may promote rapid tissue ingrowth. Most polyester mesh is braided as opposed to a true monofilament.

Both polypropylene and polyester mesh are available in coated and uncoated forms. In coated form, a hyaluronic acid, omega 3 acid or similar substance is applied to one side of the mesh. The coating allows for intra-abdominal mesh placement and is designed to prevent the formation of visceral adhesion to the mesh. Uncoated mesh is designed to promote tissue ingrowth and should not be placed against the intra-abdominal viscera.

PTFE represents a third type of permanent mesh prosthesis. It is available in flat sheets (microporous), or as mesh weave (macroporous). PTFE encapsulates rather than integrates into tissue and is less resistant to bacterial load. In its microporous form, it can be placed against the abdominal viscera without an adhesion barrier. PTFE has a high tensile strength but is prone to contracture and should not be placed in contaminated fields.

In general, the use of permanent prosthesis should be avoided in a contaminated setting. The risk of infection varies with the degree of wound contamination and the layer of the abdominal wall into which the mesh is implanted. There have been several studies demonstrating the safety and efficacy of macroporous PPP mesh in contaminated fields when the mesh is placed in the retromuscular space. Placement of mesh in this, however, requires specialized techniques that may not be feasible in the acute setting.

There are a number of bioabsorbable meshes on the market today. Bioabsorbable mesh can be divided into biologic and synthetic categories. Biologic mesh is derived from human, bovine, porcine, or ovine sources. These meshes are costly and offer inferior results to permanent mesh prosthesis in terms of hernia recurrence. They are however suitable for placement against viscera, can be used in contaminated fields and may be used as bridging repairs in the emergency setting when the abdominal wall cannot be closed primarily.

Synthetic bioabsorbable mesh is also available. The most common materials used are polyglycolic acid (PGA), polyglycolic acid with trimethylene carbonate (PGA-TMC), or poly-4-hydroxybutyrate. Polyglycolic acid is less costly and can be placed against the viscera. Poly-4-hydroxybutyrate is more costly and is available in uncoated form or is coated on one side with a hydrogel barrier to allow for placement against viscera. PGA mesh is rapidly degraded and loses its tensile strength quickly. It is suitable for temporary abdominal closure but generally results in hernia at the site of mesh implantation. PGA-TMC is more slowly resorbed and can be used as a means of tissue reinforcement. Poly-4-hydroxybutyrate has shown promising results in terms of hernia recurrence.

Hybrid meshes composed of both absorbable and permanent prostheses are available. The surgeon should be familiar with the various products available at their institution and should develop an algorithm for use based on the degree of contamination, patient comorbidities, and the tissue layer in which the mesh is to be implanted. As the degree of contamination increases, the trend is towards usage of a bioabsorbable mesh. A word of caution, however, is that even bioabsorbable mesh can become infected. Biologic mesh may degrade more rapidly in contaminated fields. Lastly, the hydrogel barrier placed on coated mesh changes the characteristics of the mesh. Coated mesh may be less likely to clear a bacterial load than uncoated mesh.

Inguinal Hernia Repair

The incidence of inguinal hernia increases with age. The management of asymptomatic inguinal hernia in the elderly remains a subject of debate. Asymptomatic inguinal hernias in men can be safely observed with a low risk of incarceration. Femoral hernias, on the other hand, have a high risk of strangulation and should be repaired. At least 20% of groin hernias in females will be femoral in nature. For this reason, female patients with asymptomatic groin hernias should be counseled to undergo elective repair. All symptomatic inguinal hernias should be repaired.

The overall mortality for emergent inguinal hernia repair in the geriatric population is <3%. Morbidity rates are approximately 20%. Impaired mental status, heart and lung dysfunctions, and oral anticoagulant therapy have been identified as factors increasing the risk of major complications and mortality. Ischemic related bowel resection may increase mortality up to 20%. Therefore, prompt reduction of incarcerated viscera is important. If there are no secondary signs of ischemia on examination (wound erythema, crepitus, systemic inflammatory response), an attempt at manual reduction of the hernia contents with or without sedation should be made. If complete reduction of the hernia contents is successful, the patient can be observed and scheduled for elective or semi-elective repair based on clinical course.

For elderly patients undergoing emergency surgery for groin hernia, approximately 20% of patients will require laparotomy and bowel resection. A similar number will have a non-mesh repair and may therefore be subjected to a higher risk of hernia recurrence. Although there are no randomized trials comparing the outcomes of elective versus urgent hernia repair in the elderly, the morbidity of urgent repair makes one question the idea of watchful waiting in asymptomatic groin hernia.

Studies have shown that mesh repair of inguinal hernia offers the lowest risk of hernia recurrence. Open mesh repair and MIS repair offer similar risk of recurrence (1%). Many consider the Lichtenstein repair to the gold standard of open inguinal repair. Mesh-related complications such as inguinodynia are minimized by placing a flat piece of mesh, preserving the cremasteric fascia, and avoiding manipulation of the neuroanatomy. The risk of chronic groin pain felt to be less than 1% in expert hands. The plug and patch technique popularized by Gilbert is a useful tool to have in the armamentarium of the acute care surgeon. Because of the three-dimensional mesh, it has an associated incidence of inguinodynia and foreign body sensation of up to 6% and should therefore be used only if other options are not feasible.

Tissue-based repair avoids the morbidity of mesh prosthesis. In the elective setting, mesh infection after inguinal repair is a rare event. In the emergency setting, some authors have reported mesh infection rates of up to 60% in the elderly population. In general, mesh complications after concomitant bowel resection are felt to be around 38%. For this reason, it is important for the general surgeon to be familiar with various tissue repairs. The Shouldice repair offers the lowest recurrence rate of all tissue-based repairs, with reported recurrence rates in the literature ranging between 0.2 and 2.7%. It is currently regarded as the gold standard for tissue repair. The technique of the repair is complex, and outcomes may not be as favorable in obese patients or those with a high BMI. Bassini repair is a similar technique and involves suturing the conjoined tendon to the iliopubic tract. Recurrence ranges between 2.9 and 25.0%, and the repair does not address femoral hernias. In contrast, the McVay repair addresses the femoral space by suturing the triple layer (conjoined tendon) to the pectineal (Cooper's) ligament. It is a tension repair often requiring a relaxing incision. Hernia recurrence rates vary between 1.5 and 15.5%.

MIS inguinal repair is safe and effective in the elderly population. Laparoscopic and robotic approaches are both feasible. MIS repairs offer the advantage of decreased acute and chronic pain as compared to open mesh repair. Both Transabdominal Preperitoneal (TAP) and Total Extraperitoneal approaches (TEP) offer similar outcomes in terms of hernia recurrence and chronic pain. TAP affords the ability to assess the intrabdominal viscera and evaluate for contralateral hernias. It may be associated with a higher risk of trocar site hernia and postoperative bowel obstruction.

Anesthetic approach may influence outcomes in the geriatric population. Local anesthesia and sedation provide several advantages. It avoids the risk of general anesthesia, which is associated with hemodynamic variability, increased risk of postoperative delirium and long-term cognitive dysfunction in the elderly. It affords the ability to perform nerve block for postoperative analgesia and decreases the risk of urinary retention. In the elective setting, open inguinal repair under local anesthesia and sedation may be a gentler approach for the frail elderly patient with comorbid illness. Alternatively, the patient may undergo minimally invasive repair under general anesthesia. The choice depends upon the patient's comorbidities, tolerance for general anesthesia, and a discussion on the goals of surgical intervention. When patients present with acute incarceration, the algorithm changes. In this instance, endotracheal intubation and general anesthesia is often required. This provides airway protection to minimize the risk of aspiration in patients with bowel obstruction. It provides muscle relaxation which may help in the reduction of the hernia contents and affords the ability to convert to exploratory laparotomy without changing the anesthetic plan mid surgery.

The choice of MIS versus open repair will depend on the clinical scenario, hernia characteristics, and the surgeon's skill set and comfort level. From an MIS approach, TAP offers the ability of prompt reduction and inspection of the abdominal viscera. If bowel is viable, the myopectineal orifice is then accessed via a peritoneal flap and a mesh prosthesis is placed. If bowel viability is questionable, immunofluorescence angiography may be used as an adjunct in assessment. The need for bowel resection may prompt conversion to an open inguinal approach followed by a tissue-based repair. Or alternatively, the patient may be re-prepped and draped, and separate gowns, gloves, and instruments used to allow for mesh placement via open inguinal approach in a clean field.

TEP in the emergent setting offers direct access to the myopectineal orifice without entering the peritoneal sac. This may facilitate reduction of femoral hernias by allowing direct access for division of the lacunar ligament. Alternatively, direct and indirect hernias can be reduced using external pressure and careful enlargement of the hernia orifice as necessary. Post reduction, if there is no evidence of purulence, the hernia sac is not necrotic and the peritoneum has not been violated, one can proceed with hernia repair and mesh placement can ensue in a "clean" environment. The preperitoneal space is deflated and the laparoscope is then redirected into the peritoneal cavity via a separate incision to allow for inspection of the viscera. Bowel resection, if necessary, can proceed via an open or laparoscopic approach. If the preperitoneal space is found to be grossly contaminated, the hernia should be repaired using an open tissue-based repair.

Open repair is also a feasible approach in the acute setting. If an inguinal approach is used, care is taken to avoid reduction of the contents of the hernia sac prior to inspection of its contents. If the bowel is found to be necrotic, it can be resected via the hernia sac followed by appropriate tissue repair of the hernia defect. Alternatively, the contents can be returned to the abdomen, the hernia repaired, and a separate laparotomy incision made to proceed with visceral resection. If the contents of the hernia sac reduce unexpectedly prior to inspection, the hernia should be repaired with or without mesh as deemed appropriate, followed by diagnostic laparoscopy to assess bowel viability. Necrosis of the hernia sac and bloody ascitic fluid within the hernia sac are often predictors of bowel necrosis. These findings alone are not contraindications to mesh placement if the operative field has otherwise remained uncontaminated.

Another open approach that is sometimes useful in the emergent setting is the Stoppa repair, via a lower midline incision. The preperitoneal space is accessed via a lower midline incision without violating the peritoneum. Similar to what has been described with the MIS TEP repair above, the contents of the hernia sac are reduced and a mesh prothesis placed in a "clean" field. Once the hernia is repaired, the peritoneum is opened in the midline and the viscera inspected.

Parastomal Hernia Repair

At least 50% of patients with stomas will develop parastomal hernias. The most effective technique for repairing parastomal hernia in the elective setting is reversal of the stoma when feasible. This approach is not appropriate in the emergent setting. The general surgeon should be familiar with techniques for parastomal repair and their associated outcomes.

The morbidity and mortality of emergent parastomal hernia repair is significant. Patient presenting with bowel necrosis of the entrapped segment or associated conduit will require resection. The addition of bowel resection in this scenario increased the perioperative risk. In this scenario, it is often most appropriate to perform a primary tissue repair of the parastomal hernia. Recurrence rates for primary repair approach 100%; however, the technique is simple, carries little wound morbidity, and allows rapid temporary correction of the hernia defect in the unstable patient.

Some studies have suggested decrease wound morbidity with laparoscopic repair over open repair. The European Hernia Society Consensus Guidelines made no recommendation as to superiority of either repair technique. Sugarbaker technique of hernia repair has been associated with the lowest hernia recurrence rates (6.4–18.0%). Recurrence rates for keyhole techniques are reported to range between 13.1 and 60.3%. There are no well powered randomized trials comparing the two techniques, and the EHS guidelines made only weak recommendation of the preference of a flat piece of mesh over a keyhole technique.

As far as selection of mesh prosthesis, permanent synthetic mesh without an adhesion barrier should be avoided in the intraperitoneal location. There have been reports of bowel erosion and the development of bowel obstruction as well as entero-prosthetic fistula in this scenario. Generally, if there is no contamination, the placement of a permanent prosthetic mesh suitable for intraperitoneal positioning is the preferred approach. Bioabsorbable mesh may be preferable in the contaminated setting. However, the use of bioabsorbable mesh with a Sugarbaker technique is generally discouraged as hernia recurrence rates are reported to be high ranging between 16 and 90%.

Postoperative Management and Complications

Elderly patients in the acute setting are often less tolerant of surgical complications. Additionally, the physiologic response to complications may be blunted in the geriatric population. Tachycardia, fever, leukocytosis, and other signs of systemic inflammatory response may not be present. The practitioner should have a high index of suspicion and be cognizant that lethargy, delirium, and failure to thrive in the postoperative period may be indicative of ongoing infection.

A team approach to rehabilitation of the geriatric patient is preferred. Elderly patients often have poor reserve and are more likely to require discharge to a skilled nursing facility after acute hospitalization. Particular attention should be paid to nutritional status and early mobilization in the postoperative period. All patients should have physical therapy consultation initiated in the immediate postoperative period. Patients with renal insufficiency, cardiac disease, diabetes, or other medical comorbidities may benefit from consultation with medical specialists. Delirium carries significant mortality in the postoperative period. Patients with delirium may benefit from psychiatric consultation and review of polypharmacy as a potential cause. Social services consultation may be beneficial in transitioning to post-hospital care.

Hernia-specific complications may arise in the postoperative period. Diabetes mellitus, COPD, intestinal necrosis, and general anesthesia have been identified as risk factors for postoperative wound complications after incarcerated hernia repair. Wound seroma is a common scenario. Generally, seroma is managed expectantly and more than 80% will resolve spontaneously without the need for intervention. Wound abscesses require drainage. Patients with infected collections around mesh often require surgical wound exploration. Mesh explanation and rates of mesh salvage in the acute setting will depend on the type of mesh, the tissue layer into which it is implanted and the degree of tissue ingrowth that has occurred. Mesh that is poorly incorporated should be debrided or removed. If tissue ingrowth has occurred, most macroporous meshes can be salvaged with antimicrobial therapy, aggressive wound debridement, pulse lavage irrigation techniques and negative pressure wound therapy. The role of suppressive antibiotics and long-term salvage rates remain unclear.

Summary

Emergency hernia repair in the geriatric patient is a growing challenge that will increase in prevalence over time. The morbidity and mortality of emergent hernia repair in the elderly is significant, and one should consider elective repair in this patient population as a preventative measure. Patient acuity and hernia-specific factors dictate the urgency of intervention. A damage control concept or staged approach should be used when faced with an unstable patient, complex anatomy, or a patient who is otherwise not adequately optimized for definitive repair. Utilization and selection of mesh prosthesis is influenced by wound class, hernia characteristics, patient factors, and degree of contamination. In all instances, a suboptimal repair with increased risk of hernia recurrence should be favored in lieu of attempting a complex repair in an unstable patient. It is better to have an alive patient with a hernia recurrence than a surgical mortality.

References

1. Miller KE, Zylstra RG, Standridge JB. The geriatric patient: a systematic approach to maintaining health. Am Fam Physician. 2000;61(4):1089–104. Erratum in: Am Fam Physician 2000 Oct 1;62(7):1519–20
2. Ceresoli M, Carissimi F, Nigro A, Fransvea P, Lepre L, Braga M, Costa G, et al. Emergency hernia repair in the elderly: multivariate analysis of morbidity and mortality from an Italian registry. Hernia. 2022;26(1):165–75. https://doi.org/10.1007/s10029-020-02269-5.
3. Surek A, Gemici E, Ferahman S, Karli M, Bozkurt MA, Dural AC, et al. Emergency surgery of the abdominal wall hernias: risk factors that increase morbidity and mortality-a single-center experience. Hernia. 2021;25(3):679–88. https://doi.org/10.1007/s10029-020-02293-5.
4. Bal J, Ilonzo N, Spencer P, Hyakutake M, Leitman IM. Loss of independence after emergency inguinal hernia repair in elderly patients: how aggressive should we be? Am J Surg. 2022;223(2):370–4. https://doi.org/10.1016/j.amjsurg.2021.03.063.
5. Yee J, Kaide CG. Emergency reversal of anticoagulation. West J Emerg Med. 2019;20(5):770–83. https://doi.org/10.5811/westjem.2018.5.38235.
6. Bellolio MF, Heien HC, Sangaralingham LR, Jeffery MM, Campbell RL, Cabrera D, et al. Increased computed tomography utilization in the emergency department and its association with hospital admission. West J Emerg Med. 2017;18(5):835–45. https://doi.org/10.5811/westjem.2017.5.34152.
7. HerniaSurge Group. International guidelines for groin hernia management. Hernia. 2018;22(1):1–165. https://doi.org/10.1007/s10029-017-1668-x.
8. Kroese LF, Sneiders D, Kleinrensink GJ, Muysoms F, Lange JF. Comparing different modalities for the diagnosis of incisional hernia: a systematic review. Hernia. 2018;22(2):229–42. https://doi.org/10.1007/s10029-017-1725-5.
9. Verdaguer M, Jofra M, Rodrigues V, Rosselló-Jiménez D, López-Cano M. Parastomal hernia. Emergency repair. Cir Esp (Eng Ed). 2021;99(8):619–20. https://doi.org/10.1016/j.cireng.2020.07.016.
10. Antoniou SA, Agresta F, Garcia Alamino JM, Berger D, Berrevoet F, Brandsma HT, et al. European hernia society guidelines on prevention and treatment of parastomal hernias. Hernia. 2018;22(1):183–98. https://doi.org/10.1007/s10029-017-1697-5.
11. Birindelli A, Sartelli M, Di Saverio S, et al. 2017 update of the WSES guidelines for emergency repair of complicated abdominal wall hernias. World J Emerg Surg. 2017;12:37. https://doi.org/10.1186/s13017-017-0149-y.
12. Carpenter CR, Bromley M, Caterino JM, Chun A, Gerson LW, Greenspan J, et al. Optimal older adult emergency care: introducing multidisciplinary geriatric emergency department guidelines from the American College of Emergency Physicians, American Geriatrics Society, emergency nurses association, and Society for Academic Emergency Medicine. J Am Geriatr Soc. 2014;62(7):1360–3. https://doi.org/10.1111/jgs.12883.
13. Dai W, Chen Z, Zuo J, Tan J, Tan M, Yuan Y. Risk factors of postoperative complications after emer-

gency repair of incarcerated groin hernia for adult patients: a retrospective cohort study. Hernia. 2019;23(2):267–76. https://doi.org/10.1007/s10029-018-1854-5.
14. Vacas S, Cole DJ, Cannesson M. Cognitive decline associated with anesthesia and surgery in older patients. JAMA. 2021;326(9):863–4. https://doi.org/10.1001/jama.2021.4773.
15. Compagna R, Rossi R, Fappiano F, et al. Emergency groin hernia repair: implications in elderly. BMC Surg. 2013;13(Suppl 2):S29. https://doi.org/10.1186/1471-2482-13-S2-S29.

Lower Genitourinary Tract Trauma 24

Charles D. Best

Bladder Injuries

The urinary bladder is generally protected from external trauma due to its deep location in the bony pelvis. Most blunt bladder injuries are the result of rapid deceleration motor vehicle accidents, but also can occur with falls, crush injuries, and assaults to the lower abdomen. Although disruption of the bony pelvis tends to tear the bladder at its fascial attachments, bony fragments can also directly lacerate the bladder, particularly the bladder neck. Blunt trauma may account for bladder injury in up to 85% of cases. Bladder laceration may also stem from penetrating trauma or various iatrogenic surgical complications and may occur spontaneously in patients with altered sensorium, such as the presence of intoxication or neuropathic disease. In elderly patients with cognitive impairment, minor trauma such as ground level fall in the presence of a full bladder may also potentially result in bladder disruption.

Bladder injuries that occur due to blunt external trauma are rarely an isolated injury; 80–94% of patients have significant associated non-urologic injuries. Mortality in these multiple-injury patients is primarily related to non-urologic injuries and ranges from 8 to 44%. The most common associated injury is pelvic fracture, associated with 83–95% of bladder injuries. Conversely, bladder injuries occur in 4–10% of patients with pelvic fracture. A sudden force to a full bladder may result in a rapid rise in intravesical pressure easily to rupture without the presence of pelvic fracture.

Bladder rupture does not occur as an isolated event to normal individuals. Most conscious patients have significant, nonspecific symptoms such as suprapubic or abdominal pain and inability to void. Associated abdominal pelvic injuries may mask or confound bladder symptoms. Physical signs include suprapubic tenderness, lower abdominal bruising, and muscle guarding or rigidity. Immediate catheterization should be performed because the most reliable sign of bladder injury is gross hematuria, which is present 93–100% of cases. If blood is noted at the meatus or a catheter does not pass easily, retrograde urethrography should be performed immediately because concomitant bladder and urethral injuries occur in 10–29% of patients.

Imaging of the bladder should be performed placed on suspicion and examination, and the presence of hematuria or pelvic fracture. The absolute indication for immediate cystography after blunt external trauma is the presence of gross hematuria associated with pelvic fracture. Relative indications for cystography after blunt trauma include gross hematuria without a pelvic fracture, or micro-hematuria with pelvic fracture. Other indications for suspecting bladder injury

C. D. Best (✉)
Harbor Regional Health Urology,
Aberdeen, WA, USA
e-mail: cbest@hmgcares.org

P. Petrone, C. E.M. Brathwaite (eds.), *Acute Care Surgery in Geriatric Patients*,
https://doi.org/10.1007/978-3-031-30651-8_24

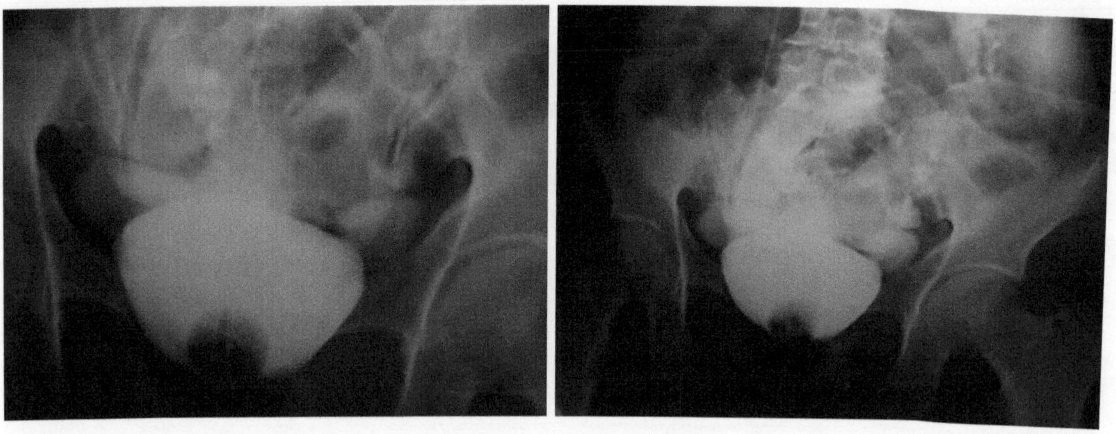

Fig. 24.1 Retrograde cystogram. Extravasation of contrast outlining bowel and paracolic gutters. Consistent with intraperitoneal bladder injury

can included penetrating injuries with pelvic trajectory, low urine output, abdominal distention, or urinary ascites seen on imaging. The diagnosis bladder rupture is extremely low in these atypical groups, 0.6% in patients with pelvic fracture and micro-hematuria, but the index suspicion should be raised by the presence of associated clinical indicators of bladder injury. Conversely, penetrating injuries of the bladder neck, pelvis, or lower abdomen with any degree of hematuria warrant cystography.

Retrograde cystography is approximately 100% accurate for bladder injury, if performed correctly. But this technique can be potentially time intensive in require some expertise in interpretation. The bladder should be filled in a conscious patient to a sense of discomfort, otherwise to 350 mL (Fig. 24.1). Traditionally, a three-film technique is recommended including precontrast image, full bladder anterior-posterior film, and a drainage film. Posterior extravasation of contrast can be missed without a drainage film. Significant bladder distention is required to visualize small lacerations.

Dense, flame-shaped collections of contrast in the pelvis are characteristics of extraperitoneal extravasation. Depending on fascial integrity, contrast may extend beyond the confines of the pelvis and can be seen in the retroperitoneum, scrotum, phallus, thigh, and anterior abdominal wall. The degree of extravasation is not always proportional to the extent bladder injury. Intraperitoneal extravasation is identified when contrast outlines loops of bowel.

Computed tomography (CT) cystography is as accurate and reliable as plain film cystography to evaluate suspected bladder injury (Fig. 24.2). It has become more of the mainstay in evaluating bladder injuries. The bladder is filled in retrograde manner using contrast dilated to 2–4% to a volume of 350–400 mL. The catheter is then subsequently clamped. Drainage films are not required after CT cystography because the retrovesical space can be well visualized. Contrast dilution is necessary because undiluted contrast material is so dense that the CT quality is compromised. Conventional abdominal CT imaging of the trauma patient may show findings suggestive of bladder injury, but is not considered to be adequate for bladder evaluation alone, and can result in incorrect or missed diagnosis in up to 13% of cases of bladder injury.

Bladder injuries can be categorized as extraperitoneal (EP), intraperitoneal (IP), or combined extraperitoneal and intraperitoneal, approximately occurring in 63%, 32%, and 4% of cases, respectively. The American Association of Surgery for Trauma (AAST) has developed an Organ Injury Scale (OIS) to provide a common language to assist with clinical decision-making (Table 24.1). The OIS is based on the degree of anatomical disruption. Grade I being mild and described as a contusion or partial laceration. Grades II-V involve complete laceration, ranging

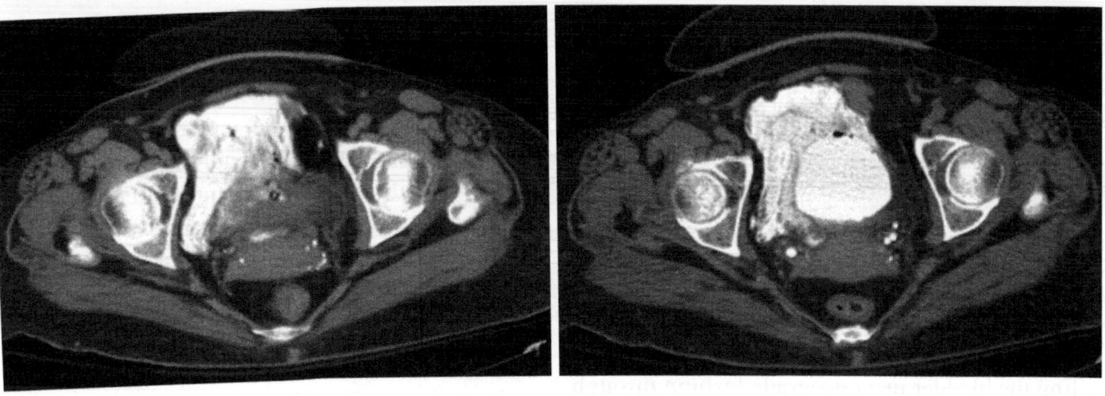

Fig. 24.2 Extraperitoneal bladder injury. Axial images from CT cystography show an accumulation of extravasated contrast solution

Table 24.1 American Association for the Surgery of Trauma-Organ Injury Scale (AAST-OIS) for bladder injury

Grade[a]	Injury type	Description of injury
I	Hematoma	Contusion, intramural hematoma
	Laceration	Partial thickness
II	Laceration	Extraperitoneal bladder wall laceration <2 cm
III	Laceration	Extraperitoneal (>2 cm) or intraperitoneal (<2 cm) bladder wall laceration
IV	Laceration	Intraperitoneal bladder wall laceration >2 cm
V	Laceration	Intraperitoneal or extraperitoneal bladder wall laceration extending into the bladder neck or ureteral orifice (trigone)

[a]Advance one grade for multiple lesions up to grade III

from less than 2 cm to the injuries involving the bladder neck and trigone.

The typical treatment for uncomplicated extraperitoneal bladder rupture, which could account for 60% of traumatic bladder injuries, is conservative management with urethral catheter drainage alone. A large-bore Foley catheter, 22 French, should be used to ensure adequate drainage. Cystography is recommended before catheter removal 7–10 days after injury to assess for persistent extravasation, in which case the catheter is maintained longer. Antimicrobial agents are instituted on the day of injury and continued for 3 days and at the time the urinary catheter is removed.

Blunt extraperitoneal injuries with complicating features require immediate open repair to prevent complications such as fistula, abscess, or prolonged leak (Table 24.2). These indications remained the same, regardless of patient age. In cases where there is a bladder neck injury, catheter drainage alone will end up requiring surgical repair in the majority. If a stable patient is undergoing exploratory laparotomy for other associated injuries, it is prudent to repair the extraperitoneal rupture; the anterior bladder wall is entered and the laceration is closed intravesically in two layers using absorbable suture. The perivesical pelvic hematoma should not be disturbed. When internal fixation of pelvic fractures is to be performed, simultaneous bladder repair is recommended because urinary leakage from the injured bladder onto the orthopedic hardware is prevented, thereby reducing the risk of hardware infection.

All penetrating or intraperitoneal injuries resulting from external trauma should be managed with immediate surgical repair. These injuries are frequently larger than suggested on cystography, and are unlikely to heal spontaneously, with continued leak of urine causing chemical peritonitis. Patients with intraperitoneal or combined intraperitoneally extraperitoneal injury have a 12.4-fold higher risk of death compared to patient's with extraperitoneal injuries alone. The laceration should be repaired with two layers of absorbable running suture. After injury has been repaired, the closure can be tested by

Table 24.2 Indications for immediate repair of bladder injury

Intraperitoneal injury from penetrating trauma inadequate bladder drainage or clot retention
Bladder neck injury
Rectal or vaginal injury
Pelvic fracture requiring open reduction and internal fixation
Stable patients undergoing laparotomy for other reasons
Bone fragments penetrating into bladder

filling the bladder in a retrograde fashion through a urethral catheter. In addition, use of methylene blue diluted in irrigation fluid may help identify any further leaks in the bladder upon filling.

When exploring bladder injuries, the ureteral orifices should be inspected for clear efflux, or ureteral integrity should be confirmed utilizing intravenous indigo carmine or methylene blue, or retrograde passage of a ureteral catheter. Any injury in close proximity to or involving the ureteral orifice or intramural ureter should be stented or reimplanted. A perivesical drain should be employed. When concurrent rectal or vaginal injury occurs, the walls of affected organs should be separated, overlapping suture lines avoided, and every attempt should be made to interpose viable tissue in between the repaired structures. Fibrin sealant injected over the bladder wall closure may help reduce complications when intervening tissue is unavailable.

In patients with intraperitoneal rupture, antimicrobials are administered for 3 days, in the perioperative period only. In cases with complex injuries or both intraperitoneal and extraperitoneal intrusive the bladder undergone repair, a cystogram has been suggested 7–14 days after surgery. For simple intraperitoneal bladder injuries, cystogram is not required prior to catheter removal.

Prompt diagnosis and appropriate management of bladder injuries allow for excellent results and minimal morbidity. Serious complications are usually associated with delayed diagnosis or treatment due to either a misdiagnosis or delayed presentation or complex injuries resulting from devastating pelvic trauma. Unrecognized bladder injuries may manifest as azotemia, sepsis, low urine output, peritonitis, ileus, urinary ascites, or respiratory difficulties. Unrecognized bladder neck, vaginal and rectal injury associated with the bladder rupture can result in incontinence, stricture, vesicovaginal or rectovesical fistula, and a difficult delayed major reconstruction. Severe pelvic fractures may cause a transient or permanent neurologic injury and results and voiding difficulties despite adequate bladder repair.

Urethral Injuries

Posterior Urethra

Pelvic fracture urethral injuries (PFUI) typically occur in conjunction with multi-system trauma. Most commonly associated motor vehicle accidents, but also from the result of falls or industrial accidents. Straddle injuries, involving all four pubic rami, open fractures, and injuries resulting in both vertical in rotational pelvic instability are commonly associated with the highest risk of urologic injury, with unstable fractures having incidence of 25% associated urethral disruption. The bulbar membranous urethral junction is more vulnerable to injury during pelvic fracture.

Urethral disruption has historically been identified by the triad of blood at the meatus, inability to urinate, and a palpably full bladder. Pelvic fracture urethral disruption is often initially identified when a urethral catheter cannot be placed by the emergency department team or when it is misplaced into a pelvic hematoma. Pelvic hematoma can often obscure the prostatic contour, resulting in misdiagnosis of impalpable prostate. The digital rectal exam has very poor sensitivity for the diagnosis of posterior urethral injuries. Females with urethral injuries can present with vulvar edema, blood or bony spiculations within the vaginal introitus, therefore indicating the need for careful vaginal examination all females with pelvic fracture.

When blood at the urethral meatus is identified, in the presence of pelvic fracture or penetrating injury to the genitals, a prompt retrograde

Table 24.3 American Association for the Surgery of Trauma-Organ Injury Scale (AAST-OIS) for urethra injury

Grade[a]	Injury type	Description of injury
I	Contusion	Blood at urethral meatus; retrourography normal
II	Stretch injury	Elongation of urethra without extravasation on urethrography
III	Partial disruption	Extravasation of urethrography contrast at injury site with Visualization in the bladder
IV	Complete disruption	Extravasation of urethrography contrast at injury site without Visualization in the bladder; <2 cm of urethra separation
V	Complete disruption	Complete transaction with >2 cm urethral separation, or extension into the prostate or vagina

urethrogram (RUG) should be performed to rule out urethral injury. Urethral instrumentation should be avoided until imaging is performed. A small-bore urethral catheter (14 F) is placed 1 cm into the fossa navicularis, and the balloon is filled with 3–5 mL of water to achieve a snug fit. Patients ideally are placed in oblique or lateral decubitus position and is preferable to perform the study under fluoroscopy if available. Twenty-five milliliters as of contrast is injected gently via a 60 mL catheter-tip syringe, and film is taken during injection. Direct inspection by flexible cystoscopy could also be performed if the expertise and equipment is available. The AAST-OIS for urethral injuries is shown in Table 24.3.

Management

Historically, immediate suprapubic tube placement was the standard of care. This can be accomplished through a small infra-umbilical incision, which allows for inspection repair of the bladder a proper placement of a large-bore catheter at the bladder dome. Alternatively, trocar suprapubic tube placement is reasonable in the bladder is distended and no other indications for surgery exist. There can be potential issues over the long term with the smaller percutaneous suprapubic tubes, as they are more likely to become obstructed with debris, but in long-term situations these can be exchanged for progressively larger bore catheters. This is often followed by delayed simultaneous cystogram and retrograde urethrogram to assess the severity and length of urethral injury.

Orthopedists frequently requested suprapubic tube not be placed if anterior pubic hardware is being used to repair pelvic fracture, due to concern that the suprapubic tube can lead to hardware infection. This complication is extremely rare and the cystostomy can be safely used even in the presence of pelvic hardware. The catheter should be placed high in the bladder and tunneled through the skin in the lower abdominal midline to keep away from the plated symphysis; this can facilitate prostatic apex identification at the time of reconstruction.

An attempt at primary endoscopic realignment of the urethral distraction injury can be reasonable in stable patients either acutely or within several days of injury. Patients with successful endoscopic realignment have significantly shorter time to spontaneous voiding compared to delayed treatment. Patients also have significantly lower stricture rate compared to suprapubic placement and delayed management (14% vs. 100%). Outcomes are improved the sooner the catheter can be placed from time of injury. We prefer performing flexible cystoscopy and advancing a guidewire across the injury into the bladder and then placing a catheter over the guidewire. This is preferable over blind placement if resources and expertise are available. This technique can be performed in the emergency room, in the operating room or in the ICU. One should remain aware that any attempt a catheterization should not delay definitive care of other traumatic injuries. Intraoperatively, a simple technique could consist of passing a catheter antegrade via a cystotomy, then tying it to another catheter which can be drawn back into the bladder in a retrograde fashion.

Incomplete urethral tears are best treated by advancing a urethral catheter across the injury. There has historically been a concern that attempt to place a catheter could convert an incomplete injury to complete transection, but there has not really been any substantial evidence to confirm this occurrence. It is imperative to assure adequate positioning of the catheter with gentle irrigation and return. Suprapubic tube placement can also be performed.

In cases with a female patient with urethral disruption associated with pelvic fracture, it is suggested to undergo immediate primary repair or at least urethral realignment over a catheter. This is to avoid subsequent urethrovaginal fistula or urethral stenosis. Associated vaginal lacerations must also be close acutely, to prevent vaginal stenosis. Delayed reconstruction can be a problem, due to the female urethra being relatively short, approximately 4 cm, to be amenable to any anastomotic repair if it becomes significantly involved with scar tissue.

Associated rectal injuries typically require open exploration, repair, irrigation, and placement of drains. Immediate suture repair of posterior urethral disruption injuries is not recommended in that scenario, due to association with unsatisfactory outcomes, as in erectile dysfunction and incontinence, stricture formation, and potential for increased operative blood loss. Patients with PFUI have an overall incidence of erectile dysfunction, ranging from 20–60%. Mostly can be related to the severity of the initial injury. Attempted urethral repair or pelvic angioembolization can contribute to higher rates of erectile dysfunction.

Anterior Urethra

As opposed to posterior urethral disruption injuries, anterior urethral injuries are typically isolated. Most occur after straddle injury and involve the bulbar urethra, which is susceptible to compression injury due to its fixed location beneath the pubic rami. A small percentage of these injuries can be result of direct penetrating injury to the penis.

Similar to posterior urethral injuries, a high index of suspicion should be maintained in all patients with blunt or penetrating trauma in the urogenital region. Retrograde urethrogram should be performed in any case of suspected urethral injury. Clinical signs of anterior urethral injuries include blood at the meatus, perineal or "butterfly" hematoma, gross hematuria, and urinary retention. In severe trauma, the Buck's fascia may be disrupted, which may result in blood and urinary extravasation into the scrotum. The significant complication of straddle injuries is the development of urethral stricture, which may become symptomatic, even up to 10 years after injury.

Anterior urethral injuries can be categorized based on radiographic findings. This can include contusion, incomplete disruption, or complete disruption. Contusions and incomplete injuries can often be treated with urethral catheter alone. Initial suprapubic cystotomy has traditionally been the treatment of choice for major straddle injuries involving the urethra. More recently, there has been success with endoscopic realignment at the time of injury.

Primary surgical repair is recommended for urethral gunshot or stab wound injuries; catheter alignment alone is associated with a significantly worse stricture rate. Debridement of the corpus spongiosum after trauma should be limited because the blood supply to the corporal bodies is usually robust, which enables spontaneous healing of most contused areas. In some cases following high velocity gunshot wounds to the urethra, initial suprapubic diversion may be recommended, followed by delayed reconstruction. Overall, patients with penetrating injuries to the anterior urethra have a relatively low incidence of delayed urethral stricture.

Genital Injuries

Penile Fracture

Penile fracture is defined as the disruption of the tunic albuginea with rupture of the corpus cavernosum and can be a surgical emergency. Fracture typically occurs during vigorous sexual activity. When the erect penis bends abnormally, the abrupt increase in intracavernosal pressure exceeds the tensile strength of the tunica albuginea, and a ventral or lateral laceration proximal or midshaft shaft usually results. The incidence of penile fracture in the United States is approximately 1.02 per 100,000 men per year. This is a

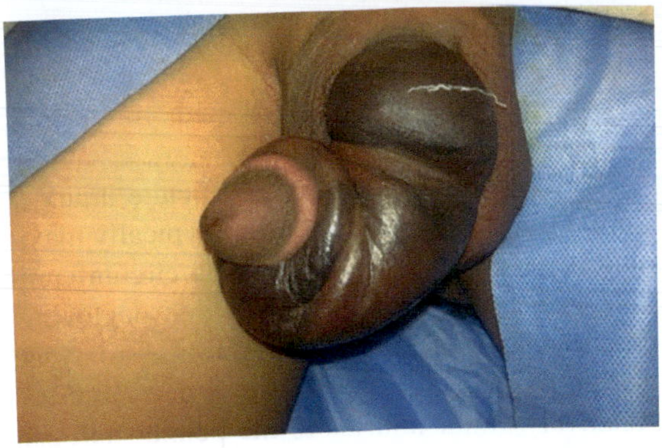

Fig. 24.3 Acute penile fracture demonstrating "eggplant" deformity

very rare injury in the geriatric patient, as erectile dysfunction as a baseline is more common.

The diagnosis of penile fractures often straightforward and can be made reliably by history and physical examination alone (Fig. 24.3). Patients usually describe a snapping or popping sound as the tunica tears, followed by pain, rapid detumescence, and discoloration and swelling of the penile shaft. If Buck's fascia remains intact, the penile hematoma remains contained between the skin and tunica, resulting in a typically described "eggplant" deformity. If the Buck's fascia is disrupted, hematoma can extend to the scrotum, perineum, and suprapubic regions, creating the "butterfly sign." Because fear and/or embarrassment are commonly associated, patient presentation to the emergency department or clinic is sometimes significantly delayed. The typical history and clinical presentation of a fractured penis usually makes initial imaging studies unnecessary. Ultrasonography is the preferred imaging modality to evaluate penile fractures, as it is fast, available, and inexpensive. Its utility may be most useful in situations when history and exam may be unclear. If ultrasound demonstrates that the tunic albuginea is not damaged, patients can potentially be treated conservatively. Magnetic resonance imaging (MRI) is reasonable in the evaluation of patients without the typical presentation and physical findings of penile fracture. MRI has 100% sensitivity and negative predictive value in detecting tunical rupture, and accuracy of localizing the lesion is 97%. It has a lower accuracy for urethral lesions, 60% sensitivity. Its use may be limited by cost and availability. The incidence of penile fractures that are associated with urethral lacerations can range from 2 to 38%, depending on underlying cause and geographical location. Urethral injuries can be associated with gross hematuria, blood at the meatus, or inability to void although the absence of these findings does not definitively rule out urethral injury. Urethral injury can be partial or complete. Given the urethral injury occurs not infrequently, and that retrograde urethrography is a simple and reliable study, clinicians should have a low threshold for urethral evaluation in all cases of penile fracture. Cystoscopy may be recommended for those patients suspected of urethral injury as the detection rate is much higher. Increased age, African-American race, and the presence of hematuria are associated with increasing risk of urethral injury.

Urgent (not emergent) exploration through distal circumcising incision is appropriate in most cases, with goals of preserving erectile function and restoring normal micturition. There is evidence that even patients with delayed presentation can have very good outcomes. Although rates of penile curvature are significantly lower in patients undergoing emergency as opposed to delayed surgery.

A circular subcoronal incision, followed by further penile degloving is the best described approach (Fig. 24.4). This allows good exposure of the corpus cavernosum and urethra and allows for separation of the neurovascular bundle if necessary. Other surgical approaches have been described including inguinoscrotal, midline ventral, and lateral. Closure of the tunical defect with interrupted 3-0 or 4-0 absorbable sutures is recommended, while deep corporal vascular ligation or excessive debridement of the delicate underlying erectile tissue should be avoided. Partial urethral injury should be oversewn using a 5-0 absorbable suture over urethral catheter. Complete urethral injury should be debrided, mobilized, and repaired in a tension-free manner over a catheter. The urethral catheter was left in for 10–21 days, depending on the severity of the injury. Broad-spectrum antibiotics and 4–6 weeks of sexual abstinence are recommended.

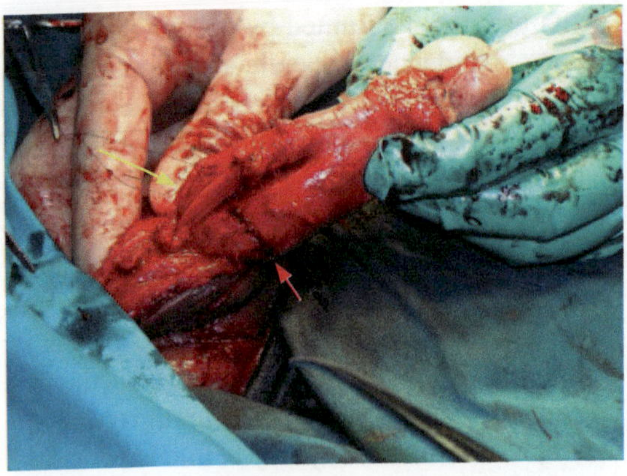

Fig. 24.4 Repair of penile fracture with urethral injury. Repaired corporal cavernosal injury (red arrow). Disrupted penile urethra with catheter in place (yellow arrow)

Immediate surgical reconstruction often results in a faster recovery and decreased morbidity, lower complication rates, and a lower incidence of erectile dysfunction or long-term penile curvature. Conservative management of penile fracture can result in penile curvature in >10% of patients, or debilitating plaques in up to 30%, and significantly higher risk of erectile dysfunction.

Gunshot and Penetrating Wounds

Most penetrating wounds to the genitalia are due to gunshots and most require surgical exploration. This type of injury accounts for roughly 45% of genital trauma. The primary objective in management is preserving the function of the genitals as well as cosmesis, while minimizing any potential long-term sequelae. Urethral injuries have been reported in 15–50% of penile gunshot wounds. Imaging is rarely required except in complex situations. Retrograde urethrography should be strongly considered in any patient with penetrating injury to the penis, especially those with high velocity missile injuries, blood at the meatus, difficulty voiding, or if bullet trajectory was near the urethra. Alternatively, intraoperative retrograde urethral injection of methylene blue or indigo carmine may identify the site of injury and adequacy of closure at completion.

Treatment principles include immediate exploration, copious irrigation, and excision of foreign matter, antibiotic prophylaxis, and surgical closure. Excellent cosmetic and functional outcomes can be expected with immediate reconstruction.

Management of a penetrating penile injury is similar to that of penile fracture. Typically maximum exposure was performed via circumferential subcoronal incision with degloving. Potentially penoscrotal infrapubic incisions can be performed for more extensive injuries. Relatively minor injuries to the penile shaft can be managed with primary.

Testicular rupture can be a result of both penetrating and blunt trauma. Blunt trauma to the testicles is typically associated with motor vehicle accidents or sports-associated activity. In all cases of blunt scrotal trauma, there should be a high index of suspicion of testicular rupture. Clinical exam can be unreliable, as many patients present with severe pain and swelling. Penetrating injuries deep to the scrotal dartos fascia should be surgically explored. Not all blunt traumatic injuries to the scrotum require exploration. Scrotal ultrasound can be an excellent addition to the physical examination, particularly if examination findings are equivocal. Ultrasound findings of a heterogeneous pattern of the testicular parenchyma, and/or loss of contour of the testis tunica can indicate testicular rupture. Clinically benign findings as well as a homogeneous echogenic testicle on ultrasound can be managed conservatively.

In cases of confirmed testicular rupture, urgent surgical exploration is essential for adequate salvage of the testicle. This is not a life-threatening injury, but can have significant repercussions, including some fertility, hypogonadism, chronic pain, and low self-esteem. There should be effort to salvage in preserve any remaining viable seminiferous tubules. In cases of blunt traumatic rupture of the testicles, exploration within 72 h has a greater salvage rate then delayed exploration.

Maximal exposure to the testicle spermatic cords can be achieved through a vertical incision of the midline scrotum. This also helps to maintain cosmesis. The tunica vaginalis can then be opened, and the testis brought out of the scrotum for inspection. Any nonviable seminiferous tubules can be sharply excised until there are only remaining bleeding edges. The tunica albuginca can then be closed with a running 3-0 absorbable suture. Testes can be then returned into the scrotum, making sure it is in proper orientation to avoid torsion. Scrotum should be closed in two layers with absorbable suture. A Penrose drain is recommended.

Urethral injury should be closed primarily utilizing standard urethroplasty principles (tension-free, watertight repair using fine, absorbable sutures, performed over small catheter). Excellent results have been reported. Patients with urethral injury in the presence of extensive tissue damage and blast effect from high velocity weapons or close-range shotgun blast usually require stage repairs and urinary diversion.

References

1. Mahat Y, Leong JY, Chung PH. A contemporary review of adult bladder trauma. J Inj Violence Res. 2019;11(2):101–6. https://doi.org/10.5249/jivr.v11i2.1069.
2. Luckhoff C, Mitra B, Cameron PA, Fitzgerald M, Royce P. The diagnosis of acute urethral trauma. Injury. 2011;42(9):913–6. https://doi.org/10.1016/j.injury.2010.08.007.
3. Myers JB, Taylor MB, Brant WO, Lowrance W, Wallis MC, Presson AP, et al. Process improvement in trauma: traumatic bladder injuries and compliance with recommended imaging evaluation. J Trauma Acute Care Surg. 2013;74(1):264–70. https://doi.org/10.1097/TA.0b013e318270df2b.
4. Anderson RE, Keihani S, Moses RA, Nocera AP, Selph JP, Castillejo Becerra CM, et al. Current management of extraperitoneal bladder injuries: results from the multi-institutional Genito-urinary trauma study (MiGUTS). J Urol. 2020;204(3):538–44. https://doi.org/10.1097/JU.0000000000001075.
5. Inaba KI, Okoye OT, Browder T, Best C, Branco BC, Teixeira PG, et al. Prospective evaluation of the utility of routine postoperative cystogram after traumatic bladder injury. J Acute Care Surg. 2013;75(6):1019–23. https://doi.org/10.1097/TA.0b013e318299b61a.
6. Hadjizacharia P, Inaba K, Teixera PGR, Kokorowski P, Demetriades D, Best C. Evaluation of immediate endoscopic realignment as a treatment modality for traumatic urethral injuries. J Trauma. 2008;64(6):1433–50. https://doi.org/10.1097/TA.0b013e318174f126.
7. Borelli J, Brandes SB. Pelvic fractures: assessment and management for the urologist. AUA Update Series. 2004;23(11):82–6.
8. Martinez-Pineiro L, Djakovic N, Plas E, Mor Y, Santucci RA, Serafetinidis E, et al. EAU guidelines on urethral trauma. Eur Urol. 2010;57:791–803. https://doi.org/10.1016/j.eururo.2010.01.013.
9. Simms A, Baradaran N, Lue TF, Breyer BN. Penile fractures: evaluation and management. Urol Clin N Am. 2021;48(4):557–63. https://doi.org/10.1016/j.ucl.2021.06.011.
10. Cozzi D, Verrone GB, Agostini S, Bartolini S, D'Amico G, Pradella S, Miele V. Acute penile trauma: imaging features in the emergency setting. Radiol Med. 2019;124(12):1270–80. https://doi.org/10.1007/s11547-019-01065-1.
11. Barros R, Ribeiro JG, da Silva HA, de Sá FR, Fosse Júnior AM, Favorito LA. Urethral injury in penile fracture: a narrative review. Int Braz J Urol. 2020;46(2):152–7. https://doi.org/10.1590/S1677-5538.IBJU.2020.99.02.
12. Pariser JJ, Pearce SM, Patel SG, Bales GT. National patterns of urethral evaluation and risk factors for urethral injury in patients with penile fracture. Urology. 2015;86(1):181–6. https://doi.org/10.1016/j.urology.2015.03.039.
13. El Assmy A, El Tholoth HS, Mohsen T, Ibrahiem E. Does timing of presentation of penile fracture affect outcome of surgical intervention? Urology. 2011;77(6):1388–91. https://doi.org/10.1016/j.urology.2010.12.070.
14. Amer T, Wilson R, Chlosta P, AlBuheissi S, Qazi H, Fraser M, Aboumarzouk OM. Penile fracture: a meta-analysis. Urol Int. 2016;96:315–29. https://doi.org/10.1159/000444884.
15. Chang AJ, Brandes SB. Advances in diagnosis and management of genital injuries. Urol Clin N Amer. 2013;40(3):427–38. https://doi.org/10.1016/j.ucl.2013.04.013.

Pelvic Trauma in Geriatric Patients

25

Pedro Yuste Garcia, José Ceballos Esparragón, Salvador Navarro Soto, M. Dolores Pérez Díaz, and Ignacio Rey Simó

Introduction

Due to the increase in life expectancy in developed countries and the improvement in its quality of life in elderly patients, there is an increase in the average age of polytraumatized patients. This average aging has been estimated at about 0.75 years/year. In 2019, the number of people over 60 years of age was 1000 milions and according to data extrapolated from the UN, an increase of 34% is expected, reaching 1.400 milions in 2030.

Although pelvic fractures are traditionally associated with younger patients and high-energy trauma, 73% of all pelvic fractures occur in patients older than 65 years (UK epidemiological study). These injuries are predominantly low-impact fractures, sustained after a fall from standing height or less, and are therefore classified as pelvic fragilty fractures (FFP). The incidence of FFP in recent decades has increased from 7.9 per 100,000 to 13.1 per 100,000 in a single study center.

Low-energy mechanisms are a frequent cause of PF, given the osteoporotic bone fragility of this type of patient. Added to this is the decrease in their physiological reserve, the presence of multiple chronic morbidities and the frequent use of anticoagulant and antiplatelet medication that will complicate bleeding control. Most of these elderly patients have multiple drug treatments, which will mask many of the clinical warning signs, so a high index of suspicion is needed in the care of these patients.

Classification of Pelvic Fractures

Most pelvic fracture classifications are based on the stability of the pelvic ring. The Tile classification (Fig. 25.1) endorsed by the Orthopedic

P. Yuste Garcia (✉)
General Surgery and Digestive System Surgery Section, University Hospital "12 de Octubre", Madrid, Spain

School of Medicine, Complutense University, Madrid, Spain

J. Ceballos Esparragón
Vithas Las Palmas Hospital Surgery Service, Las Palmas, Spain

S. Navarro Soto
Department of Surgery, University Hospital Parc Tauli, Sabadell, Barcelona, Spain

Faculty of Medicine, Autonomous University, Barcelona, Spain

M. D. Pérez Díaz
School of Medicine, Complutense University, Madrid, Spain

General Surgery and Digestive System, General University Hospital "Gregorio Marañón", Madrid, Spain

I. Rey Simó
HBP and Transplant Surgery Unit, Emergency Surgery Unit, University Hospital Complex, A Coruña, Spain

P. Petrone, C. E.M. Brathwaite (eds.), *Acute Care Surgery in Geriatric Patients*,
https://doi.org/10.1007/978-3-031-30651-8_25

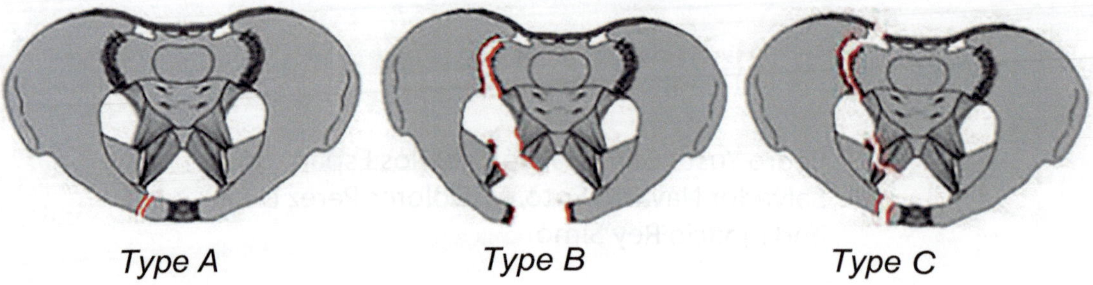

Fig. 25.1 Tile classification

Trauma Association (OTA) classifies them into three categories:

A—Completely stable
B—Partially stable, with rotational instability and partial stability of the posterior ring
C—Completely unstable, with complete disruption of the anterior and posterior ring

In the elderly, the most frequent fractures are type A and in many cases produced by low-energy trauma due to osteoporosis. In addition, unlike younger patients, this type of fracture can be accompanied by significant bleeding in 2–3% of cases. Fundamentally, due to bleeding from branches of the internal iliac or hypogastric artery. The risk also increases with atherosclerosis of the vessels, which causes greater fragility of the vessels, and also because a large number of patients are on antiplatelet or anticoagulant medication, which produces a very significant blood loss.

Assessment of the Elderly Patient with Pelvis Fracture

The initial management of pelvic trauma in the elderly does not differ from that in the young patient. This must be done following the ATLS protocol for the initial management of all polytraumatized patients, with some peculiarities or aspects to consider.

Clinical History

It is very important the evaluation of the patient's medical history, and it is necessary to know early their underlying pathologies, medications, particularly antiblockers, anticoagulants, or antiplatelet. The patient's mobility prior to the accident since it plays an important role in decision-making and treatment planning.

Physical Examination

Manual compression of the anterior iliac spines of the pelvis can guide us to the possibility of PF. It should be performed by a single explorer and should not be repeated as it may increase the risk of bleeding. We must not forget the importance of exploring the perineum, rectum, vagina, and buttocks to rule out open PF.

AP Pelvis Imaging

The clinical examination does not always reveal a PF, being necessary the early radiographic confirmation by an AP projection of the pelvis. The sensitivity of this radiological projection is around 80%, with up to 50% of all pelvic fractures being underdiagnosed.

In the hemodynamically unstable patient, the AP projection is generally the only imaging test for the initial diagnosis and allows the visu-

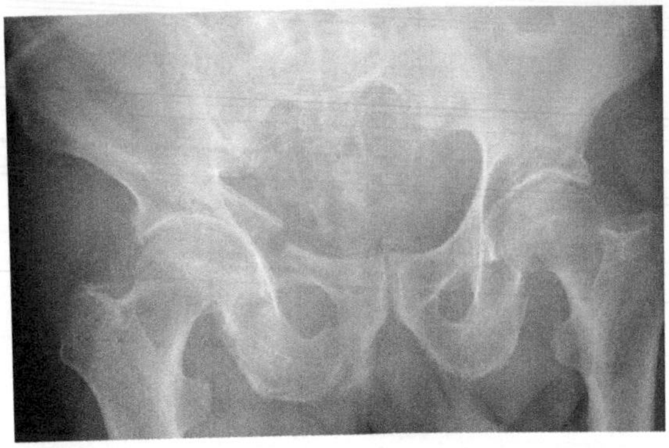

Fig. 25.2 Fracture of the pelvic branches

alization of the iliopectineal line, the ilioischial line and the highly displaced lesions of the posterior arch, although certain posterior lesions can go unnoticed, especially in the elderly population, where osteoporosis makes the detection of non-displaced fracture lines more difficult to assess.

We can ensure that conventional radiology, especially in the critical care unit with the portable device, clearly underdiagnoses bone lesions in elderly patients.

An AP radiograph of the pelvis will almost always identify the presence of pubic ramus fractures (Fig. 25.2) but will not do so in concomitant fractures of the posterior arch, nor of the sacro-iliac fractures, which tend to coexist in more than half of these patients (54%) nor in those of the sacrum, with only a sensitivity of 10.5%.

Focused Abdominal Ultrasound in Trauma (eFAST)

Many patients with pelvic fractures may have serious associated injuries. It is very important to find the source of bleeding in order to establish the action sequence. The eFAST is a rapid and non-invasive examination that has a sensitivity of 79–100% and a specificity of 95–100% for detecting intra-abdominal fluid. However, numerous publications have questioned this point, especially when the test result has been negative, advising its repetition in 5–10 min. Series with very low numbers of false positives have recently been published although certain doubts remain regarding false-negative cases. The presence of free fluid in a hemodynamically unstable patient indicates the need for urgent laparotomy.

Computerized Tomography (CT) and Magnetic Resonance Imaging (MRI)

In hemodynamically stable patients, the technique of choice is CT, which has a sensitivity of 92–97% and a specificity of 98%. It allows us to see in different projections and reconstructions the injuries of the anterior and posterior arch, ligamentous structures, and their adjacent hematomas. It also makes it possible to evaluate pelvic and/or abdominal injuries.

CT also allows us to assess the presence of active bleeding in the arterial phase ("jets" or "blush") that will force us to perform arteriographies in order to embolize the bleeding vessels, generally small branches of the hypogastric or gluteal arteries.

Elderly patients have inherent fragility of the pelvis, the arteriosclerotic rigidity of its vessels, and the possibility of taking any type of anticoagulant/antiplatelet drug means that even apparently minor fractures can cause more bleeding. The index of suspicion of concomitant arterial bleeding means that the performance of the CT and possibly the subsequent arteriography earlier than in younger patients.

As high as 80% of patients with branch fractures will associate a fracture of the posterior ring, and its diagnosis is very important in elderly patients because it can condition their subsequent functional recovery. In 2012,

Scheyerer et al. published that 96.8% of posterior ring fractures were not diagnosed in patients with rami fractures. In elderly patients, whenever a ramus fracture is diagnosed, a CT should be performed to rule out an associated fracture of the posterior ring (Fig. 25.3), and if the CT is negative but the patient continues with pain and functional impotence, an MRI should be considered, which has more sensitivity. In the case of sacral fractures in elderly patients with branch fractures, the sensitivity of MRI was 98.6% compared to 66.1% for CT. In this way, we should give more priority to CT or even to MRI for a correct staging of pelvic trauma in elderly patients following the protocol proposed by Wagner in 2015, depending on pain management and the patient's capacity for mobilization in its evaluation initial (Fig. 25.4).

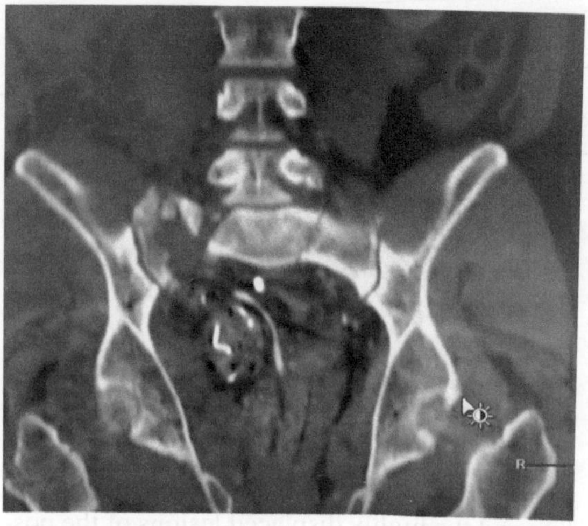

Fig. 25.3 CT Posterior pelvic ring fracture

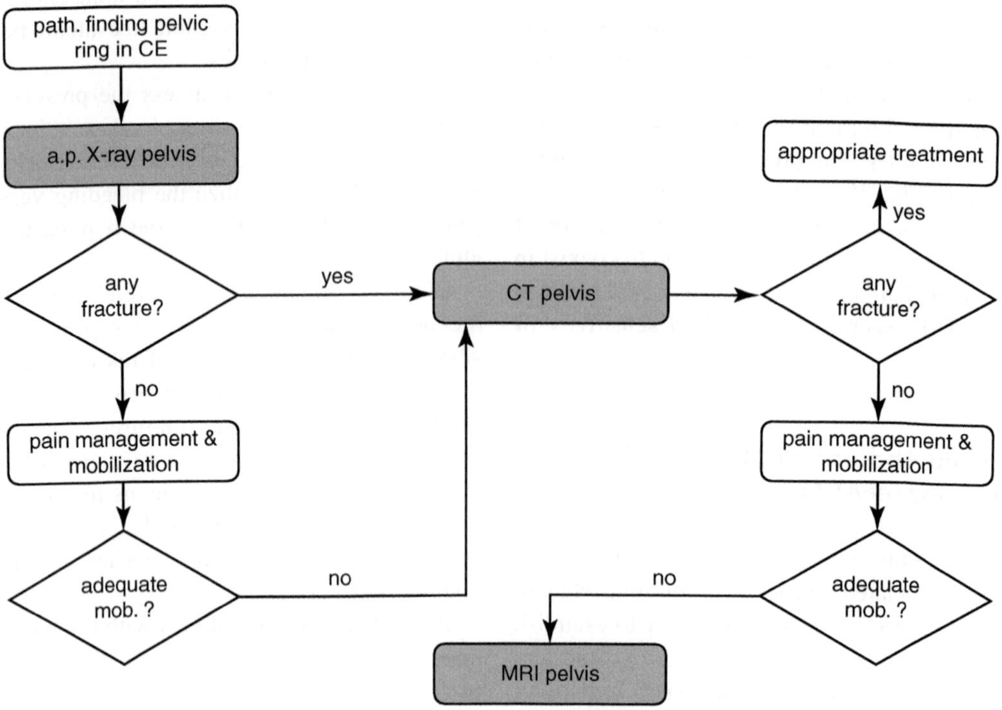

Fig. 25.4 Diagnostic algorithm for pelvic fracture in an elderly patient. (Adapted from Wagner D et al.)

Treatment

The assessment of hemodynamic stability will be the guidelines for action. The main techniques for the control of pelvic bleeding in the initial phase in hemodynamically unstable patients are pelvic fixation, angioembolization, preperitoneal packing, and REBOA (Fig. 25.5).

Most hemodynamically stable elderly patients with pelvic fractures require non-operative management (NOM) and are treated conservatively.

If a conservative treatment is decided, the three pillars are: analgesia, early mobilization, and anti-osteoporotic medication. Regarding analgesia, NSAIDs should be avoided in patients with renal insufficiency. According to the German guidelines in the PF of elderly patients, it is recommended to start with the treatment for the osteoporosis, if the patient can tolerate vitamin D and oral calcium. Furthermore, it seems that the use of bisphosphonates or osteometabolic drugs such as Teriparatide reduce the risk of new fractures and the time of consolidation.

Pelvic fixation techniques may be considered for bilateral anteriorly displaced fractures, fully displaced sacral fractures, or in patients with persistent disabling pain after 6 weeks.

The functional result is very important because prolonged immobilization will have catastrophic consequences for these patients. Whether conservative or surgical treatment is decided, patients should be mobilized as quickly as possible.

In the treatment of pelvic fractures in elderly patients, it is necessary to take into consideration some differential aspects with the younger population, such as the frequent use of anticoagulants/antiplatelet, the assessment of aggressive fluid resuscitation, and the early use of angioembolization.

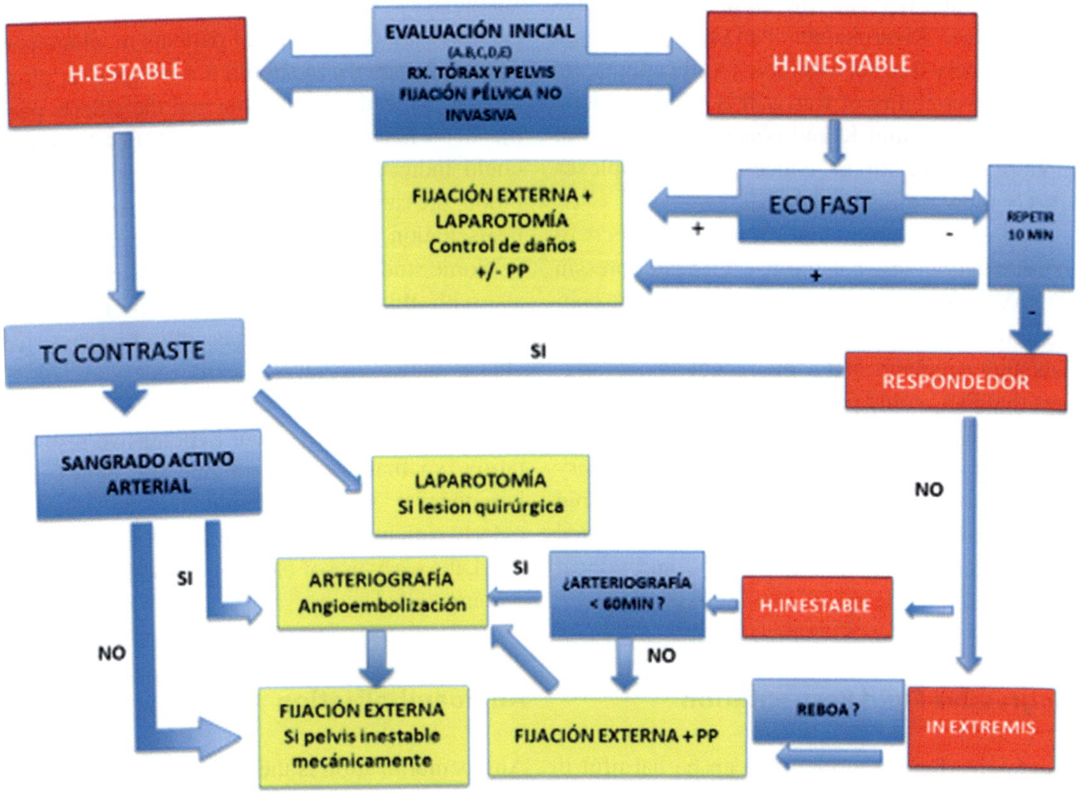

Fig. 25.5 Pelvic trauma management algorithm. (Manual de la Asociación Española de Cirujanos)

Use of Anticoagulants/Antiplatelet

One of the reasons for the complexity and peculiarity in the management of trauma in the elderly is usually polymedicated due to their underlying pathologies, and they frequently take anticoagulant and/or antiplatelet drugs at the time of trauma. Its management requires a quick investigation of the drugs the patient takes to act accordingly. On the other hand, in recent years the use of new anticoagulant such as direct thrombin or factor Xa inhibitors are becoming more frequent, offering a series of comfort and safety for the patient compared to the traditional use of warfarin. These new drugs complicate the management of these patients because there are not antidotes for these drugs that allow their effect to be immediately reversed, nor laboratory tests that give us reliable information. However, the use of the thromboelastogram is a useful tool to determine the presence of effects of both Clopidogrel-type platelet inhibitors and the new anticoagulants (Dabigatran, Rivaroxaban, Apixaban) although unfortunately it is not available in all centers.

The reversibility of warfarin is not a problem. The use of vitamin K and plasma or the use of modern prothrombin concentrate complexes (PCC) allow a quick reversal.

There are no drugs that reverse the effects of antiplatelet agents, but the use of desmopressin (DDAVP) and/or platelet transfusion can be considered. Plasma is not effective in reversing the new anticoagulants and some recent studies suggest that PCC could partially reverse the effect of Rivaroxaban.

Advances in this field are changing very quickly, so that it is recommended to have rapid conversion protocols from anticoagulation based on product availability, cost, and local preference.

Aggressive Fluid Resuscitation

Aggressive fluid resuscitation can be harmful if the bleeding is not controlled, and this is not new. In 1918, Cannon stated "if the blood pressure rises before the surgeon is prepared to control the source of bleeding, the blood that is extremely necessary can be lost"; thus, ideally, in hemodynamically unstable trauma patients, fluid resuscitation, and hemorrhage control should be performed simultaneously.

Clinical and experimental studies indicate that aggressive fluid resuscitation before the hemorrhagic focus is controlled can cause increased blood loss, clot removal, and altered coagulation factors.

Currently, the optimal volume of fluid administered should achieve acceptable tissue oxygenation without increasing blood loss in an attempt to normalize systolic pressure. This resuscitation strategy is known as "hypotensive resuscitation or permissive hypotension," fluid intake maintains a systolic blood pressure that is considered acceptable but does not reach normal values. In blunt trauma patients, it is important to maintain a low blood pressure in patients with injuries of difficult surgical control, such as pelvic fractures.

There are two groups of patients in which permissive hypotension should not be applied, those with associated head trauma and the elderly people. In the latter, blood pressure of 110–120 mmHg could indicate hypotension and try to maintain blood pressure around 90 mmHg (hypotensive resuscitation) could clearly be inadequate.

Some studies have not shown a worse prognosis with this resuscitation strategy in elderly patients, but these are basically retrospective studies with a low level of evidence.

Actually, there is no evidence on what type of patients could benefit from hypotensive resuscitation, so that we thought that the permissive hypotension strategy should not be used in elderly patients with pelvic fracture. On the other hand, the early use of blood and blood products is recommended.

Angioembolization

Angioembolization is the treatment of choice for active arterial bleeding. The technique can be performed selectively or trunkwise. The most frequent locations of bleeding are the pudendal

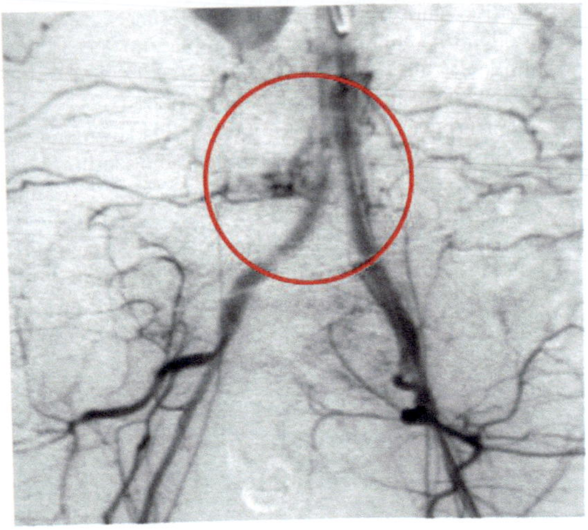

Fig. 25.6 Arteriography with angioembolization of iliac artery branches

artery, the superior gluteal artery, and multiple bleeding from small branches of the internal iliac artery (Fig. 25.6).

Traditionally its indications are:

- Lack of response to resuscitation once pelvic mechanical stability is achieved and extrapelvic sources of bleeding are ruled out.
- The presence of contrast extravasation on CT.
- Patients with PF who have undergone arteriography with or without embolization and who remain unstable once extrapelvic sources have been ruled out.
- Patients older than 60 years with severe PF, regardless of their hemodynamic status.

A prospective study evaluated the usefulness of angiography in patients with pelvic fractures, demonstrated that 94% of patients older than 60 years had pathologic angiography, versus 52% of younger patients so that the authors recommended the liberal use of angiography in patients older than 60 years with a pelvic fracture.

Conclusions

In recent decades, pelvic trauma has increased considerably in the geriatric population. These patients have a decreased physiological reserve, associated with comorbidities and polymedication (anticoagulants/antiplatelet) that can compromise life.

Pelvic fractures in the elderly people can occur with low-energy trauma, require an accurate diagnosis, trying to avoid missed injuries, so the early use of CT and even MRI should be taken into account. Due to the increased risk of bleeding, a more liberal use of angioembolization is suggested.

It is recommended to implement specific action protocols for this population in order to reduce morbidity and mortality and improve functional recovery.

References

1. Schicho A, Schmidt SA, Seeber K, Olivier A, Richter PH, Gebhard F. Pelvic X-ray misses out on detecting sacral fractures in the elderly—importance of CT imaging in blunt pelvic trauma. Injury. 2016;47:707–10.
2. Bridges LC, Waibel BH, Newell MA. Permissive hypotension: potentially harmful in the elderly? A National Trauma Data Bank Analysis. Am Surg. 2015;81(8):770–7.
3. Weber CD, Herren C, Dienstknecht T, Hildebrand F, Keil S, Pape HC, et al. Management of Life-threatening arterial hemorrhage following a fragility fracture of the pelvis in the anticoagulated patient: case report and review of the literature. Geriatr Orthop Surg Rehabil. 2016;7(3):163–7.
4. Sivapathasuntharam D, Smith G, Ashraf M, Bates P. Fragility fractures of the pelvis in the older population. Age Ageing. 2022;51:1–5.
5. Dutton RP, Mackenzie CF, Scalea TM. Hypotensive resuscitation during active hemorrhage: impact on in-hospital mortality. J Trauma. 2002;52:1141–6.
6. Ivascu FA, Howells GA, Junn FS, Bair HA, Bendick PJ, Janczyk RJ. Rapid warfarin reversal in anticoagulated patients with traumatic intracranial hemorrhage reduces hemorrhage progression and mortality. J Trauma. 2005;59(5):1131–7.
7. Jacobs DG. Special considerations in geriatric injury. Curr Opin Crit Care. 2003;9:535–9.
8. Kimbrell BJ, Velmahos GC, Chan LS, Demetriades D. Angiographic embolization for pelvic fractures in older patients. Arch Surg. 2004;139(7):728–33. https://doi.org/10.1001/archsurg.139.7.728.
9. Kudo D, Yoshida Y, Kushimoto S. Permissive hypotension/hypotensive resuscitation and restricted/controlled resuscitation in patients with severe trauma. J Intensive Care. 2017;5:11. https://doi.org/10.1186/s40560-016-0202-z.

10. Thompson CM, Maier RV. Management of shock. In: Mattox K, Moore EE, Feliciano DV, editors. Trauma. 8th ed. New York: McGraw Hill; 2017.
11. Navarro S. Hipotensión permisiva en la reanimación del paciente traumático. Cir Esp. 2007;82(6):319–20.
12. Schwed AC, Wagenaar A, Reppert AE, Gore AV, Pieracci FM, Platnick KB, Lawless RA, et al. Trust the FAST: confirmation that the FAST examination is highly specific for intra-abdominal hemorrhage in over 1,200 patients with pelvic fractures. J Trauma Acute Care Surg. 2021;90(1):137–42. https://doi.org/10.1097/TA.0000000000002947.
13. Velmahos GC, Toutouzas KG, Vassiliu P, Sarkisyan G, Chan LS, Hanks SH, Berne TV, et al. A prospective study on the safety and efficacy of angiographic embolization for pelvic and visceral injuries. J Trauma. 2002;53(2):303–8. https://doi.org/10.1097/00005373-200208000-00019.
14. Wagner D, Ossendorf C, Gruszka D, Hofmann A, Rommens PM. Fragility fractures of the sacrum: how to identify and when to treat surgically? Eur J Trauma Emerg Surg. 2015;41(4):349–62.
15. Yuste P, Gutierrez M, Hernandez H. Hematoma retroperitoneal. In: Trauma pélvico. Manual de la Asociación Española de Cirujanos, vol. 105. 3rd ed; 2022. p. 1163–70.

Geriatric Hip Fractures

26

Max Leiblein and Ingo Marzi

Introduction

Geriatric hip fractures are an entity with rising incidence due to the aging population and require urgent surgical intervention. Those fractures have an in-hospital mortality of 4.7–17.6% and a one-year mortality of 14–36%. Early surgical treatment of hip fractures is associated with a significant reduction in mortality, reduced risk of pneumonia and pressure sores. However, a lack of consent exists about what should be defined as "early" surgery.

In literature, the ideal time for surgery is shown to be less than 12 h after the accident, delaying surgery longer than 24 h increases the patient's length of stay in hospital and a delay of more than 48 h is associated with increased mortality.

Therefore, guidelines demand osteosynthesis within 24 h after admission and joint replacement with hip arthroplasty within 48 h.

Treating geriatric patients with proximal femur fractures requires knowledge about characteristics of elderly patients and an adapted management due to reduced bone quality, preexisting medical conditions and medications, such as anticoagulation. In the following, surgical treatment and management of those patients will be approached.

Epidemiology

Hip fractures are globally estimated to affect around 18% of women and 6% of men; about a third of women older than 80 years will suffer a hip fracture, one third of men over 80 years will die within 1 year after a hip fracture. Most often the femoral neck is affected, followed by intertrochanteric fractures.

While the global incidence of hip fractures in 1990 was 1.26 million, it is estimated to increase to 4.5 million in 2050 due to the increasing age of worldwide population. Thus, hip fractures represent a major burden to social services and health care systems. In 2002, costs caused by hip fractures in the United States are estimated to 17 billion US dollars.

After 1-year post-trauma, 40% of patients are not able to walk and 80% report limitations of activities of daily living, such as shopping or driving a car.

Pathogenesis

While hip fractures in younger patients typically occur after high velocity trauma, in elderly patients often a minor trauma such as a simple

M. Leiblein · I. Marzi (✉)
Department of Trauma-, Hand- and Reconstructive Surgery, University Hospital, Goethe University of Frankfurt, Frankfurt, Germany
e-mail: marzi@trauma.uni-frankfurt.de

P. Petrone, C. E.M. Brathwaite (eds.), *Acute Care Surgery in Geriatric Patients*,
https://doi.org/10.1007/978-3-031-30651-8_26

fall is leading to a fracture due to reduced bone mineral density.

This is caused by non-modifiable factors such as age, female gender, frailty, and osteoporosis as well as by modifiable factors such as medication, low calcium intake, reduced sunlight exposure, low body mass index, and comorbidities.

Classification

Multiple classifications for medial femoral neck fractures have been proposed. The classification of Garden describes the grade of dislocation of the femoral head and therefore allows assessing the risk of a femoral head necrosis. The classification of Pauwels helps to evaluate the stability of a fracture: The higher the angle of the fracture, the lower the medial stability.

A common classification for pertrochanteric fractures is the AO classification system (AO31. A1–3). Type AO31.A1 describes a simple pertrochanteric fracture with intact lesser trochanter. AO31.A2 describes a fracture involving medial cortex and lesser trochanter. Intertrochanteric and reverse fractures are described as AO31.A3.

Management of Anticoagulation

Special attention has to be paid to comorbidities and medication in geriatric patients. About 30–40% of patients with hip fractures in the United Kingdom are taking anticoagulant medications accompanied by the risk of bleeding, need for blood transfusions, infections, or revision operation due to hematoma. The risk for thromboembolic events on the other hand is increased when medication is paused. Therefore, anticoagulant medication often serves as a reason for delay of operation.

Elimination of the agent from the organism takes about five of its pharmacological half-life periods, therefore, in order to comply with the guidelines complete elimination cannot be waited for.

On the one hand, the effect of the anticoagulant agent on coagulation system has to be assessed in order to minimize surgical risk. Therefore, it has to be considered, that about two biological half-life periods for heparins (2 h) or direct acting oral anticoagulants (DOACs, 9–15 h), such as Dabigatran, Rivaroxaban, Apixaban, or Edoxaban, depending on the agent, are necessary to diminish biological effectiveness to a harmless plasma level.

The effectiveness of Vitamin K-antagonists such as Warfarin or Phenprocoumon depends on the capacity of liver synthesis, Vitamin K availability and intensity of anticoagulation.

The effectiveness of platelet inhibitors (acetylsalicylic acid, Clopidogrel, Prasugrel, Ticagrelor) depends on the synthesis of new platelets.

On the other hand, the risk of thromboembolic events must be considered and can be assessed with the CHA_2DS_2-VASC-score. Administration of tranexamic acid might help to reduce the need of blood transfusions.

These considerations lead to the following consequences concerning the timing of operation.

- *Low molecular weight heparin*: Elimination after 4 h.
- *Vitamin K-antagonists*: further measures depend on the INR-value at admission. If it is below 1.5, there is no influence on bleeding to be expected. In case of the INR being higher, administration of Vitamin K is necessary. If the INR is not sufficiently lowered, administration of platelet complex concentrate (PCC) is required (CAVE: short half-life).
- *Platelet inhibitors*: Surgery should not be delayed, as synthesis of new platelets cannot be waited for. In case of bleeding, platelet transfusion is indicated.
- *Direct oral anticoagulants (DOACs)*: In patients with regular liver function, bleeding is not to be expected after 24 h, in case of Edoxaban, which is eliminated 50% renally, renal function has to be considered. INR and PTT are no significant parameters; however, blood levels can be measured. In case of severe bleeding after 24 h, PCC should be administered. Andexanet alfa is available as an andidote for Apixaban and Rivaroxaban.

Treatment

Medial Femoral Neck Fracture

Garden I. These non-displaced and valgus-impacted fractures account for about 15–20% of all femoral neck fractures (Fig. 26.1). The compromising of blood supply of the femoral head is relatively low and the fracture situation is assessed as stable. Therefore, conservative treatment is possible. However, there is a risk of delayed ischemic necrosis due to pressure in the joint capsule caused by hematoma or secondary dislocation. Conservative treatment is successful in 44%, while 52% need secondary surgical treatment due to fracture dislocation.

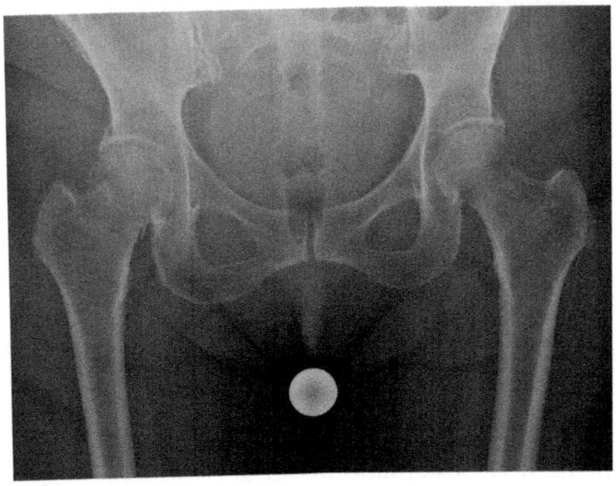

Fig. 26.1 Plain X-ray of a medial femoral head fracture on right side, type Garden I

Further risks of conservative treatment are shortening of the femoral neck and consecutive gluteal insufficiency.

Garden II–IV. While in younger patients an osteosynthesis of the medial femoral neck fracture might be favorable, in geriatric patients with frequently decreased bone mineral density or coxarthrosis, primary joint replacement is indicated (Fig. 26.2). Furthermore, in these patients, hemi-arthroplasty has advantages over a total hip replacement: shorter time of operation, less invasive surgery, lower rates of dislocations, less pulmonary complications, and lower blood loss.

In the case of decreased bone mineral density, cemented stems can improve the interface between implant and bone allowing immediate full weight bearing. Cemented implantation may lead to a higher mortality for the first 24 h; however, the difference is equaled after 7 days, and after 3 months uncemented implants show a higher mortality. Cementing technique is oriented towards the guidelines of elective hip arthroplasty. The risk of bone cement implantation syndrome (BICS) can be minimized by jet lavage, increased positive end-expiratory pressure (PEEP), vacuum-based cement preparation and retrograde cementing. Furthermore, the use of a stem centralizer is recommended.

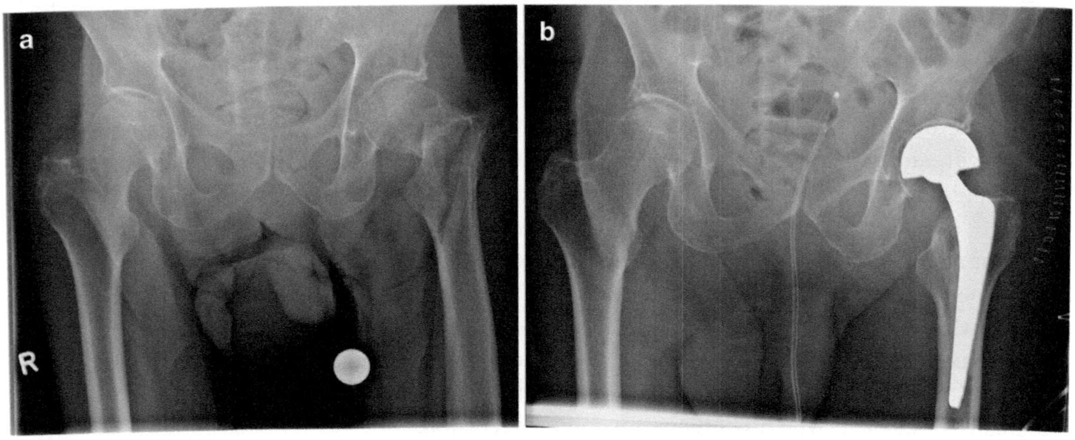

Fig. 26.2 (**a**) Plain X-ray of a medial femoral neck fracture on left side, type Garden III. (**b**) post-operative X-ray after implantation of a cemented hemiprosthesis (stem: MS-30, Fa. Zimmer, Germany, femoral head: modular-bipolar, Fa. Zimmer, Germany)

In literature, an anterolateral approach is recommended, due to lower dislocation rates compared to posterior approaches.

Lateral Femoral Neck Fracture

Lateral femoral neck fractures are commonly treated with joint replacement in geriatric patients.

Per- /Sub-Trochanteric Femoral Fracture

Therapy of per- and sub-trochanteric fractures is a domain of surgical therapy. Surgery is aiming for early total weight bearing and early mobilization, preferably achieved with osteosynthesis by a cephalomedullary nail using minimal invasive surgical technique.

Generally, an anatomic reposition is crucial in order to achieve healing. Varus malposition poses a high risk for failure of the osteosynthesis. Due to insufficient reposition and osteoporosis, 12–32% of the osteosynthesis fail and require revision. As precondition for successful cephalomedullary nailing sufficient closed reduction of the fracture might be achieved on the extension-table. If a closed reduction is not possible, open reduction must be performed.

An anatomical reposition is also helpful in order to find the correct entry point of the nail. This is crucial for the latter reaming of the medullary cavity and implantation of the nail.

Care must be taken when positioning the femoral neck screw, which should be placed "center-center," with a tendency towards the Adam's bow, positioning further cranial leads to higher risk of cut outs.

As an alternative to osteosynthesis, primary joint replacement is discussed, especially in patients with complex type AO31A2 fractures, coincidence of coxarthrosis or very poor bone quality. A technical problem is the refixation of the greater trochanter, which is crucial for joint stability and gluteal sufficiency. In case of arthroplasty, a prosthesis with long stem, or favorably a modular system with free options in concern of antetorsion, length, CCD-angle, and the opportunity of distal fixation might be chosen.

In literature, patients with extracapsular fractures treated with arthroplasty require more blood transfusion, duration of surgery is significantly longer and one-year mortality is reported to be significantly increased compared to osteosynthesis (27.6 vs 13.8%).

Furthermore, due to missing anatomic landmarks, achieving implantation with correct length and offset is complicated.

AO31A1.1–A1.3: Medial support of the femur is preserved, the lesser trochanter remains intact. In these cases, an osteosynthesis with a dynamic hip screw or a cephalomedullary implant is possible. The cephalomedullary nail carries the risk of fatty embolism and the risk of dislocation of the fracture while implanting the nail. However, the surgical approach for a dynamic hip screw on the other hand is more extended.

AO31A2.1–A2.3: In these fractures, the lesser trochanter is involved, and therefore the medial cortex weakened. Due to the increased instability, a cephalomedullary implant is recommended. In case of fractures with multifragmentary medial cortex, a long nail is recommended.

AOA3.1–3.3: In these fractures, the lateral cortex is involved, A3.1 describes a reversed oblique fracture (Fig. 26.3), A3.2 stands for an intertrochanteric transverse fracture and A3.3 runs intertrochanteric with additional lesser trochanter fragment. Those fractures account as instable fractures and closed reduction often is not possible due to tension of the pelvitrochanteric muscles. Open reposition, if necessary, with the help of a cable and osteosynthesis with a long intertrochanteric nail is recommended (Fig. 26.4). The use of too many cables however should be assessed as critical to not harm periosteal perfusion.

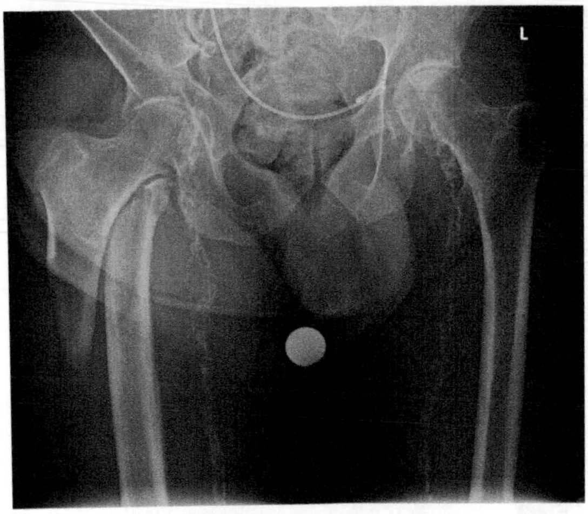

Fig. 26.3 Reversed oblique intertrochanteric fracture, type AO 31A3.1, right side with painful dislocation, shortening, and rotation. Note the arteriosclerosis of the arteries and arthritis of the left side

Periprosthetic Femoral Fracture

Periprosthetic fractures in elderly patients are reported to have an annual incidence of up to 0.13% and a mortality up to 9.8%. Lower rates of periprosthetic fractures after hip arthroplasty, notably in hemiarthroplasty, are discussed using cemented stems compared to cementless stems in elderly patients.

Periprosthetic fractures of the hip are classified according to the Vancouver classification system. Type A is located in the trochanteric region, type B is located around the stem and type C fractures are located below the stem. Type B fractures are subclassified depending on whether the stem is fixed (B1), loose with good bone quality (B2), or loose with poor bone quality or severe comminution (B3).

Treatment depends on whether the stem is considered stable or not. Basically, B1 fractures can be treated with open reduction and internal fixation, while a loose stem (B2, B3) should be changed to a longer revision-stem, preferably with a modular system. Internal fixation might be achieved, for example, with a trochanteric grip plate and cables as displayed in Fig. 26.5. Figure 26.6 shows a periprosthetic fracture Type Vancouver B2, treated with a modular revision system, providing the opportunity of distal locking. However, surgical treatment must be planned individually considering comorbidities, type of initial stem (cemented or cementless), location of the fracture, and bone quality.

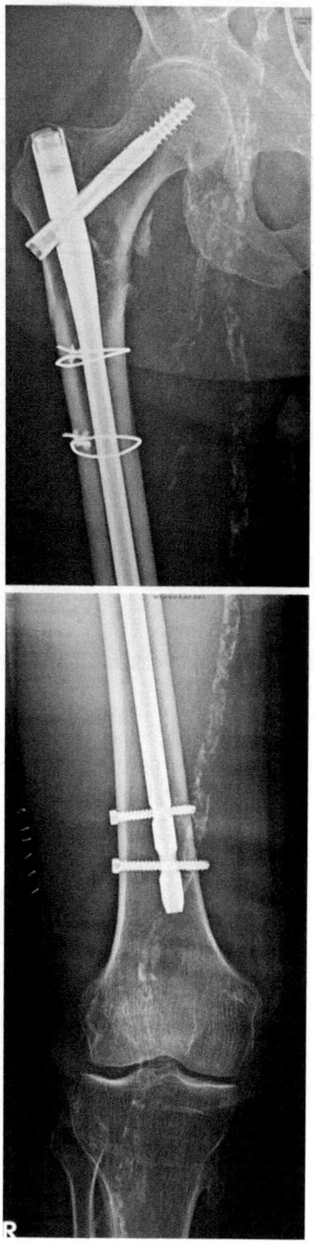

Fig. 26.4 Post-operative plain X-ray of the right femur after open reduction and fixation with two cerclages (Fa. Depuy Synthes) and cephalomedullary nail (Gamma3-nail, long, Fa. Stryker)

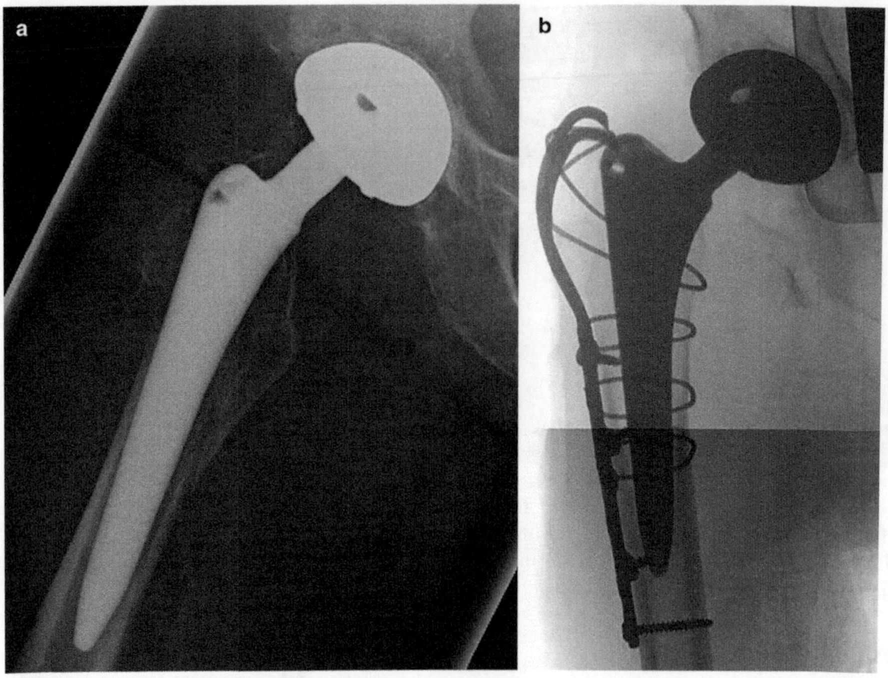

Fig. 26.5 (**a**) Periprosthetic fracture type Vancouver B1, right side in an 81-year-old female. (**b**) Plain X-ray of the post-operative result after open reduction and internal fixation with a Dall-Miles trochanteric grip plate (Fa. Stryker). Fixation is achieved with Dall-Miles cables (Fa. Stryker) and additional monocortical screws; if possible, also bicortical screws can be used around the stem

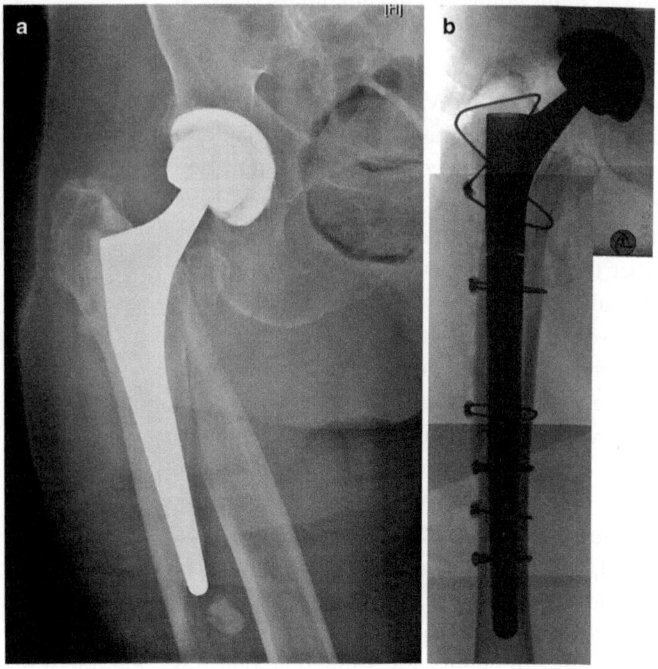

Fig. 26.6 (**a**) Periprosthetic fracture type Vancouver B2 with long oblique fracture line. (**b**) Plain post-operative X-ray after revision with a curved modular revision system (Revitan Hip System, Fa Zimmer Biomet). Note the distal locking screws, providing rotational and axial stability, giving the possibility of primary full weight bearing

Conclusions

Hip fractures of the geriatric population have an increasing incidence with a high mortality due to an aging population. Treatment is most often surgical and should aim for immediate full weight bearing and mobilization in spite of decreased bone quality. After displaced femoral neck fractures a better health status is shown when treated with total or hemi-arthroplasty compared to osteosynthesis.

Medication with anticoagulant effect is frequent in elderly patients and should not unnecessarily delay surgical treatment. Operation should be performed within the first 24 h after admission.

References

1. Bonnaire F, Bula P, Schellong S. Management of pre-existing anticoagulation for timely treatment of proximal femoral fractures. Unfallchirurg. 2019;122(5):404–10. https://doi.org/10.1007/s00113-019-0646-4.
2. Burgers PTPW, Van Geene AR, Van den Bekerom MPJ, Van Lieshout EMM, Blom B, Aleem IS, et al. Total hip arthroplasty versus hemiarthroplasty for displaced femoral neck fractures in the healthy elderly: a meta-analysis and systematic review of randomized trials. Int Orthop. 2012;36(8):1549–60. https://doi.org/10.1007/s00264-012-1569-7.
3. Coomber R, Porteous M, Hubble MJW, Parker MJ. Total hip replacement for hip fracture: surgical techniques and concepts. Injury. 2016;47(10):2060–4. https://doi.org/10.1016/j.injury.2016.06.034.
4. Cooper C. The crippling consequences of fractures and their impact on quality of life. Am J Med. 1997;103(2A):12S–9S. https://doi.org/10.1016/s0002-9343(97)90022-x.
5. Emara AK, Ng M, Krebs VE, Bloomfield M, Molloy RM, Piuzzi NS. Femoral stem cementation in hip arthroplasty: the know-how of a "lost" art. Curr Rev Musculoskelet Med. 2021;14(1):47–59. https://doi.org/10.1007/s12178-020-09681-5.
6. Griffiths R, Babu S, Dixon P, Freeman N, Hurford D, Kelleher E, et al. Guideline for the management of hip fractures 2020: guideline by the Association of Anaesthetists. Anaesthesia. 2021;76(2):225–37. https://doi.org/10.1111/anae.15291.
7. Kim S-Y, Kim Y-G, Hwang J-K. Cementless calcar-replacement hemiarthroplasty compared with intramedullary fixation of unstable intertrochanteric fractures. A prospective, randomized study. J Bone Joint Surg Am. 2005;87(10):2186–92. https://doi.org/10.2106/JBJS.D.02768.
8. Kouyoumdjian P, Dhenin A, Dupeyron A, Coulomb R, Asencio G. Periprosthetic fracture in the elderly with anatomic modular cementless hemiarthroplasty. Orthop Traumatol Surg Res. 2016;102(6):701–5. https://doi.org/10.1016/j.otsr.2016.05.013.
9. Peeters CMM, Visser E, Van de Ree CLP, Gosens T, Oudsten Den BL, De Vries J. Quality of life after hip fracture in the elderly: a systematic literature review. Injury. 2016;47(7):1369–82. https://doi.org/10.1016/j.injury.2016.04.018.
10. Sandmann GH, Biberthaler P. Pertrochanteric femoral fractures in the elderly. Unfallchirurg. 2015;118(5):447–60. https://doi.org/10.1007/s00113-015-0007-x.
11. Saul D, Riekenberg J, Ammon JC, Hoffmann DB, Sehmisch S. Hip fractures: therapy, timing, and complication spectrum. Orthop Surg. 2019;11(6):994–1002. https://doi.org/10.1111/os.12524.
12. Simunovic N, Devereaux PJ, Sprague S, Guyatt GH, Schemitsch E, Debeer J, et al. Effect of early surgery after hip fracture on mortality and complications: systematic review and meta-analysis. CMAJ. 2010;182(15):1609–16. https://doi.org/10.1503/cmaj.092220.
13. Stoffel K, Horn T, Zagra L, Mueller M, Perka C, Eckardt H. Periprosthetic fractures of the proximal femur: beyond the Vancouver classification. EFORT Open Rev. 2020;5(7):449–56. https://doi.org/10.1302/2058-5241.5.190086.
14. Veronese N, Maggi S. Epidemiology and social costs of hip fracture. Injury. 2018;49(8):1458–60. https://doi.org/10.1016/j.injury.2018.04.015.
15. Marzi I, Pohlemann T. Spezielle Unfallchirurgie. Amsterdam: Elsevier; 2017.

27 Acetabulum Fractures

Julia Riemenschneider and Ingo Marzi

Epidemiology and Pathophysiology

During the past decades the incidence of acetabular fractures in geriatric patients has increased. Per year 92/100,000 of the elderly population aged above 65 years and even 446/100,000 above 85 years suffer from an acetabular fracture.

In the younger population, those injuries are often associated with a high-energy trauma, for example a dashboard injury in the context of a car accident. Contrary to this in the elderly population, acetabular fractures are more often caused by low-energy trauma, like falls from lower heights, for example, bicycles, stairs, or even standing. Reasons for this are the increasing degeneration of bones and muscles with higher age, due to osteoporosis and inactivity. 20% of all osteoporotic pelvic fractures are acetabular fractures. Females suffer more often from a loss of bone density, which is the reason why the female gender is associated with a negative prognostic value, just like an older age.

Classification

The classification proposed by Letournel and Judet based on radiological findings is most commonly used to categorize acetabular fractures. There are two major groups—the elementary and combined fractures. Basically, five simple fractures are described only affecting a single column or wall. Associated fractures are injuries that are combined fractures with also five subgroups. Contrary to other classification systems, an overview for the need of an operative treatment based on the instability of the fracture does not exist.

Based on this, the following three acetabular fractures are most frequently seen in the elderly population: first, a fracture of both columns (26.4–28%); second, a fracture of the anterior column with affection of the posterior hemitransverse (ACPHT, 14.9–24%); and third, an isolated fracture of the anterior column (11.4–19.2%). Figure 27.1 gives an overview of the three single fracture patterns.

J. Riemenschneider · I. Marzi (✉)
Department of Trauma, Hand, and Reconstructive Surgery, University Hospital, Goethe University Frankfurt, Frankfurt, Germany
e-mail: marzi@trauma.uni-frankfurt.de

P. Petrone, C. E.M. Brathwaite (eds.), *Acute Care Surgery in Geriatric Patients*,
https://doi.org/10.1007/978-3-031-30651-8_27

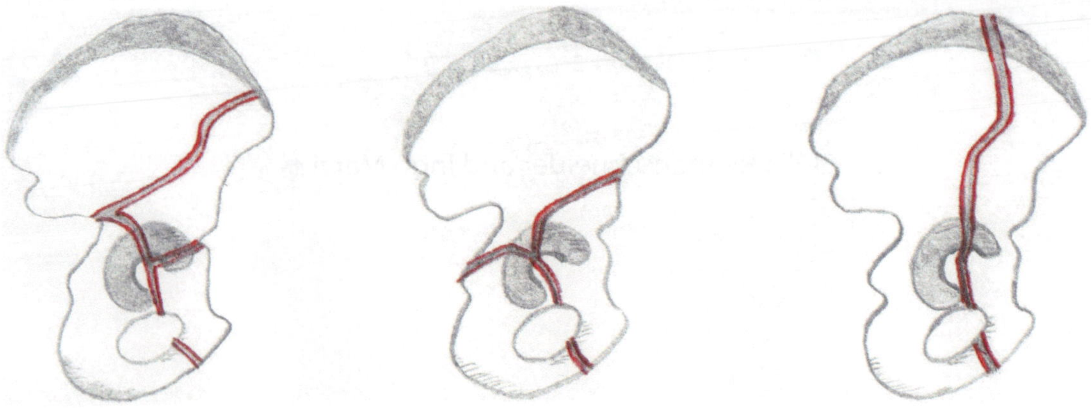

Fig. 27.1 Most frequent fracture patterns in geriatric patients based on the Letournel classification. The fracture patterns from left to right are a both-column fracture, an anterior column and posterior hemitransverse fracture (ACPHT) and a single anterior column fracture

Diagnostic

Acetabular fractures in the elderly are often caused by low-energy trauma. Clinical symptoms are unspecific. First indications can be a hematoma, or hip pain on the affected side, especially during mobilization. The first diagnostic step after the clinical survey is a plain X-ray of the pelvis with a reference ball (needs to be performed in case a Total Hip Arthroplasty (THA)). Expressions of an acetabular fracture can be incongruences of the cortex. In case of an affection of the posterior structures of the acetabulum, the dislocated fracture fragments and the rest of the acetabulum can appear as a double-curved shadow that is known as the "Gull-sign" or "Gull-wing sign" that was firstly described by Berkebile et al.

If an acetabular fracture is suspected, further diagnostic is needed for treatment decision. On the one hand additional X-rays in Ala and Obturator views can help to evaluate the affection of the anterior and posterior column (these are more often used postoperatively after osteosynthesis) or on the other hand a computed tomography (CT)-scan with 3D reconstruction.

Due to the fact, that the operative treatment options for acetabular fractures are physically demanding for the elderly, it is very important to consider the patients' individual risk factors, lifestyle, and resilience.

Therapy

For the treatment of acetabular fractures in the elderly, many options have been established. There is a range from conservative, minimal invasive, or open reconstruction to primary or secondary hip replacements. During the past decades, operative treatment methods have been developed and are more often performed.

Conservative Treatment

In case of simple, non-dislocated fractures of the acetabulum therapy is held conservatively with a combination of physical therapy and early mobilization based on a sufficient pain management. After mobilization, a radiological control needs to be performed to exclude secondary dislocation of the fracture. A conservative therapy regime will also be performed if the patient is suffering from any illness that is a contraindication for a narcosis or if the patient had been bedridden before the trauma. Figure 27.2 shows an X-ray of a conservatively treated fracture of the anterior column.

Surgical Treatment

At the moment, a guideline with precise treatment recommendations for the different acetabu-

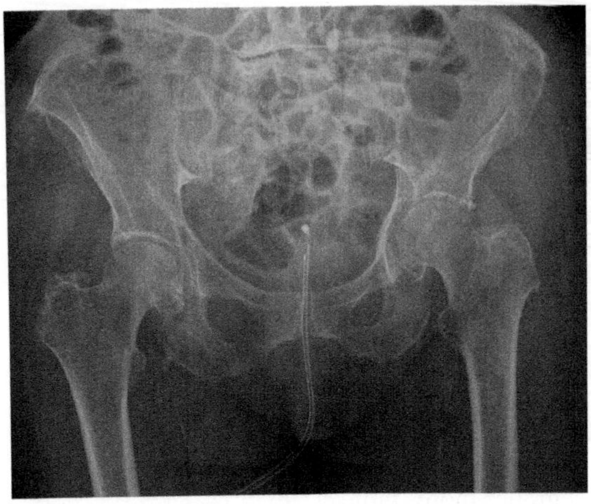

Fig. 27.2 Conservative treated acetabular fracture on the left with affection of the anterior column. Because of this patient's pre-existing condition, a therapy regime with partial weight mobilization under adequate pain management was chosen. However, this often cannot be followed by the patients, so that the fracture should be outside the weight-bearing axis

lar fracture patterns is not established. As a result, the choice of an invasive treatment method is sometimes more dependent on the clinical resources and experiences. Most common options are open reduction and internal fixation (ORIF) via different approaches, total hip arthroplasty via different approaches using reinforcement rings, combined methods or closed reduction and percutaneous pinning (CRPP). The last one is a minimal invasive procedure that performs a fracture reduction under CT guidance with pins.

Osteosynthesis is performed more frequently, especially in cases of simple fractures. After reduction, internal fixation is reached with one or more plates, either anatomically preformed or reconstruction plates. For a long time, the ilioinguinal approach has been the first choice for stabilizing fractures affecting the anterior column. For treating fractures of the posterior column, the dorsal approach is used; but this is more common in the younger population. The modified Stoppa (intrapelvic) approach or the pararectus approach are often performed in case of an impression of the quadrilateral surface with protrusion of the femoral head. Due to the great overview from the inside of the acetabulum, the modified Stoppa approach can also be used for the osteosynthesis of more complex fracture patterns. Severe intraoperative complications can be iatrogenic injuries of the bladder, the obturator vessels or nerve, and the corona mortis.

As an alternative option, a THA is possible. A THA is often chosen for more complex fractures, affection of the femoral head, severe arthrosis or if the affected side has been treated with an endoprosthesis earlier. For sufficient stability, it is often necessary to use special reinforcement rings (e.g. Burch-Schneider ring, MUTARS RS Cup system), cemented or uncemented, depending of the bone quality. This is a good additional stabilization, especially if the Os ischium is intact. Depending on the surgeon's experiences, a THA can be performed via different approaches—the most frequently used is the posterior (Kocher-Langenbeck) followed by the anterolateral and anterior (Smith-Peterson). These operations are more often associated with intraoperative higher blood losses or longer operation times.

To optimize the reduction result, in some cases a combination of THA and ORIF must be performed.

Preferred Treatment Method

Depending on the fracture pattern and the individual risk factors we recommend two different treatment options for acetabular fractures. Whenever possible from the anatomic situation and reconstruction option, we recommend to perform an ORIF via the modified Stoppa approach. This operative access gives a good overview of the fracture and is—based on various experiences—associated with less intra- and postoperative complications than a THA. Especially when the quadrilateral surface is impressed with a protrusion of the femoral head into the pelvis, plate fixation after open reduction by axial traction of the ipsilateral leg presents sufficient results. Limitations for this technique are multi-fragmentary fractures of the acetabulum, as a plate may not be able to address all fracture fragments, and affections of the femoral head or femoral neck. Regarding the postoperative treatment, patients are often only allowed to be mobilized by partial weight bearing which can be very challenging for geriatric patients, too. If a plate osteo-

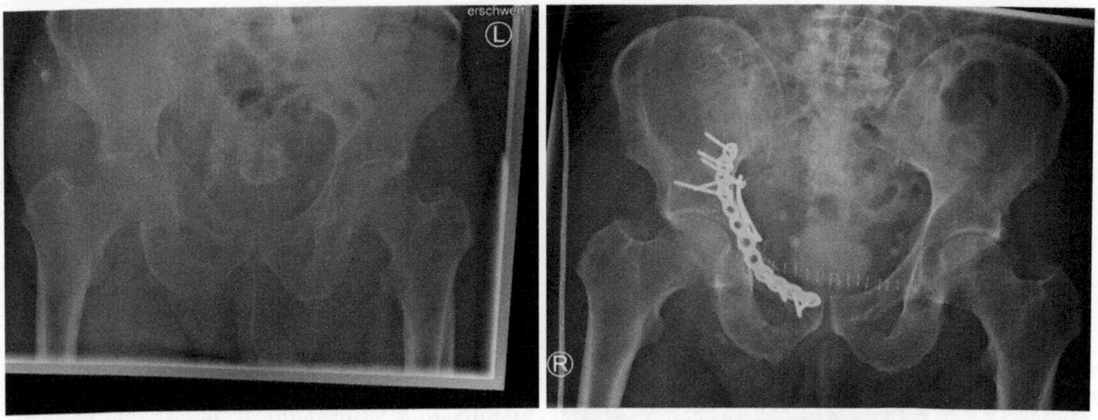

Fig. 27.3 Acetabular fracture with affection of both columns and minor dislocation of the quadrilateral surface. Via the modified Stoppa approach an open reduction and internal fixation with a suprapectineal plate (Fa. Stryker GmBH & Co. KG, Duisburg, Germany) was performed

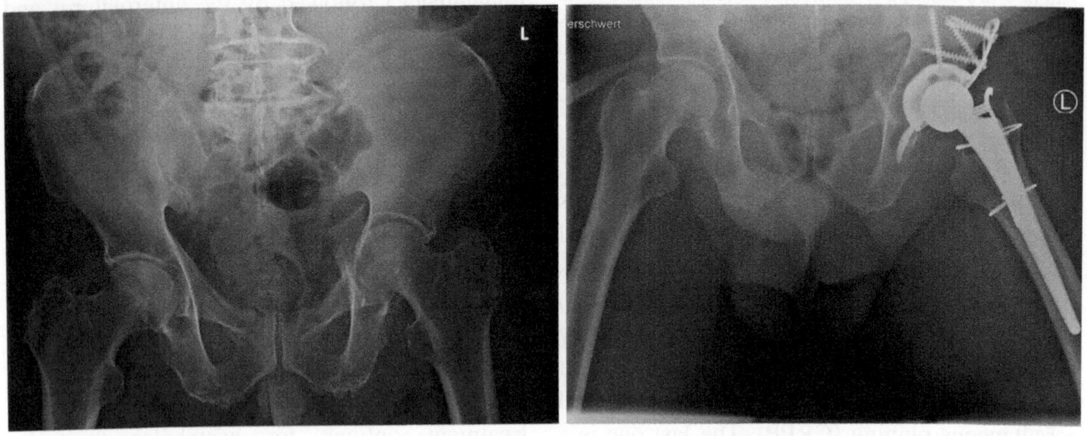

Fig. 27.4 Acetabular fracture with multi-fragmentary destruction, major dislocation of the quadrilateral surface and affection of the greater trochanter. Via the lateral approach a THA with MUTARS RS Cup System (Implantcast, Germany) and CLS stem (Zimmer Biomet Deutschland GmbH, Freiburg, Germany) was performed

synthesis does not appear to be stable enough in the preoperative planning, we perform a THA with an acetabulum enforcement ring, at best with an integrated cup (e.g., MUTARS RS cup system, Implantcast, Germany) (Figs. 27.3 and 27.4).

An advantage of this kind of operation technique is that additional fractures of the Os ilium can be overcome by a reinforcement ring. For the stability of the prosthesis, it is essential that the Os ischium is not affected. In this case or in the case of an advanced osteoporosis, a combination of both treatment methods can be necessary. After this kind of THA, patients are regularly allowed to be mobilized by full weight bearing.

Prognosis and Complications

Every treatment option has its benefits. Preoperatively, it is very important to discuss the patient's lifestyle, life expectations, and physical demands. Taking these facts in concern is helpful in order to find a patient-adapted treatment decision (ORIF or THA). The risk of a post-traumatic osteoarthrosis following an osteosynthesis with the need of a secondary THA has less relevance for geriatric patients, whose life expectation is only a few years. However, for geriatric patients who are suffering from further diseases or are bedridden shorter operation times (121 vs. 139 min), shorter hospitalization (13 vs. 21 postoperative days), and lower incidences of postoperative material failure, with the result of an operative revision (e.g., dislocations of an endoprosthesis) can be major benefits. Furthermore, comparing ORIF and THA in case of acetabular fractures the blood loss is less with 2 vs. 3 g/dL. Opposite to this, patients treated with a plate fixation via the Stoppa approach suffer more frequently from postoperative vein thrombosis which results from intraoperative trauma of greater vessels with up to 14%.

References

1. Audretsch C, Trulson A, Höch A, Herath SC, Histing T, Küper MA. Evaluation of decision-making in the treatment of acetabular fractures. EFORT Open Rev. 2022;7(1):84–94.
2. Berkebile RD, Fischer DL, Albrecht LF. The gull-wing sign. Value of the lateral view of the pelvis in fracture-dislocation of the acetabular rim and posterior dislocation of the femoral head. Radiology. 1965;84:937–9.
3. Daurka JS, Pastides PS, Lewis A, Rickman M, Bircher MD. Acetabular fractures in patients aged >55 years: a systematic review of the literature. Bone Joint J. 2014;96-B(2):157–63.
4. Ferguson TA, Patel R, Bhandari M, Matta JM. Fractures of the acetabulum in patients aged 60 years and older: an epidemiological and radiological study. J Bone Joint Surg (Br). 2010;92(2):250–7.
5. Firoozabadi R, Cross WW, Krieg JC, Routt MLC. Acetabular fractures in the senior population-epidemiology, mortality and treatments. Arch Bone Jt Surg. 2017;5(2):96–102.
6. Janko M, Verboket R, Genari M, Frank J, Marzi I. Primary or revision arthroplasty with an integrated acetabular cup-MUTARS® RS cup system. Eur J Trauma Emerg Surg. 2022;48(5):4149–55.
7. Krappinger D, Kammerlander C, Hak DJ, Blauth M. Low-energy osteoporotic pelvic fractures. Arch Orthop Trauma Surg. 2010;130(9):1167–75.
8. Letournel E. Acetabulum fractures: classification and management. Clin Orthop Relat Res. 1980;151:81–106.
9. McCormick BP, Serino J, Orman S, Webb AR, Wang DX, Mohamadi A, et al. Treatment modalities and outcomes following acetabular fractures in the elderly: a systematic review. Eur J Orthop Surg Traumatol. 2022;32(4):649–59.
10. Meermans G, Konan S, Das R, Volpin A, Haddad FS. The direct anterior approach in total hip arthroplasty: a systematic review of the literature. Bone Joint J. 2017;99-B(6):732–40.
11. Mohan K, Broderick JM, Raza H, O'Daly B, Leonard M. Acetabular fractures in the elderly: modern challenges and the role of conservative management. Ir J Med Sci. 2022;191(3):1223–8.
12. Pohlemann T, Herath SC, Braun BJ, Rollmann MF, Histing T, Pizanis A. Anterior approaches to the acetabulum: which one to choose? EFORT Open Rev. 2020;5(10):707–12.
13. Riemenschneider J, Vollrath JT, Mühlenfeld N, Frank J, Marzi I, Janko M. Acetabular fractures treatment needs in the elderly and nonagenarians. EFORT Open Rev. 2022;7(6):433–45.

Long Bone Fractures

28

Cora R. Schindler and Ingo Marzi

Introduction

Due to demographic change, the incidence of long bone fractures in older people is increasing. Comorbidities (e.g., cardiovascular disease, gait instability, or osteoporosis) predispose older people to fractures in apparently minor trauma. The most common trauma mechanism is a fall from low height, which often leads to isolated extremity fractures, particularly of the (proximal) femur, humerus, and radius. Because of their reduced physical condition, geriatric trauma patients have a higher risk of post-traumatic complications, later disability, and death. Rapid recovery is crucial for these patients, as regaining mobility and independence becomes more difficult with age but is essential to avoid the need for subsequent long-term care.

Radiological Examination After Geriatric Extremity Trauma

After clinical examination, radiological imaging is the standard method for diagnosing fractures. Conventional X-ray is both sensitive and cost-effective and remains the method of first choice. Complementary, computed tomography (CT) provides details of fracture morphology and facilitates treatment planning. Given the increased risk of occult injury and reduced concerns about the effects of radiation exposure, the threshold for performing radiological diagnostics in geriatric patients should be set low. Other imaging modalities, such as magnetic resonance imaging (MRI), have secondary relevance in geriatric extremity injuries, for example, to confirm a suspected fracture or to assess soft tissue injuries such as vessels, nerves, or ligaments.

Standard Classification of Long Bone Fractures

The AO classification was published in 1987 by Müller et al. and later supplemented by the *Arbeitsgemeinschaft für Osteosynthesefragen* (AO). While specific fracture types have their own clinical classifications, it represents the international classification standard for long bone fractures. Modern fracture treatment and guideline development are based on the 2018 version of the AO/OTA Fracture and Dislocation Classification Compendium. Radiological imaging is required for the AO classification. The affected bone itself, the localization in the bone, the fracture type, and the joint involvement result in an alphanumeric code that describes the complexity and severity of the fracture. Other classi-

C. R. Schindler · I. Marzi (✉)
Department of Trauma, Hand, and Reconstructive Surgery, University Hospital, Goethe University Frankfurt, Frankfurt/Main, Germany
e-mail: marzi@trauma.uni-frankfurt.de

P. Petrone, C. E.M. Brathwaite (eds.), *Acute Care Surgery in Geriatric Patients*,
https://doi.org/10.1007/978-3-031-30651-8_28

fications such as *Oestern* and *Tscherne* or *Gustilo-Anderson* are mainly used to classify open fractures.

Treatment of Long Bone Fractures

On the one hand, the increasing activity level of older people leads to higher expectations of the functional outcome. On the other hand, some elderly patients suffer from mental and physical deficits that make it impossible to implement more complex therapy concepts. In older trauma patients, the accompanying circumstances such as comorbidities, reduced bone quality, and the social environment play a major role. These aspects, in addition to the type of fracture itself, must be considered when choosing an appropriate treatment strategy. In any case, early reduction and immobilization of the fracture is essential to avoid secondary damage to surrounding tissues such as cartilage, nerves, and vessels and to prevent complications. Reduction is usually achieved by traction and axial alignment. Except for ankle and distal radius fractures, the associated joints should be included in immobilization and a physiological neutral position achieved. Assessment of peripheral circulation, motor function, and sensitivity before and after reduction is mandatory. The optimal time window for primary osteosynthesis is within the first 6 h. Stable fractures can be primarily splinted and, if necessary, treated by osteosynthesis after consolidation of the soft tissues (approx. 5–7 days). In the case of severely dislocated, unstable, or open fractures (grade III and above), immediate surgical reduction and stabilization is required to avoid major bleeding, soft tissue damage, perfusion deficits, and compartment syndrome. In emergencies, an external fixator can be applied and secondary definitive osteosynthesis performed within 7–14 days after soft tissue consolidation. In geriatric patients, early final treatment should always be considered to reduce the risk of post-traumatic complications due to prolonged immobilization and secondary interventions.

Oral anticoagulation should be bridged perioperatively (usually 24–48 h) with low molecular weight heparin. Depending on the urgency and risk of bleeding, coagulation should be optimized preoperatively (see Chap. 28).

Pain control is crucial in the perioperative treatment of the elderly. Inadequate analgesia increases the risk of delirium. Reduction must be performed under adequate analgesia. Fracture gap or regional anesthesia, for example, are also suitable for this purpose.

The aim is to restore functional and physical capacity, and thus independence, as quickly and painlessly as possible.

Geriatric Upper Extremity Fractures

Upper limb fractures are the second most common group of fragility fractures after hip fractures in geriatric trauma patients. Their impact on mobility and independence is severe, especially when they occur in combination with lower extremity injuries. In patients over 70 years of age, the distinction between surgical vs. conservative therapy in upper extremity fractures is becoming increasingly less defined regarding subjective and functional outcome. Therefore, non-operative therapy has a higher priority for common geriatric upper extremity fractures, such as distal radius or proximal humeral fracture.

Distal Radius Fractures

Distal radius fracture is the most common upper extremity fracture in adults over 65 years of age, with an incidence of about 350 per 100,000 person/year. The main accident mechanism is a fall onto the outstretched hand. The resulting fracture morphology depends on the position of the hand (extension or flexion) at the time of impact.

Diagnosis and Classification

Accordingly, fractures of the distal radius were historically classified as extension fractures (*Colles* fracture) or flexion fractures (*Smith* fracture). Today's standard is the *AO classification*: 2R3-A as extra-articular fractures, 2R3-B as partially articular fractures and 2R3-C as fully articular fractures. Furthermore, there are clinical terms for special forms of distal radius fracture, such as the *Barton* or *Chauffeur* fracture.

In most cases, an X-ray of the wrist in two planes, anterior-posterior and lateral, is sufficient to assess a distal radius fracture. A supplementary CT is useful especially in intra-articular fractures.

Non-operative Treatment

Non-operative treatment should be considered primarily for extra-articular fractures and stable non-displaced or minimally displaced intra-articular fractures. Relative indications for non-operative therapy are reducible fractures with instability criteria, depending on the individual constitution of the patient, especially in the presence of risk factors and contraindications to surgical treatment. Non-operative therapy includes reduction, if necessary, and immobilization in a forearm splint. The closed reduction is performed (under sufficient analgesia) either by mechanical reduction by finger-trap traction or by manual traction and countertraction via hypomochlion. It is important that the fracture can be locked in the reduced position and held in place by the splint. After the soft tissue swelling has decreased, a circular soft cast can be applied. The wrist should be immobilized in a functional position (approx. 20° dorsal extension). The metacarpophalangeal joints and the elbow remain free. The duration of immobilization depends on bone quality and fracture healing and is about 6 weeks. Disadvantage: The prolonged immobilization can be burdening for older patients and affect their independence.

Surgical Treatment

Any severely dislocated or unstable fracture of the distal radius should be treated surgically (Table 28.1). Other indications for surgical therapy are open fractures of 2° and 3°, concomitant injuries such as traumatic nerve compression or unsuccessful closed reduction. Relative indications are serial or bilateral upper limb fractures or concomitant lower limb injuries to allow early mobilization and independence.

Table 28.1 Objective criteria of a dislocated fracture of the distal radius

Radial height loss	>2 mm
Change in radial inclination	>5°
Loss of palmar inclination	>20°
Articular incongruence	>1–2 mm
DRUG incongruence	>1 mm

Most dislocated fractures of the distal radius are reduced anatomically and fixed with palmar (locking) plate osteosynthesis (Fig. 28.1). The distal plate should be fixed with locked screws for better stabilization of the articular surface and to avoid loss of alignment. With the option of polyaxial screw fixation, it is also possible to treat intra-articular fractures with dorsal comminution via the palmar approach. The dorsal approach to the wrist is mainly chosen for fractures with dorsal main fragment (e.g., *Barton* fracture) or in case of insufficient stability of the palmar fixation. Depending on the concomitant injury, compliance and bone quality, an additional splint or orthosis may be useful for a few days but should be avoided if possible. In addition to anatomical reduction, the most important purpose of surgical treatment is to achieve functional follow-up as early as possible.

Percutaneous Kirschner wire osteosynthesis allows minimally invasive reduction, which is worth the consideration in frail patients, in order to fix the reduced situation with the wires and a cast. The so-called Kapandji technique allows percutaneous reduction maneuver but fixation needs an additional cast for 4 weeks. However, there are limits to this procedure, especially in the case of multifragmentation, intra-articular fractures or osteoporotic bone, there is a risk of loosening of the wires with secondary loss of correction. This is compounded by the additional need for prolonged immobilization in a splint for protection.

In addition to emergency stabilization, a cross-wrist external fixator is also suitable in some cases for the treatment of complex fractures in the elderly. In this procedure, the fixator can remain in situ until healing. However, there is also a risk of pin loosening in osteoporotic bone. Early functional follow-up is not possible. In

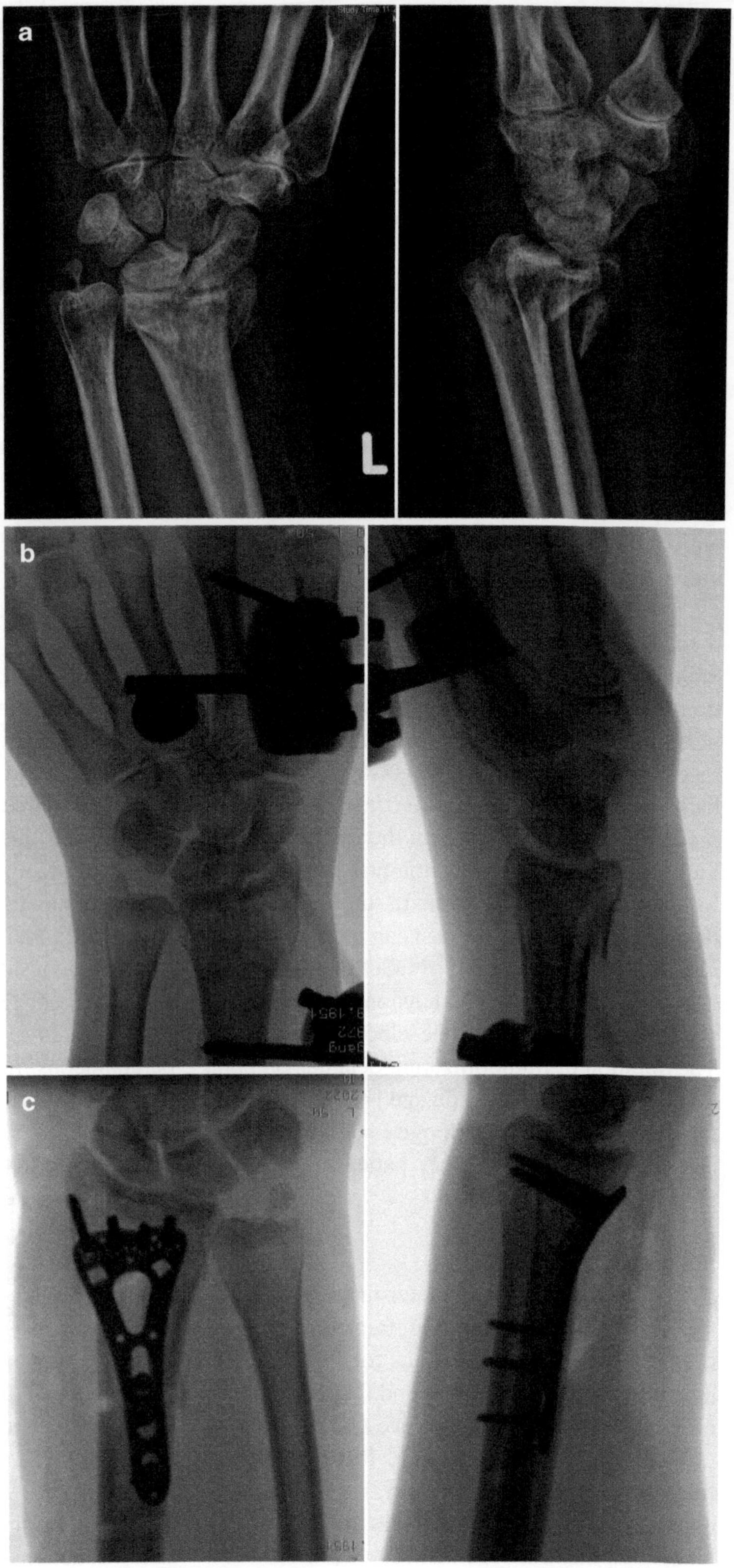

Fig. 28.1 (**a**) Two plain X-ray (a. p. left, lateral right) of the right wrist with dislocated articular fracture of the distal radius, type AO 2R3-C2.2 and avulsion of processus styloideus ulnae; (**b**) intra-operative two plain X-ray (a. p. left, lateral right) of the right distal radius after closed axial reduction and fixation with external fixator. Articular incongruence >2 mm; (**c**) after open anatomical reduction and fixation with locked plate (Fa. Depuy Synthes)

addition, elderly patients are often at risk of accidental self-injury, and ambulant pin care can be difficult.

Proximal Humeral Fracture

Proximal humerus fractures are among the most common osteoporotic fractures. Approximately 85% of these fractures occur in people over 50 years of age, with the highest incidence in the 60–90 age group and a 70:30 ratio between women and men.

The glenohumeral joint is stabilized by the articular cartilage, labrum, ligaments, rotator cuff and deltoid muscle. Interruption of the blood supply (*A. arcuata*) to the proximal humerus often results in ischemia and subsequent humeral head necrosis.

Radiography of the glenohumeral joint in two planes (a. p. and lateral Y-image) should be performed for diagnosis. Computed tomography is recommended to visualize occult fractures or to analyze complex fracture patterns. Magnetic resonance imaging (MRI) can be useful for assessing rotator cuff integrity but has secondary relevance in geriatric patients. Studies have shown that up to 40% of proximal humerus fractures are associated with rotator cuff lesions.

Classification

The *Neer* classification (1970) is the most used in clinical practice. It is based on four fracture parts: the greater tuberosity, the lesser tuberosity, the humeral head, and the humeral shaft. It clusters the non-displaced fractures as "one-part fractures" (*Neer I*), as they are considered a stable unit and can therefore be treated non-operatively. Non-displaced fractures were defined as those in which there was less than 1 cm of dislocation and 45° of angulation between the tuberosities, humeral head, and shaft. The dislocated fractures (*Neer II* +*VI*) are classified into 2-, 3-, and 4-part fractures. The anterior and posterior fracture dislocation as well as the head-split are considered as separate entities. Disadvantages of the *Neer* classification are the limited fracture morphologies and lack of derivation of a prognosis for humeral head necrosis.

Table 28.2 Non-operative treatment of proximal humerus fracture

Week	Treatment
1	Sling, mobilization of elbow and wrist/hand
2–3	Isometric mobilization of the shoulder, pendulum, passive assisted exercises max. 90° Anteversion/Abduction
4–6	Active strengthening exercises, max, 90° Anteversion/Abduction
From 7	Free mobilization, max. weight 1 kg
From 12	Full weight

Non-operative Treatment

Evidence-based guidelines for the treatment of proximal humerus fractures are still lacking. Questionable better functional outcomes with high complication rates of surgical therapy in older patients lead to controversial discussions about therapy in the current literature. This is because patients with manifest complications have an irreversible less favorable functional outcome.

It is undisputed that non-displaced fractures can be treated conservatively (Table 28.2). In these fractures, the soft tissue is usually intact, and periosteum, rotator cuff and joint capsule provide a stable fracture situation. Collapsed or minimally displaced fractures of the greater tuberosity (12–17%) and/or the *collum chirurgicum* (approximately 50–60%) can often be treated functionally. Impacted valgus fracture is also a reasonable indication for non-operative therapy.

The expected results are good, especially for non-displaced or minimally displaced fractures. Shoulder range of motion can reach about 85% of the healthy side, with good pain reduction. Possible complications of non-operative therapy include limited range of motion, humeral head necrosis, subacromial impingement due to a dislocated greater tuberosity, and pseudarthrosis.

Surgical Treatment

In case of displaced fractures, the decision must be made in discussion with the patient depending on the accompanying circumstances. 3- and 4-part and grossly dislocated fractures that do not meet special conditions for conservative therapy should be treated surgically. In addition, metaphyseal comminuted fractures, luxation fractures, open fractures, head-split, and *collum anatomicum* fractures as well as vascular and nerve injuries represent surgical indications. Basically, there are primarily joint-preserving and joint-replacing options.

Osteosynthesis

The implementation of special locking plates for the proximal humerus has significantly improved surgical therapy (Fig. 28.2). Today, osteosynthesis is the most frequently performed surgical procedure. However, the surgical treatment of geriatric fractures remains problematic. Even locked plate implants often find only poor retention in osteoporotic bone, “cutting out” occurs, whereby the screws perforate into the joint. The complication rate of locked plate osteosynthesis is about 25%, with 40% due to surgical complications, of which the most common was intraoperative screw perforation of the humeral head.

Antegrade intramedullary nailing osteosyntheses attempt to combine high stability by rigid internal fixation with soft tissue-preserving minimally invasive procedures. Indications for nailing are in cases of metaphyseal or spiral fractures that extend into the humeral shaft. Fractures of the tubercula are possible, but difficult to fix with a nail and might be better treated by plates.

Percutaneous Kirschner wire osteosynthesis can be only suitable for fractures without metaphyseal comminution. The method is technically demanding. The minimally invasive procedure avoids compromising the blood supply to the head. Disadvantages are less stable fixation and possible wire complications, such as migration.

Joint Replacement

According to current studies, joint-replacement treatment is indicated when the humeral head itself is fragmented or excavated, i.e., cancellous bone lost, in advanced osteoporosis or after failed osteosynthesis (Fig. 28.3). For a successful outcome with a total shoulder arthroplasty after fracture, the healing of the tuberosity in its correct position and the replacement of the humeral head in correct lateral offset and retroversion are crucial.

In many elderly patients, a degenerative rotator cuff lesion is pre-existing. Based on sonographic data, it can be assumed that 28% of patients over 60 years of age, 50% over 70 years of age, and 80% over 80 years of age have a rotator cuff lesion. Due to the special design, reverse total shoulder arthroplasty is particularly suitable for patients who have a relevant lesion of the rotator cuff. As the functional outcome of an inverse prosthesis depends on the deltoid muscle, the functionality of the axillary nerve must be ensured preoperatively. According to current studies, the inverse fracture prosthesis is the primary option for the treatment of non-reconstructable proximal humeral fractures in patients over 65 years of age with rotator cuff lesion.

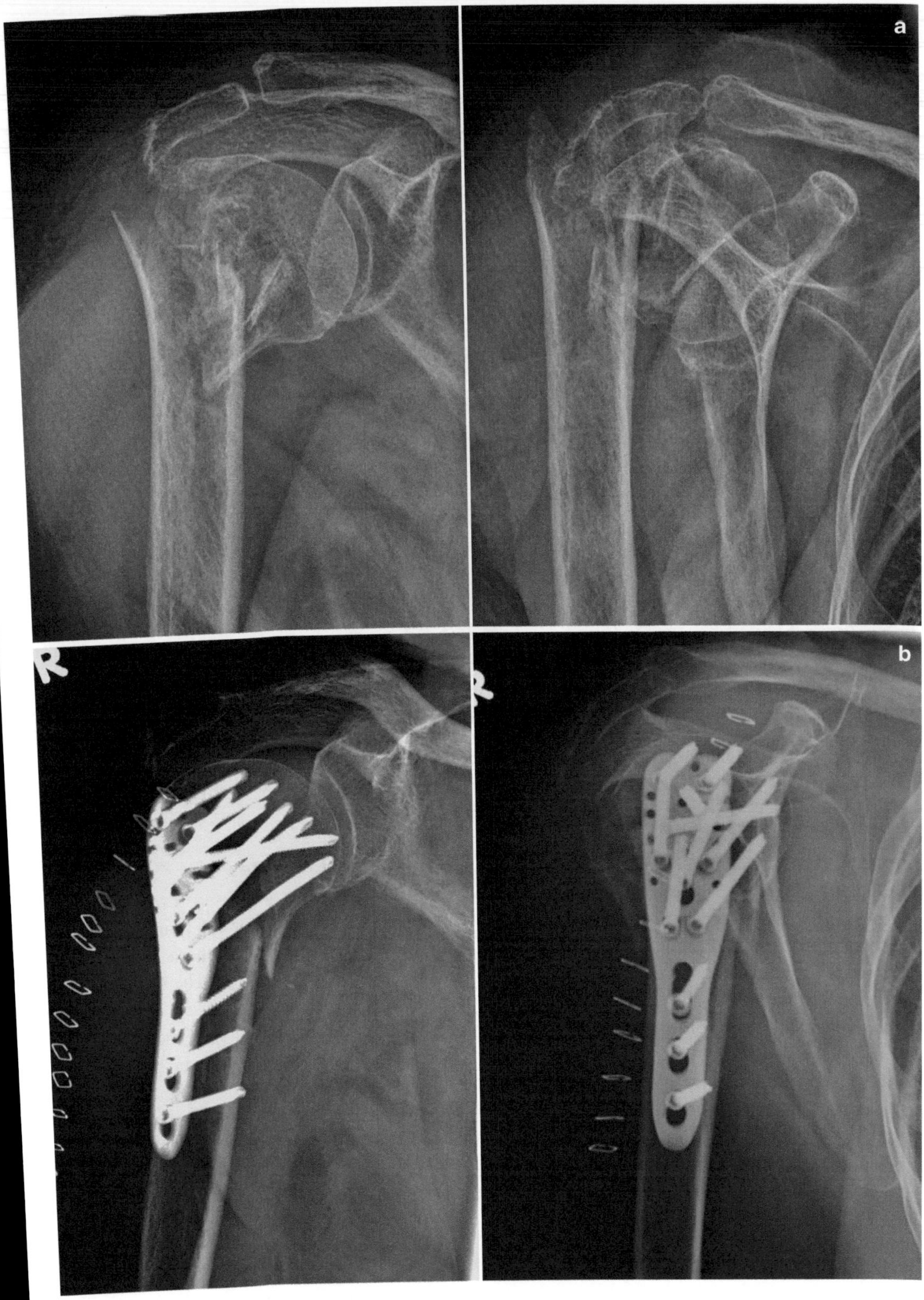

Fig. 28.2 (**a**) Two plain X-ray (a. p. left, Y right) of the right shoulder with anterior dislocated *collum anatomicum* fracture of the proximal humerus. (**b**) post-operative two plain X-ray (a. p. left, Y right) of the right humerus after open reduction and fixation with locked PHILOS plate (Fa. Depuy Synthes).

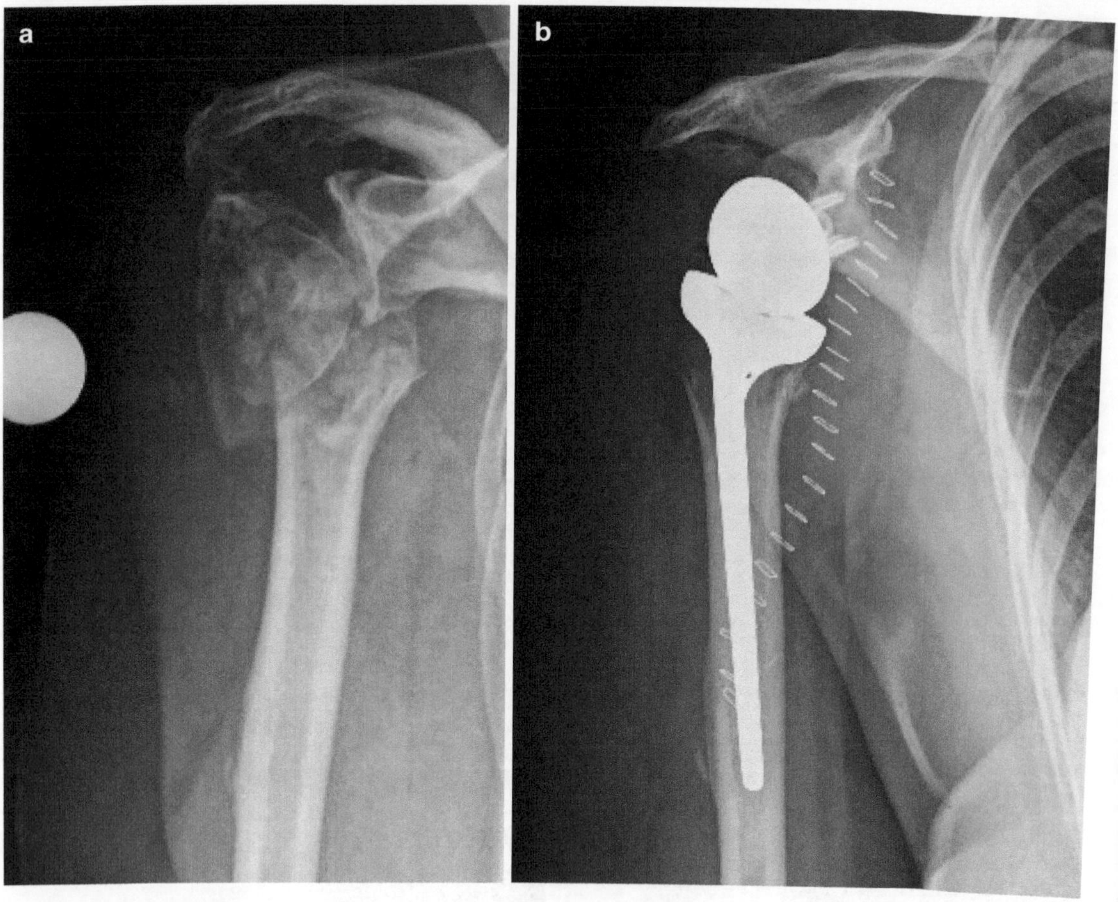

Fig. 28.3 (**a**) X-ray of a multi-fragmentary humeral head fracture with severe comminution. (**b**) joint replacement with a cemented reverse total shoulder arthroplasty (Delte Xtend, Depuy Synthes).

Lower Extremity Fractures in Old Age

The leading fractures of the lower extremities in old age are proximal femur fractures (Chap. 28). Femoral shaft fractures (approx. 10–20/100,000 person/year) and distal femur fractures (approx. 4.5/100,000 person/year) are rare but severe injuries. As with hip fractures, early surgical intervention reduces mortality by minimizing the complications associated with prolonged immobilization. Periarticular fractures, particularly distal femoral fractures, usually require surgery. While femoral shaft fractures are mainly treated with intramedullary nails, the treatment of distal femoral fractures can be more complex.

Distal Femur Fractures

Distal fractures account for 6% of all femur fractures. Approximately 50% of these injuries affect patients over 70 years of age. The 6-month mortality rate is 16% and increases to 30% after 1 year. Most fragility fractures of the distal femur are due to low-energy trauma in patients with osteopenia or osteoporosis, predominantly women. The most common mechanism of trauma is a direct axial impact or the result of torsional or rotational forces. In addition, joint stiffness due to gonarthrosis favors the genesis of this fracture.

Classification

The most used classification for distal femoral fractures is the AO classification (33–femur), which divides them into extra-articular fractures (AO 33-A), partial articular fractures (AO 33-B) and articular fractures (AO 33-C).

Non-operative Treatment

Simple, non-displaced and extra-articular fractures can be successfully treated conservatively with immobilization in casts. However, non-operative therapy of the distal femur fracture plays a minor role. The risks of associated complications by prolonged immobilization must be carefully weighed against the benefits of conservative treatment.

Surgical Treatment

Retrograde Intramedullary Nails

Surgical treatment is the main indication of distal femur fractures. Osteosynthesis with retrograde intramedullary nails is primarily indicated for AO type A fractures. The indication can be extended to non-displaced or minimally displaced intra-articular fractures in conjunction with meta diaphyseal fractures (AO type C1–C2) if a sufficient fixation of the locking screws in the distal femoral fragment is possible. The advantages of this technique are the possibility of closed reduction, minimal invasiveness, and early functional rehabilitation. Data from biomechanical studies suggest that distal locking patterns have a significant influence on the mechanical stability of the bone-implant construct and on the nature of failure in fragility fractures. In osteoporotic bone, distal locking constructions have a 38% higher load to failure compared to the conventional locking technique.

Plate Osteosynthesis

Plate osteosynthesis is indicated for all type of distal femoral fractures (AO A, B, and C). The modern trend are plates and screws with locking technique, especially in osteoporotic fractures due to the increased pull-out resistance. Locking systems behave like an internal fixator, reducing damage to the periosteum and thus optimizing the biological conditions for fracture healing. Modern plates allow the simultaneous use of locking screws (monoaxial or polyaxial) and cortical screws, maximizing the advantages of both systems. The main advantage of osteosynthesis with plates is its versatility, which allows its use in almost any fracture configuration, especially in the presence of pre-existing implants, like hip endoprosthesis or osteosynthesis devices that block the femoral shaft. Intra-articular fractures B1–C3 usually require direct visualization of the fracture and open reduction of the fragments. Fixation of the condylar mass to the shaft can be minimally invasive. For B-fractures of the distal femur, combined screw, and plate osteosynthesis can be the preferred option. After anatomical repositioning of the femoral condyles, stabilization against the shaft should be performed with a locking plate system, for example, the Less Invasive Stabilization System (LISS) (Fig. 28.4). This should be inserted minimally invasively into the stem portion. The stabilization of the medial cortex is often problematic in the treatment of distal femoral fractures. In the case of distally located and at the same time intra-articular femoral fractures, especially in older age with osteoporotic bones, stabilization with a locking plate osteosynthesis system, such as the LISS, is exclusively recommended.

Rescue Surgery of Distal Femur Fractures

More rarely, a hybrid fixator is used in which the joint fragment is stabilized, for example, by a three-quarter ring (*Ilizarov* technique). This procedure is a good alternative compared to internal implants if, for example, the soft tissues do not allow an open procedure.

In osteopenia, secondary corrective loss in the sense of axial malalignment due to sintering of the joint plateau after osteosynthesis is common. Knee arthroplasty can be secondary rescue to failed osteosynthesis or post-traumatic osteoarthritis. In severe comminuted fractures, pre-existing gonarthrosis or severe osteoporosis, primary arthroplasty appears to be attractive as the initial treatment as it reduces the risk of post-operative loss of correction and early complications. It also facilitates early mobilization of patients when compliance is limited due to cognitive deficits. The indication for primary arthroplasty must be narrow.

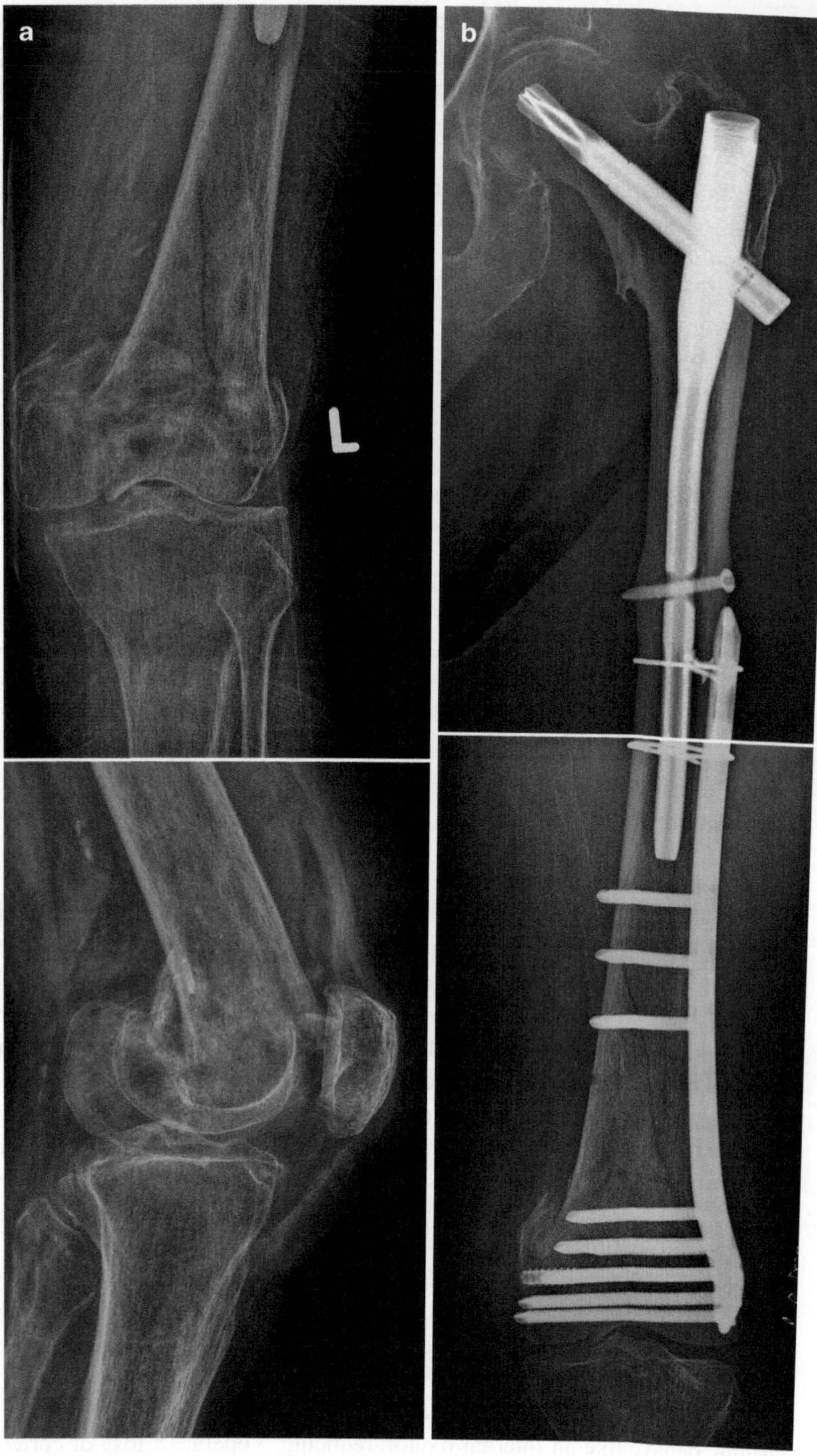

Fig. 28.4 (**a**) Two plain X-ray of the left knee with peri-implant (cephalomedullary nail) fracture of the osteoporotic distal femur, type AO 33-C1.3. (**b**) post-operative plain X-ray of the right femur after open reduction and internal fixation with ASNIS screw, LISS plate and two cerclages (Fa. Depuy Synthes)

Special Case: Periprosthetic Distal Femur Fracture

Periprosthetic knee fractures are a subgroup of distal femoral fractures. The treatment of these fractures is challenging and requires advanced skills in both trauma and prosthetic surgery. Loosen et al. described the presence of pre-existing implants in 58% of geriatric patients with a distal femoral fracture. The most used classification for periprosthetic fractures of the distal femur is that of *Rorabeck and Taylor*, which respects the extent of displacement and the stability of the prosthesis and divides fractures into three groups: fractures without displacement with stable prosthesis (type 1), fractures with displacement greater than 5 mm or angulation greater than 5° with stable prosthesis (type 2), and all supracondylar fractures with loosened prosthesis (type 3). In most cases, locked plate osteosyntheses (e.g., LISS) or directly exchange of the prosthesis is performed. Retrograde nailing osteosynthesis can also be an option, as many modern prosthesis designs have an open femoral box.

References

1. Atinga A, Shekkeris A, Fertleman M, et al. Trauma in the elderly patient. Br J Radiol. 2018;91:20170739. https://doi.org/10.1259/bjr.20170739.
2. Bliemel C, Bücking B, Ruchholtz S. Distale Femurfrakturen. Orthopädie Unfallchirurgie Up2date. 2017;12:63–84. https://doi.org/10.1055/s-0042-111298.
3. Burkhart KJ, Dietz SO, Bastian L, et al. The treatment of proximal humeral fracture in adults. Dtsch Arztebl Int. 2013;110:591–7. https://doi.org/10.3238/arztebl.2013.0591.
4. Franke S, Ambacher T. Die proximale Humerusfraktur. Obere Extremität. 2012;7:137–43. https://doi.org/10.1007/s11678-012-0171-3.
5. Kalbitz M, Gebhard F. Distale radiusfraktur. Trauma Berufskrankh. 2016;18:346–52. https://doi.org/10.1007/s10039-016-0153-6.
6. Kriechling P, Loucas R, Loucas M, et al. Primary reverse total shoulder arthroplasty in patients older than 80 years: clinical and radiologic outcome measures. J Shoulder Elb Surg. 2021;30:877–83. https://doi.org/10.1016/j.jse.2020.07.032.
7. Levin LS, Rozell JC, Pulos N. Distal radius fractures in the elderly. J Am Acad Orthop Surg. 2017;25:179–87. https://doi.org/10.5435/JAAOS-D-15-00676.
8. Müller ME, Koch P, Nazarian S, Schatzker J. The comprehensive classification of fractures of long bones. Berlin: Springer; 1990.
9. Niemeyer P, Hauschild O, Strohm PC, et al. Fracture treatment in the elderly. Acta Chir Orthop Traumatol Cechoslov. 2004;71:329–38.
10. Oestern H-J, Tscherne H. Klassifizierung der Frakturen mit Weichteilschaden. Langenbecks Archiv fer. Chirurgie. 1982;358:358. https://doi.org/10.1007/BF01271894.
11. Regel G, Bayeff-Filloff M. Diagnostik und sofortige Therapiemanahmen bei Verletzungen der Extremitäten. Unfallchirurg. 2004;107:107. https://doi.org/10.1007/s00113-004-0836-5.
12. Sanguineti VA, Wild JR, Joseph B, Fain MJ. Management of common fractures in older adults. In: Oxford textbook of geriatric medicine. Oxford University Press; 2017. p. 539–44.
13. Schumaier A, Grawe B. Proximal Humerus fractures: evaluation and Management in the Elderly Patient. Geriatr Orthop Surg Rehabil. 2018;9:2151458517750516. https://doi.org/10.1177/2151458517750516.
14. Surke C, Raschke M, Langer M. Distale Radiusfraktur: versorgungsstrategien beim älteren Menschen. OP J. 2013;28:256–60. https://doi.org/10.1055/s-0032-1327997.
15. Tampere T, Ollivier M, Jacquet C, et al. Knee arthroplasty for acute fractures around the knee. EFORT Open Rev. 2020;5:713–23. https://doi.org/10.1302/2058-5241.5.190059.

Thoracic Trauma in the Elderly

29

William Kelly, Irene Yu, Mark Katlic, and T. Robert Qaqish

Introduction

As of 2019, individuals 65 and over accounted for 16% of the US population (54.1 million), a number which has increased by 14.4 million (36%) since 2009. Further, this population is projected to approach 80 million by 2040 and 95 million by 2060. As the population continues to age, the management of the "geriatric trauma patient" has become a commonplace occurrence in emergency departments across the country and multiple studies have demonstrated a rise in volume of elderly trauma patients in this timeframe. Elderly patients experience more severe injuries when compared to their younger counterparts and demonstrate a lower threshold for sustaining traumatic injuries in low-energy mechanisms. In a report of the National Automotive sampling system/Crashworthiness Data System (1998–2007), the relationship between vehicle occupant age and the incidence of thoracic injuries was measured. The authors found that occupants 75 years or older experienced a higher percentage of moderate to severe (abbreviated injury score, AIS 2+) thoracic injuries than the three other age groups studied (25–44, 45–64, 65–74) in a tow-away crash. Moreover, the threshold for thoracic injury in older adults was lower when compared to their younger counterparts. Seventy-five percent of occupants greater than 75 years of age, sustained an AIS 2+ thoracic injuries at a crash delta-v of 37 km/h (23 mph) or less whereas the same AIS of thoracic injury in 75% of patients aged 25–44 was sustained at a crash delta-v of 46 km/h (28.6 mph). Furthermore, the ratio of thoracic injuries to other causes of death was highest in patients greater than 75. This was corroborated in a similar study that examined injury-patterns in trauma ICU patients. In this study, the authors demonstrated a strong correlation between older age and increased mortality in patients with similar levels of injury. In the elderly population, the two most common mechanisms of blunt trauma are falls and motor vehicle collisions, which are estimated to account for the majority of blunt trauma. Additionally, it is important to note that roughly 95% of geriatric trauma is resultant from blunt mechanisms.

The Thorax as We Age

Unlike other intra-thoracic or intra-abdominal organs, the lungs are in direct contact with the atmosphere. Over a person's lifetime, the lungs

W. Kelly · I. Yu · T. R. Qaqish (✉)
Division of Thoracic Surgery, Department of Surgery, University at Buffalo, Erie County Medical Center, Buffalo, NY, USA
e-mail: thamerqa@buffalo.edu

M. Katlic
Department of Surgery, Sinai Hospital, Baltimore, MD, USA
e-mail: mkatlic@lifebridgehealth.org

P. Petrone, C. E.M. Brathwaite (eds.), *Acute Care Surgery in Geriatric Patients*,
https://doi.org/10.1007/978-3-031-30651-8_29

experience numerous environmental insults, most notably, first- and second-hand tobacco smoke. The resulting oxidative stress within the airways is a key component that drives airway inflammation with the downstream effects, such as accumulation of reactive oxygen species, leading to a progressive decline in lung function with age.

With aging, the lungs, and the respiratory system, undergo both structural and physiologic changes (Fig. 29.1). The lung becomes increasingly stiff, and consequently less compliant. Moreover, lung parenchyma experiences dampening of natural elastic recoil. This is secondary to disruption of collagen and elastin fibers that

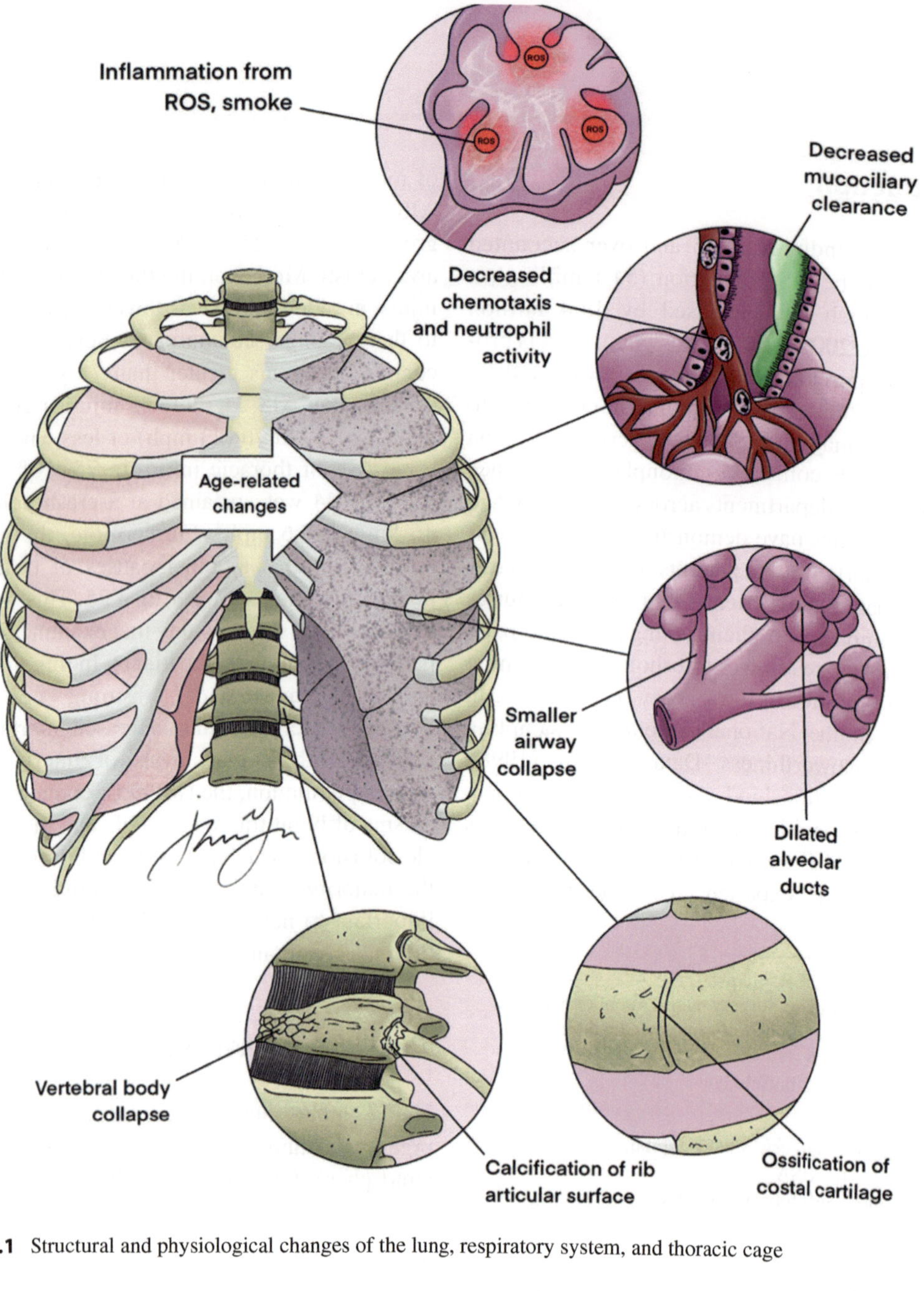

Fig. 29.1 Structural and physiological changes of the lung, respiratory system, and thoracic cage

ultimately leads to dilatation of alveolar ducts and subsequent reduction of surface area and gas exchange. As a consequence, there is a greater tendency for the small airways to collapse. In healthy elderly individuals, this may be of no consequence; however, in elderly patients who suffer acute chest trauma, pulmonary reserve is further restricted and proves less tolerant to injury.

Compliance of the chest wall is a measure of the thoracic cavity's ability to expand and contract. The compliance of an elderly patient's chest wall is decreased secondary to ossification of costal cartilages and calcification of the articular surfaces of ribs. The mobility of the chest wall is further impaired from vertebral body collapse from osteoporosis. As a consequence of osteopenia or osteoporosis, the thoracic rib cage is more brittle and less pliable during blunt trauma. This not only predisposes the chest wall to fractures (rib, sternum) but may predispose to more severe chest wall injuries (flail chest, thoracic spine fracture) and resultant morbidity and mortality. In addition, age-related changes in the geometry of the thoracic cage have been demonstrated to be a factor predisposing elderly individuals to chest wall injury.

The structural changes described above alter the chest wall dynamics and in consequence impair the respiratory cycle. Forced expiratory volume in one second (FEV1) and forced vital capacity (FVC) are reduced with age. Residual volume (RV) and functional residual capacity (FRC) increase with age as the elastic recoil of the terminal airways is compromised. The elderly adult breathes at higher tidal volumes forcing a greater energy expenditure on the muscles of respiration. Alveoli collapse at lower lung volumes in the elderly leading to greater ventilation and perfusion mismatch. Pulmonary capillary blood volume and capillary density are also decreased.

Immune-related changes are also present in the elderly lung. The elderly airway demonstrates reduced mucociliary clearance, further exposing the lung to environmental insults. Additionally, chemotaxis and the bactericidal activity of neutrophils are reduced in elderly patients. Such phenomena may predispose the lung to infection and render it more susceptible to environmental insult. Consequently, the elderly patient's respiratory system is inherently vulnerable to injury. When an elderly patient suffers trauma to the thoracic cavity, the injuries are often more severe than their younger counterparts. Furthermore, the sequelae that follow these injuries often result in a more turbulent clinical course.

Rib Fractures

Evaluation and Diagnostic Imaging

For thoracic trauma patients, the primary survey should be aimed at identifying and managing life-threatening conditions that require emergent treatment. The secondary survey can then aid in the identification of potential injuries to the chest wall prior to employing more sophisticated diagnostic modalities, such as computed tomography (CT).

It is important to palpate all aspects of the chest wall, including the costal margins and upper abdomen, when performing the secondary survey portion of the Advanced Trauma Life Support (ATLS) algorithm. The polytrauma patient often possesses distracting injuries that have the potential to prevent the provider from immediately identifying the clinical manifestations of rib fractures, such as splinting or paradoxical chest wall motion. Ecchymosis, abrasions, and seat belt injuries should alert the clinician that there may be underlying bony injury to the thorax. However, the absence of physical manifestations on the patient's chest or back does not preclude the existence of rib fractures and other injuries. Furthermore, a negative upright chest X-ray, typically taken as an adjunct to the primary survey, should not be the solely relied upon imaging modality for patients with suspected or confirmed thoracic trauma. This is because chest X-ray alone has been demonstrated to have low sensitivity in detecting rib fractures and other injuries to the thoracic cage. To encourage the judicious use of diagnostic imaging in the setting of chest trauma, various publications and consensus statements have been released offering guidance. The American College of Radiology offers a series of guidelines known as the Appropriateness Criteria for both Blunt Chest Injury and Rib Fractures. In the setting of blunt thoracic trauma from a high-energy mechanism, the authors note that Antero-Posterior (AP) chest X-ray (CXR) and chest CT are appropriate and complimentary studies. In this setting, the ease of obtaining a CXR allows for initial radiographic assessment of thoracic injuries requiring immediate intervention such as the confirmation of endotracheal tube placement or tube thoracostomy. This may also offer evidence to guide further diagnostic imaging. Conversely, CT is a more sensitive modality that allows for the detection of other injuries that might not have otherwise been detected on CXR.

In low-energy mechanisms, however, there remains some debate as to the utility of chest CT. Issues often raised surrounding the empiric use of chest CT include increased cost and radiation exposure. Another consideration in the elderly population concerns risk of nephropathy associated with IV contrast, although recent studies have raised some debate regarding contrast associated nephropathy. Further, it is worth noting that isolated rib fractures carry a relatively low morbidity/ mortality risk, and that although CT may be a more sensitive imaging modality, the detection of isolated rib fractures or lack thereof may not alter the management or outcomes in uncomplicated cases. Despite these potential drawbacks, it is important to consider the fact that low-energy mechanisms can still lead to significant injury in the elderly population.

Various studies have aimed to better define the role of chest CT in elderly patients following low-energy thoracic trauma. A 2019 study by Singleton et al. examined a population of 330 patients with an average age of 84 years. They found that chest radiographs demonstrated a 40% sensitivity relative to CT. Patients with rib fractures identified on CT were found to have a greater hospital admission rate, yet despite increased detection of radiographically occult rib fractures, there was no statistically significant difference in interventions performed, ICU admission, length of stay, or mortality.

It is important to consider that guidelines and recommendations for imaging after sustaining thoracic trauma are aimed at the general population and may not necessarily be appropriate to apply to geriatric trauma patients. It is well known that elderly patients sustain thoracic injuries with low-energy mechanisms and multiple rib fractures are associated with increased pulmonary morbidity and mortality. In addition, geriatric patients demonstrate blunted responses to hypoxia and hypercarbia which may result in a delayed clinical presentation as signs of respiratory compromise may not be immediately apparent. Thus, the use of chest CT in low-energy blunt trauma should remain a consideration in this patient population, as elderly patients may prove less able to tolerate the sequelae of missed thoracic injuries.

Epidemiology and Etiology of Rib Fractures

Rib fractures represent the most common thoracic injury following blunt chest trauma in the elderly. A study examining traumatic rib fractures utilizing the national trauma databank (NTDB) examined 564,798 patients admitted to the hospital with traumatic rib fractures between 2010 and 2016. For elderly patients in this cohort, the most common mechanisms resulting in rib fractures were falls, (51.9%, n = 67,675) followed by motor vehicle accidents (38.1%, n = 49,591). Mortality rate for the elderly subgroup in this study was 7.6% (n = 12,239). Although falls are the predominant mechanism of trauma in our elderly patients, blunt chest trauma from MVCs also represent a large portion of traumatic admissions. Moreover, seatbelts, steering wheels, armrest, and side panels are often responsible for rib and sternum fractures during motor vehicle collisions.

Rib Fracture Management

The management of rib fractures has evolved over the past two decades. Multimodal analgesia and aggressive pulmonary toilet are the fundamental tenets of rib fracture management and apply across all patient populations. In addition, the increased utilization of regional anesthesia, and the emergence of surgical rib fixation as a viable treatment option have further contributed to the clinician's armamentarium for the treatment of rib fractures.

Supportive Measures and Monitoring

Management of rib fracture-associated pain helps prevent splinting, subsequent atelectasis, and thus helps mitigate the risk of suffering pulmonary sequelae, for which the elderly are at increased risk. One modality often employed to attempt to reduce the risk of complications following rib fractures is incentive spirometry (IS). Despite its relative ubiquity, there is a dearth of high-quality evidence to support the use of IS. While the therapeutic benefit is unclear, the patient's ability or lack thereof to perform IS provides useful information to the clinician. Additionally, continuous hemodynamic monitoring, supplemental oxygen and pulse oximetry are paramount in caring for the elderly patient with bony thoracic injury as these tools allow for timely recognition of changes in clinical status.

Pharmacologic Analgesia

Currently, the effective management of rib fracture-associated pain places emphasis on the utilization of a multimodal pain regimen. This approach utilizes at least two different classes of drugs in order to target different pathways for pain control. A 2022 cohort study examining 653 patients with rib fractures found that the use of a multimodal pain regimen resulted in a significant reduction in inpatient opiate consumption. Acetaminophen is a non-opioid analgesic with a relatively benign side effect profile for patients with normal hepatic function and is commonly utilized in the treatment of pain associated with rib fractures. Non-steroidal anti-inflammatory drugs (NSAIDs) are commonly administered in younger patients with rib fractures; however, their use in elderly individuals needs to be heavily balanced in light of baseline renal dysfunction and history and risks of peptic ulcer disease. Gabapentin is a medication that has demonstrated efficacy in the treatment of neuropathic pain, and it is also utilized in the treatment of rib fracture-associated pain. While the evidence for the use of gabapentin in the treatment of rib fracture-associated pain is mixed, it is important to note that care must be taken in appropriate dose adjustment when prescribing these medications to the elderly, given the renal mechanism of excretion. Lidocaine patches are a low-risk, topical modality for rib fracture analgesia, and are another potentially useful addition to a multimodal pain regimen for rib fractures.

Oral and intravenous narcotics are the mainstays of therapy. The intravenous route has many forms including nursing administered versus patient controlled routes and both are effective; however, the potential side effects of this class of medications in the elderly population warrant close monitoring. Potential side effects of intravenous narcotic use include respiratory depression and central nervous and hemodynamic perturbations. Moreover, any underlying cognitive impairment (i.e., dementia, Alzheimer's) must be taken into consideration when prescribing narcotic therapy in the inpatient setting as these medications may increase a patient's risk of delirium.

Regional Anesthesia

In the past decade, the body of literature surrounding regional anesthesia for the treatment of rib fracture-associated pain has grown considerably. In addition to epidural anesthesia, such procedures as paravertebral block, erector spinae block, serratus anterior plane block, intrapleural anesthesia, and intercostal nerve block have all been shown to demonstrate potential benefit. Epidural anesthesia (EA) involves the injection of anesthetic agent into the epidural space at the thoracic or lumbar level. EA is able to maintain adequate analgesia while not influencing the patient's level of sedation. This allows the patient to participate more frequently in pulmonary physical therapy. Based on the most recent recommendations from the Eastern Association for the Surgery of Trauma (EAST) in conjunction with the Trauma Anesthesiology Society, authors conditionally recommend the use of epidural anesthesia in appropriate patients who have sustained blunt thoracic trauma. Contraindications to the use of epidural anesthesia include coagulopathy, unstable spinal trauma, patient refusal, infection overlying the puncture site and increased intracranial pressure. Furthermore, if there is concern for potential abdominal injury, it is important to recognize that the anesthesia may mask abdominal pain, making a patient's abdominal exam unreliable.

Thoracic paravertebral blockade involves the administration of the anesthetic agent into the paravertebral space. The injections produce unilateral somatic and sympathetic blockade without the inherited risks of spinal cord injury or need to palpate along the fractured rib segments. Erector spinae (ES) blockade is another viable option for the treatment of rib fracture-associated pain. This procedure is performed utilizing ultrasound guidance to infiltrate anesthesia into the erector spinae plane or place a catheter for continuous infusion. Similar to ES block, serratus anterior plane blockade offers another safe modality for the treatment of rib fracture-associated pain and can be performed with the patient in the supine position. Intrapleural anesthesia involves placement of a local anesthetic into the pleural space via an indwelling catheter. The diffusion of anesthetic and thus the effectiveness of the procedure, is gravity dependent. Consequently, patient positioning, presence of hemothorax or pneumothorax and tube thoracostomy may impair its effectiveness.

Intercostal nerve blocks depend on the infiltrating anesthetic agent to bathe the posterior compartment of the intercostal space. This is typically achieved via percutaneous injection or catheter placement and requires multiple anatomic injections above and below the affected rib segments. This achieves unilateral analgesia, improves peak expiratory flow rates and volumes without significant effects on hemodynamics however requires palpation overlying the fractured ribs and repeated injections.

Presently, although the preferred delivery of analgesia is epidural anesthesia, clinical factors, patient preference, and considerations of resource limitations often dictate which intervention a patient receives. The analgesic options are numerous and should often combine multiple modalities of pain control with the overarching goal of optimizing a patient's ability to participate in pulmonary physiotherapy and also facilitate patient mobility.

Surgical Management

The practice of surgical stabilization of rib fractures (SSRF) has emerged in the last two decades as a viable and important treatment option for the management of rib fractures in select circumstances. Rib fracture fixation aims to address two main problems associated with rib fractures, namely management of pain and the restoration of respiratory mechanics, which thus reduce a patient's risk of development of associated pulmonary sequelae. There are several indications for SSRF including severe pain refractory to other pain management strategies, respiratory failure, pain due to pathologic rib movement (i.e., due to flail chest or severely displaced non-flail patterns), failure to wean from mechanical ventilation, and ongoing pain from chronic nonunion or malunion of rib fractures. Another instance where patients may undergo SSRF is in an "on the way out" scenario, where a patient undergoes thoracotomy for another reason, and the decision is made to perform SSRF prior to completing the operation. Multiple studies have demonstrated the utility of SSRF for the treatment of flail chest as well as the treatment of severe, non-flail fracture patterns.

Another important consideration is whether this procedure is safe and efficacious for elderly patients with rib fractures or flail chest. A 2020 study utilizing the Trauma Quality Improvement (TQIP) database assessed outcomes of patients older than 65 who underwent SSRF. Of 758 patients older than 65 who underwent SSRF, there was a significantly lower mortality rate when compared to matched controls; however, this group had higher rates of tracheostomy and ventilator-associated pneumonia (VAP). Further analysis, however, demonstrated that early SSRF was associated with decreased ICU length of stay, hospital length of stay, and decreased rates of VAP. Moreover, a 2022 analysis by Duong et al. examined the TQIP database to analyze how rates of pulmonary complications and mortality of geriatric patients undergoing SSRF are compared to younger individuals. From 2010 to 2016, 21,517 underwent SSRF, of which 16.2% ($n = 3001$) were geriatric patients. The authors demonstrated a 7% increase in SSRF cases from 2010 to 2016. Despite being less injured based on median ISS, geriatric patients had higher rates of mortality, and this association held true even after adjusting for covariates.

Presently, there is still a paucity of data pertaining to the use of SSRF specifically in elderly patients. The decision to perform SSRF in this population should be made on an individual, case-by-case basis with the aims of reducing pain and optimizing respiratory function.

Flail Chest

Flail chest is the result of two fractures to the same rib in three or more contiguous ribs or combined sternal and rib fractures. The clinical manifestations on physical exam result in an inward displacement of the affected segment during inspiration and outward movement during expiration termed "paradoxical" chest wall movement. As a result of this gross deformity of the chest wall, the dynamics of the chest wall and diaphragm are altered compromising the respiratory parameters of lung function. Consequently, the patient's inspiratory capacity is limited, and the vital capacity may decrease by more than 50%. The deformity restricts the lung and decreases its compliance. Additionally, pain from severe rib fractures can limit deep breathing and effective cough, causing mucus plugging and atelectasis, which can further worsen the lung's ability to perform gas exchange. This is summarized in Fig. 29.2. In the elderly patient, where the reserve for respiratory compromise is already reduced, an insult such as an unstable chest wall is often devastating to the patient's respiratory

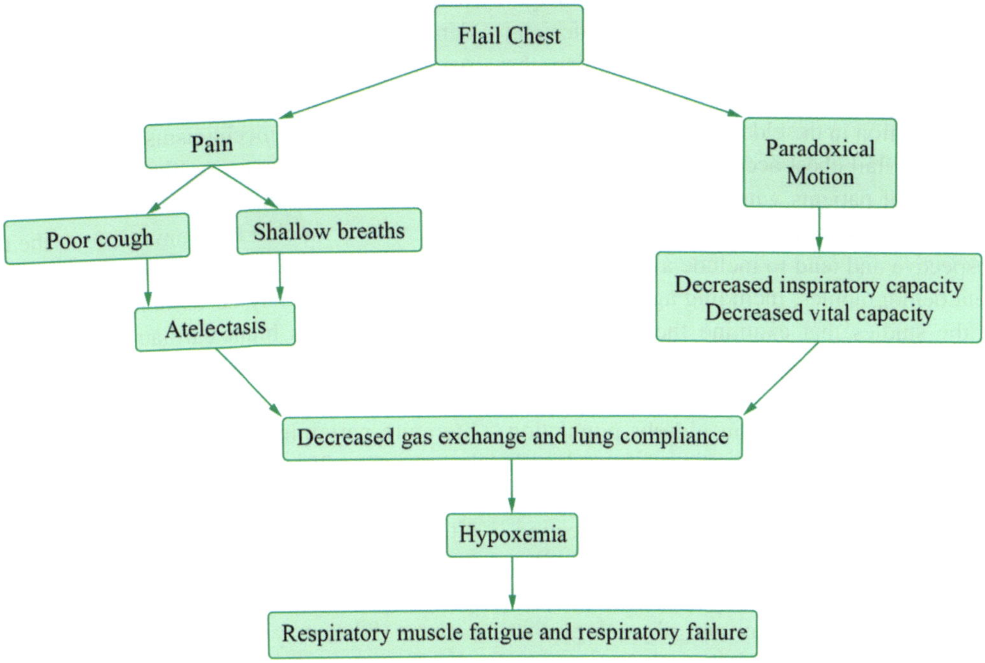

Fig. 29.2 The physiological changes and consequences of flail chest

system and is often associated with a high morbidity and mortality.

The incidence of flail chest has been estimated to range from 1 to 7% of patients who sustain blunt chest trauma. Estimated mortality rates for flail chest vary greatly; however, it is important to consider that flail chest is often associated with other serious injuries owing to the force of the blunt trauma mechanism needed to create the flail segment in the first place. Commonly associated injuries include lung contusions of varying severity and severe head injuries. For patients who are admitted to the intensive care unit and intubated, such associated injuries prolong ventilatory support times as appropriate mentation and good respiratory function are two aspects commonly required to attempt extubation. In a retrospective review by Albaugh et al., 58 trauma patients admitted with flail chest were examined. Patients above the age of 55 ($n = 26$) had a 58% mortality whereas mortality reported for patients less than or equal to 55 ($n = 32$) was 16%. Although flail chest is a relatively uncommon thoracic injury, it is a marker of more severe chest trauma and often portends a longer and more morbid hospitalization, especially in the elderly.

The current literature on the surgical management of flail chest has grown over the past decade; however, few studies specifically examine the effects of flail chest and the outcomes of operative intervention in the elderly population. Due to the fact that flail chest accounts for only a small percentage of patients with rib fractures following blunt chest trauma, existing studies are often retrospective and tend to include a wide range of patient demographics, including age. Because of this, the studies that examine the outcomes of SSRF for flail chest vary in their results and recommendations. It is unclear at this time whether SSRF for flail chest in the elderly population positively affects long-term outcomes or length of stay. To better delineate considerations such as mortality rate, appropriate candidate selection, and appropriate timing of procedure, further study is warranted. Because of the various differences in thoracic anatomy and physiology that manifest in the elderly adult, and their greater likelihood of having significant medical comorbidities, future studies should either examine these populations directly or utilize more robust sub-group analysis.

Sternal Fractures

With the introduction of seat belt legislation, the incidence of sternal fractures has risen due to increasing force from the belt against the chest during collisions. In the setting of blunt chest trauma, the rate of sternal fracture has been estimated to range from 3 to 8%. The most common fracture pattern is a transverse fracture of the sternal body, with fractures to the manubrium or xiphoid being less common. Sternal dislocation is an even rarer pathology resulting in the posterior (type 1) or anterior (type 2) displacement of the manubrium. The mortality associated with isolated SF is low, but poorer outcomes are associated with comorbidities, associated injuries, and advanced age.

The diagnostic accuracy of chest X-ray (CXR) relative to chest computed tomography (CT) in the evaluation of sternal fractures is low. Trauma algorithms are becoming increasingly CT-driven, which may also be contributing to the rising incidence of sternal fractures in blunt chest trauma patients.

Given that the most common causes of sternal fractures are blunt mechanisms such as MVC and falls, geriatric patients are likely to sustain other injuries in the setting of a sternal fracture. In the evaluation of an elderly trauma patient, the clinician should maintain a high index of suspicion for injuries that may be associated with sternal fractures such as blunt cardiac injury, rib fractures and pulmonary contusion, all of which are predictors of increased mortality. The existing literature pertaining to isolated sternal fractures is scant. One 2014 study, however, examined the association between isolated sternal fracture and blunt cardiac injury. The authors identified 88 patients with isolated sternal fracture, of which 82% ($n = 72$) were the result of MVC. Most patients (88%, $n = 77$) were admitted to the hospital for observation and only two patients demonstrated EKG changes or elevated cardiac enzymes; however, these perturbations quickly normalized and none of the patients experienced adverse cardiac outcomes. However, given the potential harm associated with a missed cardiac injury, evaluation is still warranted. While EKG alone is not sufficient to rule out blunt cardiac injury, the addition of troponin I increases the negative predictive value to 100%.

Surgical intervention for sternal fractures is a relatively uncommon procedure, and the existing data on sternal fracture repair is not exhaustive. Indications for repair include severe, intractable pain, respiratory insufficiency or ventilator dependence, sternal deformity/instability, and nonunion or hunched posture with limited range of motion. The most common complication of sternal fixation is surgical removal of hardware secondary to pain. Accordingly, further prospective studies should be conducted before guidelines and algorithms are created to assist the clinician in surgically treating patients with sternal fractures. Additionally, a concerted effort should be made in future studies to stratify geriatric patients to better characterize outcomes.

Associated Injuries and Pulmonary Sequelae

Elderly patients commonly sustain more than one injury to the thorax as a result of blunt thoracic trauma. In a retrospective cohort study by Bulger et al., trauma patients with rib fractures greater than 65 ($n = 277$) were compared to similarly injured patients less than 65 ($n = 187$). The incidence of hemothorax and pulmonary contusion in elderly patients (greater than 65) was 25% and 27%, respectively, and was not statistically significant from the incidence of hemothorax and pulmonary contusion for patients <65. Interestingly, pneumothorax in association with rib fractures occurred less frequently in patients greater than 65 (34% vs 44%).

The accepted initial management of traumatic hemothorax is tube thoracostomy. The inability of the first chest tube to adequately drain the hemothorax should not prompt additional placement of a secondary tube. Video-assisted thoracoscopic surgery (VATS) is recommended in these instances where a hemothorax is retained. Ideally, this should be performed early (3–7 days of hospitalization) to decrease the risks of empyema, although logistical and patient-related constraints can lead to this procedure being performed outside this ideal timeframe.

Post-traumatic hemothorax can be successfully treated with VATS drainage in elderly patients. A retrospective review examined 60 patients (mean age 63.2) who underwent VATS for post-traumatic hemothorax and the outcomes for elderly patients within this review (15 patients) were examined. Ninety-three percent of the elderly patients included in the study underwent successful VATS drainage of their hemothorax with no inpatient mortalities. The elderly patients were greater than 80, mostly suffered blunt thoracic trauma (87%) and had a median delay between trauma and VATS of 16 days (range 1–45 days). The outcomes reported included median hospital stay after VATS (20 days), number of patients requiring ICU level care (9/15), mean ICU stay (11.8 days) post-operative mechanical ventilation (5/15). The authors concluded that the morbidity and extended prolonged hospitalizations may be improved if patients are referred earlier for surgical management rather than later.

The management of patients with pulmonary contusions requires a careful evaluation of fluid and resuscitation status. Level 1 recommendations do not exist for the management of pulmonary contusions; however, the current guidelines support the judicious administration of fluids to maintain tissue perfusion and manage shock while simultaneously avoiding unnecessary fluid administration. Unfortunately, management guidelines for pulmonary contusions in the elderly do not exist. Consequently, a careful examination of the patient's volume status, echocardiographic findings, serial chest radiographs and laboratory surrogates for volume and resuscitation status will help the clinician tailor treatment of the elderly trauma patient accordingly.

Pneumonia is one of, if not the single most common pulmonary sequelae related to blunt chest trauma. Pneumonia was observed in 31%

of elderly patients treated over a 10-year period admitted with rib fractures and the risk of nosocomial increases by 27% for every additional fractured rib. Given that pneumonia negatively contributes to the overall morbidity and mortality of elderly patient, measures taken to prevent pneumonia offer promise in improving outcomes for geriatric patients who have sustained chest trauma.

Concluding Remarks

The elderly trauma patient is often more severely injured and consequently may have a prolonged, more volatile clinical course. This remains consistent with thoracic injuries in this age group. Our elderly patients are more vulnerable to injury and are limited in their tolerance to traumatic insult. The clinician responsible for the care and evaluation of the elderly thoracic trauma patient should maintain a high index of suspicion while judiciously assessing the patient for bony injury in all components of the chest wall. Greater attention to associated intra-thoracic injuries may also prepare the clinician for common pulmonary sequelae that accompany blunt thoracic trauma. As the geriatric trauma literature continues to grow and further emphasis is placed on tailoring care to the elderly trauma patient, outcomes in this population should hopefully continue to improve.

References

1. Llompart-Pou JA, Chico-Fernandez M, Sanchez-Casado M, Alberdi-Odriozola F, Guerrero-Lopez F, Mayor-Garcia MD, Gonzalez-Robledo J, et al. Age-related injury patterns in Spanish trauma ICU patients. Results from the RETRAUCI. Injury. 2016;47(Suppl 3):S61–5. https://doi.org/10.1016/S0020-1383(16)30608-8.
2. Hanna R, Hershman L. Evaluation of thoracic injuries among older motor vehicle occupants: technical report. NHTSA. 2009. US DOT HS 811 101.
3. Gomez CR, Boehmer ED, Kovacs EJ. The aging innate immune system. Curr Opin Immunol. 2005;17:457–62.
4. Henry TS, Kirsch J, Kanne JP, Chung JH, Donnelly EF, Ginsburg ME, Heitkamp DE, et al. ACR appropriateness criteria(R) rib fractures. J Thorac Imaging. 2014;29(6):364–6. https://doi.org/10.1097/RTI.0000000000000113.
5. Singleton JM, Bilello LA, Canham LS, Levenson RB, Lopez GJ, Tadiri SP, Shapiro NI, et al. Chest computed tomography imaging utility for radiographically occult rib fractures in elderly fall-injured patients. J Trauma Acute Care Surg. 2019;86(5):838–43. https://doi.org/10.1097/TA.0000000000002208.
6. Peek J, Ochen Y, Saillant N, Groenwold RHH, Leenen LPH, Uribe-Leitz T, Houwert RM, et al. Traumatic rib fractures: a marker of severe injury. A nationwide study using the National Trauma Data Bank. Trauma Surg Acute Care Open. 2020;5(1):e000441. https://doi.org/10.1136/tsaco-2020-000441.
7. Burton SW, Riojas C, Gesin G, Smith CB, Bandy V, Sing R, Roomian T, et al. Multimodal analgesia reduces opioid requirements in trauma patients with rib fractures. J Trauma Acute Care Surg. 2022;92(3):588–96. https://doi.org/10.1097/TA.0000000000003486.
8. Galvagno SM Jr, Smith CE, Varon AJ, Hasenboehler EA, Sultan S, Shaefer G, To KB, et al. Pain management for blunt thoracic trauma: a joint practice management guideline from the Eastern Association for the Surgery of trauma and Trauma Anesthesiology Society. J Trauma Acute Care Surg. 2016;81(5):936–51. https://doi.org/10.1097/TA.0000000000001209.
9. Chen Zhu R, de Roulet A, Ogami T, Khariton K. Rib fixation in geriatric trauma: mortality benefits for the most vulnerable patients. J Trauma Acute Care Surg. 2020;89(1):103–10. https://doi.org/10.1097/TA.0000000000002666.
10. Duong W, Grigorian A, Nahmias J, Farzaneh C, Christian A, Dolich M, Lekawa M, et al. An increasing trend in geriatric trauma patients undergoing surgical stabilization of rib fractures. Eur J Trauma Emerg Surg. 2022;48(1):205–10. https://doi.org/10.1007/s00068-020-01526-7.
11. Albaugh G, Kann B, Puc MM, Vemurlapalli P, Marra S, Ross S. Age-adjusted outcomes in traumatic flail chest injuries in the elderly. Am Surg. 2000;66:978–81.
12. Klei DS, de Jong MB, Oner FC, Leenen LPH, van Wessem KJP. Current treatment and outcomes of traumatic sternal fractures-a systematic review. Int Orthop. 2019;43(6):1455–64. https://doi.org/10.1007/s00264-018-3945-4.
13. Dua A, McMaster J, Desai PJ, Desai SS, Kuy S, Mata M, Cooper J. The association between blunt cardiac injury and isolated sternal fracture. Cardiol Res Pract. 2014;2014:629687. https://doi.org/10.1155/2014/629687.
14. Clancy K, Velopulos C, Bilaniuk JW, Collier B, Crowley W, Kurek S, Lui F, et al. Screening for blunt cardiac injury: an eastern Association for the Surgery of trauma practice management guideline. J Trauma Acute Care Surg. 2012;73(5 Suppl 4):S301–6. https://doi.org/10.1097/TA.0b013e318270193a.
15. Bulger EM, Arneson MA, Mock CN, Jurokovich GJ. Rib fractures in the elderly. J Trauma. 2000;48(6):1040–7.

Esophageal Injuries and Esophageal Emergencies in Geriatric Patients

30

Matthew Zeller, T. Robert Qaqish, and Mark Katlic

Anatomy and Physiology of the Esophagus

The esophagus is a tubular organ within the gastrointestinal system that connects the pharynx to the stomach. Anatomically, it travels caudally through the neck, superior mediastinum, and posterior mediastinum into the abdominal cavity. The proximal esophagus is at the level of the 6th cervical vertebra, and the gastroesophageal (GE) junction is at the level of the 11th thoracic vertebra spanning 20–30 cm in length. The esophagus spans the mediastinum and is closely approximated to the heart, major vessels, and lungs but is protected anatomically by the rigid spine dorsally, mediastinal organs, and rib cage ventrally. Three anatomic areas of narrowing within the native esophagus occur naturally from the compression of adjacent structures. From cranial to caudal, these include the upper esophageal sphincter (UES) created from the cricopharyngeus muscle and inferior pharyngeal constrictor (thyropharyngeus), the crossing of the left main-stem bronchus, and finally, the esophageal hiatus at the diaphragm.

Histologically, the layers of the esophagus include the mucosa, lamina propria, muscularis mucosa, submucosa, muscularis propria, and adventitia. The mucosal layer is comprised of stratified squamous epithelia with a distinct transition distally to secretory gastric columnar mucosa (Z-line). The muscularis propria layer includes the inner circular muscle, outer longitudinal muscle, and Auerbach plexus. The esophagus differs from other intra-abdominal gastrointestinal and mediastinal organs as it does not have a serosal layer. The lack of an esophageal serosal layer decreases natural defenses against the spread of infection and metastatic disease.

The esophagus has a rich blood supply and network of interconnecting vasculature receiving blood from the inferior thyroid arteries, aorta, bronchial arteries, left gastric artery, and inferior phrenic arteries. Venous drainage includes inferior thyroid, azygous, hemiazygous, bronchial, and coronary veins. The upper third of the esophagus is innervated somatically by the superior laryngeal nerves, whereas the lower third is innervated autonomically by the vagus nerve.

The function of the esophagus is to transfer a food bolus to the stomach. It accomplishes this task through coordinated contraction and relaxation of the esophageal muscles, creating a peristaltic motion propelling content caudally. The

M. Zeller · M. Katlic
Department of Surgery, Sinai Hospital, Baltimore, MD, USA

T. R. Qaqish (✉)
Division of Thoracic Surgery, Department of Surgery, University at Buffalo, Erie County Medical Center, Buffalo, NY, USA
e-mail: thamerqa@buffalo.edu

P. Petrone, C. E.M. Brathwaite (eds.), *Acute Care Surgery in Geriatric Patients*,
https://doi.org/10.1007/978-3-031-30651-8_30

tonic resting pressure of the UES keeps air from entering the stomach and prevents gastric contents from entering the airway during swallowing. Relaxation of the UES allows the release of gastric contents during vomiting and passage of a food bolus during eating. The resting tonic nature of the Lower Esophageal Sphincter (LES) prevents reflux of gastric contents into the esophagus. There are three types of esophageal contractions: primary, secondary, and tertiary. Primary contractions are stimulated by the initiation of swallowing and occur caudally with rhythmic peristaltic motion. Secondary contractions are reflexes that occur from the dilation and irritation of the esophagus and occur independently and are localized. Tertiary contractions are individual contractions without peristaltic character and may be uncoordinated, monophasic, or multiphasic.

Changes to the Esophagus in Older Adults

With a projected one-fifth of the population over the age of 65 by 2050, the surgical population is becoming older. Age alone is a well-known risk factor for worse outcomes with traumatic injury though the decision to undergo surgery should not be solely based on age but rather on individualized risk stratification and goals of care. The higher disease burden, decrease in physiologic reserve, and the anatomical and physiological changes seen with aging substantially impact the older adult's response to traumatic injury and must be considered when caring for this population.

The key physiologic change of the esophagus with aging occurs in the esophageal neuromusculature and sphincters. The aging esophagus may exhibit a decreased rate and amplitude of primary peristaltic contractions (measured by the distal contractile integral (DCI), and decreased distal latency (DL)), complete aperistalsis, absent or decreased secondary peristalsis with distention, or an increase in tertiary contractions. The UES shows decreased resting pressure and decreased relaxation with aging. The changes to the LES with aging are not as well understood. Recent studies using high-resolution manometry show no significant difference in LES tonic pressure but rather show a significant correlation between age and increased mean integrated relaxation pressure (IRP), DCI, and DL. These changes may be due to decreased neuron innervation to the LES and lower compliance observed in the aging esophagus. Anatomically, type one hiatal hernia and esophageal diverticula show a higher prevalence within the older adult population. Additionally, this population is at risk for polypharmacy impacting the physiological function of the esophagus and pill-induced esophagitis (Table 30.1).

Table 30.1 Common medications prescribed to older adults and the physiologic impact on esophageal function

Medication class	Physiologic impact on the esophagus
Anticholinergics	Decrease esophageal peristalsis, decrease LES tone
Nitrates	Decrease LES tone
Calcium channel blockers	Decrease LES tone
Benzodiazepines	Decrease LES, UES tone
Tricyclic antidepressants	Decreased LES tone
Theophylline	Decrease LES tone

Advanced age, frailty, systemic disease, and other comorbidities impact fitness and increase the risk of complications and poor outcomes for older adults undergoing esophageal procedures or experiencing esophageal trauma. Comorbid conditions contribute to decreased fitness and may predispose this population to greater risks for iatrogenic esophageal injury.

- The following list represents a non exhaustive list of esophageal diseases that the elderly population may possess:
  - GERD
  - Achalasia
  - Hiatal hernia
  - Nutcracker esophagus
  - Diffuse esophageal spasm
  - Fibrovascular polyps
  - Esophageal diverticula
  - Esophageal cancer
  - Benign esophageal stricture
  - Barrett's esophagus

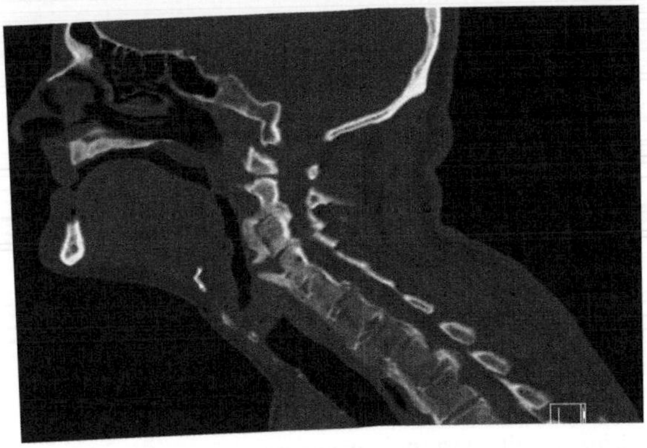

Fig. 30.1 CT Cervical Spine showing anterior cervical osteophytes impinging the hypopharynx in an older adult. (Image courtesy of T. Robert Qaqish, MD)

When complications or injury occur, the decreased muscle mass seen in older adults contributes to lower physiologic reserve, impacting the ability to withstand significant trauma and systemic infection. The increased colonization of the oropharyngeal tissues, specifically Gram-negative organisms, seen in aging individuals may increase the risk of mediastinitis in the presence of perforation or penetrating injury. Furthermore, coagulopathy is more likely to be present due to medication or platelet dysfunction secondary to renal insufficiency or failure or hepatic disease. Osteophytic changes within the cervical and thoracic vertebrae have been implicated in traumatic and iatrogenic esophageal injury leading to perforation of the esophagus (Fig. 30.1). Finally, liver disease, such as hepatitis, which is seen in higher prevalence within the older adult population, carries an increased risk for mortality in adult trauma patients.

Iatrogenic Esophageal Injury Epidemiology

As the majority of patients undergoing esophageal instrumentation are older adults, iatrogenic esophageal injury accordingly impacts the older adult population. Age is an independent risk factor for 30-day mortality in instrument-related esophageal perforations. Accounting for nearly half of the perforations to the esophagus, esophageal instrumentation is the most common cause of iatrogenic injury to the esophagus. The mechanism of injury may occur mechanically from direct insult, indirectly from procedures on adjacent structures, or secondarily from medications or radiation treatment.

Table 30.2 Common procedural interventions performed within the older adult population and the associated iatrogenic esophageal injuries

Intervention	Potential esophageal injury
Esophagogastroduodenoscopy (EGD)	Perforation, dissection, hematoma
Thoracic radiation	Esophagitis, esophageal stricture
Left atrial ablation	Esophagoatrial fistula, perforation
Thoracic Endovascular Aortic Repair (TEVAR)	Stent erosion into esophagus
Anterior cervical vertebral surgery	Perforation, ulceration, hematoma
Naso or orogastric tube placement, endotracheal intubation	Dissection, perforation, hematoma
Myotomy, fundoplication and/or wrap, hiatal hernia repair, vagotomy, mediastinoscopy, thyroidectomy, tracheostomy	Perforation, hematoma
Transesophageal echocardiography	Perforation, dissection, hematoma
Esophageal dilation	Perforation, dissection, hematoma

There are three main categories of mechanical iatrogenic injury that present acutely, which include dissections, hematomas, and perforations. Late-onset mechanical injuries may present weeks following the index procedure, such as a thermal burn leading to fistulous disease. The mechanism of insult for esophageal injury and resultant injury varies according to the procedure undertaken (Table 30.2).

Of the mechanical iatrogenic injuries, esophageal perforation is the most common, which occurs in roughly 1 in 3000 upper endoscopies. Perforation is characterized by full-thickness injury to the esophagus and usually occurs at the areas of anatomical narrowing, areas of disease within the thoracic esophagus, or following therapeutic intervention. Esophageal dissections leading to the creation of a false lumen occur less often but often do not require operative intervention. Hematomas develop within the submucosal layer and are self-limited unless they cause a mass effect on surrounding structures. Fistulous disease is often not recognized during the index procedure but in the weeks following with varying presentations based on the involved mediastinal structures. Fistulas may form between the trachea, left atrium, pericardium, or aorta, and the esophagus.

The presence of pathologic esophageal narrowing from achalasia, Schatzki's rings, peptic esophageal strictures, extraluminal compression, or areas of increased weakness such as Killian's triangle occur in higher prevalence in the older population. Additionally, diseases of the esophagus seen in higher prevalence within the older adult population, such as Zenker's diverticula, friable masses, and radiation changes, increase the risk of injury from esophageal instrumentation. Extrinsic compression of the esophagus can cause an increased risk for esophageal injury during instrumentation. Compression may be secondary to comorbid conditions in the older adult, such as thoracic aortic aneurysms, mediastinal masses, or left atrial enlargement from mitral valvular disease.

Presentation and Diagnosis of Iatrogenic Esophageal Injury

Iatrogenic esophageal injury is suspected when a patient complains of new-onset symptoms (i.e., chest pain) in the postoperative period from a procedure requiring esophageal instrumentation. While chest pain is the most common complaint, patients may also report dysphagia, dysphonia, odynophagia, dyspnea, and abdominal, back, neck, or shoulder pain. On exam, the patient may show signs such as subcutaneous emphysema or hematemesis. The degree to which patients will experience these symptoms is based on the anatomical location of the perforation, the containment of the perforation, and the time since the injury occurred. As the time from initial perforation increases, so does the severity of the systemic inflammatory response. Tachycardia may occur early as a result of this inflammatory response, and hypotension denotes a worse prognosis as the spillage of esophageal contents worsens the degree of systemic inflammation. It is important to consider that the older adult population commonly does not present with the classic signs and symptoms. Due to lower physiologic reserve or the presence of beta-blocker therapy, older adult patients may present with altered mental status rather than tachycardia and signs of sepsis. Therefore, there should be a higher index of suspicion and a lower threshold for diagnostic evaluation in older adult patients.

Prompt diagnosis and management of the perforation are key to decreasing morbidity and mortality. While there is significant mortality, approximately 13%, following perforation, there remains no standard approach to managing perforations, but accurate and rapid diagnosis often requires multiple imaging modalities. Contrast esophagography remains the gold standard for diagnosing esophageal perforation and identifying the anatomic location of the perforation but has a high false-negative rate. Adjunctive imaging such as CT esophagogram may show additional pathology and the extent of contamination within the pleural cavity and mediastinum. Endoscopic evaluation allows direct visualization of the esophagus to categorize the perforation further. Endoscopy may be the most important diagnostic tool for ruling out further pathology or contributions to the perforation.

Traumatic Esophageal Injury Epidemiology

Traumatic injury of the esophagus (TIE) is very uncommon, accounting for a minority of all injuries to the esophagus and less than 0.01% of the injuries as a result of trauma. Over half of TIE are secondary to penetrating trauma, with roughly a third to one-tenth occurring from blunt trauma. Additionally, TIE shows a predominance in young males and results in more severe injury than other traumatic injuries. Of the penetrating mechanism, gunshot injury is the most common mechanism. Motor vehicle crash accounts for the most common mechanism of blunt TIE. Falls account for a significant portion of blunt cervical esophageal injury in the older adult population. A review of the National Trauma Registry showed a 12% overall mortality of patients with traumatic esophageal injury. In this review, roughly a quarter of the 944 patient samples were over the age of 50, which was an independent risk factor for mortality. Additional independent risk factors for mortality included hypotension in the emergency department, esophageal perforation, severe head injury, and GCS <9.

Traumatic injury to the esophagus is rare due to the anatomically protected nature of the esophagus. As it courses through the neck attached to the prevertebral fascia, the esophagus lies ventral to the bony cervical vertebrae and dorsal to the cartilaginous trachea. Upon entering the thoracic cavity, it is protected by the rigid thoracic chest wall and thoracic vertebrae. The thoracic esophagus remains ventral to the thoracic vertebrae and medial to the descending thoracic aorta. Throughout its caudal course in the thorax, it is closely surrounded by structures that are key to preserving life and, if injured, lead to rapid decompensation and morbidity. Thus, isolated TIE is exceedingly rare, but rather, TIE often occurs in the setting of significant polytrauma to the neck, mediastinum, and/or the abdomen. Cervical TIE is associated with lower mortality than thoracic TIE and is more prevalent with blunt trauma. This lower mortality is likely due to the lack of communication to the mediastinum and containment of perforation within the cervical region.

Penetrating Injury to the Esophagus

Penetrating injury to the esophagus most commonly results from a gunshot or stabbing injury to the neck, thorax, or, less commonly, the epigastrium. A solitary injury to the esophagus from a penetrating mechanism is uncommon due to the close proximity of the heart, lungs, and major vessels within the neck and thorax. Consideration of the trajectory of the projectile or penetrating object is important in understanding the risk of esophageal involvement. High morbidity and mortality are seen in penetrating TIE due to concomitant injury and spread of esophageal contents within the mediastinum when the diagnosis is delayed greater than 24 h. If death does not occur from injury to vital organs first, mortality may result from the spread of bacteria to the mediastinum leading to sepsis and potential multi-organ failure. When penetrating TIE occurs in older adults, this population experiences high esophageal-related complications compared to younger populations.

Blunt Injury to the Esophagus

Blunt esophageal trauma comprises up to 37% of traumatic esophageal injuries. There is a paucity of epidemiological studies exploring the incidence of blunt esophageal injury in the older adult population. In blunt pharyngoesophageal injuries, older adults comprise only 6.7%. Of the patients with blunt pharyngoesophageal trauma, only a quarter require neck exploration. Similar to penetrating TIE, blunt TIE outcome is determined by the injury burden and location, prompt diagnosis, and early management.

When blunt traumatic injury to the esophagus does occur, it most commonly occurs secondary to motor vehicle accidents, falls, and assaults, including strangulation. The proposed mechanisms of esophageal injury and perforation in the setting of blunt trauma involve intraluminal pressure changes leading to tissue injury, direct compression injury, or shearing from the acceleration/deceleration of tissues during trauma. The acceleration/deceleration motion and rapid changes in pressure seen in the esophageal lumen can cause tearing of the esophageal tissue. During the acceleration or deceleration seen with motor vehicle accidents, the weight of the stomach, especially when full of gastric contents, may lead to shearing injuries at the gastroesophageal junction. The theorized mechanism of perforation to the thoracic and cervical esophagus occurs when the UES is closed and rapid pressure changes within the esophageal lumen, creating a high-pressure environment. Additionally, external compression from surrounding structures such as osteophytes may be implicated in the risk for esophageal injury following blunt trauma (Fig. 30.1).

Diagnosis of Traumatic Injury of the Esophagus

Initial care of the trauma patient does not differ between the older adult and the adult population. The initial evaluation of the trauma patient begins with the primary survey, assessing the patient's airway, breathing, and circulation. If an unstable patient is taken to the operating room, esophageal intervention should only be undertaken following control of bleeding and any other life-threatening injury. Once stable, esophagoscopy should be performed in the operative room or ICU if there is a high suspicion of injury. If an esophageal injury is suspected, a nasogastric tube should be placed at the time of endoscopy, as blind placement may lead to worsening of the esophageal injury.

Chest radiography obtained as an adjunct to the primary survey may show widened mediastinum, subcutaneous air, or pneumothorax but has low sensitivity for TIE and should not be relied on for TIE diagnosis. For stable patients with blunt or penetrating traumatic injuries to the neck, thorax, or abdomen, computed tomography (CT) is commonly obtained to evaluate for life-threatening traumatic injuries. Without oral contrast, CT has a low sensitivity for esophageal injury. Findings such as periesophageal fluid, pneumomediastinum, pleural effusions, esophageal wall thickening, and pneumothorax on CT should increase the suspicion of TIE. If an esophageal injury is seen on the initial CT or if there is high suspicion for TIE despite negative CT, a fluoroscopic esophagography with contrast should be performed. This remains the gold standard diagnostic imaging for esophageal perforation. Classically, a water-soluble contrast agent would be the first line contrast agent. If negative, the study may be repeated with barium, which is more radio-opaque and offers higher specificity for esophageal perforation though this algorithm varies amongst institutions. Dedicated thoracic CT esophagography is becoming more common in the acute setting to evaluate esophageal injury. Following a positive fluoroscopic or CT esophagography, an esophagoscopy should be performed to visualize the injury directly.

Cervical esophageal injuries that occur between the UES to the sternal notch, differ from thoracic or abdominal esophageal injuries because they are more contained. Additionally, cervical injuries are not subject to the negative pressure from inspiration seen in thoracic perforations, contributing to an increased risk for mediastinal contamination in the chest.

If esophageal perforation is suspected, the provider must resuscitate the patient, ensure appropriate intravenous access as well as administer broad-spectrum antibiotics and antifungal agents prior to a discussion of the operative or endoscopic management. This is especially important in older adults to avoid the progression of sepsis.

Principles of Surgical Management of Traumatic Esophageal Injury

The American Association for the Surgery of Trauma (AAST) Esophageal Injury Scale can be used to guide the operative management of TIE.

- Grade I – Contusion or hematoma, partial thickness laceration
- Grade II – Less than 50% laceration
- Grade III – Greater than 50% laceration
- Grade IV – Less than 2 cm disruption of tissue or vasculature
- Grade V – Greater than 2 cm disruption of tissue or vasculature

Low-grade injuries (AAST grades I-III) can be addressed with debridement of devitalized tissue and primary repair or repair over a drain or addressed endoluminally with thoracic drainage. High-grade injuries (AAST IV-V) include those with a significant loss of esophageal tissue or inflammation and may require esophageal exclusion and diversion with the creation of a cervical esophagostomy or repair over a T-tube. Despite injury grade, it is imperative to drain the contamination to prevent mediastinitis and overwhelming sepsis. When repair is contraindicated due to patient instability or significant mediastinitis, wide local drainage should be performed until the patient can tolerate repair. In some instances, esophagectomy may be required.

For thoracic esophageal traumatic injuries, management is commonly determined on the containment of the perforation to the mediastinum or extension to the pleural space. If the perforation does not violate the pleura and is contained, conservative management may be possible. For non-contained thoracic esophageal perforations, despite AAST grading, operative drainage is indicated. A wide debridement of devitalized tissues is performed with primary repair in two layers if anatomically possible. Upper and mid thoracic esophageal perforation may be approached via the right chest. Distal esophageal perforations requiring repair be approached via the left chest. The repair is then covered with a pedicled soft tissue flap of intercostal muscle, inflamed pleura, or pericardial fat. Feeding needs to be established in the operating room, either via PEG or jejunostomy tube placement via laparotomy or laparoscopy, depending on the patient's clinical stability. The patient should be kept nil per os, started on enteral feeding, when clinically appropriate, and initiated on broad-spectrum antibiotics. An antifungal agent should be added to the antibiotic therapy.

For traumatic cervical esophagus injuries, operative intervention is performed when there is a clearly identified perforation on imaging. If no clear perforation is identified, surgical drainage may be performed. Primary repair is performed in two layers buttressed with a muscular flap from the omohyoid, strap, or sternocleidomastoid (SCM) muscles.

Surgical exploration is required with any penetrating injury to the abdomen or blunt injury with pneumo- or hemoperitoneum. When there is perforation of the abdominal esophagus following TIE, an upper midline laparotomy is indicated. Once the perforation is identified, there should be debridement of devitalized tissues, primary repair with omental or gastric buttress, and a drain left postoperatively to monitor for an anastomotic leak.

Endoluminal Management of Esophageal Perforation

Traditionally, open surgical management has been the standard of care in the management of esophageal perforation from iatrogenic and traumatic causes. Recent practice has increased the use of endoluminal therapies for specific indications. For TIE, the use of esophageal stents varies widely, with 2–10% of patients receiving stents. Endoluminal therapy is much more common for managing esophageal perforation from iatrogenic injuries. Close to a quarter of all-cause esophageal perforation is managed with endoluminal methods, and 67% of perforations managed with stents do not require additional interventional treatment. The use of endoluminal therapies for iatrogenic esophageal perforation in older adults has not been determined though studies are suggesting improved patient-reported long-term outcomes.

The use of endoluminal therapy remains nuanced. The choice to perform endoluminal therapy is based on the presence of comorbid injuries, the stability of the patient, the time since the injury occurred, and the characteristics of the perforation (size, location, contamination). A traumatic mechanism may preclude the use of endoluminal therapies if there is significant polytrauma that requires operative intervention. Covered stents restore continuity of the esophageal lumen rapidly (Fig. 30.2) but rely on adequate drainage of the extraluminal contents (i.e., thoracostomy drainage or thoracoscopy for mediastinal/pleural drainage/decontamination on the affected side) and require endoscopic stent exchange. Thoracoscopy may either be performed immediately after stent deployment or shortly after, depending on the patient's clinical status. Stent placement may be ideal in patients with small perforations with comorbid diseases

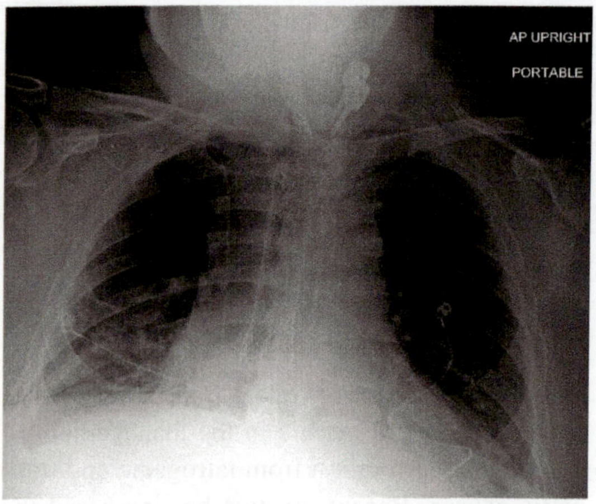

Fig. 30.2 Radiographic view of an esophageal stent placed for an upper esophageal perforation. (Image courtesy of T. Robert Qaqish, MD)

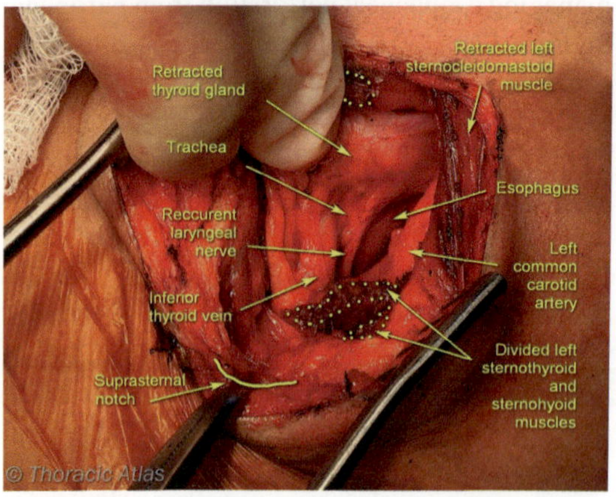

Fig. 30.3 Relevant anatomy during left neck exploration after division of the strap muscles and inferior thyroid artery. Note that the finger rather than a metal retractor is used to displace the thyroid gland to avoid injury to the recurrent laryngeal nerve. (Image accessed from https://medicine.uiowa.edu/iowaprotocols/exposure-cervical-esophagus. Arshava EV)

who are unfit for surgical treatment. Stents are not ideal for perforations within the cervical esophagus or GE junction due to their migration risk. Simple drainage of cervical esophageal perforations is often all that is required. This can usually be performed via a left neck incision (Fig. 30.3).

Endoscopic clips may be used for smaller perforations with minimal or no extraluminal spillage. More recent developments such as endoscopic suturing and endoscopic vacuum therapy are possible alternatives to operative, stent, or clip management but remain understudied.

Conclusion

Esophageal injury from iatrogenic and traumatic causes is associated with significant morbidity and mortality. The older adult population carry risk factors for poor outcomes when affected by esophageal injury. Early diagnosis and treatment are paramount when esophageal injury is suspected. Recognition of the lower reserve and increased comorbidities of the older adult must be considered when caring for esophageal injuries in this population.

References

1. Rosenthal R, Zenilman M, Katlic M, editors. Principles and practice of geriatric surgery. 3rd ed. Cham: Springer; 2020.
2. Djinbachian R, Marchand E, Yan W, Bouin M. Effects of age on esophageal motility: a high-resolution manometry study. J Clin Med Res. 2021;13(8):413.
3. Christmas AB, Wilson AK, Franklin GA, Miller FB, Richardson JD, Rodriguez JL. Cirrhosis and trauma: a deadly duo. Am Surg. 2005;71(12):996–1000. https://doi.org/10.1177/000313480507101202.
4. Biancari F, Saarnio J, Mennander A, Hypén L, Salminen P, Kuttila K, et al. Outcome of patients with esophageal perforations: a multicenter study. World J Surg. 2013;38(4):902–9.
5. Sdralis EIK, Petousis S, Rashid F, Lorenzi B, Charalabopoulos A. Epidemiology, diagnosis, and management of esophageal perforations: systematic review. Dis Esophagus. 2017;30(8):1–6.
6. Gambhir S, Grigorian A, Swentek L, Maithel S, Sheehan BM, Daly S, et al. Esophageal trauma: analysis of incidence, morbidity, and mortality. Am Surg. 2019;85(10):1134–8.
7. Aiolfi A, Inaba K, Recinos G, Khor D, Benjamin ER, Lam L, et al. Non-iatrogenic esophageal injury: a retrospective analysis from the National Trauma Data Bank. World J Emerg Surg [Internet]. 2017;12(1):19.
8. Patel MS, Malinoski DJ, Zhou L, Neal ML, Hoyt DB. Penetrating oesophageal injury: a contemporary analysis of the National Trauma Data Bank. Injury. 2013;44:48–55.

9. Barmparas G, Navsaria PH, Serna-Gallegos D, Nicol AJ, Edu S, Sayari AA, et al. Blunt pharyngoesophageal injuries: current management strategies. Scand J Surg. 2018;107(4):336–44.
10. Sargent T, Al-Katib S. Computed tomography imaging of iatrogenic esophageal injuries. J Comput Assist Tomogr. 2022;46(3):355–62.
11. Moore EE, Jurkovich GJ, Knudson MM, Cogbill TH, Malangoni MA, Champion HR, et al. Organ injury scaling. VI: Extrahepatic biliary, esophagus, stomach, vulva, vagina, uterus (nonpregnant), uterus (pregnant), fallopian tube, and ovary. J Trauma. 1995;39(6):1069–70.
12. Raff LA, Schinnerer EA, Maine RG, Jansen J, Noorbakhsh MR, Spigel Z, et al. Contemporary management of traumatic cervical and thoracic esophageal perforation: the results of an eastern Association for the Surgery of trauma multi-institutional study. J Trauma Acute Care Surg. 2020;89(4):691–7.
13. Axtell AL, Gaissert HA, Morse CR, Premkumar A, Schumacher L, Muniappan A, et al. Management and outcomes of esophageal perforation. Dis Esophagus. 2022;35:1.
14. Brinkmann S, Knepper L, Fuchs H, Hoelscher A, Kuhr K, dos Santos DP, et al. Short- and long-term follow-up of patients with non-neoplastic esophageal perforation. Langenbeck's Arch Surg. 2022;407(2):569–77.

Pulmonary Injury

31

John O. Hwabejire, Jefferson A. Proaño-Zamudio, and George C. Velmahos

Introduction: Aging of the Lungs and the Chest

There are major physiologic changes that occur in the pulmonary system in geriatric patients that make this system particularly prone to injuries. These include loss of alveolar units and surface area, decrease in chest wall compliance and decreased chest wall muscle mass. These changes render the chest wall and the lungs in elderly individuals very brittle and slow to recover from blunt or penetrating trauma. The presence of pre-injury respiratory comorbidities such as chronic obstructive pulmonary disease (COPD), malnutrition, sarcopenia, and pre-existing frailty can make even minor pulmonary trauma have major clinical consequences. Given that, elderly patients often present late, prompt diagnosis, and treatment of pulmonary injuries, while taking into consideration the peculiarities of geriatric patients, is essential for good clinical outcomes.

J. O. Hwabejire (✉) · J. A. Proaño-Zamudio · G. C. Velmahos
Harvard Medical School, Boston, MA, USA

Division of Trauma, Emergency Surgery and Surgical Critical Care, Department of Surgery, Massachusetts General Hospital, Boston, MA, USA
e-mail: jhwabejire@mgh.harvard.edu

Epidemiology

The most common pulmonary injury is pulmonary contusion associated with rib fractures. A recent retrospective review performed exclusively on patients at least 65 years old by Bader and colleagues reported an incidence of lung contusion of 28% in elderly patients with blunt chest trauma. Hemothorax and pneumothorax can complicate up to 25% and 34% of admissions for rib fractures, respectively. Penetrating thoracic trauma in the elderly in general has a low incidence.

Mechanisms of Injury

A recent review of the Trauma Quality Improvement Program (TQIP) dataset by Naar and colleagues identified falls as the most common (77.4%) mechanism of blunt chest wall trauma, followed by motor vehicle collision (22.6%). A large nationwide study using the Medicare analytic files found that ground level falls account for the most common trauma mechanism in geriatric trauma patients. Penetrating mechanisms constitute less than 5%.

P. Petrone, C. E.M. Brathwaite (eds.), *Acute Care Surgery in Geriatric Patients*,
https://doi.org/10.1007/978-3-031-30651-8_31

Initial Trauma Evaluation and Resuscitation

As in any trauma patient being evaluated in the emergency department, Advanced Trauma Life Support (ATLS) principles should be followed. It should be noted, however, that the geriatric patient presents an additional challenge. Normal vital signs in elderly patients are notoriously deceptive, as these patients may have baseline hypertension or blunted sympathetic response due to being on beta-blockers. An age-adjusted shock-index (SI) might be a more useful alternative for initial clinical hemodynamic evaluation than heart rate or blood pressure alone. Zarzaur and colleagues reported an age-adjusted shock-index (age multiplied by SI) to have a predictive performance measured by area under the receiver operator characteristics curve (AUROC) of 0.693, outperforming heart rate (AUROC 0.626), systolic blood pressure (AUROC 0.857), and unadjusted SI (AUROC 0.684).

Assuming a patent airway or a definitive airway has been established, the next step in evaluation of a thoracic trauma patient is breathing. In the context of pulmonary injury, it is the time to examine the patient for signs of life-threatening tension pneumothorax. Tension pneumothorax results when air is forced into the pleural space and intrathoracic pressure increases to the point of obstructing circulation. Signs include hypotension, tracheal deviation away from the affected hemithorax, neck vein dilation, and absent breath sounds on the affected hemithorax. Extended Focused Assessment with Sonography in Trauma (eFAST) can be a useful adjunct in the trauma bay, especially if obtaining a chest film might delay intervention. If a tension pneumothorax is diagnosed or suspected, current ATLS guidelines recommend immediate decompression using a 5–8 cm over the needle catheter at the fifth intercostal space, slightly anterior to the midaxillary line. Direct placement of a chest tube or finger thoracostomy are also alternatives.

If chest tube insertion is required, the output should be examined. If an immediate output of 1500 mL of blood or more is obtained, massive hemothorax is then diagnosed, which is an indication for blood transfusion and a thoracotomy in the operating room.

Chest computed tomography (CT) is a fundamental tool in the evaluation of the chest trauma patient and should be pursued in all hemodynamically stable polytrauma patients with a suspected chest injury, either based on clinical examination or initial chest X-ray. In the elderly, there should be a high index of suspicion for hidden or silent injuries and chest computed tomography should be performed liberally. If there is concern for a concomitant cardiac or vascular injury (for example, in a high-energy mechanism such as a motor vehicle collision) intravenous contrast should be given during the CT examination.

Management of Specific Injuries

Rib Fractures and Pulmonary Contusions

Rib fractures are the most common injury pattern in the elderly with a thoracic injury. They are associated with significant morbidity and mortality. In the classic study by Bulger and colleagues, they showed that each additional rib fracture in an elderly patient increases mortality by 19% and pneumonia risk by 27%. The cardinal symptom is pain upon breathing or moving. An algorithm developed by the Western Trauma Association (WTA) suggests that all patients aged 65 years and older should be admitted to the Intensive Care Unit (ICU) or other monitored or step-down unit; however, a recent analysis by Naar and colleagues showed that patients with isolated rib fractures admitted to a hospital floor have a low rate of unplanned ICU admission.

The cornerstone of the management of isolated rib fractures is pain control. A multimodal analgesia strategy should be used routinely. An oral or intravenous regimen consisting of acetaminophen and non-steroidal anti-inflammatory (NSAID) agents is a reasonable first choice. The use of narcotic opioid medications should be minimized as much as possible to avoid well-known adverse effects such as somnolence, constipation, or respiratory depression, as well as the unintended consequence of opioid dependence. Regional analgesia modalities such as epidural analgesia, paraspinal block, intercostal and, more recently, anterior serratus block have emerged as important components of any multimodal pain control strategy, but specific guidance in the rib fracture patient is lacking. A reasonable strategy is for the clinician to evaluate pain control and breathing difficulty in a continuous fashion and consider more invasive interventional management as soon as ineffective pain management becomes apparent. The issue of rib fixation for the management of rib fractures represents an ongoing controversy, as data regarding the effectiveness remains sketchy at best.

A common complication of blunt chest wall injury and rib fractures in the elderly patient is pulmonary contusion (PC). It is well-known that clinical manifestations of PC evolve over time. They become clinically and radiologically apparent within the first hours after injury and resolve over the first week. They should always be suspected in the blunt trauma patient with rib fractures. Clinical manifestations include chest pain, cough, hemoptysis, and decreased oxygen saturation. Respiratory impairment can range from mild to severe respiratory distress, stemming from impaired gas exchange in the contused lung parenchyma superimposed on decreased ventilation from pain due to the chest wall component. Management is mostly supportive with adequate pain control, judicious fluid resuscitation (to avoid worsening pulmonary edema), pulmonary toilet, and supplemental oxygen. Noninvasive ventilation (NIV) has been suggested as an alternative to endotracheal intubation and mechanical ventilation in patients who do not have another indication for intubation. A recent meta-analysis of five studies estimated a pooled relative risk of 0.26 (0.09–0.71) for NIV compared to mechanical ventilation, but only one of the studies was a randomized trial and no distinction was made between the different NIV modalities (continuous positive airway pressure [CPAP], bi-level positive airway pressure [BiPAP]). In patients requiring mechanical ventilation, a lung protective strategy should be emphasized.

In the elderly patient, medical comorbidities need to be reviewed at every point during clinical decision-making. COPD and other respiratory diseases can complicate ventilatory support. Anticoagulation is a primary concern when evaluating the use of regional analgesia.

Traumatic Hemothorax

For small hemothorax, if there is no other indication for placement of a chest tube, tube thoracostomy may be deferred initially, provided that the patient is hemodynamically stable and has no evidence of respiratory compromise. If there is a need for thoracic drainage, the EAST guidelines recommend considering a pigtail catheter (14 Fr or less) instead of a thoracostomy tube (20 Fr or larger) in hemodynamically stable patients due to similar risk of retained hemothorax and the theoretical potential for decreased pain at the insertion site, but more high-quality studies are needed. The EAST guideline recommends early (within the first 4 days of the hospitalization) video-assisted thoracoscopic surgery (VATS) to drain the retained hemothorax and decrease risk of subsequent fibrothorax or empyema.

The patient with a massive hemothorax, defined as an initial drainage of 1500 mL or 200 mL/h output for 2–4 h should be diagnosed in the trauma resuscitation area in the emergency department. Emergent thoracotomy in the operating room is indicated in these cases.

Delayed Hemothorax

An increasing number of elderly patients is on anticoagulation for multiple reasons. Following pulmonary trauma with rib fractures, these patients may present with delayed hemothorax. This often occurs after they have been discharged from the hospital, and their anticoagulation is restarted. The incidence of delayed hemothorax in geriatric patients was reported in one study to be about 1.3%. There is no consensus on the definition of delayed hemothorax, but in the authors', they may occur up to 1–2 weeks after the initial trauma and many require chest tube placement. Having a vigilant geriatric trauma follow-up is essential in these patients on anticoagulation.

Traumatic Pneumothorax

Small pneumothoraces can be observed if there are no other indications for tube thoracostomy. Recent literature supports that a pneumothorax with a distance between the edge of the parietal pleura and the edge of the visceral pleura of 35 mm of less as measured by CT can be safely observed. In the event of clinical deterioration, evacuation by pigtail catheter or tube thoracostomy can be instituted.

Sternal Fractures

Isolated sternal fractures by themselves are not associated with major complications. The management is mostly conservative unless they contribute significantly to chest wall instability in the setting of other injuries (multiple rib fractures, sterno-manubrial dislocation/fracture), are severe (comminution, sternal discontinuity) or are associated with persistent symptoms (deformity, pain, clicking).

Penetrating Trauma

The incidence of penetrating trauma in elderly patients is quite low in general. Penetrating thoracic trauma is managed in a similar manner as penetrating trauma in other age groups. However, given the morbidity associated with procedures such as thoracotomy and median sternotomy, as much as possible, it is important to clarify whether these kinds of procedures are within the goals of care for geriatric patients prior to performing them.

Conclusion

Rib fractures are the most common type of chest trauma in geriatric patients. They are associated with increased morbidity and mortality. The cornerstone of management is adequate pain control. Traumatic pneumothorax and hemothorax are managed similarly as in other patients. However, delayed hemothorax can be a major problem in geriatric patients requiring a vigilant follow-up system for patients on anticoagulation.

References

1. Howard F, Rockwood K, Young JB, editors. Brocklehurst's textbook of geriatric medicine and gerontology. 8th ed. Philadelphia: Elsevier; 2017.
2. Bader A, Rahman U, Morris M, McCormack JE, Huang EC, Zawin M, et al. Pulmonary contusions in the elderly after blunt trauma: incidence and outcomes. J Surg Res. 2018;230:110–6.
3. Bulger EM, Arneson MA, Mock CN, Jurkovich GJ. Rib fractures in the elderly. J Trauma Acute Care Surg. 2000;48(6):1040–7.
4. Naar L, el Hechi MW, van Erp IA, Mashbari HNA, Fawley J, Parks JJ, et al. Isolated rib cage fractures in the elderly: do all patients belong to the intensive care unit? A retrospective nationwide analysis. J Trauma Acute Care Surg. 2020;89:1039–45.
5. Fakhry SM, Shen Y, Biswas S, Duane TM, McBride KM, Elkbuli A, et al. The public health burden of geriatric trauma: analysis of 2,688,008 hospitalizations from Centers for Medicare and Medicaid Services inpatient claims. J Trauma Acute Care Surg. 2022;92:984–9.
6. American College of Surgeons Committee on Trauma. ATLS advanced trauma life support student course manual. 10th ed. Chicago: American College of Surgeons; 2018.
7. Zarzaur BL, Croce MA, Magnotti LJ, Fabian TC. Identifying life-threatening shock in the older injured patient: an analysis of the national trauma data bank. J Trauma. 2010;68:1134–8.
8. Brasel KJ, Moore EE, Albrecht RA, de Moya M, Schreiber M, Karmy-Jones R, et al. Western trauma association critical decisions in trauma: management of rib fractures. J Trauma Acute Care Surg. 2017;82:200–3.
9. Ho AMH, Ho AK, Mizubuti GB, Klar G, Karmakar MK. Regional analgesia for patients with traumatic rib fractures: a narrative review. J Trauma Acute Care Surg. 2020;88:e22–30.
10. Feliciano DV, Mattox KL, Moore EE, editors. Trauma. 9th ed. McGraw-Hill; 2021.

11. Chiumello D, Coppola S, Froio S, Gregoretti C, Consonni D. Noninvasive ventilation in chest trauma: systematic review and meta-analysis. Intensive Care Med. 2013;39:1171–80.
12. Patel NJ, Dultz L, Ladhani HA, Cullinane DC, Klein E, McNickle AG, et al. Management of simple and retained hemothorax: a practice management guideline from the eastern Association for the Surgery of trauma: Hemothorax management guideline. Am J Surg. 2021;221:873–84.
13. Choi J, Anand A, Sborov KD, Walton W, Chow L, Guillamondegui O, et al. Complication to consider: delayed traumatic hemothorax in older adults. Trauma Surg Acute Care Open. 2021;6:e000626.
14. Eddine SBZ, Boyle KA, Dodgion CM, Davis CS, Webb TP, Juern JS, et al. Observing pneumothoraces: the 35-millimeter rule is safe for both blunt and penetrating chest trauma. J Trauma Acute Care Surg. 2019;86:557–62.
15. Yeh DD, Hwabejire JO, Demoya MA, Alam HB, King DR, Velmahos GC. Sternal fracture - an analysis of the National Trauma Data Bank. J Surg Res. 2014;186:39–43.

Tracheobronchial Injuries

32

Peep Talving, Sten Saar, and Lydia Lam

Introduction

Airway integrity is imperative for cellular respiration thus any given tracheobronchial injury may potentially result in airway obstruction, significantly reduced tidal volumes, life-threatening hypoxia, cardiorespiratory compromise, and fatal outcomes.

Schneider and colleagues reported overall distribution of tracheobronchial injuries at 58% and 42% as iatrogenic and traumatic in origin, respectively. The majority of iatrogenic tracheobronchial injuries occur during emergency endotracheal intubation, direct-, flexible- or rigid bronchoscopy, percutaneous tracheostomy placement, endotracheal airway dilatation, stent placement or at surgical procedures in the neck, mediastinum or thoracic cavities. The majority of these iatrogenic injuries occur in the posterior tracheal membrane.

In trauma settings, both penetrating and blunt injuries to the neck and chest raise suspicion of tracheobronchial injury particularly when airway compromise, subcutaneous emphysema, hemoptysis, or pneumothorax is present. Cervical trachea is readily exposed to penetrating insults including stab wounds and gunshot injuries (Fig. 32.1a, b). Blunt insults to the neck may occasionally disrupt cervical trachea in high-speed motor vehicle accidents or in direct blows. Thoracic tracheobronchial injuries are caused mainly by high-impact motor vehicle crashes and occasionally by thoracic gunshot injuries.

In this chapter we delineate contemporary iatrogenic and traumatic epidemiology, anatomy with relevant features, clinical investigations, imaging, management and complications following iatrogenic and traumatic tracheobronchial injuries.

P. Talving (✉) · S. Saar
Division of Acute Care Surgery, Department of Surgery, North Estonia Medical Center, Tallinn, Estonia

Department of Surgery, University of Tartu, Tartu, Estonia
e-mail: peep.talving@ut.ee; sten.saar@ut.ee

L. Lam
Division of Trauma and Surgical Critical Care, Department of Surgery, Keck School of Medicine, University of Southern California, LAC + USC Medical Center, Los Angeles, CA, USA
e-mail: lydia.lam@med.usc.edu

P. Petrone, C. E.M. Brathwaite (eds.), *Acute Care Surgery in Geriatric Patients*,
https://doi.org/10.1007/978-3-031-30651-8_32

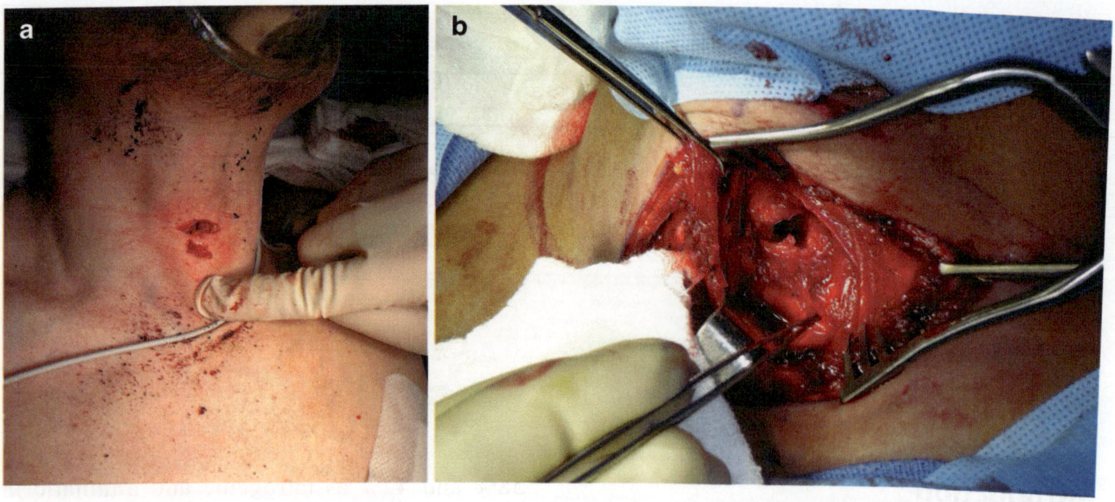

Fig. 32.1 (**a, b**) Images demonstrating patients with tracheal injuries secondary to a stab wound (1a) and a gunshot wound (1b), respectively

Epidemiology

Iatrogenic Injuries

Considering millions of endotracheal intubations, bronchoscopies, endoluminal airway dilatations, and tracheostomies worldwide on an annual basis compared to the limited number of scientific reports on iatrogenic lesions, the iatrogenic tracheobronchial injuries are rare and remain underreported in the literature. The incidence of iatrogenic tracheobronchial injuries is estimated to be at 0.005% after single-lumen endotracheal intubations. However, following emergency intubations, iatrogenic lesions have been reported in up to 15% of cases in postmortem series. After double-lumen intubations, the iatrogenic lesions occur more frequently than single lumen intubations ranging between 0.05 and 0.19% of interventions. Following percutaneous dilatational tracheostomies, tracheobronchial injuries occur in about 1% of cases. Most iatrogenic tracheal injuries are confined to the low-resistance posterior membranous portion of the trachea and have a longitudinal course. Injuries caused by the endotracheal tube or bougie-tip are located in mid third of the trachea and extent between 5 and 130 mm in most severe cases. In transmural tracheal injuries, esophagus may protrude into the tracheal lumen and in extreme instances the lesion may be associated with esophageal injury. Cardillo and colleagues stratified injury severity in iatrogenic injuries depicted in Table 32.1. Modifiable risk factors for iatrogenic tracheobronchial insults during airway management and interventions are procedural and instrumentational while nonmodifiable risk factors comprise anatomic properties including advanced age, tracheal malignancy, female gender, long-term steroid inhalation, and presence of tracheal diverticuli.

Table 32.1 Morphologic classification of a tracheal wall injuries (data from Cardillo et al.)

Level I	Mucosal or submucosal lesion without mediastinal emphysema and esophageal injury
Level II	Injury extending to the muscular wall with subcutaneous or mediastinal emphysema without mediastinitis or esophageal injury
Level IIIa	Complete laceration with esophageal or mediastinal soft-tissue herniation without mediastinitis or esophageal injury
Level IIIb	Any laceration with esophageal injury or mediastinitis

Traumatic Injuries

The true population-based incidence of traumatic tracheobronchial injuries is poorly documented as the majority of patients with major airway injuries expire in prehospital settings. In a large autopsy study including 1178 trauma victims, Bertelsen et al. reported a low incidence at 0.03% (33/1178) of tracheobronchial injuries with 82% fatal outcomes almost instantaneously after injury. In this study, tracheobronchial injuries were located to mainstem bronchi and trachea at 70% and 30%, respectively. Among victims sustaining isolated thoracic injuries, tracheobronchial injuries occurred in 2.8% of cases. Other authors have collectively reported an incidence of 2.5–3.2% of tracheobronchial lesions in subsequent autopsy series. It has been estimated that approximately 0.5% of victims of major trauma surviving to trauma centers suffer a tracheobronchial injury. Schibilsky and co-authors observed a population-based incidence at 0.4% of traumatic tracheobronchial injuries among all hospital admissions with Injury Severity Score ≥9 per DGU Trauma Registry in Germany. Penetrating mechanisms accounted for 16% of all tracheobronchial injuries in this series. The reported incidence of 561 tracheobronchial injuries at 640 healthcare facilities during 14 years of patient recruitment provides an annual incidence of 0.06 tracheobronchial injuries per institution across acute care facilities in Germany. Traumatic tracheobronchial injuries were located to subglottic and supraglottic locations at 70% and 29%, respectively, following both penetrating and blunt insults. Rossbach and colleagues reported a proportion of penetrating mechanisms at the University of Texas Health Science Center, San Antonio at 59% in a cohort of 28 patients with tracheobronchial injuries during 32 years, translating into one penetrating tracheobronchial traumatic injury annually. Also, Demetriades and co-authors prospectively collected 223 patients with penetrating neck injuries documenting only 2 tracheal injuries (0.8%) in their clinical series. The incidence of tracheal injuries following blunt mechanisms is estimated to be at 0.4% with 70–80% of injuries confined to the thoracic tracheobronchial tree.

Traumatic tracheobronchial tears can be longitudinal confined mostly to the posterior membranous trachea, transverse between the tracheal rings, or spiral. In about 8–10% the lesions can be complex with multiple injury sites or a combination of injury patterns. The vast majority of tracheobronchial injuries are associated with a significant overall injury burden including pneumothoraces, lung contusions, multiple rib fractures, hemothoraces, lung lacerations, diaphragmatic injuries, and esophageal injuries at 41%, 32%, 30%, 23%, 8%, 2%, and 1%, respectively.

Following penetrating trauma to the neck, it has been reported by Demetriades et al. a total of 137 injuries to the cervical structures in 233 patients comprising 35%, 39% and 25% of concomitant vascular, visceral, and nervous system injuries, respectively, associated with less than 1% of tracheal lesions. Transmediastinal gunshot injuries are a distinct entity with particularly high mortality and incidence of concomitant injuries to the heart, great vessels, and airways. Okoye et al. studied 133 patients with transmediastinal gunshot injuries who survived to the hospital and observed an incidence of tracheobronchial injuries at 1%. Overall, tracheobronchial injuries are associated with 25% in-hospital mortality in a population-based large series.

Tracheal and Bronchial Surgical Anatomy

The trachea, consisting of cervical and thoracic segments, is a 10–13 cm long tubular-shaped structure consisting of 15–20 horseshoe-shaped rings of cartilage interconnected with ligaments and covered with respiratory epithelium. The thickness of the tracheal wall averages 3 mm with a diameter of about 2.3 cm. The trachealis muscle forms the posterior membranous wall comprising the vast majority of iatrogenic lesions. Strong peritracheal connective tissue may contain minor lesions and leave them unnoticed.

The cervical trachea begins at the lower edge of the cricoid cartilage at the level of C6 and ends at the level of the aortic arch at the level of thoracic outlet. The cervical trachea with a length of 3–5 cm comprises 70–80% of penetrating tracheal injuries. Thoracic trachea starts at the level of thoracic outlet and descends to the level of carina at the level of T4 dividing further into right and left mainstem bronchi. Overall, 70–80% of blunt tracheobronchial injuries occur in the thoracic segment of the tracheobronchial tree.

The upper part of trachea derives blood from inferior thyroid arteries and lower part through bronchial arteries. Blood vessels run laterally on both sides of the trachea in a segmental fashion.

The trachea has a close relationship with many vital structures, thus, tracheal injuries are often associated with vascular, digestive and nervous system lesions. The right and left lobe of the thyroid gland are located on the anterolateral sides of the proximal cervical trachea connected with the thyroid isthmus at the level of the second or third tracheal ring. The isthmus is divided during an open surgical tracheostomy placement. The esophagus begins at the level of cricoid cartilage and courses posteriorly but may be positioned slightly to the left lateral side. The right and left recurrent laryngeal nerves, which are branches of the vagus nerve, course alongside with the trachea in a posterolateral location. The left recurrent nerve loops under the aortic arch and right recurrent nerve under the right subclavian artery before coursing cranially towards vocal cords. Also, there are a number of large blood vessels surrounding the trachea. The brachiocephalic trunk courses anterolaterally from left to right across the distal and mid trachea. The left common carotid artery runs over the distal and mid trachea left to the midline of the trachea. The pulmonary trunk is located anterior and to the left of the tracheal carina. Superior vena cava courses along the right anterior part of the trachea and the azygos vein joins the superior vena cava just above the right mainstem bronchus. Azygos vein ligation at this particular location via a right posterolateral thoracotomy provides an ample surgical access to the entire intrathoracic tracheobronchial tree except the distal left mainstem bronchus. The trachea divides into the right and left main bronchi on the level of the carina as mentioned above. About 75% of blunt tracheobronchial tree injuries are located at this pericarinal location that is best accessed via right thoracotomy. The right main bronchus courses slightly more cranially and is more vertical and shorter (about 2.5 cm) compared to the left main bronchus. The left mainstem bronchus is about 5 cm long and more horizontal. Mainstem bronchi divide into the lobar bronchi and subsequently into segmental bronchi accessed surgically via right or left thoracotomies, respectively (Fig. 32.2).

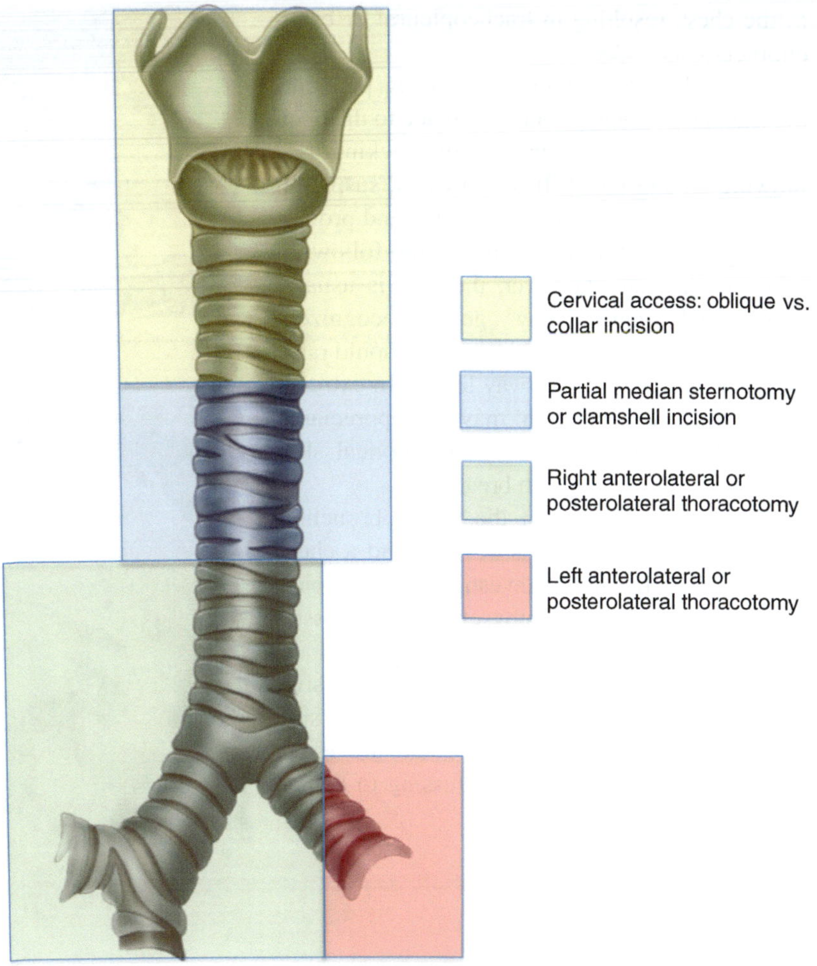

Fig. 32.2 An illustration depicting a surgical access depending on the injury site (Illustration by T. Veršinina, MD)

Clinical Findings

Tracheobronchial injuries are divided clinically into obvious and occult injuries. Most frequent and obvious clinical and radiological sign of tracheobronchial injuries is subcutaneous emphysema that may occasionally raise to the upper eyelids (Fig. 32.3) and caudally to the extraperitoneal pelvic cavity. Subcutaneous emphysema has been noted in 87% of tracheobronchial lesions. Tracheobronchial lesions are frequently associated with pneumomediastinum, pneumothorax, dyspnea, respiratory distress, and hemoptysis. Respiratory compromise may occur when airway obstruction evolves or when significant tidal volumes are lost due to pleural breach

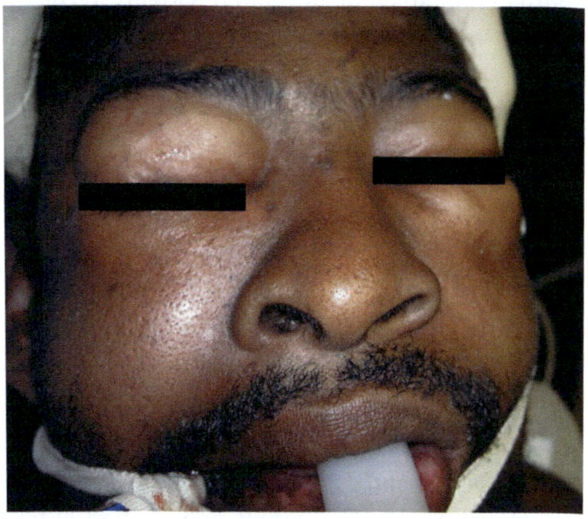

Fig. 32.3 An image of a patient with a gunshot injury to the chest with a significant facial epmhysema

to the chest, resulting in tracheopleural or bronchopleural air leaks.

Cervical tracheal injuries following penetrating trauma are obvious and visible due to the open wound in the neck, occasionally sucking and blowing air and blood. If not obvious, suspicion for airway injury must be maintained and prompt investigation for tracheal injury should follow. In blunt mechanisms, however, the skin is usually intact and injury may go unrecognized. Ecchymosis or hematoma in the neck should raise a clinical suspicion for airway lesion. In extreme cases, tracheal separation may be appreciated with palpable tracheal defect and cervical skin fluctuations in concert with breathing.

In thoracic segment of the tracheobronchial tree, the injuries are not as obvious and a chest radiograph is the initial investigation of choice depicting mediastinal emphysema besides associated lung and chest wall lesions. When mediastinal pleura is not breached, massive pneumothorax may not develop. Patients in stable respiratory and hemodynamic state are asked to cough and spit on a gauze dressing to depict blood contained sputum.

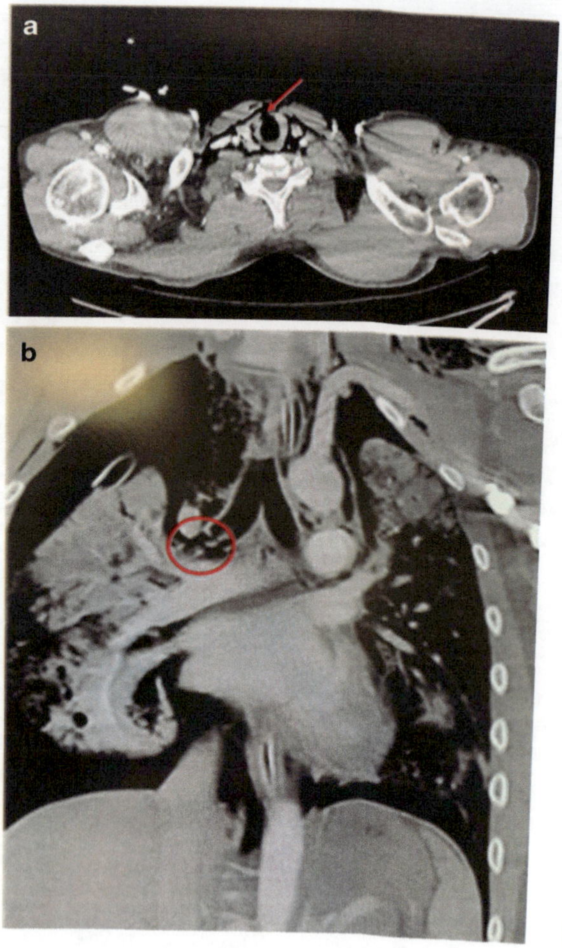

Fig. 32.4 (**a, b**) Computed tomography images of a with transmural cervical tracheal injury (4a, red arrow pointing to the tracheal injury) and right mainstem bronchial injury (4b, the red circle encompassing a total bronchial injury), respectively

Investigations

During the primary survey, the chest X-ray is routinely obtained in all injured patients to rule in or out radiological signs of tracheobronchial injuries including subcutaneous and mediastinal emphysema, pneumothorax, tension pneumothorax and occasionally, when major main stem bronchial injury is present, a "fallen lung" can be observed in addition to concomitant chest wall and lung injuries.

Chest computed tomography (CT) is widely available in contemporary settings and provides excellent imaging to rule in or exclude tracheobronchial injuries in concordance with clinical suspicion. CT findings demonstrate the presence of mediastinal and subcutaneous emphysema and pneumothoraces. CT may also depict partial tracheobronchial wall injuries and transmural tracheal lesions with high accuracy (Fig. 32.4a, b). Likewise, CT depicts mediastinal fat or esophageal herniation into tracheal lumen in transmural lesions thus associated esophageal injury must be ruled out with subsequent CT esophagography. In a population-based European investigation, esophageal injuries were associated with 1% of tracheobronchial injuries. However, in the US trauma settings, 11% of tracheobronchial injuries were associated with esophageal injuries. In iatrogenic injuries, associated esophageal injuries are infrequent entities.

Bronchoscopy is the investigation of choice to diagnose tracheobronchial injury location and extent if patients' clinical condition permits

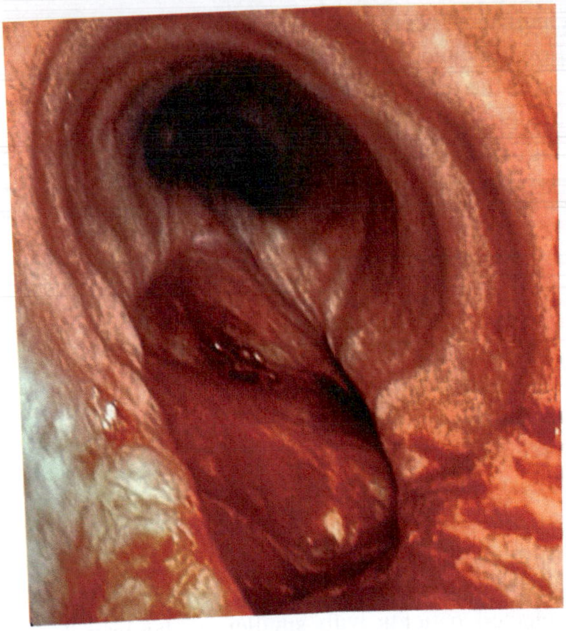

Fig. 32.5 A bronchoscopic view of an iatrogenic injury of posterior wall of trachea at emergency intubation with bougie (Courtesy of T. Vanakesa, MD)

(Fig. 32.5). Bronchoscopy can be performed with conscious sedation without endotracheal intubation or with sedation in intubated patients. The tracheobronchial lumen is cleared of blood and secretions and the tracheobronchial tree is carefully inspected. The vast majority of blunt injuries are located within 2 cm distal to carina with preponderance to the right mainstem bronchus. Bronchoscopy may act as an interventional modality to locate the injury site and pattern and to guide endotracheal cuff placement to cover smaller lesions in selected patients. Likewise, bronchoscopy-guided intubation facilitates placement of the endotracheal tube cuff distal to injury site for improved ventilatory effort in tracheal injuries.

Management

Airway Management

The initial clinical management follows Advanced Trauma Life Support® principles to ensure airway patency, adequate oxygenation,

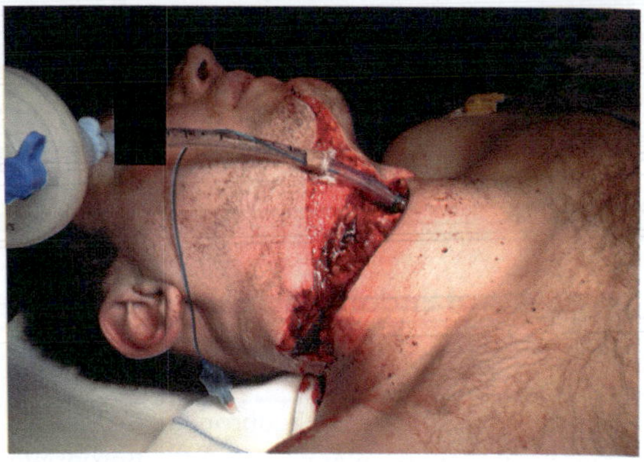

Fig. 32.6 An image of a patient with complete transection of sublaryngeal trachea with direct intubation via the defect

ventilation, and circulation. Cricothyroidotomy and fiberoptic capabilities must be available in emergency settings. In occasional instances, cervical trachea can be intubated through the exposed tracheal wound after grasping the distal trachea with a clamp to avoid tracheal retraction into mediastinum at intubation (Fig. 32.6). Whenever the patient can spontaneously maintain patent airway in suspected laryngotracheal injuries, spontaneous ventilation is supported to prevent disastrous airway loss at emergency intubation. When conscious sedation is not an option, the preferred method of securing the airway is endotracheal intubation with video laryngoscope. Videolaryngoscopic intubation is augmented by flexible bronchoscope for post-glottic tube guidance when vocal cords can be passed. The procedure is performed in a fully monitored setting by two providers; one provider handling the bronchoscope and the second one ensures safe monitoring and sedation. Fiberoptic attempts are made to clear the airway from blood and secretions and to pass the endotracheal tube distal to tracheal injury. In smaller injuries near the carina, the cuff may be inflated over the lesion to occlude the defect and to maintain tidal volumes. Airway management in injuries distal to carina includes attempts of single lung ventilation by mainstem intubation into uninjured bronchial lumen. In peri-carinal injuries, bronchoscopy-guided selective right and left bronchial intubation is attempted with two small-sized endotracheal tubes connected via appropriate Y-connector to the ventilatory circuit. The final rescue option in advanced facilities is veno-venous Extracorporeal Membrane Oxygenation (ECMO) following cannulation of femoral vessels by trained providers.

Surgical and Endobronchial Management

Surgical repair of tracheobronchial injuries requires judicious planning and appropriate access. Injuries proximal to aortic arch are accessed with an oblique cervical incision that can be extended to a partial or complete sternotomy for access to mid trachea. Wide exposure for cervical trachea is obtained by collar incision with an appropriate-sized skin flap for extensive injuries or in through-and-through lesions. Tracheal injury site is debrided and sutured with interrupted absorbable sutures placing a viable pedicled tissue-flap between injury site in proximity lesions. In extensive injuries, we recommend a distal tracheostomy for improved airway access and for early weaning from the ventilator.

Access to intrathoracic trachea is best achieved through a right posterolateral thoracotomy. In multicavity injuries, the access to contralateral thoracic cavity or abdominal cavity may be necessary, thus an anterolateral thoracotomy is the preferred option in these settings. Double-lumen intubation is preferred, if feasible, allowing the lung to be deflated for surgery. The azygos vein is seen crossing over the right mainstem bronchus into the superior vena cava and can be ligated and divided thus providing ample access to the entire intrathoracic trachea from thoracic inlet to the carina. The proximal left mainstem bronchus can likewise be accessed via aforementioned surgical approach. With this approach also the esophagus is readily available for repair posterior to the trachea. The transmural mainstem bronchus laceration is digitally closed and repaired with interrupted absorbable sutures. When full circumferential injury is encountered, the endotracheal tube can be digitally guided into distal mainstem bronchus and repair is performed following appropriate debridement of the tissues over the endotracheal tube. Following repair, the endotracheal tube can be pulled back to preferred site which is 1–2 cm proximal to carina and air leak is controlled.

Left distal mainstem bronchus access requires extension to the left chest across the sternum and the repair is performed in similar fashion. Following repair, the chest is closed and chest tubes are inserted as warranted. The airway pressures and end-expiratory pressures should be kept at minimal and chest tube will monitor for potential suture insufficiency seen as air leaks. Chest tubes are removed when there is no sign of suture insufficiency and the patient is weaned off from the mechanical ventilation.

Non-operative management is subjected to selected patients with smaller tracheobronchial lacerations, i.e., <2 cm and tolerate spontaneous breathing or minimal ventilator support. Likewise, conservative management is applied to poor surgical candidates due to underlying conditions and comorbidities. These patients, however, may qualify for endobronchial interventions including self-expanding metallic stent placements.

Overall, 61% and 39% of iatrogenic injuries are subjected to surgical and conservative or endobronchial management, respectively. Management of iatrogenic injuries is determined by the clinical condition of the patient and the extent of the injury. Iatrogenic injuries are predominantly located to posterior tracheal membrane and can be accessed surgically as delineated above. Lesions larger than 2 cm are universally subjected to a surgical repair. Lesions <2 cm with mild emphysema and maintained tidal volumes can be managed conservatively on spontaneous or mechanical ventilation. Non-operative management includes serial chest radiographs, low airway pressures, and antimicrobial prophylaxis for mediastinitis. Distal cuff placement is preferred to isolate the injury and to avoid air leak under mechanical ventilation. Endobronchial stenting of trachea or carina with Y-stent are evolving options in these instances. Endoluminal surgical repair of iatrogenic posterior membrane injuries is likewise evolving.

Postoperative Management

The vast majority of patients subjected to isolated tracheobronchial surgical repair can be extubated after surgical repair. Non-invasive ventilation is attempted in patients with minor associated injuries requiring some ventilatory support. It is important to maintain good pulmonary toilet and humidify the air to maintain airway moisture. When invasive ventilatory support is required due to extensive injury burden, a large-bore endotracheal tube is placed at the end of the procedure to allow adequate airway toilet and bronchoscopy-surveillance. Ventilatory management is determined by the underlying condition of the patient in addition to the location and frailty of the repair. Airway pressures are maintained as low as possible that provide adequate oxygenation and ventilation. Endotracheal cuff is placed distal to the injury or surgical repair to avoid disruption of the repair. Pressure control mode on a conventional ventilator can assure that peak airway pressures remain controlled. If patient condition allows, rapid wean to pressure support mode will further decrease any unnecessary stress on the repair to allow for optimal outcome of repair. Consider high flow oxygen as the spontaneous breathing benefit the healing of the airway repair. Blunt tracheobronchial rupture patients would be expected to sustain a large force leading to associated pulmonary contusions and lacerations. Sound respiratory management including judicious fluid administration to decrease pulmonary edema, and utilizing positive end expiratory pressure (PEEP) for recruitment of alveoli will further expedite the possibility of early extubation.

Empiric broad-spectrum antimicrobial treatment covering Gram positive, Gram negative, and anaerobic agents is provided in tracheobronchial injuries for 1 week. In a review by Pastene et al., the authors separated the etiology of mediastinitis into three groups: deep sternal wound infection (DSWI), descending necrotizing mediastinitis (DNM), and esophageal perforation. DSWI was associated with mostly Gram positive and Gram negative, whereas the other two included anaerobic bacteria. The recommended antibiotic of choice is piperacillin/tazobactam or a third-generation cephalosporins with metronidazole. Antifungals are recommended should an associated esophageal perforation be involved. Cultures should be obtained early and de-escalation of antibiotics to the specific cultures would be an appropriate antibiotic stewardship.

Outcomes and Complications

In 40–100% of cases with tracheobronchial injuries are associated with a significant overall injury burden contributing to detrimental outcomes. Consequently, it has been estimated that traumatic tracheobronchial injuries result in a prehospital mortality in up to 80%.

Mortality in patients sustaining penetrating and blunt tracheobronchial injuries subjected to surgical repair ranges between 6–18% and 25%, respectively. Independent risk factors for fatal outcomes in these instances are need for emergent airway access and blunt injury patterns. Mortality following iatrogenic tracheobronchial lesions are mainly associated with underlying disease process.

Anastomotic stenosis or dehiscence occur in 5–6% following surgical repair of tracheobronchial injury. Stenosis may manifest usually 1–4 weeks later in three different scenarios. Firstly, the patient may have sustained a minor injury that has been initially overseen. Secondly, the overall injury burden may have prevented early treatment of tracheobronchial injury. Lastly, the surgical repair itself may complicate with stenosis. Bronchoscopy remains the gold standard diagnostic modality in these settings. The first line treatment is balloon-dilatation under direct visualization. Surgical treatment is preserved for stenotic lesions with dyspnea, stridor, or recurring pneumonias. Surgical reconstruction includes resection and end-to-end anastomosis. Airway stents are likewise evolving in treatment of airway stenosis.

Conclusion

Tracheobronchial injuries constitute a heterogenous entity of life-threatening airway lesions that require clinical suspicion, prompt airway management in respiratory insufficiency and thorough investigations with chest X-ray, CT scan, and bronchoscopy in that order. The majority of injuries require surgical management in the neck for cervical tracheal lesions or through a right thoracotomy for thoracic tracheobronchial lesions, respectively. In iatrogenic injuries and in poor surgical candidates, non-operative management with metallic stents is evolving.

Important Points

- Overall, iatrogenic tracheobronchial injuries predominate.
- Spontaneous breathing in patients with patent airway allows CT- and bronchoscopy-guided highly accurate diagnosis.
- High-risk airway is secured with endotracheal intubation facilitated by direct laryngoscopy, video laryngoscopy, or bronchoscopy-guided endotracheal intubation.
- Major tracheal injuries in the neck are explored via collar incision.
- Tracheobronchial injuries in the chest are explored through a right thoracotomy.
- Tracheobronchial injuries are repaired with interrupted absorbable sutures.

References

1. Schneider T, Volz K, Dienemann H, et al. Incidence and treatment modalities of tracheobronchial injuries in Germany. Interact Cardiovasc Thorac Surg 2009;8:571–6.
2. Bertelsen S, Howitz P. Injuries of the trachea and bronchi. Thorax. 1972;27(2):188–94.
3. Boutros J, et al. Multidisciplinary management of tracheobronchial injury. Eur Respir Rev. 2022;31:1–10.
4. Cardillo G, et al. Tracheal lacerations after endotracheal intubation: a proposed morphological classification to guide non-surgical treatment. Eur J Cardiothorac Surg. 2010;37(3):581–7.
5. Chu CPW, Chen PP. Tracheobronchial injury secondary to blunt chest trauma: diagnosis and management. Anaesth Intensive Care. 2002;30(2):145–52.
6. Demetriades D, et al. Evaluation of penetrating injuries of the neck: prospective study of 223 patients. World J Surg. 1997;21(1):47–8.
7. Gómez-Caro Andrés A, et al. Successful conservative management in iatrogenic tracheobronchial injury. Ann Thorac Surg. 2005;79(6):1872–8.
8. Johnson SB. Tracheobronchial injury. Semin Thorac Cardiovasc Surg. 2008;20(1):52–7.
9. Karmy-Jones R, et al. Traumatic injury to the trachea and bronchus. Thorac Surg Clin. 2007;17:35–46.
10. Koletsis E, et al. Surgical decision making in tracheobronchial injuries on the basis of clinical evidences and the injury's anatomical setting: a retrospective analysis. Injury. 2012;43(9):1437–41.
11. Grewal HS, et al. Treatment of tracheobronchial injuries. Chest. 2019;155(3):595–604.
12. Miñambres E, et al. Tracheal rupture after endotracheal intubation: a literature systematic review. Eur J Cardiothorac Surg. 2009;35(6):1056–62.
13. Okoye OT, et al. Transmediastinal gunshot wounds in a mature trauma Centre: changing perspectives. Injury. 2013;44(9):1198–203.
14. Pastene B, et al. Mediastinitis in the intensive care unit patient: a narrative review. Clin Microbiol Infect. 2020;26(1):26–34.
15. Schibilsky D, et al. Traumatic tracheobronchial injuries: incidence and outcome of 136.389 patients derived from the DGU trauma register. Sci Rep. 2020;10:1–7.
16. Welter S. Repair of tracheobronchial injuries. Thorac Surg Clin. 2014;24(1):41–50.

Geriatric Cardiac Trauma

33

Alberto García, Isabella Caicedo-Holguín, Daniela Burbano, Diego Peña, and Carlos Alberto Ordoñez

Introduction

As the world population grows older, major trauma in geriatric patients becomes more prevalent. The percentage of geriatric patients reported by the Pennsylvania Trauma Outcomes (PTO) was 30.75%. Trauma in the geriatric population, specifically cardiac trauma, is uncommon. The Pennsylvania Trauma Outcomes Registry reported 14.19% of cardiac injuries in patients older than 65 years. Heart injury in the elder represents 20% of overall heart injuries, with a mortality of 35%.

In the Trauma Registry of Fundación Valle del Lili, in Cali, Colombia, 161 cardiac injuries were managed from 2010 to 2021. Twenty-seven percent of them were in patients over 45 years old, and 13% in patients older than 65. The most common trauma mechanism in the group older than 45 was blunt, compared to those younger than 45 years, who presented more commonly penetrating mechanism. While trauma severity was less in older patients, mortality was higher (Table 33.1).

The main concern with geriatric patients undergoing trauma is a low physiologic reserve, which added to an underlying heart disease, contributes to a higher number of cardiac complications after trauma. The PTO reports that 2.9% of geriatric patients developed myocardial infarction after heart injury, with a 50% mortality rate when it occurs.

Different anatomic and physiologic changes occur with age: a drop in the number of myocytes has been reported, bringing a decline in cardiac function of 50% between the ages of 20 and 80. The atrial pacemakers suffer apoptosis, with 50–75% of cells lost by 50 and fibrosis of the bundle of His. Additionally, there is fibrosis and calcification of the fibrous skeleton of the heart. The elasticity of the aorta and great arteries

A. García (✉) · C. A. Ordoñez
Division of Trauma and Acute Care Surgery, Department of Surgery, Fundación Valle del Lili, Cali, Colombia

Department of Intensive Care, Fundación Valle del Lili, Cali, Colombia

Division of Trauma and Acute Care Surgery, Department of Surgery, Universidad del Valle, Cali, Colombia

Universidad Icesi, Cali, Colombia
e-mail: alberto.garcia@correounivalle.edu.co; alberto.garcia@fvl.org.co; carlos.ordonez@fvl.org.co

I. Caicedo-Holguín
Centro de Investigaciones Clínicas, Fundación Valle del Lili, Cali, Colombia
e-mail: isabella.caicedo@fvl.org.co

D. Burbano
Department of Surgery, Universidad de Caldas, Manizales, Colombia

D. Peña
Universidad Icesi, Cali, Colombia

Cardiovascular Surgery, Fundación Valle del Lili, Cali, Colombia
e-mail: alvaro.pena@fvl.org.co

P. Petrone, C. E.M. Brathwaite (eds.), *Acute Care Surgery in Geriatric Patients*,
https://doi.org/10.1007/978-3-031-30651-8_33

Table 33.1 Fundación Valle del Lili. Cardiac trauma 2010–2021. Characteristics according to age. (Personal communication. Caicedo Y, 2022)

Age years	Patients n (%)	Penetrating *n* (%)	ISS median (IQR)	Mortality *n* (%)
<45	117 (73)	106 (91)	20 (13–26)	13 (11)
45–64	22 (14)	13 (62)	16 (9–25)	2 (9)
≥65	21 (13)	2 (10)	9 (9–9)	4 (19)
Total	160 (100)	121 (77)	16 (9–25)	19 (12)

decrease, affecting the compliance, making the vessels stiffer, resulting in increased afterload, causing ventricular hypertrophy. The inotropic ventricular reserve decreases, generating reduced exercise tolerance. A process of β-adrenoceptor desensitization takes place with aging, which affects the adrenergic modulation.

Additionally, the effects of frailty, comorbidities, and medications may mask the manifestations of shock, make diagnosing a cardiac injury challenging, or reduce the tolerance to trauma.

Trauma Mechanisms

Ground level falls are the most common mechanism of injury in the elderly population, motor vehicle crashes and pedestrians struck by a motor vehicle represent second and third most common mechanism of injury in the elderly population respectively.

Regarding thoracic trauma, it is slightly more common in the elder than the young population, and it is the second most commonly injured body region in the elder after head injury. Cardiac trauma is rare in the geriatric population, blunt trauma is the main mechanism of trauma, accounting for 90% of geriatric cardiac injury and it represents 20% of all cardiac injury with a mortality between 25% and 50%.

The cardiac injury most likely results from compression of the thoracic cage due to blunt forces or rapid acceleration and deceleration. Energy transfer is augmented due to the sarcopenia and decreased bone density of the thoracic wall in the aged patient. This mechanism affects the right ventricle primarily, although more than 50% of the patients have lesions of multiple heart chambers. The result of the energy transference is a broad spectrum of injuries, ranging from arrhythmias or conduction defects to valvular damage or rupture of cardiac chambers (Table 33.2).

A more limited energy transference causes the lesion in penetrating trauma, directly damaging the structures. In most cases, hemorrhage is the predominant physiopathologic alteration (Table 33.2).

In the following sections, we will present the approach in the management of blunt and penetrating cardiac trauma in the geriatric population.

Blunt Cardiac Trauma

As previously mentioned, blunt trauma can cause a broad range of alterations (Table 33.3.):

Myocardial Injury

Myocardial injury is more common in the right ventricle and atrium than in the left ventricle and atrium, and it is defined as the development of a laceration or tear in the walls of the atria, ventricles, or papillary muscles. It can be due to direct impact of the anterior chest wall, indirect pressure caused by forces applied to the abdominal veins, increasing preload, and intracardiac pressure, leading to myocardial rupture, compression of the thoracic cage due to forces applied to the sternum and the vertebral bodies, acceleration and deceleration forces, blast forces and penetration of the myocardium due to displaced rib or sternal fractures. Patients usually present with acute cardiac tamponade, pericardial effusion, hypotension, tachycardia, and have a high mortality, up to 80% which require emergent surgical treatment. Surgery principles will be presented in the penetrating trauma section.

Table 33.2 American Association for the Surgery of Trauma-Organ Injury Scale (AAST-OIS) for heart injury

Grade	Description
I	Blunt cardiac injury with minor ECG abnormality (nonspecific ST or T wave changes, premature atrial or ventricular contraction or persistent sinus tachycardia)
	Blunt or penetrating pericardial wound without cardiac injury, cardiac tamponade, or cardiac herniation
II	Blunt cardiac injury with heart block (right or left bundle branch, left anterior fascicular, or atrioventricular) or ischemic changes (ST depression or T wave inversion) without cardiac failure
	Penetrating tangential myocardial wound up to, but not extending through endocardium, without tamponade
III	Blunt cardiac injury with sustained (>6 beats/min) or multilocal ventricular contractions
	Blunt or penetrating cardiac injury with septal rupture, pulmonary or tricuspid valvular incompetence, papillary muscle dysfunction, or distal coronary arterial occlusion without cardiac failure
	Blunt pericardial laceration with cardiac herniation
	Blunt cardiac injury with cardiac failure
IV	Penetrating tangential myocardial wound up to, but extending through, endocardium, with tamponade
	Blunt or penetrating cardiac injury with septal rupture, pulmonary or tricuspid valvular incompetence, papillary muscle dysfunction, or distal coronary arterial occlusion producing cardiac failure
	Blunt or penetrating cardiac injury with aortic mitral valve incompetence.
	Blunt or penetrating cardiac injury of the right ventricle, right atrium, or left atrium
	Blunt or penetrating cardiac injury with proximal coronary arterial occlusion
	Blunt or penetrating left ventricular perforation
	Stellate wound with <50% tissue loss of the right ventricle, right atrium, or of left atrium
V	Blunt avulsion of the heart; penetrating wound producing >50% tissue loss of a chamber

Table 33.3 Blunt cardiac injury. ECG alterations and anatomic lesions

Alteration/lesion	*n*	%
ECG alteration	204	83
Sinus tachycardia	172	56
Abnormal ST	126	41
Bundle branch block	55	18
T change	46	15
Abnormal Q	21	7
Atrioventricular block	20	7
Ventricular fibrillation	7	7
Lesion	43	100
Cardiac chamber rupture	28	65
Hemopericardium without chamber rupture	5	12
Pneumopericardium without cardiac herniation	3	7
Pericardial hernia	3	7
Intrapericardial phrenic hernia	4	9

Septal injuries, should be considered as a type of myocardial injury, but due to its characteristics they are diagnosed in later evaluations. They are very rare, more commonly ventricular septal than atrial septal injuries, and patients usually present with dyspnea, chest pain and anxiety, similar to myocardial infraction clinical presentation.

Pericardial Injuries
They are very rare in blunt trauma. Injuries range between pericardial lacerations, rupture or pneumopericardium.

When they are isolated, they usually do not have clinical significance. However, cardiac herniation should be considered if the injury is of a considerable size because it poses high mortality in the next minutes. A cardiac herniation presents as sudden hypotension, loss of pulse, and severe hypoperfusion. Usually associated with changes in the position of the patient. Additionally, if there is myocardial injury, these patients are at higher risk of exsanguination and death.

On rare occasions, a pericardial effusion has a delayed presentation, similar to a postpericardiotomy syndrome. Mild cases can be treated with NSAIDs. Severe cases require drainage, which, in older patients, is better performed by ultrasound-guided percutaneous techniques.

Valvular Injury
The most common causes are due to papillary muscle rupture, chordae tendineae rupture, tearing of valve leaflets, and contusion of papillary muscles leading to delayed necrosis and eventual rupture. Papillary muscle rupture usually has an acute onset, while the other injuries tend to have a more insidious presentation. Generally, it initiates with signs and symptoms of valvular regurgitation of the affected valve.

Myocardial Contusion
There is no consensus to define this entity. Therefore, the spectrum is broad. It ranges from a mild elevation of cardiac biomarkers to significant myocardial dysfunction. The most common presentation is a chest discomfort and bruising, with electrocardiographic abnormalities such as alterations of the ST segment, ventricular tachycardia, heart blocks, and other arrhythmias.

Commotio Cordis
This Latin term refers to sudden cardiac death resulting from ventricular fibrillation caused by a fast-moving non-penetrating blow to the precordium, like a baseball. It is rare in the elder population and common youngsters and athletes.

Evaluation

The initial evaluation should focus on the principles of systematic assessment, based on priorities, proposed by the ATLS®. It is important to consider the physiological implications of an elderly patient as mentioned previously.

The FAST examination is a key element to rapidly identify pericardial fluid in the primary survey. Additionally, EKG monitoring and chest X-ray should be obtained. Further, a thorough physical examination is required.

As described in the guidelines for blunt cardiac trauma, when a normal EKG and normal troponin are present, blunt cardiac trauma can be ruled out.

It is important that isolated sternal fractures are not correlated with cardiac injury. Therefore, not all of these patients require further examination over the initial evaluation if clinically there is no suspicion.

In selected cases, in patients who require further evaluation, computed tomography, magnetic resonance, or a formal echocardiography can be performed, this last one being de image of choice.

Treatment

Usually, patients who manage to arrive to the hospital are those with less severe injuries.

Blunt cardiac trauma is usually self-limited and is treated with supportive care. Some patients might require vasopressors, inotropic, or mechanical support.

Surgery is extremely rare, usually associated with a mortality between 40 and 70% and it should be restricted to patients with structural abnormalities, such as ruptured papillary muscle, valvular injury, or myocardial rupture. In the cases of pericardial effusions, a pericardial window can be performed, to determine further interventions. But most injuries which require surgical repair, can be performed by a cardiovascular surgeon after patient stabilization and after ruling out life-threatening pathologies.

According to an analysis performed by Norri et al., they suggest that contrary to what people may think, elderly patients with blunt traumatic cardiac arrest have a good survival rate, and clinicians should not be discouraged to perform cardiopulmonary resuscitation (CPR) only because of the their age.

Penetrating Trauma

Although penetrating cardiac trauma is ten times less frequent in subjects older than 65, it carries a high mortality rate. Trauma services must be aware to properly detect and manage the entire spectrum of cardiac injuries.

Grossly, two-thirds of the patients with a significant hemopericardium after a penetrating precordial trauma arrive to the emergency department with shock or tamponade. The remaining third are asymptomatic or have mild, subtle manifestations.

Unstable patients must be operated on immediately (Fig. 33.1). Depending on the degree of instability, the available resources, and the surgeon's training, a left anterolateral thoracotomy or a median sternotomy must be performed. After accessing the pleural cavity, the surgeon must check the lung expansion. If an accidental esophageal or monobronquial intubation is not corrected, every therapeutic effort will be futile.

The descending aorta must be cross-clamped if systolic blood pressure is less than 70 mm Hg; the pericardium opened longitudinally and anterior to the phrenic nerve, to avoid its damage. Bleeding from the cardiac wound is transiently controlled by digital compression. A Satinsky clamp can achieve this objective on low-pressure cavities such as the atriums or the right ventricle. In selected cases, transient control can be achieved with a Foley catheter. Time must be given to the physiological recovery, and then the definitive management may be executed. Meanwhile, additional bleeding sources are identified and transiently controlled by clamping, compressing, or packing.

The cardiac wound is sutured with a 4/0 monofilament vascular suture supported by teflon pledgets (Fig. 33.2a, b). The stitch must follow the curve of the needle and the second surgeon must be prepared to retrieve the needle with a second needle holder to prevent its dislodgement, which can cause additional trauma and loss of blood. If available, a mechanical stabilizer should be used to avoid unnecessary cardiac mobilization and further damage to the myocardium.

Wounds adjacent to a coronary artery must be closed with horizontal mattress sutures placed beneath the artery. Distal coronary artery injuries can be ligated. Nevertheless, proximal injuries must be treated with a CABG, which can be performed under cardiopulmonary bypass or off-pump with a cardiac mechanical stabilizer.

In the initial scenario of extreme bradycardia or hypotension, the cardiac wound must be expeditiously sutured so that the open bi-manual cardiac massage can be made. Direct defibrillation must be performed using the internal paddles to deliver 20–50 joules if ventricular fibrillation occurs.

Resuscitation must be stopped if the patient fails to recover a perfusion rhythm or if after volume expansion and vasopressor support, systolic blood pressure cannot be maintained higher than 70 mmHg without unclamping.

Rarely do cardiac trauma patients require damage control procedures. When it occurs, the extra-cardiac sources of bleeding are quickly controlled, oozing surfaces are gently packed, and the surgical incision is temporarily closed.

In most cases, the surgery can be finished regularly. Before closing the thorax, the surgeon must check four aspects. First, a posterior wound of the heart must be ruled out. Sometimes, it does not bleed during the first operation, and it does in the immediate postoperative period (Fig. 33.2a).

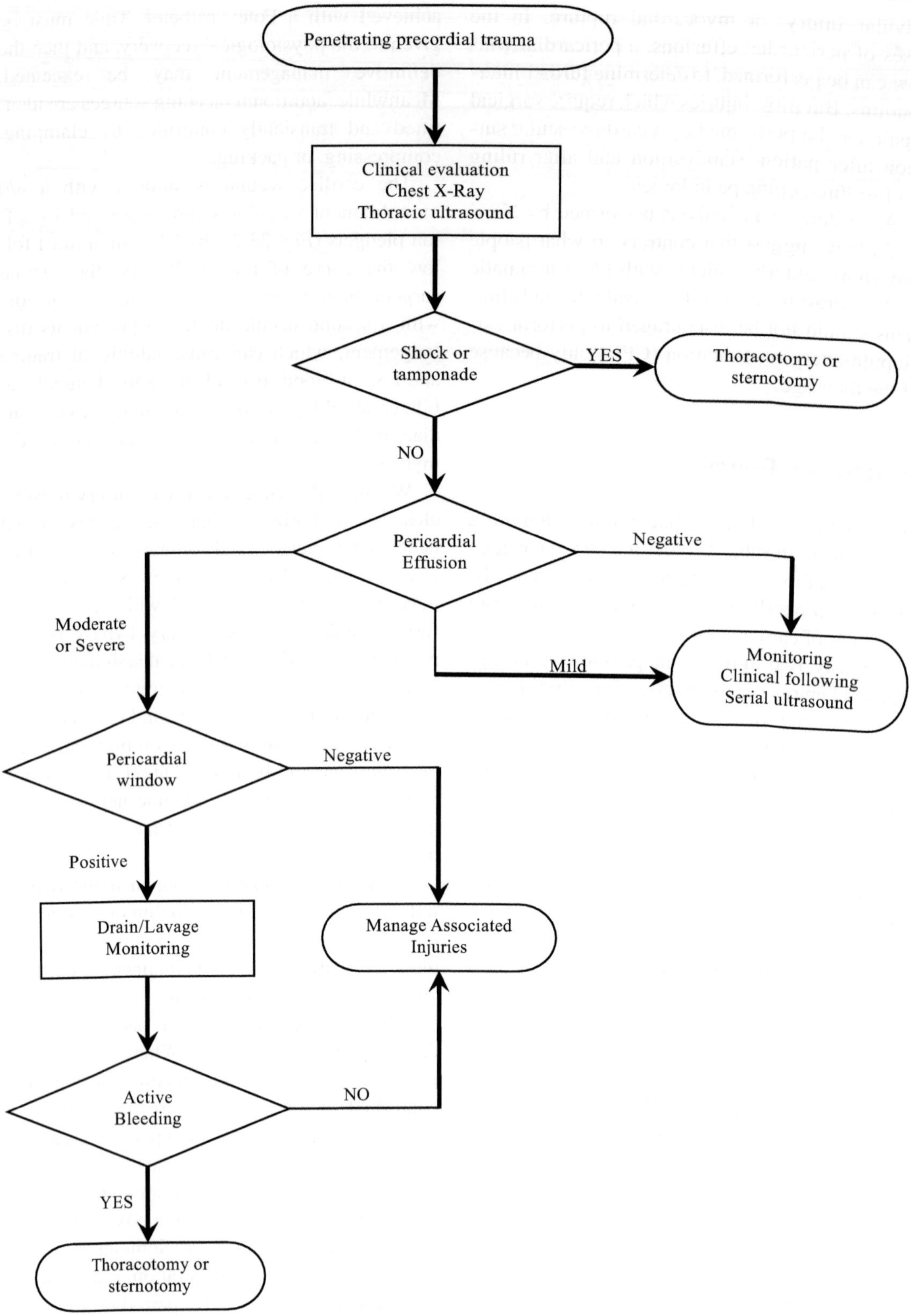

Fig. 33.1 Algorithm for the surgical decisions in penetrating precordial trauma. (Modified from Gonzalez-Hadad, et al.)

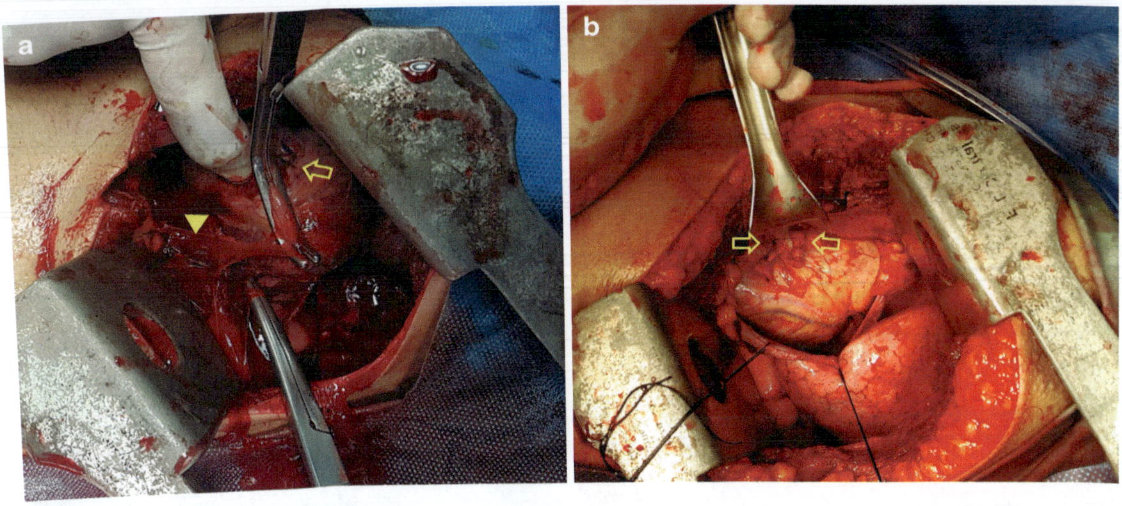

Fig. 33.2 Photographs were taken from the left side of the patients. A left anterolateral thoracotomy was performed. The head of the patient is on the right side of the image. (**a**) Anterior and posterior stab wounds of the right ventricle. The anterior wound was already sutured (open yellow arrow). The surgeon exposed the posterior wall (yellow triangle) by grasping the apex with a Satinsky clamp. His index finger controls the wound in preparation for suturing. This maneuver allows the safe and quick exposition of the posterior wall and avoids unnecessary manipulation and blood loss. (**b**) Anterior wound of the right ventricle. The pericardial sac was longitudinally opened, parallel to the phrenic nerve. The myocardium was sutured with horizontal mattress stitches, supported by teflon pledgets

Second, the surgeon must palpate the heart to detect a thrill that heralds a communication between chambers or a valvular lesion. These must be investigated and treated after the first surgery. Third, the surgeon must avoid closing the pericardium under tension. It will produce a scenario similar to a cardiac tamponade. If that is the case, the sac must be left wide open. Fourth, the traumatic and surgical wounds must be inspected carefully to identify and ligate bleeding vessels and prevent a potentially lethal postoperative hemorrhage.

Around 25% of stable patients with a precordial penetrating wound have hemopericardium. The approach to this condition has evolved after recognizing that most of them have self-limited injuries not requiring surgical correction. The ultrasound performed during the initial evaluation guides further decisions (Fig. 33.1).

If the ultrasound is negative, the patient will be observed clinically with monitorization, for 24 h with ultrasonographic vigilance every 6 h (Fig. 33.1).

If the exam is positive for hemopericardium, the examiner must search for tamponade signs and measure the hemopericardium volume. Subjects with small volumes (<1 cm) without any tamponade sign will be followed and monitored as the negative patients (Fig. 33.1).

If any sign of tamponade is found or the hemopericardium is bigger than 1 cm, a pericardial window must be performed promptly. It can be executed by subxiphoid (Fig. 33.3) or by minimally invasive routes. During the procedure, the hemodynamic stability is monitored, the pericardial space is drained, and lavaged with 500 c.c. to 1 L of warm saline is performed. A sternotomy or thoracotomy is indicated if instability appears or active bleeding is documented (Fig. 33.1).

In observed patients, surgery is indicated if clinical deterioration or an increase in the size of the effusion occurs.

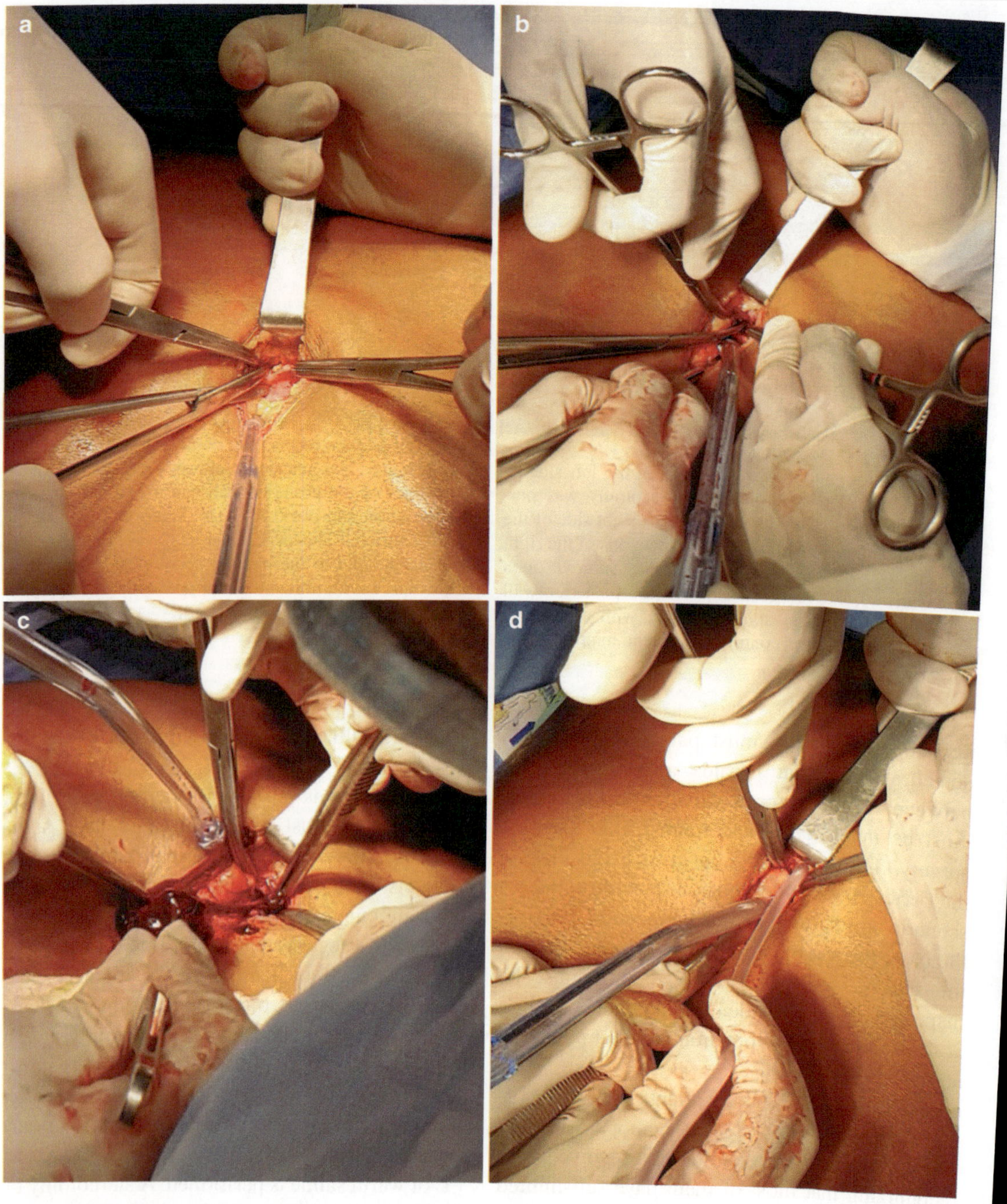

Fig. 33.3 Lavage of the pericardial sac after a positive subxiphoid pericardial window. (**a**) The surgeon made an eight cm subxiphoid incision that includes the skin, the subcutaneous fat and the fascia. The surgeon has located the pericardium behind the sternum and grasps it with two Rochester clamps. (**b**) A 1 cm incision is performed in the pericardium. The drainage of blood indicates that the window is positive. (**c**) The pericardial sac is thoroughly drained, including some clots. (**d**) After ensuring no ongoing bleeding, a 16 Fr Nelaton is used to lavage the sac

Prognosis

Information regarding prognostic factors in cardiac trauma in the elderly is limited.

Given the low proportion of penetrating injuries, specific information about this subset is not reported. Available information from adult cohorts identified variables associated with higher death probability such as gunshot wounds, multiple chambers compromise, and physiologic deterioration manifested as undetectable blood pressure, diminished Glasgow Coma Scale, need for airway in the emergency department, emergency room thoracotomy, or aortic cross-clamping.

Blunt trauma patients with cardiac injuries had longer hospital and ICU stay and worse mortality outcomes when compared with subjects without cardiac injuries.

Reports of traumatic cardiac arrest and blunt cardiac injury identified higher mortality with advanced age. However, survival was described even in octogenarians.

Blunt cardiac injury patients who experienced disruption of anatomic structures had a longer hospital stay and a higher risk of death than individuals with arrhythmias or conduction defects.

The severity of the thoracic trauma, the magnitude of the associated trauma, the extent of physiologic deterioration, and the need for massive transfusion were associated with mortality.

Functional status at discharge worsened as trauma severity and age increased. 53% of the patients between 65 and 79 years returned home at discharge compared to 29% of the octogenarians. Octogenarians most often required skilled nursing facilities (37% vs. 15%).

Summary

Cardiac trauma is uncommon among the geriatric population. Subjects with a cardiac injury have a higher probability of multiorgan failure, longer hospital stay, and a higher risk of death. Blunt mechanisms are the most frequent. Rhythm, frequency, conduction, and hemodynamic alterations, common in blunt cardiac injuries, must be distinguished from the cardiovascular alterations related to age and medications' effects. Specific diagnoses will indicate specific treatments. Rupture of a cardiac chamber will indicate an emergent surgical procedure.

Penetrating cardiac injuries are rare in the geriatric population. Specific protocols do not exist. The approach must follow protocols developed for younger patients.

Unstable patients must be operated on immediately. Stable individuals with penetrating precordial trauma will be selected with an ultrasound. If negative, or positive with <1 cm effusions can be safely observed. Symptomatic patients or subjects with larger effusions will be submitted to a pericardial window with drainage and lavage of the pericardial sac. A thoracotomy or sternotomy must be performed if instability or persistent bleeding occurs.

Survival is possible at advanced ages with good chances of recovery with a good functional status.

References

1. Barraco R, Rodriguez A, Ivatury R. Geriatric trauma and acute care surgery. Why this book and why now? A rational and systems impact for geriatric trauma and acute care surgery. Cham: Springer; 2018.
2. Clare D, Zink KL. Geriatric Trauma. Emerg Med Clin North Am. 2021;39(2):257–71.
3. Cheitlin MD. Cardiovascular physiology-changes with aging. Am J Geriatr Cardiol. 2003;12(1):9–13.
4. Da Costa JP, Laing J, Kong VY, Bruce JL, Laing GL, Clarke DL. A review of geriatric injuries at a major trauma Centre in South Africa. S Afr Med J. 2019;110(1):44–8.
5. Stroda A, Thelen S, M'Pembele R, Adelowo A, Jaekel C, Schiffner E, et al. Incidence and prognosis of myocardial injury in patients with severe trauma. Eur J Trauma Emerg Surg. 2021;48:3073–9.
6. Gao JM, Li H, Wei GB, Liu CP, Du DY, Kong LW, et al. Blunt cardiac injury: a single-center 15-year experience. Am Surg. 2020;86(4):354–61.
7. El-Andari R, O'Brien D, Bozso SJ, Nagendran J. Blunt cardiac trauma: a narrative review. Fortschr Med. 2021;5:28.
8. Tenzer ML. The spectrum of myocardial contusion: a review. J Trauma. 1985;25(7):620–7.
9. Brathwaite CE, Rodriguez A, Turney SZ, Dunham CM, Cowley R. Blunt traumatic cardiac rupture. A 5-year experience. Ann Surg. 1990;212(6):701–4.

10. Norii T, Matsushima K, Miskimins RJ, Crandall CS. Should we resuscitate elderly patients with blunt traumatic cardiac arrest? Analysis of National Trauma Registry Data in Japan. Emerg Med J. 2019;36(11):670–7.
11. Gonzalez-Hadad A, Ordonez CA, Parra MW, Caicedo Y, Padilla N, Millan M, et al. Damage control in penetrating cardiac trauma. Colomb Med (Cali). 2021;52(2):e4034519.
12. Gonzalez-Hadad A, Garcia AF, Serna JJ, Herrera MA, Morales M, Manzano-Nunez R. The role of ultrasound for detecting occult penetrating cardiac wounds in hemodynamically stable patients. World J Surg. 2020;44(5):1673–80.
13. Asensio JA, Ogun OA, Petrone P, Perez-Alonso A Wagner M, Bertellotti R, et al. Penetrating cardia injuries: predictive model for outcomes based o 2016 patients from the National Trauma Data Bank Eur J Trauma Emerg Surg. 2018;44(6):835–41.
14. Tyburski JG, Astra L, Wilson RF, Dente C, Steffe C. Factors affecting prognosis with penetratin wounds of the heart. J Trauma. 2000;48(4):587–90 discussion 90–1
15. Grossman M, Scaff DW, Miller D, Reed J 3rd, Hoey B, Anderson HL 3rd. Functional outcomes in octoge narian trauma. J Trauma. 2003;55(1):26–32.

Vascular Trauma and Vascular Emergencies in the Elderly

34

Julia R. Coleman and Ernest E. Moore

Introduction

As life expectancy increases and people over the age of 65 years account for a growing proportion of our population, the modern day surgeon must be equipped for handling the unique challenges of caring for injured geriatric patients. First, the consequence of injury is more pronounced in the aging population, with significantly higher rate of admissions and mortality after injury compared to trauma patients ages 15–40, even after controlling for degree of injury. Secondly, the physiology of the geriatric trauma patient is substantially different than their younger counterparts, with diminished physiologic reserve, greater cardiac fragility, more sensitive respiratory mechanics, and progressively impaired renal function, all of which must be contextualized within a greater burden of comorbidities.

Vascular trauma remains one of the most challenging tenants of care of critically injured patient. While many of the principles of vascular trauma care translate across age groups, there are special considerations for the geriatric trauma which will be elaborated in this chapter.

J. R. Coleman
University of Colorado-Denver, Denver, CO, USA
e-mail: Julia.coleman@cuanschutz.edu

E. E. Moore (✉)
University of Colorado-Denver, Denver, CO, USA

Ernest E Moore Shock Trauma Center, Denver, CO, USA
e-mail: ernest.moore@dhha.org

The Effect of Aging on Vascular Biology, Physiology, and Injury Outcomes

Before discussing approach to vascular trauma emergencies in geriatric patients, one must understand how aging affects the cardiovascular system and how this ultimately results in poorer outcomes after vascular injury. Cardiovascular dysfunction is prominent in the elderly, characterized by functional decline in myocardial and electrical conducting performance and progressive atherosclerotic disease. As a result, many elderly patients are prescribed medications, such as beta blockers, which affect cardiac performance. Furthermore, many elderly trauma patients have a higher baseline blood pressure and relative hypoperfusion may occur at seemingly "normal" blood pressures. Ultimately, these factors can skew perception of a trauma patient's physiology and lead to erroneous perception of normal hemodynamics. Failing to recognize hemorrhagic shock in elderly trauma patients is one of the leading causes of preventable death due to delayed resuscitation. Recognizing that the threshold for a diagnosis of shock should be different in geriatric patients, there is a growing adoption of age-adjusted shock index in geriatric

P. Petrone, C. E.M. Brathwaite (eds.), *Acute Care Surgery in Geriatric Patients*,
https://doi.org/10.1007/978-3-031-30651-8_34

trauma patient triage ([heart rate/systolic blood pressure] × age).

Beyond cardiac dysfunction, the systemic arterial system in geriatric patients is more likely to be diseased or chronically occluded, posing a greater vulnerability to injury, decreased tolerance to acute ischemia, and difficulty in assessing pulse quality on examination. Further, the degree of arterial disease can be a proxy for assessing injury risk; metrics of arterial stiffness (such as cardio-ankle vascular index) have been associated with higher risk of fall-related injuries. Progressive calcification and loss of elasticity in the vascular system not only changes the physiologic responses to trauma, injury, and hemorrhagic shock, but can complicate management. For example, one of the principal tenants of vascular trauma of proximal and distal control must be approached with a greater degree of caution in the setting of vascular calcific disease in geriatric patients, in which clamping across calcified vessels may lead to embolic complications. Ultimately, peripheral vascular disease in geriatric surgical patients independently predicts complications and mortality.

Outcomes after vascular injury and repair in geriatric patients, whether in a post-traumatic or elective setting, are also strongly influenced by frailty. Frailty, a multifactorial state of decreased physiologic reserve, is present in up to 50% of geriatric surgical patients and is associated with poor postoperative outcomes after vascular injury, including increased complications, readmission, disposition to facilities, and mortality. As a result of the unique physiology and anatomy of aging, trauma patients greater than 65 years old must be approached with a different strategy than their younger counterparts.

Initial Assessment of the Geriatric Trauma Patient

Regardless of location of vascular injury, the initial assessment of the trauma patient remains the same. Upon arrival to the trauma bay, traditional Advance Trauma and Life Support (ATLS) algorithmic care should be pursued, with particular attention to airway, vascular access, blood pressure restoration with whole blood resuscitation (when available), normothermia, and rapid assessment of a patient's physiologic and coagulation status. In patients who are hypotensive, we insert a 7 French catheter into the common femoral artery to both serve as a mechanism for monitoring arterial blood pressure, but also as potential access for Resuscitative Endovascular Balloon Occlusion of the Aorta (REBOA). In elderly patients, however, there may be a greater risk of vascular complication. Additionally, in patients with blunt mechanism and hypotension, there should be a low threshold for pursuing empiric pelvic compression.

Following blunt trauma, an Extended Focused Assessment for the Sonographic Evaluation of the Trauma Patient (E-FAST) should be expeditiously performed to rule out an associated cardiac injury with secondary tamponade or hemothorax. A "Big Two" (plain film of pelvis and chest) can assist in ruling out severe thoracic and pelvic pathology which may merit expeditious intervention. In penetrating trauma, a routine flat-plate X-ray of the involved body region to ascertain missile trajectory and location. In patients who are hemodynamically stable, a computed tomography (CT) scan with triple phase contrast is helpful in ascertaining sites of active extravasation which may merit interventional radiology consultation for embolization or a pelvic hematoma which may need placement of a zone III REBOA. In the case of extremity trauma, a dedicated pulse exam is mandatory; however, this may be compromised in geriatric patients who may have chronically occluded vessels and baseline examinations which are different from the younger trauma patient.

General Operative Approach to Vascular Trauma

If an operative intervention is indicated for vascular trauma, planning is paramount. For torso injuries, the entire trunk from the chin to the knees should be prepared and draped in the standard fashion. Before induction of general anesthesia, the surgeon should assure the necessary resuscitation resources (blood, autotransfusion apparatus) and emergency vascular supplies (emergency thoracotomy tray, aortic clamp, REBOA) are ready.

As in a trauma patient of any age, the same principles of damage control exist in the setting of major abdominal vascular trauma and significant hemodynamic compromise. A midline laparotomy incision should be made, all clots and blood removed, and any sites of active bleeding identified. This may merit packing or focused pressure with the operating surgeon's finger, laparotomy pad, sponge stick, or Alice clamps. If a vessel injury has been identified, the operating surgeon and assistant should perform expeditious dissection to isolate the proximal and distal vessel for control to accommodate a temporary shunt. In the setting of geriatric patients, the burden of calcific arterial disease is greater, posing a challenge when attempting to identify areas of undiseased vessel for clamping. When possible, clamping onto calcified vessel should be avoided to prevent embolic consequences, however if this is not possible, often digital pressure alone can be effective and mitigates embolic risk.

Abdominal Vascular Trauma

Major abdominal vascular trauma can be a life-threatening crisis which must be immediately addressed by a trauma surgeon. While penetrating trauma accounts for a higher percent of major abdominal vascular injury, blunt trauma, which is more common in the geriatric population, accounts for 10–15% of total traumatic cardiovascular injuries. Further, after motor vehicle collisions, geriatric patients are more likely to have severe pelvic injuries with concomitant vascular involvement, more likely to require massive transfusion due to their injuries, and are three times more commonly found to have blunt aortic injuries compared to patients less than 65 years old. While rare in younger trauma patients, rupture of a pre-existing aortic aneurysm or distal embolization from an aneurysm secondary to blunt abdominal trauma can be seen in geriatric patients.

Abdominal vascular hemorrhage sources include the viscera, mesentery, or blood vessels. Retroperitoneal hematomas are organized into three zones: zone 1 is the midline retroperitoneum (abdominal aorta, proximal renal arteries, superior mesenteric artery, infrahepatic IVC), zone 2 is the upper lateral retroperitoneum (renal artery and vein), and zone 3 is the pelvic retroperitoneum (iliac artery and vein). The zone of hematoma guides the approach, as outlined below.

Abdominal Aortic Injury

If a Zone 1 midline supramesocolic hematoma is encountered, proximal control is achieved via a left medial visceral rotation by reflecting all left-sided intra-abdominal viscera, including the colon, spleen, pancreatic tail, and gastric fundus to the midline, allowing for visualization of the abdominal aorta from hiatus to aortic bifurcation. This medial mobilization maneuver allows for clamping of the supraceliac aorta. Alternatively, to this approach, if active hemorrhage is identified, one may expeditiously divide the gastrohepatic ligament, retract the stomach to the left, and divide the right crural muscle to access the supraceliac aorta for clamping. Either of these maneuvers, depending on the exact location of the injury, also allows access for distal control. In contrast, the inframesocolic aorta can be exposed by retracting the transverse mesocolon cephalad, eviscerating the small bowel to the right, and then opening the midline retroperitoneum until the left renal vein. A proximal aortic clamp can then be placed inferior to the left renal vein, and the distal aortic clamp can be placed at the level of the bifurcation, sometimes requiring sacrifice of the inferior mesenteric artery. More recently, resuscitative aortic occlusion of the aorta (REBOA) has been employed to achieve proximal aorta control of aortic injuries and is particularly useful for supra-renal injuries.

In the setting of aortic injury with segment loss and profound shock, the use of intraluminal shunting or rapid insertion of an albumin-coated

Dacron, or polytetrafluoroethylene (PTFE) interposition graft is acceptable. However, if the anatomy and physiology allow, definitive aortic repair should be pursued with lateral aortorrhaphy with polypropylene suture, patch aortoplasty with bovine pericardium, or end-to-end anastomosis. This may be more challenging in a geriatric patient with tethered vessels and calcific disease. It is also worth noting that the young trauma patient has a smaller aortic caliber and therefore, the operating surgeon should be prepared for a larger potential tube graft for aortic repairs (16 mm in diameter or larger) in the elderly.

Inferior Vena Cava Injury

An inferior vena cava (IVC) injury should be suspected when significant hemorrhage or hematoma is observed in the right inframesocolic area or near the mesenteric root. Exposure of the infrahepatic IVC is best achieved through a right medial visceral rotation in which the right colon is released through incising the white line of Toldt and performing a Kocher maneuver to release the C-loop of the duodenum. This allows for visualization of the IVC from the iliac veins to the inferior edge of the liver. Temporary hemorrhage control should be achieved with digital pressure and sponge sticks, Satinsky clamps may be appropriate for anterior wounds of the vena cava, but cross-clamping should be avoided because of the risk of avulsing lumbar veins. It is important to prioritize inflow into the vena cava because outflow occlusion may increase bleeding. Difficulties in control of IVC bleeding at venous confluences may merit temporary ligation clamping of the common femoral veins via inguinal incisions. When physiology and anatomy allow, IVC injuries should be repaired transversely with polypropylene suture; however, in a damage control setting, the IVC may be ligated, which should prompt bilateral below-knee, four-compartment fasciotomies (and possibly thigh fasciotomies as well).

Mesenteric Vessel Injury

Injury to the celiac axis or its proximal branches is best exposed with the aforementioned medial visceral rotation, but often require a left eighth rib thoracoabdominal incision for adequate exposure. Celiac branch vessels injuries are more difficult to repair due to the dense neural and lymphatic tissues and small vessel caliber and can be treated with ligation although there is a risk of major hepatic necrosis following common hepatic artery ligation. In contrast, SMA injuries pose cannot be ligated, and exposure may be more difficult. If SMA injury is found beneath the pancreas, this may require pancreatic neck transection for best visualization. In the case of damage control surgery, an intraluminal shunt can be inserted into the debrided ends of the SMA, but if physiology and anatomy allow, primary repair or a saphenous vein on the distal infrarenal aorta should be pursued. Retroperitoneal tissue should be placed over the suture line to avoid future aortoenteric fistula. This may be more difficult in the geriatric patient, in which there may be less retroperitoneal fat or more thickened retroperitoneal tissue; in such a setting, an omental pad is preferred. Similar to the SMA, exposure and repair of the superior mesenteric vein (SMV) can be challenging. If the injury is near its junction with the splenic vein, the pancreatic neck may need to be transected, with medial to lateral mobilization of the pancreatic body. The SMV should be repaired via lateral venorrhaphy or end-to-end anastomosis with polypropylene suture, assuring to also control and/or ligate posterior collateral branches.

Porta Hepatis Injuries

Hematoma or hemorrhage in the right upper quadrant near the portal triad should raise concern for injury to the portal vein or hepatic artery. Before a hematoma or hemorrhage is explored, proximal control is achieved with a Pringle maneuver, encircling the hepatoduodenal ligament with vascular tape or a non-crushing vascular clamp. Distal control, located at the edge of the liver, may not be possible, given the short length of the porta, but manual compression will suffice. Given its diminutive size, primary repair of the hepatic artery is difficult, however left or right hepatic artery ligation is usually well tolerated due to significant collateralization; hepatic resection may be required if ischemic necrosis develops, and cholecystectomy should be pursued in the case of right hepatic artery ligation. In contrast to the hepatic artery, the portal vein is generally larger in size but can be difficult to fully expose and should be repaired. In the case of a posterior injury, medialization of the common bile duct and cystic duct with a full Kocherization of the duodenum may be necessary; further, a retropancreatic portal vein injury may require transection of the pancreatic neck. Options for portal vein repair include lateral venorrhaphy with polypropylene suture, resection with end-to-end anastomosis, interposition grafting, transposition of the splenic vein to the SMV, venovenous anastomosis from the SMV to the distal portal vein or end-to-side portacaval shunt. Portal-systemic shunts, however, can be associated with hepatic encephalopathy.

Renal Vasculature Injury

Zone 2 retroperitoneal hematomas do not always merit exploration, especially following blunt trauma. However, if expanding or penetrating mechanism, the hematoma should be explored. Exposure of the left renal artery and vein is achieved through the left medial visceral rotation, whereas the right renal artery and vein is exposed through the right medial visceral rotation and Kocher maneuver. In some cases, lateral arteriorrhaphy or resection with end-to-end anastomosis for arterial injuries or lateral venorrhaphy for venous injuries can be performed; however, salvage rates with attempted arterial revascularization and repair are low if there has been >4 h delay (ranging 25–30%). While nephrectomy may be required for destructive injuries the degree of postoperative renal failure is higher in the geriatric patient. More recently, renal artery stenting has been employed.

Pelvic Vasculature Injury

Zone 3 retroperitoneal hematomas do not always mandate exploration, however in the setting of an expanding hematoma and hemodynamic compromise, an injury to the iliac artery or vein should be suspected and exploration should be pursued. Proximal control of the iliac arteries can be achieved by eviscerating the small bowel to the right and dividing the midline retroperitoneum over the aortic bifurcation. In contrast to younger trauma patients, in geriatric patients, there is common adherence between the common iliac artery and vein at this location, which can make for difficult isolation of the artery. Distal vascular control can be achieved just proximal to the inguinal ligament where the external iliac artery exits the pelvis. When massive pelvic arterial hemorrhage in zone 3 is encountered, zone III REBOA should be placed. Alternatively if no REBOA is available, Fogarty balloon catheter for temporary control of internal iliac arteries, followed by into injection of a flurry of autologous clot, microfibrillar collagen, topic thrombin, and calcium chloride into the distal internal iliac artery. Ligation of the common and external iliac arteries should be avoided, with a concerted effort to repair these injuries through lateral arteriorrhaphy, resection and end-to-end anastomosis or saphenous vein or PTFE grafting, or transposition. In a damage control setting, temporary intraluminal shunt is the preferred choice with delayed reconstruction. In contrast, unilateral internal iliac artery ligation can be done with relative impunity.

In terms of pelvic venous injuries, exposure is the same as for arterial injuries, with the exception that temporary right common iliac artery transection may be required to access the right common iliac vein. In contrast to the arterial injuries, proximal and distal control can typically be achieved through digital pressure. Lateral venorrhaphy can be performed with polypropylene suture, but ligation can also be pursued for common or external iliac vein injuries. When massive pelvic venous hemorrhage is encountered, strategies include packing the missile tracks with vaginal packs, inserting fibrin glue, placing a Foley catheter, inserting sterile tacks directly into visible defects, or suturing omental patches into obvious areas of perforation. For persistent bleeding venovenous bypass may be required to access the bleeding sites.

While penetrating iliac arteries should be approached rapidly during a laparotomy, an initial strategy for pelvic hematoma due to venous bleeding or associated osseous injury is preperitoneal pelvic packing (PPP). This operative strategy for hemostasis can be done exclusively or concomitantly with a separate laparotomy incision, in which six laparotomy pads are inserted through a preperitoneal dissection around the pelvic space; when done in conjunction with external fixation, this strategy can often be definitive management.

Thoracic Vascular Trauma

The majority of thoracic great vessel injuries are due to penetrating trauma, and as such, are less frequently encountered in the geriatric patients. High mechanism blunt trauma has been associated with blunt thoracic aortic injury, most classically in a rapid deceleration event in which injury occurs at tethering points like the ligamentum arteriosum. Additionally, iatrogenic injury remains a relevant etiology of great vessel injury, related to percutaneous central venous catheter placement, trocar chest tubes, use of Swan-Ganz balloons, and esophageal self-expanding metal stents. Given the significant number of geriatric patients who are hospitalized and undergo aforementioned procedures, it is worth reviewing thoracic vascular trauma and its relevant exposures and repair.

Patients with thoracic great vessel injuries may present with signs of intrapericardial vascular injury including pericardial tamponade (Beck's triad of distended neck veins, pulsus paradoxus, and muffled heart sounds), hypotension, upper extremity hypertension, discordant extremity blood pressures or pulses, heart murmur, expanding thoracic outlet hematoma, unstable fractures of the sternum, or flail chest. While these signs of chest trauma are worth knowing, it is important to remember that only 50% of patients with thoracic vascular injury due to blunt trauma present with external physical signs of injury.

Patients who incur injury to the thoracic great vessels, in particular after penetrating mechanism, may present to the trauma center with signs of life followed by hemodynamic collapse. In such a setting, it is the authors' institutional practice to pursue an emergency department thoracotomy (EDT) if cardiopulmonary resuscitative (CPR) has been ongoing for <10 min after blunt trauma, <15 min after penetrating thoracic trauma, and <5 min after non-torso penetrating trauma. This allows not only for aortic cross-clamping, but quick identification and temporizing measures of great vessel injuries, such as apical packing for subclavian injuries or hilar clamping for pulmonary vessel injuries. In addition to physiologic collapse tube thoracostomy placement for hemothorax with immediate output of >1500 mL of blood should prompt thoracotomy.

Plain film radiography in the trauma bay may also have clues to great vessel injury include hemothorax, widened mediastinum, loss of aortic knob, depression of left mainstem bronchus, loss of perivertebral pleural stripe, deviation of nasogastric tube, or leftward tracheal deviation. A Spiral CT scan of the chest is ideal for screening for mediastinal hematoma and great vessel injury.

The likelihood of a geriatric patient, with diminished reserve and likelihood of underlying cardiovascular disease, surviving to the hospital and operating room with a great vessel injury is highly unlikely, and as such, discussion of repairs will be brief.

Ascending Thoracic Aortic Injury

While nonoperative may be an initial approach to temporize a patient, it also may be definitive management in patients with minor aortic lesions such as intimal tears or small pseudoaneurysms. Medical management of these patients consists of intensive hemodynamic monitoring, beta blockade, and selective nitroprusside. For patients with substantial descending thoracic aortic injuries, endovascular stenting is generally well tolerated.

For patients with hemodynamic instability and suspected thoracic great vessel injury of unknown location, left anterolateral thoracotomy should be performed first. Damage control principles for thoracic vascular trauma include partial or complete pneumonectomy for severe hilar vascular injuries, temporary ligation, shunting, and packing and temporary chest closure. For patients with known ascending aortic injury, a median sternotomy, and anterior ascending aortic injuries can often be repaired primarily; however, cardiopulmonary bypass may be required for posterior injuries. In the case of a transverse aortic arch injury, the median sternotomy may need to be extended to the neck for exposure of the arch and brachiocephalic branches.

Innominate Artery Injury

Median sternotomy is the ideal approach for uncontrolled bleeding from an innominate artery injury. A right cervical extension and division of the innominate vein may be required. Running lateral arteriorrhaphy should be attempted, however if this is precluded, repair may mandate bypass exclusion grafting with Dacron tube graft. Prosthetic grafts are the repair of choice, in particular in geriatric patients with enlarged, stiff vessels. After bypass is completed, the hematoma associated with the injury can be explored for more definitive repair. Endovascular treatment, however, is the preferred treatment for a contained injury.

Descending Thoracic Aortic Injury

The current management of blunt descending thoracic aortic rupture is endovascular stent placement. In the past, the standard treatment was operative repair with partial left heart bypass to avoid paraplegia.

Thoracic Vena Cava Injury

Injuries to the thoracic vena cava are uncommon, but when they do occur, they are often accompanied by other devastating injuries and may produce hemopericardium with cardiac tamponade. Exposure is classically difficult and typically requires total cardiopulmonary bypass with inferior cannula insertion in the inferior vena cava via the groin and intracaval balloon occlusion via right atriotomy. While superior vena cava injuries are repaired by lateral venorrhaphy, inferior vena cava is repaired via the right atrium.

Pulmonary Artery and Vein Injury

As with the other great vessel injuries, median sternotomy is the approach of choice, which provides ready visualization and access to the main and proximal left pulmonary artery. The intrapericardial right pulmonary artery can be exposed between the superior vena cava and ascending aorta. Anterior injuries can typically be repaired primarily, but posterior injuries may require cardiopulmonary bypass. More distal pulmonary artery injuries should be accessed through posterolateral thoracotomy, often necessitating tractotomy for exposure and partial or complete pneumonectomy. Access to pulmonary veins may be difficult via median sternotomy. To temporize massive bleeding, the hilar vessels can be controlled with a looped umbilical tape snared with a Rumel tourniquet or partial occlusion with a large-angled Satinsky clamp. If ligation is required, the corresponding lobe is resected.

Subclavian Artery Injury

For subclavian injuries located in the thoracic outlet or cavity, cervical extension of the median sternotomy is typically required for right-sided injuries and left anterolateral thoracotomy in third intercostal space for left-sided injuries (with a supraclavicular incision for distal control). This exposure may require resection of the medial clavicle for proximal control and division of the anterior scalene muscle; care should be taken to avoid injury to brachial plexus and phrenic nerve during exposure. Repair of an arterial or venous injury is accomplished through lateral arteriorrhaphy, or graft interposition.

Axillary Artery and Vein Injury

Exposure is obtained at the inferior edge of the center of the clavicle, running laterally in the groove between the deltoid and pectoralis major muscle. The pectoralis major muscle can be split or divided 2 cm from its humeral insertion, followed by division of the pectoralis muscle, to allow access to the underlying axillary vessels. Exposure and manipulation of the vessels should be done with caution to avoid injury to the intimately associated brachial plexus. The distal axillary artery warrants reconstruction due to the risk of arm ischemia.

Peripheral Vascular Trauma

The incidence of peripheral vascular trauma is low, representing less than 5% of civilian trauma and mainly occurs with penetrating mechanisms in young males. However, with increasing frequency of endovascular procedures, there is possibility of iatrogenic injuries in geriatric patients undergoing catheterization and angiography. Physical exam should be focused on a thorough pulse exam proximal and distal to an injury. In particular in the setting of penetrating injury or bone fracture, the arterial pressure index (also known as "A:A"), a measurement of the systolic blood pressure in the injured extremity divided by that in the uninjured extremity, can help to screen for injury, with a threshold of <0.9 prompting further radiologic evaluation. Further, attention should be directed to "hard" and "soft" signs of vascular injury, included but no limited to large, expanding, or pulsatile hematoma, absent pulses, palpable thrill or audible bruit, injury to adjacent nerves, and proximity of penetrating wounds to major vessels. If a patient is hemodynamically stable, CT angiography with run off to the extremities can be helpful in both diagnosis and operative approach, particularly in the elderly with likely pre-existing vascular disease.

While specific exposures will be discussed below, the principles of vascular repair are the same regardless of site. REBOA may be useful for inguinal junctional injuries. The immediate first step in extremity hemorrhage is pressure, applied digitally, with packing, or with a compressive device. While tourniquets may be used in the field with great success, these should be used selectively in the trauma bay management and may exacerbate venous bleeding. However deep injuries which cannot be controlled with pressure should have a tourniquet placed. Much like thoracic and abdominal vascular trauma, as in a trauma patient of any age, the same principles of damage control exist in the setting of extremity vascular trauma and hemorrhage shock. Wide prepping and draping of the involved and uninvolved extremities allow for wide exposure to injury and access to contralateral venous graft harvesting if required. Incisions should be made accounting for location of required proximal and distal control of anticipated site of injury, ensuring an "S" incision across flexor creases. Prioritization should proceed as follows: hemorrhage control, proximal control, distal control, arterial repair, and venous repair. Once the hemorrhage has been controlled, intraluminal thrombus burden should be removed (via Fogarty catheter) proximally followed by distally to maximize collateral blood flow and both limbs flushed with heparinized saline. This is followed by an intraluminal Pruitt-Inahara shunt insertion to preserve distal flow. The T on this shunt can be used for confirmation of flow, angiography, and tissue plasminogen activator (tPA) infusion. This temporizing measure allows for ongoing resuscitation, additional emergent procedures including craniotomy, thoracotomy or laparotomy, and stabilization of open fractures which may preclude definitive vascular repair. If shunts are not available, short segments of IV tubes. Robust inflow and backflow should be ensured, and proximal and distal control should be in place to allow for a blood-free working area during repair. 5-0 polypropylene suture should be used for subclavian, axillary, and femoral arteries in a circumferential fashion, whereas smaller caliber (6-0 and 7-0) polypropylene suture for veins. A parachute technique is particularly helpful for smaller or deeper vessels. Upon completion of repair, the arteriotomy or venotomy should be flushed, releasing the distal occlusion last. Systemic heparinization is not mandated for vascular injury repairs, though antiplatelet therapy has been associated with decreased thrombotic complications postoperatively. It is prudent to remain highly vigilant of need for fasciotomy following reperfusion injury as patient undergo continued resuscitation.

Upper Extremity Arterial Injuries

Any vascular injury of the upper extremity can be exposed along an incision from the superior edge of the sternal notch, running along the superior aspect of the clavicle, crossing mid-clavicle to the infraclavicular border, tracing the deltopectoral and bicipital groove, crossing the elbow obliquely, and running along the radial side of the volar forearm to the wrist crease. The length and location of the incision along this line should be dictated by the location of injury, ensuring approximately 6 cm proximal and distal to site of injury.

The brachial artery is the most commonly injured peripheral arterial injury. Exposure is obtained with an incision in the medial groove between the biceps and triceps muscle, which may be extended obliquely across the antecubital crease laterally and through a dense fibrous extension of the biceps tendon to expose the bifurcation and proximal radial and ulnar artery. This same exposure will allow for access to the brachial or basilic vein if needed as an autologous conduit during repair. Care should be taken to preserve the median nerve throughout the upper arm, as it courses intimately with the brachial artery.

For the radial artery, exposure is obtained with an incision along the radial side of the volar forearm, which can be extended proximally across the antecubital fossa. The flexor muscles can be retracted inferomedially to optimize exposure. Exposure of the ulnar artery is through a separate incision anterior to the medial epicondyle and running down the ulnar side of the volar forearm to the wrist. The flexor muscles can be retracted superolaterally to optimize exposure. Care should be taken to avoid injury to the ulnar nerve, which is intimately associated with the mid-ulnar artery. The ulnar and radial arteries can be respectively ligated with impunity as long as single vessel flow to the hand is documented.

Lower Extremity Arterial Injuries

The external iliac artery and vein can be approached via the aforementioned transabdominal approach, but a retroperitoneal approach above the inguinal ligament is a useful exposure for proximal control of the external iliac artery A "hockey stick" incision (or two separate incisions traversing inguinal ligament vertically and laterally along the iliac crest) allows for exposure to the iliac and femoral structures. It is worth noting that due to visceral adiposity and laxity of the skin which occurs with age, the groin crease should not be confused for the location of the inguinal ligament in geriatric patients; the pubic tubercle should serve as the landmark for both the inguinal incision and approximated location of the femoral artery. The hockey stick is followed by division of the external and internal oblique muscles and arrival into the retroperitoneal space, retracting the peritoneum medially to expose the psoas muscle and iliac vessels. Care should be taken to avoid injury to the ureters during this component of the dissection.

For femoral artery and vein, proximal exposure can be obtained through a longitudinal incision along the medial sartorius muscle, starting two fingerbreadths lateral to the pubic tubercle. This incision can be extended into the hockey stick incision as needed, which includes division of the inguinal ligament. In this case, injury to the inferior epigastric or circumflex iliac branches should be avoided. After the longitudinal or hockey stick incision, dissection then proceeds through the deep fascia and femoral sheath, opening widely for proximal and distal control. The profunda artery, which can be ligated with impunity, is located approximately 4–6 cm inferior to the inguinal ligament in the posterolateral location, most noticeably identified where the femoral artery caliber changes. Medial and lateral circumflex arteries subsequently branch off the profunda within 2–3 cm of its origin. Care should be taken when dissecting the profunda artery to avoid the "vein of woe," the lateral circumflex vein as it crosses the profunda origin. The entirety of the ensuing superficial femoral artery can be exposed by continuing dissection medially along the sartorius, retracting the muscle to expose the roof of the adductor canal. Care should be taken during this dissection to avoid injury to the femoral and saphenous nerves.

For the popliteal artery and vein, the medial approach is generally recommended, though we prefer a posterior approach with CTA confirmation of the injury site. For the medial approach, positioning includes flexing the knee 30° and rotating the leg laterally. Exposure to the popliteal artery and vein can be made through a single incision, traversing the knee, or two separate incisions for proximal and distal control. This includes incising between the vastus medialis and sartorius muscle, extending inferior 1 cm posterior to the posterior border of the tibia, completing the dissection toward the medial head of the gastrocnemius, and detaching the tibial attachments to the soleus muscle; the pes anserus (semitendinosus, semimembranosus, and sartorious) is divided into unroof the popliteal artery. This exposure allows for visualization of the entire neurovascular bundle. The vein will be encountered first and needs mobilization to fully visualize the artery. Care should be taken to avoid injury to the saphenous vein and the tibial nerve, located posteromedial to the popliteal artery. Once the popliteal artery is identified, this can be traced distally to the trifurcation by the soleal attachments. The first anterior branch is the tibial artery, which courses lateral and anterior to the interosseous membrane. The tibioperoneal trunk continues under the soleus muscle to branch into the peroneal (fibular) artery laterally and the posterior tibial artery medially. If the tibial artery is the area of suspected injury, it can also be accessed through a standard anterior fasciotomy incision. For injuries along this vascular bundle, the popliteal artery should be repaired, whereas the vein can be ligated, and similarly, the tibial artery can be ligated with impunity as long as single vessel flow to the foot is ensured. The posterior approach is via a curved incision across the popliteal space. The first vascular structure encountered is the lesser saphenous vein which leads to the subfascial popliteal vein. The tibial nerve is in proximity to the popliteal artery. The advantages of the posterior approach include a less extensive incision and shorter interposition graft.

Conclusion

Vascular injury management remains a critical skill for trauma surgeons. As the population of patients greater than 65 years old grows and represents an increasing proportion of the trauma patient population, surgeons must appreciate the distinct physiology and anatomy of aging as it pertains to the vascular system. While the tenants of vascular injury, such as proximal and distal control, remain the same for geriatric patients, there are unique considerations which must be included in the care of the elderly. While geriatric patients are less likely to survive to the hospital after vascular injuries, they are more likely to have ensuing complications and mortality if they do. As such, the trauma surgeon must be ready for expeditious recognition of vascular injuries, exposure and control, and a wide variety of damage control and definitive treatment options.

References

1. Morris JA, MacKenzie EJ, Damiano AM, et al. Mortality in trauma patients: the interaction between host factors and severity. J Trauma. 1990;30:1476.
2. Banning LBD, Moumni ME, Visser L, et al. Frailty leads to poor long-term survival in patients undergoing elective vascular surgery. J Vasc Surg. 2021;73(6):2132–9.

3. Eichinger M, Robb HDP, Scurr C, et al. Challenges in the PREHOSPITAL emergency management of geriatric trauma patients–a scoping review. Scand J Trauma Resusc Emerg Med. 2021;29:100.
4. Ho VP, Schiltz NK, Reimer AP, et al. High-risk comorbidity combinations in older patients undergoing emergency general surgery. J Am Geriatr Soc. 2019;67(3):503–10.
5. McRae PJ, Walker PJ, Peel M, et al. Frailty and geriatric syndromes in vascular surgical Ward patients. Ann Vasc Surg. 2016;35:9–18.
6. Turuscheva A, Frolova E, Kotovskaya Y, et al. Association between arterial stiffness, frailty, and fall-related injuries in older adults. Vasc Health Risk Manag. 2020;16:307–16.
7. Visser L, Banning BD, El Moumni M, et al. The effect of frailty on outcome after vascular surgery. Eur J Vasc Endovasc Surg. 2019;58(5):762–9.
8. Feliciano DV, Moore EE, Mattox KL. Trauma. 9th ed. New York: McGraw-Hill; 2021.
9. American College of Surgeons Committee on Trauma. Advanced surgical skills for exposure in trauma. Chicago: American College of Surgeons; 2010.

Injury Due to Extremes of Temperature

35

Patrizio Petrone

Introduction

Hypothermia occurs when the human body cannot generate more endogenic heat than is lost to the surrounding environment. This is caused by external environmental conditions or medically-induced internal thermal regulation difficulties acting singly or in concert. Human beings are homeotherms, functioning within a narrow range of body temperature between 36.4 °C and 37.5 °C. Core temperatures outside this range are poorly tolerated. This optimal temperature is maintained by physiological mechanisms that involve retention or loss of heat; failure of thermoregulation is associated with pathophysiological consequences.

Primary accidental hypothermia is defined as a core temperature equal to or less than 35 °C or 95 °F. The causes of hypothermia are multifactorial and include excessive exposure to snow, wind, water, or altitude.

There are a number of risk factors that increase an individual's risk to hypothermia: old age, male gender, and minority ethnic status. The level of risk can be reduced by behavioral changes, including wearing clothing appropriate to the outside conditions.

P. Petrone (✉)
Department of Surgery, NYU Long Island School of Medicine, NYU Langone Hospital—Long Island, Mineola, New York, USA
e-mail: patrizio.petrone@nyulangone.org

Cold exposure hypothermia is a winter season contributor to morbidity and mortality in the northern hemisphere's middle-high latitudes, with most morbidity and mortality research coming from the United States and Scandinavia. Hypothermia has also been reported in tropical and sub-tropical environments during local cool seasons. Cold exposure hypothermia deaths and hospitalizations have been previously demonstrated to have some association with reported ambient weather conditions. Patients affected with hypothermia are not infrequently seen in every emergency department, regardless of the location or season of the year. In the United States, there are more than 650 deaths per year due to accidental hypothermia. However, the true number of deaths due to hypothermia remains unknown because a large number of patients who die are never seen in the emergency department. When compared to other atmospheric hazard events, this exceeds the observed fatality range for tornadoes, hurricanes, lightning, and floods, and itself is only exceeded by heat-related mortality.

The rate of hypothermia-related death in the United States has fallen during the last 20 years, but it is unclear whether this is because of changes in reporting, the implementation of improved preventive measures, or weather patterns.

Hypothermia can happen in any environment, and its effects on patients are dependent on the presence of existing comorbidities. Interestingly,

P. Petrone, C. E.M. Brathwaite (eds.), *Acute Care Surgery in Geriatric Patients*,
https://doi.org/10.1007/978-3-031-30651-8_35

the states with the highest incidence of hypothermia-related deaths are those with milder weather and sudden temperature changes and western states with high elevations and significant diurnal temperature excursions.

Factors contributing to the risk of accidental exposure to hypothermia include impaired behavioral responses to cold exposure from compromised cognition, such as dementia, drug induced (alcohol and sedatives), encephalopathies, and metabolic disorders. Other predisposing factors include lack of adequate clothing, homelessness, poverty, exposure in the wilderness, and immobility, as seen in patients with neuromuscular failure (e.g., stroke, hip fracture, and spinal cord injury).

Maintenance of a normal core temperature is achieved from a balance between heat production and heat loss. The most important mechanisms of heat loss include radiation, evaporation, and conduction, with convection accounting for minimal heat loss. Radiation is the transfer of radiant energy, and it contributes to 55% of heat loss. This is the route of heat loss in fully exposed patients. Evaporation is the conversion of a liquid into vapor and usually accounts for 30% of total body heat loss, 25% of which occurs from the skin surface, and the other 5% from the lungs. Conduction is the transfer of heat between two masses and accounts for 15% of the total heat loss. Water can increase the conductive losses by 25-fold being one of the fastest ways to lose body heat. Convection is defined as the transfer of heat due to the flow of liquids or gases over a surface. Heat loss by convection is minimal, but it can be increased up to fivefold in windy conditions, as it can occur during transport of the patient in helicopter.

Based on the etiology, the differential diagnosis for patients with hypothermia can be divided as follows: (1) increased heat loss (cold exposure, iatrogenic [cold fluid infusions], toxins, dermatologic [dermatopathies and burns]); (2) decreased heat production (extremes of age, hypoglycemia, malnutrition, hypopituitarism, hypothyroidism, fatigue/trauma); (3) impaired thermoregulation (peripheral vascular failure, neuropathies or spinal injury, diabetes, central nervous system trauma, and cerebrovascular accidents).

Alternatively, hypothermia can be classified from a functional stand point as: (1) controlled hypothermia (the active cooling of patients, which has been shown to improve neurological outcomes after cardiac arrest); (2) endogenous hypothermia (intrinsic dysfunction in thermoregulation, metabolic disorders, or increased heat losses); (3) accidental hypothermia (a primarily extrinsic problem, with no secondary pathologies). Taking into consideration the grade of severity, accidental hypothermia can further be classified as mild hypothermia with core temperatures ranging between 32 °C and 35 °C (90 °F–95 °F), moderate hypothermia between 28 °C and 32 °C (82 °F–90 °F), and severe hypothermia temperature less than 28 °C (82 °F).

Patients with primary hypothermia who are healthy usually survive, with aggressive rewarming techniques indicated in selected patients. In cases of mild hypothermia, noninvasive external rewarming is sufficient to restore the desired temperature. In cases of moderate hypothermia, more aggressive external rewarming is indicated. Finally, in cases of severe hypothermia invasive rewarming techniques are indicated, including cardiopulmonary bypass or arteriovenous rewarming. Elderly or malnourished patients are less likely to be able to rewarm spontaneously, and therefore they are candidates for more aggressive rewarming methods.

Hypothermia has profound systemic effects. The initial effect of hypothermia involves a sympathetic response that causes vasoconstriction, tachycardia, and increased myocardial oxygen consumption. In mild hypothermia, patients have vigorous shivering and cold white skin. Patients with moderate hypothermia may have mental status changes, such as amnesia, confusion, and apathy, in addition to reduced shivering, slurred speech, hyporeflexia, and loss of fine motor skills. Most severely hypothermic patients have no shivering and present with cold edematous skin, hallucinations, areflexia, oliguria, fixed dilated pupils, bradycardia, hypotension, and pulmonary edema.

The management strategies of hypothermia are either passive or active. The passive techniques include drying the patient, warming the environment, using blanket or clothing insulation and head cover, and the patient's shivering itself; in contrast, the active techniques include external (heating pad, warm water blankets and bottles, etc.), internal (heated intravenous solutions, cavities lavage, etc.), and extracorporeal rewarming (hemodialysis, continuous arteriovenous rewarming, and cardiopulmonary bypass).

Localized hypothermia can be classified into freezing injuries, known as frostnip or frostbite, and nonfreezing tissue injury, such as trench or cold immersion foot. Frostbite is defined as freezing of tissues due to crystal formation in the extracellular space, causing osmotic pressure and severe cellular dehydration with destruction of the membranes.

The nose, ears, hands, and feet are the areas most richly invested with arteriovenous anastomoses; therefore, they are the most sensitive and predisposed areas to frostbite, mainly due to rapidity of the circulation. Factors that can influence this condition include tight garments, nicotine, and Raynaud phenomena. Classification of frostbite should be done after demarcation occurs, which usually happens 3–4 weeks after the injury.

Accidental Hypothermia

Demographic and Risk Factors

Demographics of hypothermia reveal that adults between the ages of 30 and 49 years are most commonly affected, with men being at risk 10 times more often than women are. However, the true incidence of hypothermia in the elderly living in urban areas is probably underreported. Approximately 50% of all deaths in the United States attributed to hypothermia occur in individuals who are 65 years and older. The elderly have been shown to be at considerable risk for developing hypothermia. Thacker et al. found that the age group of 75 years and greater had crude death rates of approximately 0.7 per 100,000, with the rate increasing to 1.52 per 100,000 for ages greater than 85. Furthermore, prior research in Ireland has indicated that the elderly (defined as 65 years of age or greater) have a higher case fatality rate for hypothermia when compared to other age groups or other causes of death.

One of the largest contributors to the high level of elderly hypothermia vulnerability is the decreased efficiency of the thermo-regulation system as humans age. Additionally, actual temperature sensation of the cold is diminished in elderly persons, meaning conditions are not perceived to be as cold. Many elderly have a smaller body mass index than middle-aged adults. Smaller bodies lose radiative heat more quickly than larger bodies, and many elderly have less subcutaneous fat providing insulation against the cold because of malnutrition. Age-related mental decline also contributes to their vulnerability.

There are several other factors that confound elderly hypothermia vulnerability. The elderly often live in social isolation, which has been shown to increase vulnerability to natural hazard events, as in, for example, the 1995 Chicago Heat Wave. This isolation combined with inefficiencies of the thermo-regulation system can produce a situation in which hypothermia risk is greatly increased, even when indoors. Indoor hypothermia has been noted in several studies and the associated outcome is suggested to be worse for vulnerable groups such as the elderly. Eighty-one cases of hypothermia were identified during the period 1981–1998 in a hospital located in Paris, France. Twenty-nine of the 81 afflicted individuals perished, with a high percentage of the decedents found indoors. It is thought that indoor hypothermia victims can fare worse than outdoor victims for the following reasons: they are not likely to be found as quickly, there is exposure to moderately cold temperatures for a longer period of time, the victims are more likely to be lightly clothed, and many of these indoor victims are found lying on the ground, which can promote cooling. Evidence also suggests if elderly hypothermia victims are in a comatose state at the time of hospital admission survival is less likely.

The elderly appear to have distinct perceptions of natural hazard events that confounds their vulnerability. While there are almost no studies examining the elderly response to cold temperatures, studies examining elderly perception of heat indicate a general "known everything" attitude. Oftentimes they underestimated the danger, thought that dangerous situations were not as hazardous as they seem, or they simply did not self-identify as elderly, so took fewer precautions.

Based on a study performed by Petrone et al. they conclude that for hypothermic ED patients increased severity of illness was associated with older age and found indoors but not associated with initial rectal temperature, gender, alcohol or trauma.

Management

The management strategies of hypothermia are either passive or active (Table 35.1). Passive rewarming is recommended in a mildly hypothermic patient with a core temperature greater than 32 °C. Passive rewarming modality reduces convective, conductive, and radiant heat loss. It is initiated by removing wet clothing, insulating the patient, and protecting him or her from the environment. The patient should be in an ambient temperature of at least 21 °C.

Table 35.1 Rewarming techniques for hypothermia

Passive
Dry patient
Warm environment
Shivering
Blanket or clothing insulation
Head cover
Active
External
Heating pad, warm water blankets, and warm water bottles
Immersion in warm bath
External convection heaters (i.e., lamps and radiant warmers)
Internal
Heated intravenous solutions
Gastric or colonic lavage
Peritoneal lavage
Mediastinal lavage
Warmed inhalational agents
Extracorporeal rewarming
Hemodialysis
Continuous arteriovenous rewarming (CAVR)
Continuous venovenous rewarming (CVVR)
Cardiopulmonary bypass

Warmed and humidified air is indicated to reduce heat loss from respiration. Insulation is accomplished with the use of blankets and foil insulators covering the body, including the head.

If the thermoregulatory mechanisms and normal endocrine function are intact, and if shivering is also present, this method increases the core temperature by 0.5–2 °C/h. If not, active rewarming methods are indicated.

In patients with mild hypothermia not responding to passive rewarming or patients with moderate hypothermia, active external rewarming is indicated. It involves applying heat directly to the skin with consequent core rewarming from the warmed blood in the setting of normal circulation. The use of low-dose vasodilators such as nitroglycerin facilitates convective rewarming with a Bear Hugger (3M (®) Bair Hugger (® TM) Therapy, St. Paul, Minnesota, USA) by facilitating heat transfer; this modality can expedite convective rewarming by 0.8 °C–1 °C/h.

The American Society of Anesthesiologists recommends the use of forced air rewarming devices to treat hypothermia in postoperative patients during recovery, and these devices warm the patient by 1–2.5 °C/h. Warm water blankets, warm water bottles, heating pads, and warm water immersion are other methods of active external rewarming.

Active Internal Rewarming

Warm Intravenous Fluid Rewarming Technique

Although warm intravenous fluids are important, they are not an effective means of treating hypothermia because of the small difference in temperature and large difference in mass between the body and the infused fluid. Consequently, 1 L of crystalloid solution warmed to 40 °C infused into a patient with a

32 °C temperature would be equivalent to transfusing 8 kilocalories (kcal) into the patient, which will only increase the body temperature by 0.14 °C. Despite this limitation, warm intravenous fluids can be particularly useful in the treatment of hypothermic patients with large fluid resuscitation requirements. This can be achieved using a fluid warmer or alternatively, a regular microwave oven. One liter of crystalloid at room temperature can be heated in a microwave to 40 °C in 2.5 min. Of special note, dextrose-containing solutions cannot be heated in the microwave because glucose caramelizes at 60 °C. Moreover, safety restrictions prevent microwaving solutions stored in glass because of potential shattering of the container. The American Association of Blood Banks recommends that blood not be heated above 42 °C. Microwaved blood warming should not be performed, as this results in morphologic changes in the red blood cells and subsequent hemolysis.

Body Cavity Lavage Rewarming Techniques

Body cavity lavage is a process in which warm fluid is circulated in the thoracic or abdominal cavities to facilitate direct core warming. Pleural irrigation results in cardiac rewarming and may be the method of choice if an arrhythmia is present. The pleural cavity can be instilled with large volumes (10–120 L/h) of 40–45 °C fluid through a thoracostomy tube placed in the second or third anterior intercostal space in the midclavicular line, and then drained via a second tube in the fourth, fifth, or sixth intercostal space in the posterior axillary line. Alternatively, peritoneal lavage has a dual effect: it can be used to diagnose occult abdominal trauma in hypothermic patients and can rewarm the peritoneal cavity, through a placement of 2 or more catheters, with direct irrigation of the liver, which is believed to restore its synthetic and metabolic properties, and can facilitate the clearance of toxins and lactic acid. The stomach, colon, and bladder are poor sites for body cavity lavage because of the small surface area for heat exchange.

Extracorporeal Rewarming Techniques

Hemodialysis is the most readily available extracorporeal rewarming technique. It can raise the core temperature 2–3 °C/h, but it requires adequate blood pressure. Alternatively, many emergency centers now have available commercial fluid warmers to heat-infused crystalloids and blood. The rate of rewarming that can be achieved with most commercially available warming devices is significantly lower when compared with cardiopulmonary bypass (3 °C–4 °C/h). Continuous arteriovenous rewarming (CAVR) with mechanical devices is much faster than the rate of rewarming that can be achieved with peritoneal, gastric, pleural, or bladder irrigation or active airway rewarming. This technique uses a simple modification of the level 1 warmer system [Level 1 (R) Fast Flow Fluid Warmer system, Smiths Medical, Rockland, Massachusetts, USA] by moving the vertical arm to a horizontal orientation, thereby repositioning the heat exchange element. It is relatively simple and uses the patient's blood pressure to send the blood through a small counter current heat exchange device. CAVR uses femoral arterial and venous lines placed percutaneously or by cutdown to create an arteriovenous fistula that runs continuously through the external warming system pumped by the patient's blood pressure. A canine model evaluation of the system demonstrated that CAVR was capable of exceeding the rewarming rate of other external rewarming systems by 1.5–2.5 times.

Although not as efficient as cardiopulmonary bypass for rewarming, the greatest advantage of CAVR is that it does not require heparinization as heart bypass does. Continuous venovenous rewarming is technically easier to set up and also less invasive, CARV is more rapid in rewarming patients, but both methods are superior to less invasive techniques. Cardiopulmonary bypass is the most effective method of rewarming, but it is not uniformly available in hospitals without an open-heart surgery program. It raises the core body temperature by 7–10 °C/h, supports the circulation, and avoids cardiac trauma when performing CPR.

Table 35.2 Potential complications from rewarming the severely hypothermic patient

Core temperature afterdrop
Rewarming-related hypotension
Hypoglycemia
Bladder atony, paralytic ileus
Bleeding diathesis
Rhabdomyolysis
Changes in electrolytes
Ventricular fibrillation
Hyperkalemia and hypophosphatemia

Patients who have sustained asphyxia before hypothermia (e.g., submersion in water or avalanches) have a poorer prognosis because of hyperkalemia, whereas patients with non-asphyxiation hypothermia have better prognosis. The Alaska guidelines state that an adult patient should not be resuscitated if they have been submerged for more than 1 h. In children, resuscitation should be continued until they are rewarmed, even in submersion injuries.

The decision to defer rewarming must be made taking into consideration that the lowest initial temperature recorded in an adult was 13.7 °C, whereas in a child, it was 14.2 °C, with recovery after 45 min of submersion in 41 °C water.

Besides the rewarming method chosen, the patient should be monitored during and after rewarming, paying special attention to the potential complications of rewarming the severely hypothermic patient (Table 35.2).

Cold Injury

For many years, cold injury was almost exclusively reported in military personnel. Baron Larrey, surgeon-in-chief of the Napoleon's army, was the first to describe the pathophysiology of frostbite and introduced the concept of friction massage with ice or snow. He was also the first to describe the similarities between hypothermia and burns while recognizing the beneficial effects of rewarming. The effects of cold on ground troops became evident during the wars of the twentieth century. Cold injuries were caused by prolonged immersion in cold water (1.6–4.4 °C), during World Wars I and II. During the Korean War, "tropical immersion foot" was noted in soldiers exposed to constant wetness at comparatively warm water temperatures. More recently, during the Malvinas (Falklands) Islands conflict in 1982, both Argentinean and British troops reported injuries after exposure to both freezing and nonfreezing water temperatures.

Currently, cold injury is more prevalent in the civilian population. Ambient temperature and length of exposure are the most important factors in determining the extent of heat loss.

The presence of both wind chill and wet clothing is a major contributing factor to heat loss and the development of cold injury. Other risk factors include alcohol consumption, because of its impairment of judgment and vasodilatatory effects, and smoking, because of its vasoconstrictive effect. Chronic medical conditions such as atherosclerosis and diabetes mellitus that result in peripheral vascular disease and neuropathy are also important predisposing medical conditions. Psychiatric illness and homelessness by virtue of inappropriate behavior or inadequate shelter or clothing are also considered risk factors. Recreational and extreme winter sports such as high-altitude climbing, hiking, and skiing can all lead to hypothermia partly because of fatigue, inappropriate clothing or equipment, or unexpected changes in weather conditions. The extremities are the most frequently affected, with 90% of hypothermic injuries affecting either the hands or feet. Other common sites include ears, nose, cheeks, and male genitalia. The freezing of the corneas has been reported.

Classification and Clinical Manifestations of Frostbite

Most frostbite injuries appear similar during initial evaluation. For this reason, the classification of frostbite is applied only after rewarming. Frostbite has been categorized into four degrees of severity (Table 35.3). On physical examination, the sensitivity of the affected part should be tested. The

Table 35.3 Classification of frostbite

Superficial frostbite
First degree
Partial skin freezing
Erythema, edema, and hyperemia
No blisters or necrosis
Occasional skin desquamation (5–10 days later)
Second degree
Full-thickness skin freezing
Erythema and substantial edema
Vesicles, desquamation, and black eschar (gangrene) formed
Deep frostbite
Third degree
Full-thickness skin and subcutaneous freezing
Violaceous or hemorrhagic blisters
Skin necrosis
Blue-gray discoloration
Fourth degree
Full-thickness skin, subcutaneous tissue, muscle, tendon, and bone freezing
Little edema
Initially mottled and deep red or cyanotic
Eventually dry, black, and mummified

ability to sense light touch and noxious stimuli helps to determine the prognosis. Favorable prognostic indicators suggesting superficial injury are normal skin color, development of clear fluid in the blisters, and the ability of the skin to deform under pressure. Dark color, hemorrhagic blisters, cyanosis, and hard nondeforming skin suggest deep injury. There is often a discrepancy between the limit of the skin lesions and the extent of damage to deeper structures. Several radiological techniques have been used in an attempt to provide an accurate early assessment of tissue viability. These include plain film radiographs, venous radioisotope scanning (^{131}I, ^{133}Xe, and ^{99}Tc), angiography, and digital plethysmography for the assessment of tissue perfusion. Magnetic resonance imaging and magnetic resonance angiography appear to be superior techniques because they can directly visualize the occluded blood vessels and provide definite delineation of ischemic soft tissue. These findings may allow earlier surgical intervention. However, currently, no technique is sufficiently accurate to guide excision of tissue during early stages, and therefore, definitive treatment should be delayed for at least 3–4 weeks.

Surgical and Nonsurgical Management of Frostbite

There are 3 phases of frostbite treatment: (1) prethaw field care phase or prehospital treatment, (2) immediate hospital (rewarming) phase, and (3) post-thaw care phase, which continues for several weeks or months. The pre-thaw field care phase takes place before reaching a health care center and consists of primarily protecting the injured part from mechanical trauma, avoiding thawing until definitive rewarming can be performed. The extremity should be padded for protection, and elevate the affected part(s) with splinting as indicated; however, no other treatment should be initiated. The affected part should also not be rubbed or placed near a heat source. If possible, the frostbite patient should be admitted to a specialist unit.

Immediate hospital care is directed at reducing the progressive dermal ischemia. Rewarming should be done at 40–42 °C for 15–30 min or until thawing is complete. Thermal injuries occur when rewarming is performed outside a narrow temperature range, such that rewarming at too low temperature reduces tissue survival and rewarming at high temperatures produces increased thermal damage. A red or purple appearance of the involved part indicates the end of vasoconstriction and immersion rewarming can then be discontinued. The therapeutic approach is based on the knowledge of the pathophysiology of the frostbite. White blisters are debrided to reduce the wound's contact with the high levels of prostaglandin F2α and thromboxane A_2 in the blister fluid. Hemorrhagic blisters are best left intact to prevent desiccation by exposure if debrided. In both cases, topical aloe vera is used every 6 h as an inhibitor of thromboxane, which also reduces tissue necrosis. An alternate dressing utilizing Silvadene ointment to open wounds is equally acceptable.

A history of tetanus immunization should be obtained to determine the need for further immunization. In terms of analgesia utilize opioid, intramuscularly or intravenously as indicated.

Ibuprofen administered at 400 mg every 12 h, and benzyl penicillin 600 mg every 6 h for 48–72 h can be considered. Daily hydrotherapy for 30–45 min at 40 °C and wound care allow debridement of the wounds and encourage active and passive range of motion in an effort to preserve function. For documentation and legal purposes, photographic records on admission, at 24 h and serially every 2–3 days until discharge must be obtained. Smoking and drinking alcoholic beverages are prohibited during recovery as both can interfere with blood circulation.

Early surgical care consists of limited debridement of blisters and necrotic tissue. Fasciotomy is necessary if compartment syndrome develops. Amputation and more aggressive debridement are delayed until the progressive ischemia is complete and final demarcation is achieved, which might happen starting after the third week, but usually after 1 month and up to 3 months.

Other therapeutic modalities have been investigated. These include infusion of low molecular-weight dextran to reduce blood viscosity, anticoagulation with heparin to reduce thrombosis of the superficial dermal plexus, thrombolysis with streptokinase, hyperbaric oxygen, intra-arterial injection of vasodilator such as reserpine and, finally, sympathectomy. None of these modalities has been reported to improve tissue viability over that seen with rapid rewarming alone. However, they have shown some promise in animal models and further clinical studies are ongoing.

Morbidity and Mortality

If the physiological problems that occur during the rewarming in the cases of systemic hypothermia are corrected, there is a relative balance between oxygen supply and demand allowing for local tissue survival. The underlying cause of hypothermia, the reversibility of the process, and the presence of comorbid conditions are consistent predictors of outcome. Serum potassium level greater than 10 mEq/L is a marker of extensive cell death and was associated with 100% mortality avalanches and climbing accidents. All reversible causes of hyperkalemia (e.g., renal failure, drug toxicities, rhabdomyolysis, and adrenal insufficiency) should be excluded before attributing the elevated potassium levels to irreversible cell death. Other markers of poor outcome include advanced age, acidosis on admission, renal insufficiency, ammonia level greater than 250 mmol/L, fibrinogen levels less than 50 mg/dL, coagulopathy, cardiac arrest, need for mechanical ventilation, Glasgow Coma Scale score equal to or less than 5, vasopressor requirement, absence of outdoor exposure, and greater duration of exposure.

In clinically ambiguous situation and in the absence of clear signs of irreversible injury, there is a consensus to follow the American Heart Association recommendations to rewarm patients to at least 35 °C before declaring futility of life-sustaining measures and deciding about withdrawing support.

The overall mortality rate depends on the associated comorbidities. In the largest multicenter study consisting of 428 patients with a mean core temperature of 30.61 °C, a 17% mortality rate was reported, with most deaths occurring because of underlying diseases rather than the hypothermia itself.

For patients who sustain frostbite, late sequelae include cold insensitivity, sensory loss, and hyperhidrosis. Less commonly, osteoarthritis, chronic pain, and heterotopic calcification have been reported as long-term sequelae of frostbite.

Conclusion

Increased participation in outdoor activities and the epidemic of homelessness have caused the incidence of cold injuries in the civilian population to rise dramatically over the last 20 years.

Knowledge of the treatment is crucial for emergency room physicians in both rural and urban areas. Recent developments have significantly advanced the understanding of the pathophysiology of hypothermic and frostbite injuries. Together with improved rewarming techniques and utilization of radiological assessment of tissue viability, future advancements should allow a more aggressive and active approach to the management of these injuries.

References

1. Silfvast T, Pettilä V. Outcome from severe accidental hypothermia in Southern Finland—a 10-year review. Resuscitation. 2003;59:285–90.
2. Walpoth BH, Walpoth-Aslan BN, Mattle HP, Radanov BP, Schroth G, Schaeffler L, Fischer AP, von Segesser L, Althaus U. Outcome of survivors of accidental deep hypothermia and circulatory arrest treated with extracorporeal blood warming. N Engl J Med. 1997;337(21):1500–5.
3. Van der Ploeg GJ, Goslings JC, Walpoth BH, Bierens JJLM. Accidental hypothermia: rewarming treatments, complications and outcomes from one university medical centre. Resuscitation. 2010;81:1550–5.
4. Brown DJA, Bruuger H, Boyd J, Paal P. Accidental hypothermia. N Engl J Med. 2013;367:1930–8.
5. Kempainen RR, Brunette DD. The evaluation and management of accidental hypothermia. Respir Care. 2004;49(2):192–205.
6. Petrone P, Asensio JA, Marini CP. Management of accidental hypothermia and cold injury. Curr Probl Surg. 2014;51(10):417–31.
7. Petrone P, Kuncir EJ, Asensio JA. Surgical management and strategies in the treatment of hypothermia and cold injury. Emerg Med Clin N Am. 2003;21(4):1165–78.
8. Baumgartner EA, Belson M, Rubin C, Patel M. Hypothermia and other cold-related morbidity emergency department visits: United States, 1995–2004. Wilderness Environ Med. 2008;19:233–7.
9. Danzl DF. Hypothermia. Semin Respir Crit Care Med. 2002;23(1):57–68.
10. Roeggla M, Holzer M, Roeggla G, Frossard M, Wagner A, Laggner A. Prognosis of accidental hypothermia in an urban setting. J Intensive Care Med. 2001;16(3):142–9.
11. Lim C, Duflou J. Hypothermia fatalities in a temperate climate: Sydney, Australia. Pathology. 2008;40:46–51.
12. Danzl DF, Pozos RS, Auerbach PS, Glazer S, Goetz W, Johnson E, Jui J, Lilja P, Marx JA, Miller J, et al. Multicenter hypothermia survey. Ann Emerg Med. 1987;16(9):1042–55.
13. Megarbane B, Axler O, Chary I, Pompier R, Brivet F. Hypothermia with indoor occurrence is associated with worse outcome. Intensive Care Med. 2000;26:1843–9.
14. Dharmarajan T, Wijidada D. Hypothermia in the geriatric population. Aging Health. 2007;3(6):735–41.
15. Petrone P, Marini CP, Miller I, Brathwaite CEM, Howell RS, Cochrane D, Rodríguez-Velandia W, Rahn C, Allegra JR. Factors associated with severity of accidental hypothermia: a cohort retrospective multi-institutional study. Ann Med Surg (Lond). 2020;55:81–8. https://doi.org/10.1016/j.amsu.2020.04.018.

Plastic Surgery and Soft-Tissue Injury Trauma

36

Hilliard T. Brydges, Bachar F. Chaya, and Pierre B. Saadeh

Introduction

Soft-tissue trauma in the geriatric population is both common and uniquely challenging. Judicious management of soft-tissue injuries in an acute setting is paramount in this population, as age is a significant risk factor for many associated complications, including the development of chronic wounds and rapid deconditioning followed by often-irreparable functional and psychosocial decline. Often, timely reconstitution of damaged tissue can serve as the only bulwark against these many negative externalities. However, despite best clinical efforts, unique physiologic considerations in the elderly makes the management of wounds often inconsequential in a younger cohort, into a prolonged and often herculean effort. Hence, prevention is perhaps as paramount as management.

In this chapter, we will outline factors that contribute to the propensity and severity of acute soft-tissue trauma in the elderly and discuss unique management and prevention considerations. We finish with a discussion of soft-tissue trauma as an indicator of abuse in the elderly.

H. T. Brydges (✉) · B. F. Chaya · P. B. Saadeh
Hansjörg Wyss Department of Plastic Surgery, NYU Grossman School of Medicine, New York, NY, USA
e-mail: Hilliard.Brydges@nyulangone.org; Bachar.Chaya@nyulangone.org; Pierre.Saadeh@nyulangone.org

Soft-Tissue Changes and Unique Considerations in the Elderly

Geriatric patients undergo many age-related physiologic changes which result in an increased propensity for and severity of soft-tissue injuries and present unique challenges in the management of these defects. Factors contributing to these changes are both intrinsic (naturally occurring) and extrinsic factors (are due to "wear-and-tear," lifestyle factors outside of the body).

Skin changes common among the geriatric population include a thinner dermis, disorganized epidermis and flattening of the dermal-epidermal junction. Reduction in lipid production within the stratum corneum weakens barrier functions of the epidermis and may contribute to infection and desiccation of wounds. Further, reduction in dermal appendages (i.e., hair follicles) limits re-epithelialization, as these serve as a major source of stem cells following injury. At the level of the dermis, there is a reduction in immunologic and dermal cells required for wound healing. Elastin becomes fragmented while collagen changes in composition, density, and organization. Physiologic changes are not relegated to superficial soft-tissue structures and notable changes to deeper structures include decreased density and functionality of muscle and adipose tissue. Cumulatively, these changes reduce the skin's

P. Petrone, C. E.M. Brathwaite (eds.), *Acute Care Surgery in Geriatric Patients*,
https://doi.org/10.1007/978-3-031-30651-8_36

barrier function, decrease its resistance to force (shear in particular), and make the elderly more prone to superficial soft-tissue trauma.

Exacerbating skin-related changes, nearly all immune cells decline in both function and number with age, placing the geriatric populations at increased risk soft-tissue infections. Further, the normal wound healing process relies heavily on immunologic cells and thus loss of these cells increases the risk for delayed or aberrant wound healing. Vasculature decreases in density and angiogenesis becomes increasingly disordered with age. Thus, waning of immune cells is exacerbated by the physiologic decreases in blood flow experienced in this population, resulting in reduced delivery of lymphocytes following injuries. In addition to decreased immune support for infection prevention and wound healing, decreased delivery of platelets and erythrocytes decreases the intrinsic hemostatic capacity and limits oxygen delivery to healing tissue. Further, thinning of vasculature increases subcutaneous bleeding and decreased lymphatic function makes this population more prone to postoperative edema.

While changes in soft tissue contribute to the severity of wounds and challenges with wound management; naturally occurring neuropathic changes, place this population at increased risk for soft-tissue trauma. Neuropathic changes may be age related or secondary to medical comorbidities. These changes result in decreased sensation and motor responsiveness, with a notable decline in pain sensation and reflexes. Neuropathy, in conjunction with decreased muscle and bone density, make geriatric patients less capable of responding to noxious stimuli and as a result, these patients experience a greater incidence and severity of injury following falls and other classically benign traumas.

Many of the changes outlined above may be exacerbated by lifestyle choices and medical commodities common among elderly patients. Prolonged ultraviolet light (sun) exposure results in connective tissue and cellular dysfunction and contributes to skin laxity. While common comorbidities in this population including diabetes and atherosclerosis greatly limit vascular function increasing the risk of wound-related complications. Neurologic disorders such as dementia and peripheral neuropathy, both increase the incidence of injuries and worsen their severity by limiting patient's capacity to identify and mange wounds. In geriatric patients with neurologic decline, incontinence is also common and when combined with a decreased capacity for self-care, presents a considerable risk to the soft tissue of the pelvic region.

Nearly all soft-tissue changes are exacerbated by malnutrition (of both micro- and macronutrients) which, owing to decreased intake and absorption, is increasingly common among the elderly. Notable micronutrients include vitamin C and A, which when deficient impair soft-tissue repair. While minerals such as zinc, copper, and magnesium, if deficient, impair connective tissue production. From a macronutrient perspective, while elderly individuals often require lower caloric intakes, profound caloric deficiency (marasmus) and protein-specific deficiency (kwashiorkor), particularly arginine and glutamine, both contribute to poor wound healing outcomes. Malnutrition is increasingly common among patients with active malignancies, those with comorbid substance use disorders, elderly patients who struggle with activities of daily living and are dependent on caregivers, as well as those with decreased neurologic function/communication capacity.

Management

Like all acute/traumatic injuries, management should begin with stabilization of vital functions. In the management of soft-tissue injuries, hemostasis is paramount, and uniquely important among geriatric patients who have decreased autonomic capacity and delayed blood pressure homeostasis.

Non-surgical Wound Management

Once stabilization and hemostasis are achieved, clinicians can turn their attention to soft-tissue injuries and their associated externalities. History and physical exam are crucial to elucidate factors that may impact wound healing and thus management. Information regarding the etiology of soft-tissue trauma can help distinguish acute from chronic injuries and determine additional workup/interventions (i.e., CT scan for significant wounds or suspicion of deeper infection, tetanus vaccine in contaminated wounds, etc.). In addition to the trauma history, clinicians should garner a clear understanding of any underlying comorbidities, active medications, and past interventions as these are crucial to planning primary and secondary reconstructive options. On physical exam, the wound should be evaluated for potential contamination, including retained foreign bodies, any signs of infection as well as the potential involvement of deep tissues and nearby functional structures.

Many common medical comorbidities greatly influence soft-tissue trauma management. In the elderly, diabetes is common and glycemic optimization is crucial for wound healing. Blood flow to the injured area (as well as overall cardiac function) should be evaluated to ensure appropriate oxygenation of wounds. Of note, arterial insufficiency is common among geriatric patients, particularly in distal lower extremities and common clinical signs include hair loss, shiny/dry skin, thickened nails, color changes, cool skin, and diminished pulses. Further testing may be needed to evaluate for peripheral arterial disease (PAD) including ankle-brachial index (ABI), noninvasive vascular studies, CT angiography, and angiography (which can be concurrently therapeutic and diagnostic). Any decline in partial pressure of oxygen in the arterial blood (PaO_2) will increase risk of wound healing complications. As a rule of thumb, PaO_2 less than 40 mmHg increases infectious risk, while PaO_2 less than 20 mmHg makes healing unlikely to occur. If peripheral arterial disease is suspected, vascular surgery should be consulted to assess the need for revascularization prior to reconstruction. Chronic venous stasis is another vascular comorbidity common among the elderly, symptoms include dilated veins, swelling, tan or a reddish-brown skin, and venous ulcers. Non-surgical management includes Unna boots and compression stockings.

In addition to assessing comorbidity severity, lab tests may also be employed to evaluate for nutritional deficits, blood dyscrasias, and electrolyte abnormalities. Much contention exists regarding laboratory values as indicators of nutritional status and while the physical exam can provide clues to a patient's caloric nutritional status, many obese patients are found to be malnourished and thus should be closely evaluated as well. Finally, while macronutrient deficiencies can be difficult to address acutely, micronutrients and electrolytes can often be rapidly supplemented and thus should be considered in the acute setting.

In addition to medical disease and nutritional status, many medications impact wound healing, and clinicians should consider temporary holds in the acute setting. Glucocorticoids are common and well documented to negatively affect soft-tissue healing. These medications reduce immune cell prevalence and functionality as well as connective tissue formation. Despite these negative effects, great care should be taken prior to reduction of steroid medications, to avoid potential adrenal insufficiency or exacerbation of underlying disease. A medical history notable for active malignancy should raise a red flag for clinicians, as cancer leads to metabolic aberrations which exacerbate malnutrition and directly impact wound healing. Further, many malignancy treatments can be particularly pernicious in soft-tissue trauma, as systemic chemotherapeutics negatively impact cellular replication necessary for wound healing/infection management and radiation impairs local tissue repair and may lead to chronic wound formation.

As with all patients, geriatric patients with soft-tissue trauma should be evaluated for social and behavioral factors which can impact wound healing. Notable social determinants of health in geriatric soft-tissue trauma include capacity for self-care, presence of social support, as well as food/housing insecurity. Finally, alcohol, substance, and tobacco use disorders remain high among geriatric cohorts and when present, should raise a clinician's index of suspicion for malnutrition and potential wound healing complications.

Finally, past surgical history can play a role in planning primary and backup reconstructive options. Previous traumatic injuries and reconstructive procedures should guide the selection of available tissues for reconstruction, while a history of surgical/anesthetic adverse events can alter risk-benefit calculations for operative interventions. When planning reconstruction, a staged approach should be considered, and non-urgent reconstructive options may be delayed while the patient's overall health status and wound bed are optimized.

Wound Optimization

Once the patient is stabilized, a clear history is taken and related factors are assessed, management of the wound can proceed. The first and most crucial step in the management of soft-tissue injuries is infection prevention and treatment. Visibly contaminated wounds should be washed out extensively and examined for foreign bodies. The removal of foreign bodies while crucial (as these can impact healing and serve as a nidus for infection), should be done with great care, as large foreign bodies may impinge on crucial local structures and contribute to compression hemostasis. Infectious complications and necrotic tissue are less likely to be found in the acute setting; however, management via local/systemic antibiotics as well as sharp/medical debridement is crucial to prepare a wound bed for closure. Accurate assessment of blood flow to determine the viability of the tissues is equally paramount. SPY Elite laser angiography (Indocyanine green) can be used in conjunction with physical exam to assess blood flow. These data can guide debridement through accurate real-time assessment of local tissue perfusion.

Reconstructive Surgery

Depending on severity, closure of open wounds is often the first step in acute reconstructive management. Closure can be conducted by either primary or secondary intention. Minor/superficial wounds can be left to heal by secondary intention, as the skin laxity often present in the elderly can promote closure. However, if there is concern that secondary closure will fail, the threshold for primary closure in this population should be lower than in younger cohorts as greater skin laxity allows for easier approximation of wounds, and the aforementioned physiologic deficiencies decrease wound contracture necessary for secondary closure. If closure cannot be achieved primarily/secondarily and/or a wound is not optimized for closure, wound debridement and vacuum-assisted closure (VACs) can be valuable tools for both reducing infectious risk and promoting wound healing (via stimulating granulation tissue formation). Hyperbaric oxygen therapy (HBOT) has emerged as a valuable adjunct therapy that should be considered when treating traumatic wounds. Hyperbaric oxygen mitigates the effects of acute traumatic ischemia through four main mechanisms: vasoconstriction, hyperoxygenation, decreased neutrophil activation (reducing the production of free radicals and preventing reperfusion injury) and reduced blood viscosity.

In reconstructive surgery, the reconstructive ladder (Fig. 36.1) is often employed as a useful heuristic in designing reconstructive protocols. Treatments lower down on the ladder are employed before those above, unless otherwise indicated.

In addressing soft-tissue defects, which cannot be closed by primary or secondary intention, autologous grafts, and dermal scaffolds can be employed. These options are most useful for patients with trauma that impacts a significant portion of body surface area but are largely relegated to superficial, non-functional structures, i.e., burn injuries. Skin grafts are broadly categorized into full-thickness (including all dermal or epidermal layers) or partial thickness which includes variable amounts of dermis.

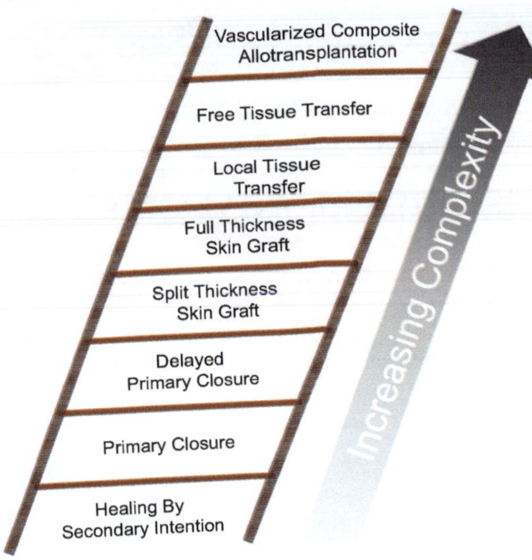

Fig. 36.1 Reconstructive ladder for soft-tissue defects. Generally, reconstructive options lower on the ladder should be employed before those higher up

Full-thickness skin grafts are useful for small defects; whereas, partial-thickness grafts have the benefit of great take and availability. Further, unlike full-thickness grafts, partial-thickness leave stem cell containing dermal appendages intact at the harvest site. This enables rapid reepithelization and gives the potential to reuse the same donor site for future grafts. Overall, grafts are useful options in patients with extensive superficial injuries and a good stock of available healthy tissues; however, they should not be employed if there is a concern for further complications at the donor site (from which the graft is taken) or if grafting will be insufficient to address the area/volume of defect. In cases where the defect requires full-thickness grafting but is too large for available donor tissue, acellular dermal matrices (ADM) be employed. ADMs serve as connective tissue scaffolds for vascular ingrowth, upon which partial-thickness skin grafts can be placed. ADMs are also useful for thicker coverage around joints especially when "stacking" is performed. However, these tools are costly and should be used judiciously.

The next rung on the reconstructive later is tissue flaps. Flaps refer to the movement of tissues that include native blood supply and are broadly categorized by the type of tissue included in the flap. Fasciocutaneous flaps include skin and underlying non-muscular soft tissue. Flaps are referred to as musculocutaneous if muscle is included as well. When based on blood supply from surrounding skin, flaps are considered random pattern. When based on intact named blood supply they are considered axial flaps (which include pedicle flaps). In general, axial flaps offer greater reliability given knowledge of supported soft-tissue territories. Perforator flaps are designed based on the watershed area of a particular perforator vessel. Finally, free flaps refer to pedicle flaps that are disconnected from their native vasculature and anastomosed, via microsurgical techniques, to vasculature at a distant recipient defect site. Of note, flaps can also include hard tissue/bony structures where necessary. Plastic surgery should be consulted for all wounds for which any form of complex reconstruction is warranted, or if tissue loss results in major functional impairment (including the face, hands/upper extremity, lower extremity, or sphincters) (Fig. 36.2).

Finally, in the cases of limb trauma, where hemostasis cannot be achieved, infection/necrosis cannot be debrided/continues to spread, or reconstruction cannot be conducted—amputation may be necessary. Given the geriatric population's propensity for deconditioning, recovery following limb salvage should be balanced with the quicker recovery but functional impact of amputation. Unless emergently necessary the decision to amputate a limb should be made through a multidisciplinary team approach with shared decision-making from the patient.

Complications of Acute Soft-Tissue Trauma in the Elderly

Following reconstruction, patients should be closely followed and repeatedly evaluated for would healing complications. Table 36.1 highlights some of the more common complications, including signs of disease onset and a brief overview of management considerations.

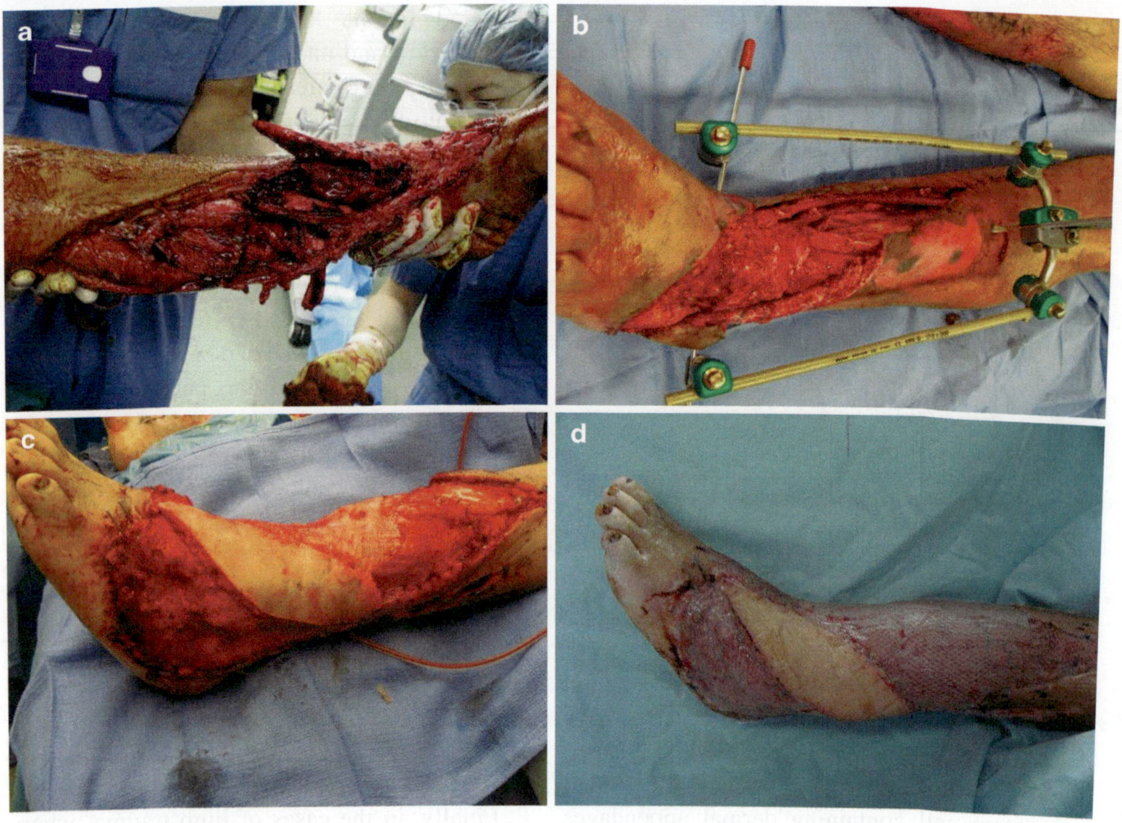

Fig. 36.2 Representative case of lower extremity reconstruction: (**a**) open tibia and fibula fracture with extensive soft-tissue trauma. (**b**) Remaining soft-tissue defect following external fixation and serial debridement. (**c**) Defect following myocutaneous latissimus dorsi-free flap. (**d**) Final reconstruction following skin grafting

Table 36.1 Overview of common potential complications of acute soft-tissue injury in the elderly

Complication	Signs/diagnosis	Management
Necrosis/flap loss	Dusky tissues, decreased oxygenation, diminshed bleeding to pin pick	Debridement (medical or surgical). Reoperation
Local infection (cellulitis, erysipelas, necrotizing fasciitis)	Erythema, edema, pain, purulent drainage	Repeated local tissue debridement, PO/IV antibiotics
Osteomyelitis	Soft necrotic bone, MRI to suggest, biopsy to confirm	Debridement, IV antibiotics
Sepsis/systematic inflammatory response	Fever, hypotension, tachycardia	Identification of the source, culture-directed IV antibiotics, pressors as indicated
Deconditioning/delirium	Decreased movement, sleepiness, waxing, and waning cognition	Preventative measures, opening windows, engaging with patient, maintaining sleep wake cycle
Chronic wound formation	Non-advancing wound edge, hyper-/de-pigmentation, friable/lack of granulation tissue	Complex and multimodal

Prevention

While many effective options have been developed for the treatment and reconstruction of acute soft-tissue wounds, management is often challenging and prevention of trauma remains paramount. Key considerations in the prevention of soft-tissue trauma in this population involve many of the issues discussed above—particularly comorbidity management and lifestyle optimization.

One issue more common in the geriatric population is prolonged hospital stays/bed rest, which predisposes patients deconditioning as well as pressure injuries. Pressure injuries are challenging to manage and can greatly complicate recovery following soft-tissue trauma. These injuries can be prevented by moving the patient when possible (ideally of their own volition) and offloading for patients who may not be sensate in areas predisposed to pressure ulcer formation (sacrum, heel, etc.). Various types of support surfaces, including pneumatic beds and Roho cushions, have been developed to mitigate pressure and shear forces experienced by sedentary patients. These support structures reduce pressure injuries by sensing and redistributing the patients' weight (to maximize surface area/localize pressure to resilient regions) or mechanically alternating the pressure against the various contact points. Identification of the optimum support surface from the variety of available options should be driven by evidence of their relative effectiveness in prevention of given pressure injuries and overall, should be tailored to unique patient needs. Further, in the inpatient and critical care settings, ensuring patients' beds remain uncluttered and they are not laying on wires can greatly reduce their risk.

Soft-Tissue Trauma and Elder Abuse

Due to many age-related changes outlined above, elderly patients are prone to soft-tissue trauma. However, elder abuse is both common and difficult to recognize; therefore, irrespective of injury pattern clinicians should maintain a high index of suspicion. Table 36.2 is adapted from Lachs et al. and highlights important clues to abuse including atypical patterns of injury, common presentations, and associated risk factors.

When clinicians have concerns about elder abuse, they should assess the patient for risk factors. Clinicians should take a thorough history from the caregiver and patient separately where possible, looking for discrepancies (however, a discrepancy does not indicate the caregiver is aware of/is the perpetrator, rather the victim may be unwilling to disclose in their presence out of protective instincts/cultural norms). Throughout the interview, it is crucial to maintain a supportive and non-judgmental tone and indirect questions (i.e., "do you feel safe at home?") should be used before direct questions (i.e., "does anyone hit you?") when possible. Given the increased risk associated with cognitive decline and mental illness, a formal assessment for both is strongly recommended.

Of note, the factors outlined above should increase a clinician's index of suspicion for abuse but should not be taken as diagnostic. If abuse is uncovered, effort should be taken to remove the patient from the abuser and the police and/or adult protective services should be contacted. If abuse is not uncovered but concern remains following the initial assessment, involving experts and referral to adult protective services may be an appropriate next step.

Finally, discussion in this chapter centers around signs of physical abuse; however, this is not the most common form of abuse in this population, and clinicians caring for geriatric patients should take care to educate themselves on forms of abuse outside the scope of this chapter (verbal/psychosocial and financial abuse, etc.).

Table 36.2 Highlights of heuristics, which may increase clinicians' index of suspicion for elder abuse when evaluating a geriatric soft-tissue injury

Category	Clue	Notes
Injury patterns	Associated hard tissue trauma	Facial fractures (malar, zygomatic, mandibular), dental fractures, and atypical long bone fractures
	Atypical bruising patterns	Facial bruising, bruising to the lateral aspect of the right arm, and posterior torso, including back, chest, lumbar, and gluteal regions
	Anogenital abrasions	May be indicative of sexual abuse
Presentations	Diffuse injuries at different stages of healing	Important to distinguish from injuries related to normal function
	Unaddressed injuries/injuries found incidentally	Lacerations healing by secondary intention, multiple unset fractures
	Depression/behavior health issues	Manifestation of unaddressed abuse, geriatric-specific psychometric instruments should be used to assess
Risk factors	Cognitive decline	Inability to recognize abuse or voice concerns
	Inappropriate dress/poor hygiene	Indicates the patient may be unable to care for themselves, increasing risk for neglect related injuries
	"Young old" woman	Both female sex and early geriatric years are risk factors for abuse
	Lives with/dependent on young children/spouse	Most common perpetrators of abuse

Table adapted from Lachs et al.

Conclusion

Soft-tissue trauma is common in geriatric populations. Natural age-related changes (both to soft tissue and other body systems) increase the risk for and severity of these injuries. Like the non-geriatric population, stabilization is the first step in management, after which engagement of reconstructive and wound management experts may be necessary. Issues related to medical comorbidities and lifestyle are common among the elderly and can complicate soft-tissue trauma management. Even with appropriate care, wound management, and reconstruction are challenging, and this population is at increased risk of complications or progression to chronic wounds, therefore prevention is paramount. Finally, while not diagnostic, soft-tissue trauma is a common sign of elder abuse and clinicians should maintain a high index of suspicion, particularly when atypical patterns are present.

Disclosures These authors have no relevant disclosures.

References

1. Ramos-e-Silva M, Boza JC, Cestari TF. Effects of age (neonates and elderly) on skin barrier function. Clin Dermatol. 2012;30(3):274–6.
2. Bonifant H, Holloway S. A review of the effects of ageing on skin integrity and wound healing. Br J Community Nurs. 2019;24(Sup3):S28–33.
3. Kohl E, Steinbauer J, Landthaler M, Szeimies RM. Skin ageing. J Eur Acad Dermatol Venereol. 2011;25(8):873–84.
4. Andersen JL. Muscle fibre type adaptation in the elderly human muscle. Scand J Med Sci Sports. 2003;13(1):40–7.
5. Borgoni S, Kudryashova KS, Burka K, de Magalhães JP. Targeting immune dysfunction in aging. Ageing Res Rev. 2021;70:101410.
6. Tsuchida Y. Age-related changes in skin blood flow at four anatomic sites of the body in males studied by xenon-133. Plast Reconstr Surg. 1990;85(4):556–61.
7. Jakic B, Kerjaschki D, Wick G. Lymphatic capillaries in aging. Gerontology. 2020;66(5):419–26.
8. Bouche P. Neuropathy of the elderly. Rev Neurol. 2020;176(9):733–8.
9. Gosain A, DiPietro LA. Aging and wound healing. World J Surg. 2004;28(3):321–6.
10. Baumann L. Skin ageing and its treatment. J Pathol. 2007;211(2):241–51.
11. Pirlich M, Lochs H. Nutrition in the elderly. Best Pract Res Clin Gastroenterol. 2001;15(6):869–84.
12. Stechmiller JK. Understanding the role of nutrition and wound healing. Nutr Clin Pract. 2010;25(1):61–8.
13. Cleophas TJ, van Marum R. Age-related decline in autonomic control of blood pressure: implications for the pharmacological management of hypertension in the elderly. Drugs Aging. 2003;20(5):313–9.
14. Gottrup F. Oxygen in wound healing and infection. World J Surg. 2004;28(3):312–5.
15. Lachs MS, Pillemer KA. Elder abuse. N Engl J Med. 2015;373(20):1947–56.

Wound Healing in the Geriatric Population

37

Scott Gorenstein, Kenneth Droz, and Brian Gillette

The problem with aging is not that it's one damn thing after another—it's every damn thing, all at once, all the time.

—John Scalzi, Old Man's War

Introduction

Some of the earliest accounts of medical treatment relate to caring for open wounds. There are clay tablets dating from 2200 BC that portray basic wound care such as cleaning and bandaging wounds. The use of various topical agents such as honey have been described in Egyptian scrolls. Pressure injuries have been found on Egyptian mummies. In the nineteenth century, the British surgeon Joseph Lister began placing carbolic acid into open fractures and noted that sepsis was often prevented. It was also during this time that hand washing, and sterilization of instruments became common practice. In times of war, wound care is critical and during the Civil War of the United States over 17,000 soldiers succumbed to sepsis due to contaminated wounds. In World War 1, a Belgian surgeon, Depage described the process of wound debridement and delayed closure which is still standard practice today.

The most recent publication of the World Population Databank has current population of 7.96 billion people with 10% over 70 years of age. Due to the recent COVID 19 pandemic, there have been some decreases in life expectancy with the United States having an average life expectancy of 73 for men and 79 for women. Worldwide the population is expected to continue to increase with an expected population of 9.7 billion people in mid-2050. Life expectancy is also expected to continue to rise and therefore the number of people over age 70 that will be seeking medical care will also increase. The elderly population is generally more active than prior generations and is therefore subject to more injury leading to acute and often chronic wounds. All these factors are leading to an increasing

S. Gorenstein (✉) · B. Gillette
NYU Langone Hospital—Long Island Wound Healing Center, Mineola, NY, USA

NYU Long Island School of Medicine, Mineola, NY, USA
e-mail: scott.gorenstein@nyulangone.org

K. Droz
NYU Langone Hospital—Long Island Wound Healing Center, Mineola, NY, USA

P. Petrone, C. E.M. Brathwaite (eds.), *Acute Care Surgery in Geriatric Patients*,
https://doi.org/10.1007/978-3-031-30651-8_37

prevalence of wounds and wound-related complications in the geriatric population. This chapter aims to provide an overview of the rapidly evolving basic science of wound healing in older adults, best practices for preventing and treating various acute and chronic wound types in the geriatric population, and guidelines for optimal coordination of care.

The Biology of Aging Skin

Skin is the body's largest organ with the average male adult having approximately 3.6 kg and 2 square meters of it. Our skin protects us against dehydration, provides a barrier against harmful agents, is responsible for production of vitamin D, among many other functions. Skin homeostasis is maintained and restored after damage through a complex interplay involving a multitude of cell types, extracellular matrix components, soluble factors, and microbes. As we age, the most obvious skin changes that occur, such as wrinkling, loss/graying of hair, thinning/fragility, and development of pigmented spots, are driven by changes at the cellular and molecular level such as mitochondrial DNA damage, telomere shortening, immunosenescence, oxidative stress, extracellular matrix (ECM) remodeling, and changes in secretion of inflammatory cytokines. Such age-related changes contribute to slow healing of surgical incisions, increased incidence of wound dehiscence and susceptibility of skin to infections and the development of chronic wounds. Here we review some of the basic biology underlying skin changes with aging and their impact on wound healing.

Stem Cell Dysfunction and Senescence

Stem cells are responsible for maintaining tissue homeostasis throughout the lifetime by replacing cells lost to normal wear and tear or injury. As humans age, many stem cell reservoirs become depleted due to cellular senescence driven by alterations in the stem cell microenvironment. There are several pools of stem cells within different compartments in adult skin, including (but not limited to) keratinocyte stem cells (KSC) in the epidermal basal layer, hair follicle stem cells (HFSC), and melanocyte stem cells (MSC) within the hair follicle (HF) bulge, adipose mesenchymal stem cells (ADMSC) within the hypodermal adipose tissue, and pericytes associated with the dermal microvasculature that all play important roles in skin maintenance and wound healing. Intriguingly, the reduced ability for stem cells to maintain and regenerate healthy tissue with aging is not purely intrinsic to stem cells themselves, but also involves dysfunction of other cell types that support the stem cell niche. For example, it has been shown that aged HFSC show impaired hair follicle generation after injury within aged dermis but could still regenerate hair follicles when transplanted in young dermis, while young HFSC also could not regenerate HF in aged dermis, suggesting that alterations in supportive cells with aging prevent proper orchestration of HF regeneration by HFSC.

Perturbations in Inflammatory Cells and Cytokines

During the course of normal wound healing, an initial inflammatory phase recruits immune cells including neutrophils and proinflammatory macrophages to help clear pathogens and devitalized tissue, which then transitions to an anti-inflammatory state during the proliferative phase when re-epithelialization occurs (Fig. 37.1). Pathologic persistence of a proinflammatory state in the wound environment is associated with delayed wound healing in chronic wounds. Aging is associated with an increase in proinflammatory cytokine levels by immunosenescent cells, which can be an important factor in the disruption of wound healing and in inflammatory dermatoses.

Degradation of Extracellular Matrix

The skin ECM is important for establishing appropriate mechanical properties and for

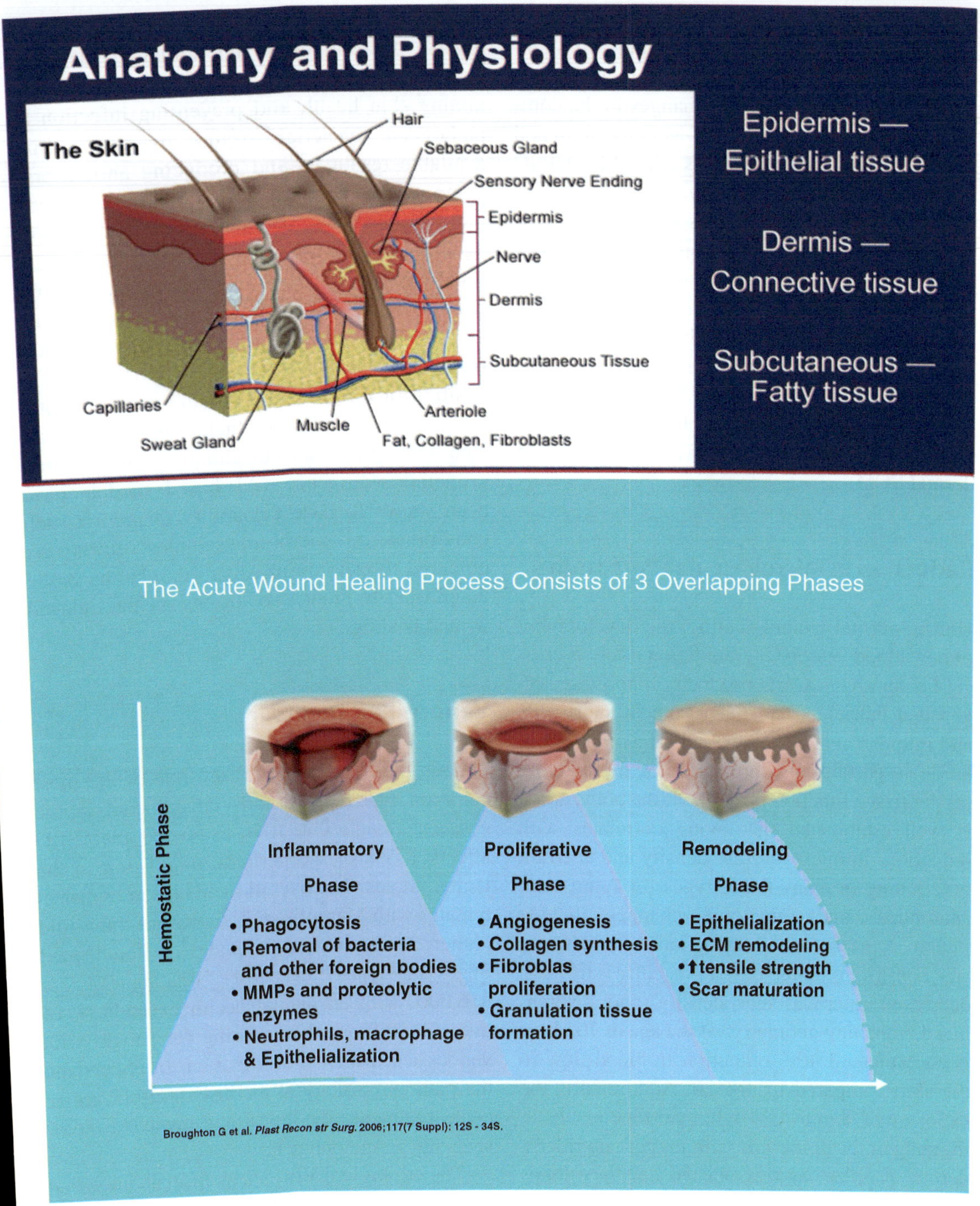

Fig. 37.1 Skin anatomy and the wound healing process

supporting the proper functioning of stem cells and other cell types. For example, collagen XVII, a transmembrane protein that mediates adhesion between keratinocytes and other skin stem cells to the surrounding ECM and is essential for supporting proper HFSC and KSC function, is reduced with aging and UV exposure which negatively impacts wound healing capacity. The extracellular matrix molecule fibulin 7 regulates basement membrane integrity and supports stem cell maintenance during aging by protecting them against impacts from inflammation. Changes in the composition and stiffness of the ECM in the stem cell niche with aging silences genes critical for HFSC activation in response to injury. Aging fibroblasts reduce expression of genes responsible for ECM production and become more similar to preadipocytes, which contributes to decreased dermal thickness and likely increases susceptibility to infection and impaired wound healing. Aging dermal fibroblasts also acquire a "senescence-associated secretory phenotype" (SASP) in which they secrete proinflammatory cytokines and matrix metalloproteinases (MMPs) which degrade the dermal ECM.

Reduction in Microvascular Perfusion

During normal wound healing, the development of new blood vessels in granulation tissue is critical for removing waste products, supplying oxygen and nutrients, and trafficking of stem cells and immune cells to the wound. The microcirculation is particularly important for maintaining proper tissue function throughout the body, and it is well established that aging correlates with reductions in microvascular density and aberrant functioning in many tissue types. In aging skin, anatomical and functional changes include impaired microvascular vasodilation and chronic vasoconstriction, increased vascular stiffness, decreased microvascular density, and disorganized branching geometry. At the age of 70, there is an estimated 40% reduction in blood flow to the skin compared to age 20. Additionally, the exposure of skin to UV light over time results in thinning of the epidermis with loss of rete ridges, dermal papillae, and associated capillary loops responsible for maintaining epidermal supply.

Alterations of the Microbiome

Human skin is colonized by a complex ecosystem of microbes, with approximately one-million bacteria per square centimeter, and has the most diverse microbiome of all human tissues. The skin microbiome plays important roles in maintaining skin health and preventing infection by pathogenic bacterial strains by constraining available resources and producing antibacterial compounds. The composition of the skin microbiome generally becomes more diverse with aging, driven by age-related changes in immune function and a decrease in sweat and sebum production. Such changes in microbial communities vary by body site according to changes in host factors such as skin lipid composition. The composition of the skin microbiome also correlates with specific conditions, including those associated with aging, and intriguingly methods using artificial intelligence (AI)-based models have been shown to have the ability to predict such conditions from microbiota samples, offering the potential to use non-invasive microbiome-based diagnostics to predict conditions such as delayed wound healing.

Venous Leg Ulcers

Venous Leg Ulcers (VLU) are one of the most common types of wounds encountered in the geriatric population. It is estimated that VLU affects 1–3% of the geriatric population in the United States. The overall incidence in higher in females with Margolis et al. showing a three-fold higher incidence than in males. In the United States that approximate cost of treating a VLU is $16,000, with an annual health expenditure of over $14 billion. When caring for patient with venous leg ulcers, it is important to understand the pathophysiology of the disease itself, utilize clear treatment algorithms, and involve a multi-specialty team approach.

The etiology of VLU stems from an increased hydrostatic pressure in the normally low-pressure venous systems of the lower extremities. The epidemic of morbid obesity is the largest cause of venous insufficiency is the United States. The incidence of chronic venous insufficiency (CVI) increases with age, obesity, and a sedentary lifestyle; however, VLU only occurs in approximately 5% of patients with CVI. The lower extremity venous system is composed of a superficial and deep system—see Fig. 37.1. The normal anatomy of the vein includes the presence of valves (made of elastic tissue). Once these valves are damaged the flow of blood is reversed leading to congestion, extravasation of RBC, decreasing oxygen diffusion and hemosiderin deposition in the subcutaneous tissue causing an inflammatory response. Mast cells degranulate causing a histamine release which explains why patients with CVI with or without ulceration often complain of itching of the lower extremities. This inflammatory response involves leukocyte recruitment, increased matrix metalloprotease inhibition, changes to the myofibroblasts and development of varicosities. Macrophage phenotype is shifted to the M1 type with the release of IL-1α, IFN-1ÿ, and TGF-β1. These changes cause a delay in healing upon wound and/or development of spontaneous ulcerations.

When evaluating a patient with a wound of the lower extremity the differential diagnosis includes pressure injury, arterial insufficiency, malignancy, vasculitis, and VLU. Characteristics that favor a diagnosis of VLU include edema, presence of varicosities, hyperpigmentation, lipodermatosclerosis, and obesity. The typical appearance of a VLU is a shallow ulcer with irregular borders often on the lateral aspect of the midcalf. Typically, the ulcer with have a beefy red appearance although with chronicity the presence of slough and thick fibrotic scar tissue becomes more apparent. Without treatment these ulcers can become circumferential and are often associated with large amount of clear drainage which severely impairs patients' ability to perform activities of daily living and adversely affects their quality of life.

The Venous Clinical Severity Score is a derivative of the prior CEAP (clinical great, etiology, anatomic location, and pathophysiology) which has been in use for over 20 years. This classification ranges from C0 to C6 and is based on physical examination with qualifiers for symptomatic (CS) vs asymptomatic (CA) disease (Table 37.1). Diagnostic workup should include assessment of arterial status (pulses, ABI/PVR, CTA, etc.), venous duplex to r/o DVT and evaluate for reflux, laboratory workup including CBC, CMP, Hgb A1c, ESR, and CRP. If pulses are palpable consider debridement and application of antimicrobial dressing under compression. For patients with non-palpable pulses and/or ABI <0.65 or PVR with flattened waveforms referral to vascular surgery for possible intervention is mandatory. If the patient has adequate arterial circulation and the wound does not decrease in size by 50% or more with 4–6 weeks of compression, biopsy, and use of regenerative medicine is recommended. The various types of regenerative products used by these authors are presented in Table 37.2.

The use of various extracellular matrices (ECM) or skin substitutes has significantly improved healing rates in chronic venous

Table 37.1 Venous clinical severity score

Classification	Description
C0	No Visible or palpable signs of venous disease
C1	Telangiectaslas or reticular veins
C2	Varlcose veins
C3	Edema
C4a	Milder skin changes due to enous disorders (pigmentation, eczema)
C4b	Severe skin changes due to venous disorders (dermatosclerosis, atrophie blanche)
C5	C4 along with healed ulcers
C6	Skin changes with active ulcers

Table 37.2 Example regenerative medicine products

Generic name	Description	Mechanism of action	Trade name
Porcine urinary bladder matrix	Lyophilized sheet of intact basement membrane and subadjacent lamina propria of the porcine urinary bladder ECM	Guides wound healing response by providing a complex molecular architecture that aids in biologic tissue repair[20]	MatriStem Burn Matrix and MicroMatrix
Granulocyte-macrophage colony-stimulating factor	Pleiotropic cytokine	Promotes proliferation and differentiation of bone marrow-derived monocyte precursors into macrophages[21]	Leukine
Cryopreserved placental membrane	Source of MSCs, collagen matrix, growth factors (preserved structural and cellular integrity)	Anti-inflammatory, antimicrobial, angiogenic activities Create a moist environment[22,23]	Grafix
Bilayered bioengineered living skin substitute	Type I bovine collagen dermal layer fibroblasts with overlying epidermal layer keratinocytes	Produces a great number of cytokines and growth factors that stimulate differentiation and proliferation in the nonhealing wound bed[24-26]	Apligraf
Acellular matrix scaffold	Porcine small intestine submucosa ECM	Contains collagen, elastin, glycosaminoglycans, proteoglycans, and growth factors Numerous cell types attach and migrate into the matrix Reduces level of MMPs[27]	Oasis
Dehydrated human amnion/ chorion membrane allograft	Dehydrated human amnion/chorion membrane allograft	Provides matrix, nonimmunogenic, reduces inflammation/scar tissue/ pain, antibacterial, contains GF and cytokines[28,29]	Epifix
Bilayered cross-linked type I bovine tendon collagen combined with chondroitin-6-sulfate and a semi-permeable silicone membrane	Bilayered cross-linked type I bovine tendon collagen combined with chondroitin-6-sulfate and a semi-permeable silicone membrane	Guides growth of the neo-dermis with silicone as a temporary epidermal barrier[30-32]	Integra
Purified type I collagen with polyhexamethylenebiguanide	Purified type I collagen with polyhexamethylenebiguanide	Selectively binds and condenses bacterial DNA chromosomes[33-35]	Puraply

ECM, extracellular matrix; GF, growth factor; MSC, mesenchymal stem cell; MMP, matrix metalloproteinase.

insufficiency ulcers. The underlying principle of wound bed preparation is paramount to the success of whichever product is chosen. It is critical to maintain at least 20–30 mmHg of graduated compression after the application. Often patients require more than one application, however if after three applications of any given product there is not significant (>20%) healing going back to the diagnostic tree is indicated. Circumferential chronic venous ulcers present for over 1 year frequently demonstrate poor response to treatment and palliative care should be considered after a comprehensive discussion with patient/family regarding the goals of care.

Pressure Injuries

The National and International Pressure Injury definition is: "A pressure injury is a localized injury to the skin and/or underlying tissue, usually over a bony prominence or related to a medical device. The injury occurs, as a result of intense or prolonged pressure, or pressure in combination with shear and/or friction." The term pressure injury replaced pressure ulcer at the National Pressure Ulcer Advisory Panel (NPUAP) meeting in 2016. Pressure injuries (PIs) have a high prevalence among adult inpatients. In the United States, 4.5% of admitted Medicare patients will experience a PI during any given admission. The prevalence of PUs varies widely between institutions and among patient populations. PU prevalence is approximately 15% in many acute care facilities but can exceed 40% in some long-term care settings. Pressure ulcer rates have increased over the last decade despite efforts to improve wound treatment and nursing care.

PIs result in significant morbidity, mortality, and cost to the patient and the healthcare system. PI development is correlated with increased re-admission rates, increased inpatient lengths of stay, and both same-admission and 30-day mortality. Advanced stage PIs, particularly stage IV ulcers, have dramatic effects on mortality, with 180-day mortality as high as 68.9%. In addition, these ulcers incur a potential cost to hospitals of $124,000 per episode and cost the US healthcare system $10.2 billion in 2019. Although many of these wounds are preventable the center for Medicare services has declared hospital acquired pressure injuries (HAPI) as a never event. For the surgeon caring for the geriatric patient, it is therefore critical to understand the preventive measures and treatment modalities for pressure injuries.

The first step in preventing a pressure injury is recognizing the risk factors for developing one. There are many screening tools available and the most widely used is the Braden Scale. The Braden Scale was developed by Barbara Braden and Nancy Bergstrom in 1988 and has since been used widely in the general adult patient population. The scale consists of six subscales and the total scores range from 6 to 23. A lower Braden score indicates higher levels of risk for pressure ulcer development. A score of 18 or less indicates a patient at high risk. For these patients, active prevention is mandated and requires offloading surfaces (table), moisture control, use of skin barriers and repositioning. In the operating room (OR), all bony prominences need to be adequately padded and extra care should be taken when transporting the patient to and from the operating table.

As early as the 1840s, Robert Graves advocated repositioning immobile patients twice daily to treat PUs. In the intervening centuries, patient repositioning has become a widely accepted practice in the prevention and management of PIs despite a paucity of evidence supporting an optimal regime of repositioning. Repositioning temporarily redistributes interface pressures on sites prone to ulceration, relieving the microcirculatory ischemia that continuous pressure induces. However, excessive turning or extremes of positioning (i.e., 90° head-raised, or lateral decubitus positions) can increase shearing forces and friction, as well as promote ulceration at additional sites. Early studies in rats demonstrated that pressure-induced muscle ischemia begins in less than 2 h, which supported the longstanding clinical tradition of patient repositioning every 2 h.

Less frequent positioning of up to once every 4 h or a specific pattern of positioning has not been found to adversely affect PI development. The failure to identify an ideal repositioning protocol is due in part to the multifactorial nature of PIs; a 2-h turning frequency may be ideal on a static, cold foam bed but suboptimal on an alternating pressure bed. The lack of large, prospective randomized controlled trials of patient positioning has forced us to rely on clinical experience and expert opinion to pragmatically construct a protocol for repositioning. In concert with currently accepted practice, we endorse turning patients laterally to 30° every 2 h. In addition, avoid positioning patients with the head of the bed elevated more than 30°, or rotated laterally 90° for extended periods of time. We feel that this protocol maximizes the potential benefit of repositioning while minimizing risks of excess friction or shear, is comfortable to patients, and minimizes excess workload on the nursing team.

Once a pressure injury is identified a treatment algorithm must be initiated (Fig. 37.2a) which depends on the NPUAP Stage of the PI (Fig. 37.2b). For Stage 1 and Stage 2 lesions, local care is often all that is needed. There are various types of dressing, ointments, and creams which can be used. Our preference is cadexomer iodine for Stage 2 ulcers unless the patient is not tolerant to iodine, in which case a silver antimicrobial is recommended. For Stage 3 and 4 wounds surgical debridement is often required. Debridement of pressure ulcers includes special attention to removal of nonviable tissue and undermining or tunneling down to the level of grossly viable tissue. This can include removal of underlying periosteum or bone (Fig. 37.3a, b). The entire wound is thoroughly probed and irrigated to ensure removal of purulent pockets. Areas of tunneling or undermining are unroofed by triangulation (Fig. 37.3c, d) to stimulate healing of the wound bed from the base and decrease epithelialization forming over dead space with the potential to become infected. It is particularly important to consider the home care or facility nurse and their ability to pragmatically apply the

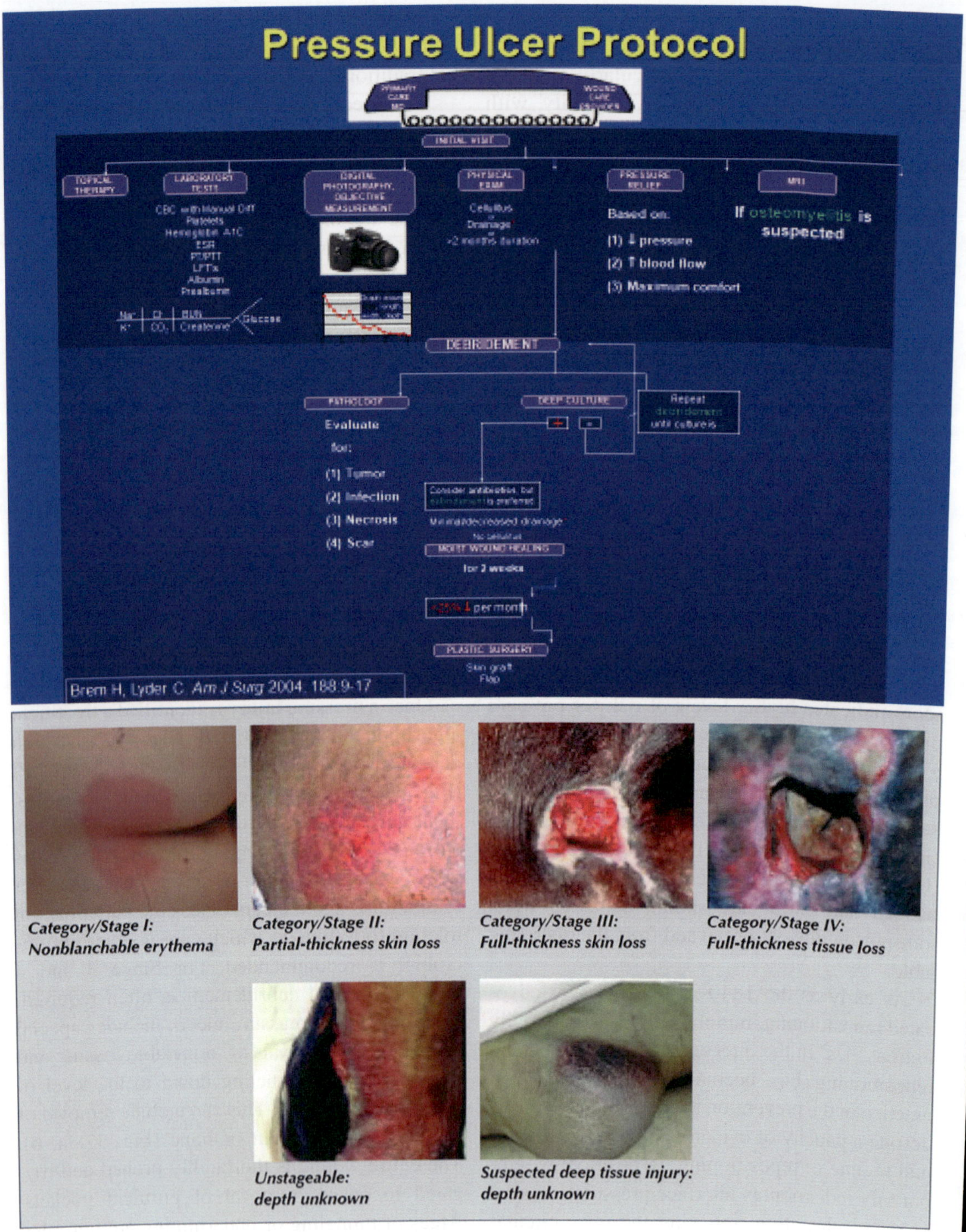

Fig. 37.2 Pressure injury protocol and NPUAP classification system

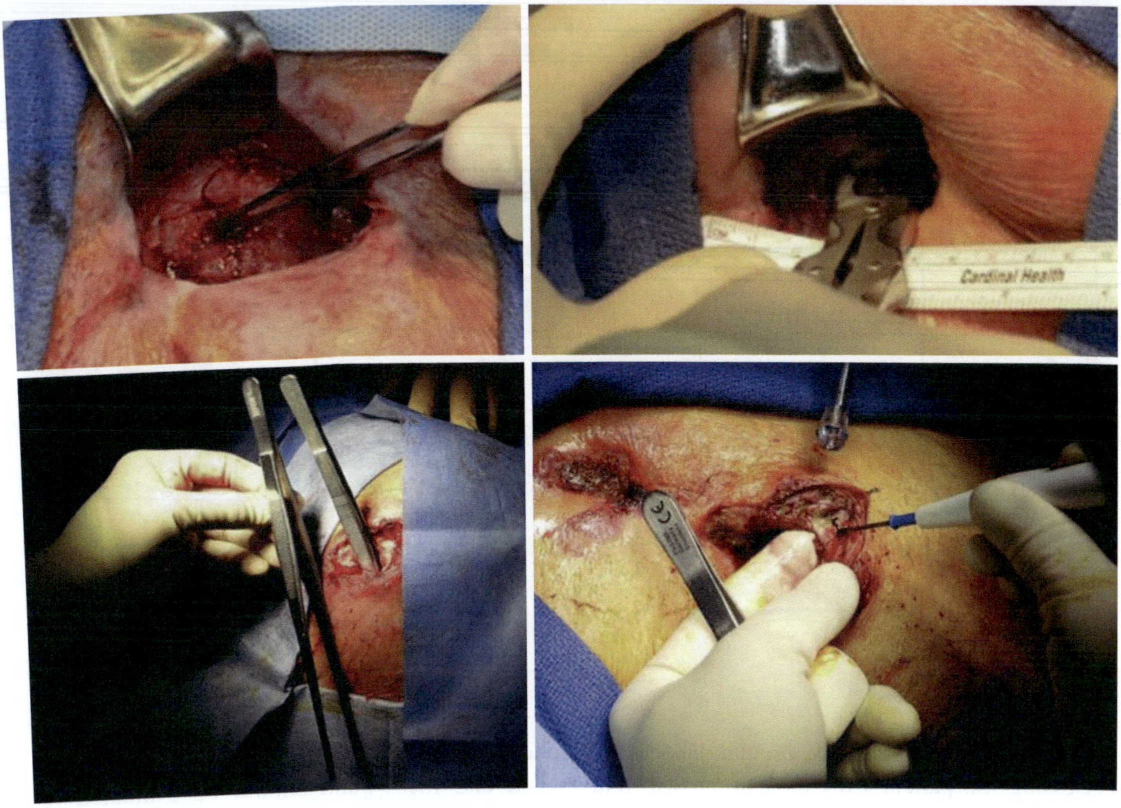

Fig. 37.3 Debridement of pressure injuries

secondary dressing. For example, if the patient receives negative pressure therapy, the wound would be extended to accommodate the vacuum sponge. In our experience, the application of a vacuum-assisted wound closure device was performed 2–3 days postoperatively instead of at the time of operation to decrease bleeding occurrences.

Diabetic Foot Ulcers

Foot ulcerations in patients with diabetes is a major source of healthcare expenditures worldwide. The International Diabetes Federation (IDF) estimates that in 2019 463 million people were diagnosed with diabetes. The lifetime risk of a developing diabetic foot ulcer (DFU) is approximately 25%. Approximately 67% of all lower extremity amputations in the United States are related to diabetes. An estimated 33% of adults aged 65 or older have diabetes, and this population is at higher risk for complications such as DFU. With proper care it has been shown that elderly patients with diabetes can heal at the same rate as younger patients.

The first step in assessing a patient with a diabetic foot ulcer is a good history and physical (Fig. 37.4). The physical examination should include a complete vascular assessment with ankle brachial index (ABI) measurements as well as a good neurological exam to assess neuropathy. The ABI can be obtained easily with the use of a standard blood pressure cuff and measuring the systolic blood pressure at the brachial and posterior tibial artery. If this ratio is less than 0.9, it suggests the presence of PAD. In patients with diabetes, this ratio is often greater than 1 which suggests medial calcinosis. Often using a combination of ABI and peripheral vascular resistance is performed, and this provides more information about the arterial circulation; however, this test

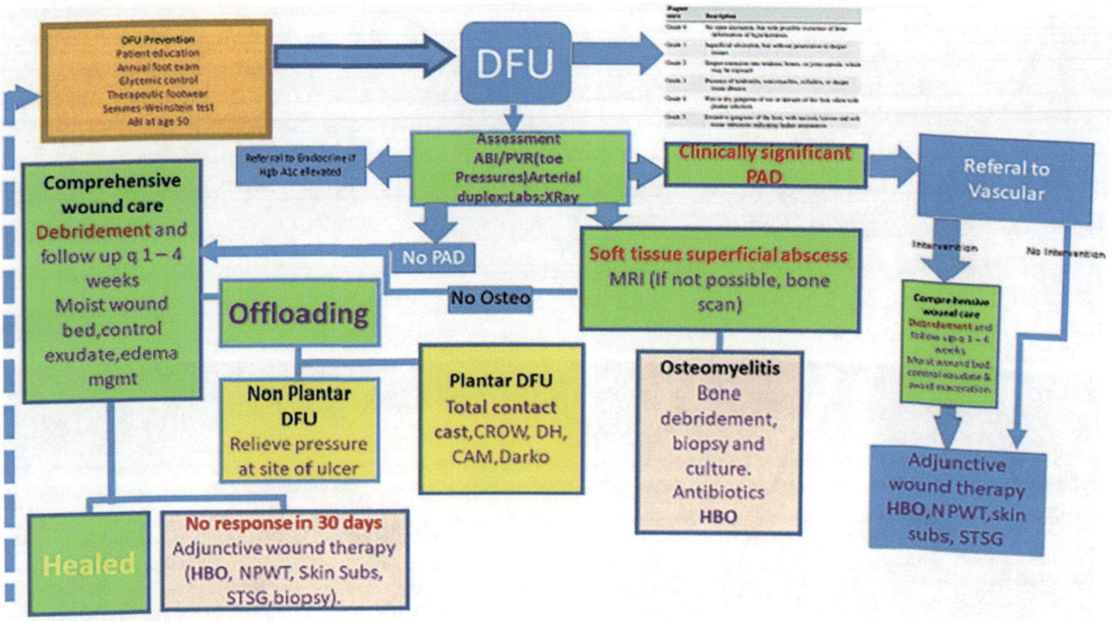

Fig. 37.4 DFU algorithm

needs to be performed in a vascular laboratory. Assessing the patient's digital hair growth and skin condition also provides valuable information about the patient's circulation. The presence of digital hair and normal skin quality is consistent with adequate circulation. Another option is the use of a pulse oximeter to compare the SaO_2 of the fingers to the toes. A difference of 2% or more is as accurate as ABI testing to diagnose lower extremity arterial disease.

After assessment of vascular status, a thorough neurological examination must be performed. Using a monofilament, the Semmes–Weinstein monofilament exam is performed by placing the monofilament perpendicular to the skin and applying pressure until the filament buckles (Fig. 37.5). This should be performed on the plantar surface of the hallux, sub first, third, and fifth metatarsal sites. Absence of sensation at any of these sites is considered a positive test for neuropathy. Evaluating the foot for the presence of any callous formation, deformity, fungal nails, hammer toes, and plantar/dorsi flexion is also a critical part of the exam.

After a thorough exam of both feet attention should then be focused on the wound. Wound photography and measurements are taken at each visit, and the wound should be evaluated for probe to bone. If the wound probes to bone, the presence of osteomyelitis is highly likely. Imaging starting with plain films of both feet followed by advanced imaging such as MRI, CT, or bone scan is required. At this point, surgical debridement needs to be planned if adequate circulation is present and the patient is not in extremis. For patients presenting with sepsis surgical debridement and/or amputation is required. Consultation with foot and ankle surgery or podiatry is recommended to plan debridement and maximize functional outcome. During the debridement pathology and tissue cultures of the deepest level of tissue left behind should be taken with clean instruments in order to guide antibiotic therapy.

Care Coordination

According to the Agency for Healthcare Research and Quality (AHRQ), care coordination is the intentional management of patient care by the individual(s) coordinating the care with the

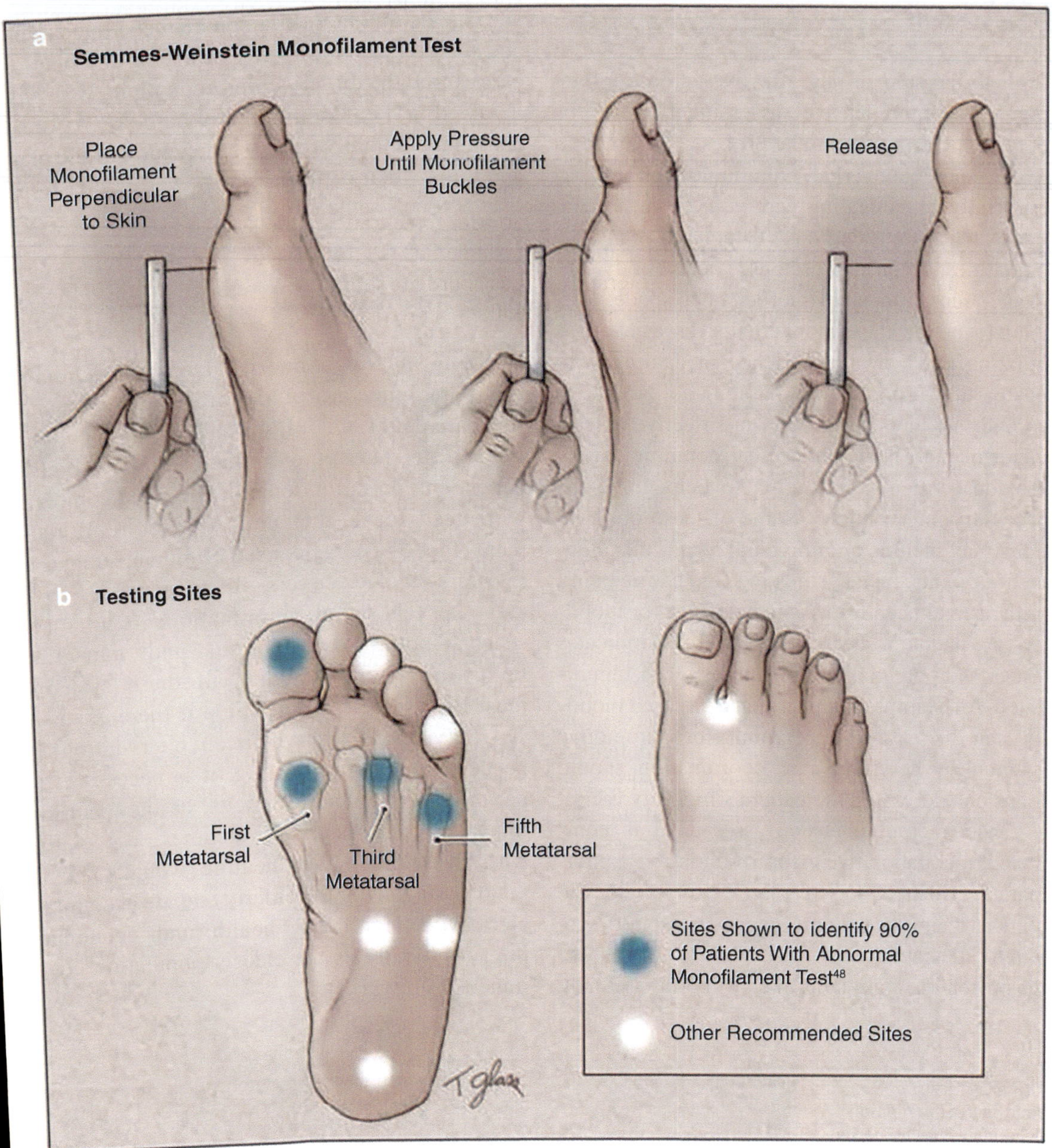

Fig. 37.5 Semmes–Weinstein monofilament exam

patient, and other healthcare personnel or agencies to deliver safe, high-quality care. This can be accomplished by licensed clinicians such as a nurse navigator, case manager. Nurse manager, staff nurse, or nurse coordinator. In the absence of a licensed clinician, a non-licensed individual may be assigned the role such as a navigator, care coordinator, or an individual familiar to clinical workers on the role of care coordination. Regardless of the care coordination model, care coordination remains a high priority area for quality improvement throughout all of healthcare.

Assessment

Prior to the start of any effective care coordination, a comprehensive assessment must be obtained. During the intake process, it is imperative to note nonverbal communication (NVC) especially when dealing with vulnerable populations such as the elderly. NVC includes many cue modalities, facial expressions, vocals, body language, sensation, and interpersonal space. It is vital to notice these nonverbal cues as well as utilizing one's own experience in dealing with this particular population that may not be able to verbally let their needs known. Effective assessment, of both NVC and verbal communication, provides critical information to help guide the necessary interventions. Some of these observations may include an individual's gait, misalignment of joints, facial grimacing (indicating pain), or their total need for assistive devices for mobility. A patient's decreased mobility indicates issues and potential complications when unmitigated. An example of this is that decreased mobility can increase the potential for automotive accidents. Therefore, care coordination should focus on addressing the patient's mobility issues.

Once a comprehensive assessment is completed, a collaborative effort of choosing a pragmatic, evidenced-based plan occurs with the clinical team, the patient, and their support system to alleviate many of these issues and resolve the presenting complaint. A care coordinator may act as a facilitator and liaison between the patient and the clinical team(s) by verifying the plan of care through direct communication with all involved in the patient's direct care. The coordinator should finally reinforce teaching of the plan and utilize their expertise in answering questions to everyone's satisfaction.

Assessment Tool

Utilizing nursing theorist Dorothea Orem's metaparadigm concept, definition of person and self-care deficit model, we can focus on patient systems to determine if the patient is totally dependent, partially dependent, or independent with need for further education or reinforcement (Fig. 37.6). A licensed clinician, such as a registered nurse, covers all the patient's systems: psychosocial, elimination, regulatory, sensory-motor, oxygenation, and nutrition. Following Orem's model, all these systems must be assessed to determine if there exists a self-care deficit for which an intervention is needed. For wound healing, it is necessary to pay attention to these deficits, as they can all impact wound healing outcomes, especially with the elderly. Non-healing wounds are a major issue facing the elderly and are accompanied with significant health and economic impact globally as the elderly population continues to grow.

Fig. 37.6 Care coordination in relation to patient self-care needs

Patient self care	Care Coordination
Totally dependent	Identify patient's support system and include them in the patient's plan of care. Determine available long term care options and discuss what is pragmatic and evidenced based. Involvement of the primary care physician and other specialists.
Partially dependent	Implementation of collaborative team(s) of other allied health care agencies and ancillary specialists. Communicate with patient and all caregivers and reinforce plan of care.
Independent	Reinforce patient education and plan of care. Communicate with involved care teams and needed heath care agencies and DME companies. Prepare patient for discharge self care.

Case Study

An 82-year-old male presents to the wound care clinic with a complaint of multiple traumatic wounds due to a fall. Vitals: 180/98, R-20, P-88, afebrile. Noted is the patient's imbalance and unsteady gait. Patient lives alone and admits they have no support system. Here a focused approach will only be concerned with the presenting complaint but unless the self-care issues are properly addressed, the patient will continue to have recurring falls and injuries. Therefore, treatment should be multifaceted rather than focused whereby the plan of care includes employment of healthcare agencies, fall prevention strategies, physical and occupational therapy, involvement of primary care physician, and other allied specialists. This is not to suggest that the wound healing clinician should undertake every detailed aspect of care outside their purview. But as the saying goes, if you see something say something.

Psycho-Social

The focus in assessing psychosocial aspects is to determine the patient's mental capacity and the ability to adhere to the plan of care and to understand the patient's available support system at home and in the community. A self-care deficit could prompt the need for family/significant other involvement and allied healthcare agencies for many reasons. This can be accomplished through a family meeting or over the phone, where the plan of care is delineated and determines what is pragmatic for the family to undertake. Not only will this type of coordination be most beneficial to secure a plan of care, but it is also necessary from a legal standpoint. Who is legally responsible for all the decision-making and who is legally able to consent for the patient? It is vital to determine the health care proxy (HCP) for all care coordination must go through that individual. What if the patient is alert and oriented but demonstrates deficits in comprehension, which in part can be caused by patient anxiety? Care coordination would focus on education reinforcement, or the patient may appoint a designee to assist in comprehending the plan, which does not necessarily have to be a legal HCP. In most instances, it is the spouse or significant other, the next-door neighbor, religious leader, friend, or another healthcare professional. It is essential for effective care coordination to identify the responsible individual that can help convey, and even support, the plan of care. What if the patient has little to no support system at all? What if they are living in someone else's residence and are not allowed to have ordered home health services? What if they are homeless, uninsured, or undocumented? Caring for these vulnerable groups is challenging to successfully deliver quality care. A perfect evidenced-based treatment plan may not be pragmatic for these individuals and quite possibly be harmful, as in the example of a limb compression dressing turning into a tourniquet. These patients are in danger of limb loss or worse. In these cases, involvement of social services, government agencies, and other health agencies may be a necessary part of the plan of care. It is the care coordinator's responsibility to be aware of services that are available to these patients so that they can provide optimal care coordination.

Care coordination must be safe for both patient and clinician. An unsafe environment does not foster trust between the patient and caregiver. If the home health service provider does not feel safe within the patient's environment, delivery of care of these services will be most challenging and not optimal for quality care. At this point, it may be necessary to visit a clinic more frequently than if the home services were in place. If clinic visits are not available or within reason for the patient to travel more frequently, then a long-term solution must be brought up for discussion with the patient, their support system (or lack thereof), and the healthcare team. Delivery of home services to shelters and hotels may be more readily available to the patient than in their current living conditions. If after every effort and opportunity has been afforded to the patient and the team, and still the pragmatic evidenced-based plan of care has not been able to effectively execute, then choices for the patient must be presented to them for palliative care or in some instances, hospice care. If there is no reasonable expectation for adequate wound healing to take place, then the focus of advanced therapies and the risks, time, and costs that each brings, are no longer necessary and there must be a paradigm shift in our model from wound healing to optimization of the patient's quality of life as the primary focus.

Elimination

Addressing a patient's elimination deficits can be as simple as a referral to a continence nurse, or as complex as having a discussion with them regarding surgical intervention addressing incontinence issues. Most common pressure injury sites are proximal to fecal contamination and erosive urinary incontinence. Optimal wound healing for pressure injuries occurs when wound bioburden, drainage, offloading, continence management, nutrition, and hydration are properly managed. Management of bioburden and infection are challenging when the wound is continually exposed to excrement and/or if the surrounding healthy skin is slowly eroded away from excessive moisture from urine.

Regulatory

Determination of a patient's difficulty in adherence to prescribed therapies by other specialists is primarily the thought process in care coordination for regulatory issues. An elevated HgbA1C can indicate a patient's struggle in maintaining an adequate diabetic regimen. All too quickly we can mistakenly judge the patient as noncompliant. Care coordination should be focused on determining if the patient is first knowledgeable of their diagnosis and the treatment plan. Any deficits can signal point of contact education and a referral to a specialist or healthcare program. Additionally, it needs to be determined whether the patient can afford his prescribed medication or a specialist visit or not. For the care coordinator, this challenge can be met through research of available programs for the vulnerable population that cannot afford costly medications. Many of these programs can be offered by the manufacturer themselves through coupons or hardship requests. It has been shown that uncontrolled diabetes does have an effect on wound healing and vascular circulation. Mismanagement or no management of these underlying diseases leads to poor outcomes for the patient and wound healing.

Sensory-Motor

Determination of a patient's mobility and sensation is necessary to establish before any plan can be implemented. If the patient cannot reach their wound to adequately care for themselves, then implementation of the patient's support system in conjunction with outside health services such as physical therapy (PT) to help improve physical mobility and muscle strength, occupational therapy (OT) to improve function and activities of daily life (ADLs), home health attendants/aides to assist with patient ADLs, home health nursing to carry out the plan of care and be the teams extra set of eyes of the patient in the community. Implementation of assistive devices to improve mobility and function may be necessary to help improve the patient's mobility. Such devices are referred to as durable medical equipment (DME) and range from walking canes to motorized wheelchairs, from simple offloading seat cushions to a hospital bed with a group I, II, or III sleep surface. Much of care coordination is utilized in assisting the patient in obtaining such needed devices. Ordering a DME can be challenging when it comes to determining what the patient's health care coverage will cover or deny. Each request of a DME must be justified as medically necessary in regard to this patient and their particular issue and need. Patience is needed for both the healthcare team and the patient when DMEs are ordered but the coverage does not cover the need. Each patient should be encouraged to determine what each of their policies will cover. Unfortunately, this can be laborious for the patient as well as the healthcare team if there is not a dedicated person working solely on these issues. These coordinators come in the shape of case managers, social workers, navigators, nurses, or unlicensed office staff. Whoever the designated care coordinator is, they must have an excellent knowledge of the diagnoses, treatment protocols, team members, and excellent communication skills with the team, the patient, the support system, outside agencies, and other health care organizations (HCOs), must have an adequate knowledge of insurance coverage and an ability to communicate effectively with them. In summary, most private offices cannot afford the luxury of retaining a licensed professional to accomplish all of this effectively; therefore, the physician must take on this role, even if the office secretary is doing some of these things, and they may even be more knowledgeable, still the onus lies upon the licensed professional.

Oxygenation

Adequate circulation and oxygenation of tissue is vital for wound healing. Many patients have respiratory issues like chronic obstructive pulmonary disease (COPD) to poor peripheral circulation. No oxygen means tissue death. As a care coordinator, the focus would be on whether the patient has proper follow-ups with specialists that are treating the patient issues. If not, then a referral to a specialist can be suggested. Does the patient have care coordination for delivery of oxygen DME? If not, a care coordinator can communicate with the specialist's office and determine if they will care for the patient's oxygen needs. Poor circulation is highly prevalent among the diabetic population. Lack of circulation, arterial or vascular or both, necessitates an immediate referral to vascular specialists to determine if an intervention can be performed to improve this. Care coordination would focus on assisting patients with making their appointment, confirmation of said appointment, and return follow-up after the appointment. Another intervention that can potentially improve circulation or perfusion to the wound is hyperbaric oxygen therapy (HBOT). Coordination would then focus on the ability for the patient to obtain access to HBOT as prescribed by the physician. The patient is again encouraged to determine what their insurance policy covers, such as transportation benefits. Some coverages allow for transportation to and from treatments. Many insurances require letters of medical necessity with corroborating clinical documentation as well as their referral form. Keep in mind, each patient must be transported to their destination safely and without contraindication to their diagnosis. For example, it would be inappropriate for the patient to be transported to their appointments in a wheelchair if they have pressure injuries that they will be resting on during transport. Transportation can take longer than anticipated leaving the patient placing additional unneeded pressure to their wounds. Likewise transporting a patient via stretcher when their wound does not qualify them for ambulance (stretcher) transportation is inappropriate and the cost of the total trip can fall upon the patient if the transportation need could not be supported with documentation. Or worse, qualifying a patient for a Medicare covered service, when the guideline strictly states they do not, then fraudulently ordering these services can have repercussions upon our licenses if it is determined that Medicare or Medicaid fraud was committed.

Nutrition and Hydration

It is evident that poor nutrition leads to poor outcomes multisystem wide. It comes as no surprise that adequate nutrition and hydration is therefore vital to wound healing. After determination through nutrition screening, physical exam, and supporting labs, and malnutrition or dehydration has been established, coordination of care should focus on whether the patient has adequate nutrition available to them. Can they afford nutritious healthy choices or do they find themselves making poor choices because of economic determinants. Do they have a need for a referral to a speech and swallow specialist? Maybe they need a referral to correct any dental issues impeding their ability to masticate or swallow? Do they have their cultural foods available to them? Do they have meal assistance? Do they have the ability to obtain groceries? What is their knowledge regarding proper nutrition? After determining the deficit areas, the care coordinator may make a referral to a nutritionist. Supplements can be ordered by the physician, but do they have the ability to obtain these?

Conclusion

Due to the inevitable biological dysfunctions that accrue with advancing age, the skin of elderly patients is prone to develop wounds of various etiologies which can prove difficult to heal. Ensuring optimal wound prevention and treatment is a multidisciplinary endeavor involving a multitude of wound care and other specialists adhering to evidence-based protocols. Care coordination for the elderly wound care patient is challenging and requires a multifaceted approach by a knowledgeable licensed professionals with excellent communication skills, collaboratively involved in the patient's care and ensuring care needs and goals are being met.

References

1. Russell-Goldman E, Murphy GF. The pathobiology of skin aging: new insights into an old dilemma. Am J Pathol. 2020;190(7):1356–69. https://doi.org/10.1016/j.ajpath.2020.03.007.
2. Ge Y, Miao Y, Gur-Cohen S, et al. The aging skin microenvironment dictates stem cell behavior. Proc Natl Acad Sci U S A. 2020;117(10):5339–50. https://doi.org/10.1073/pnas.1901720117.
3. Liu N, Matsumura H, Kato T, et al. Stem cell competition orchestrates skin homeostasis and ageing. Nature. 2019;568(7752):344–50. https://doi.org/10.1038/s41586-019-1085-7.
4. Honnegowda TM, Kumar P, Udupa EGP, Kumar S, Kumar U, Rao P. Role of angiogenesis and angiogenic factors in acute and chronic wound healing. Plast Aesthet Res. 2015;2(5):243–9. https://doi.org/10.4103/2347-9264.165438.
5. Bentov I, Reed MJ. The effect of aging on the cutaneous microvasculature. Microvasc Res. 2015;100:25. https://doi.org/10.1016/J.MVR.2015.04.004.
6. Howard B, Bascom CC, Hu P, et al. Aging-associated changes in the adult human skin microbiome and the host factors that affect skin microbiome composition. J Investig Dermatol. 2022;142(7):1934–1946.e21. https://doi.org/10.1016/J.JID.2021.11.029.
7. Larson PJ, Zhou W, Santiago A, et al. Associations of the skin, oral and gut microbiome with aging, frailty and infection risk reservoirs in older adults. Nat Aging. 2022;2(10):941–55. https://doi.org/10.1038/s43587-022-00287-9.
8. Carrieri AP, Haiminen N, Maudsley-Barton S, et al. Explainable AI reveals changes in skin microbiome composition linked to phenotypic differences. Sci Rep. 2021;11(1):1–18. https://doi.org/10.1038/s41598-021-83922-6.
9. Margolis DJ, Bilker W, Santanna J, Baumgarten M. Venous leg ulcer: incidence and prevalence in the elderly. J Am Acad Dermatol. 2002;46(3):381–6. https://doi.org/10.1067/MJD.2002.121739.
10. Vasudevan B. Venous leg ulcers: pathophysiology and classification. Indian Dermatol Online J. 2014;5(3):366–70. https://doi.org/10.4103/2229-5178.137819.
11. Howell RS, Gorenstein S, Castellano M, et al. Wound care center of excellence: guide to operative technique for chronic wounds. J Am Coll Surg. 2018;226(2):e7–e17. https://doi.org/10.1016/J.JAMCOLLSURG.2017.11.002.
12. Brem HH, Tomic-Canic M, Tarnovskaya A, et al. Healing of elderly patients with diabetic foot ulcers, venous stasis ulcers, and pressure ulcers. Surg Technol Int. 2003;11:161–7.
13. Schultz EM, McDonald KM. What is care coordination? Int J Care Coord. 2014;17(1–2):5–24. https://doi.org/10.1177/2053435414540615.
14. Hall JA, Horgan TG, Murphy NA. Nonverbal communication. Annu Rev Psychol. 2019;70:271–94.
15. Hartweg DL. Dorothea Orem: self-care deficit theory. Thousand Oaks: Sage; 1991. p. 58.

Necrotizing Soft Tissue Infections 38

Dennis J. Zheng and Areti Tillou

Case Presentation

A 78-year-old man with a history of hypertension, diabetes mellitus, and heart failure presented to the emergency department with altered mental status. History was obtained from the patient's caregiver because he was non-verbal on arrival. The caregiver reported that the patient had begun to complain of left leg pain 4 days prior to presentation; gradually he stopped walking and grew incoherent.

Upon initial evaluation, vital signs were notable for heart rate 85 beats/min, blood pressure 169/140 mmHg, respiratory rate 21 breaths/min, temperature 97.4 °F (36.3 °C), and oxygen saturation 95%. Physical examination displayed bilateral lower extremity edema with patches of erythema, scattered ecchymoses, and multiple non-hemorrhagic bullae most prominent in the left lower extremity. Initial laboratory testing showed white blood cell count 19×10^9/L, creatinine 3.4 mg/dL, pH 7.32, lactic acid 8.2 mg/dL. Intravenous fluids were administered and broad-spectrum antibiotics were initiated. Computed tomography of the left lower extremity revealed soft tissue swelling of lower segments, obliteration of subcutaneous fat planes, and significantly thickened deep fascia, with imaging findings interpreted as uncomplicated soft tissue infection.

Following admission to the intensive care unit, the patient was treated with high-flow oxygen, correction of electrolyte imbalance, and other supportive measures while comprehensive infectious workup was performed. Over the next 12 h, the patient's left lower extremity worsened in appearance, with discoloration progressing from red to dark purple and spreading to the foot. The patient became hemodynamically unstable, requiring increased intravenous fluid resuscitation and vasopressor support. General surgery was consulted, and given increasing suspicion for necrotizing soft tissue infection, the patient was taken urgently to the operating room.

Intra-operatively, necrotic skin over the anterolateral and posterior surfaces of the left calf was excised and copious yellow-gray discharge was released. The underlying fascia was clearly non-viable and were easily separated from surrounding tissues upon palpation. All necrotic tissue was debrided and a sample was sent for pathological analysis. The wound was thoroughly irrigated with normal saline and hydrogen peroxide before it was dressed with gauze soaked in Dakin's solution. The patient was transported still intubated and mechanically ventilated back to the intensive care unit. The following day he returned to the operating room for additional

D. J. Zheng · A. Tillou (✉)
Department of Surgery, David Geffen School of Medicine at UCLA, Los Angeles, CA, USA
e-mail: dzheng@mednet.ucla.edu; atillou@mednet.ucla.edu

P. Petrone, C. E.M. Brathwaite (eds.), *Acute Care Surgery in Geriatric Patients*,
https://doi.org/10.1007/978-3-031-30651-8_38

debridement, wash-out, and placement of negative pressure wound therapy. Over the next several days, the patient's hemodynamics and mental status improved significantly as antibiotic treatment was tailored to microbial culture results. Two weeks following the first debridement, a split-thickness skin graft was applied to the wound, and he was eventually discharged home without issue. At 6-month follow-up, his surgical areas appeared fully healed and he was able to walk with a slight limp.

Introduction

Necrotizing soft tissue infection (NSTI) is a severe condition characterized by rapidly progressive local tissue damage and powerful systemic inflammatory response. It may occur in any or all layers of skin and soft tissue in any part of the body and always necessitates prompt recognition, appropriate antimicrobial therapy, and timely surgical intervention. No discrete laboratory value or imaging study can definitively exclude the presence of necrotizing infection, which remains a difficult clinical diagnosis due to its rarity and diversity of presentations. Surgical exploration is the gold standard for both confirmation and treatment of NSTI. Although they are associated with significant morbidity and mortality in patients of all ages, NSTIs are of particular importance in the geriatric population. Older patients are more susceptible to challenges in early diagnosis, acute management, and optimization of long-term healing. When appropriate, strong clinical suspicion must be maintained to avoid delays in care and maximize the likelihood of favorable outcomes.

Epidemiology

NSTI is one of many types of skin and soft tissue infections (SSTIs), a broad grouping of pathologies that may involve the skin, underlying subcutaneous tissue, superficial or deep fascia, and/or muscle. Many classification systems function to further categorize SSTI by variables such as anatomic location, depth of extension, or presence of purulence. Of the millions of SSTI cases occurring each year, a small proportion (1000, according to some estimates) are categorized as NSTI, based on the presence of necrosis in any layer of the soft tissue compartment. Though relatively imprecise, the estimated incidence of NSTI overall has increased over the past several decades worldwide. The annual incidence of necrotizing *fasciitis*, the most common type of NSTI, range from 0.3 to 15 cases per 100,000 persons per year. By comparison, the necrotizing forms of SSTI at the level of muscle (*myositis*) or skin (*cellulitis*) are much less common. Advancing age is a well-documented predisposing factor for SSTI, the incidence of which increases with each decade of life. Over 25% of all NSTI patients are over the age of 60.

Etiology/Risk Factors

NSTIs may originate primarily (without apparent site of entry) or as a secondary event following a break in the skin barrier. After invasion, bacteria (or their spores) proliferate and release enzymes and toxins that damage local vasculature and lead to ischemic necrosis of tissues. Toxins may also cause systematic manifestations of sepsis through mechanisms such as massive cytokine release, potentially leading to multisystem organ dysfunction. Thus, risk factors for NSTI include any event leading to breaching of skin, such as penetrating trauma, blunt trauma (muscle strain or sprain), burns, insect bites or injection drug use, recent surgical incision, or mucosal injury such as hemorrhoids. Other known risk factors include immunosuppressive conditions including diabetes, cirrhosis, neutropenia, and HIV. Inadequately treated SSTI such as decubitus ulcer or perirectal abscess can also progress to NSTI.

Understanding NSTI through this framework helps explain why the elderly are particularly at risk for infections of the skin and soft tissue; as humans age, the skin thins and wounds heal more poorly, becoming a more vulnerable site of entry for bacteria. Older adults are more likely to contend with chronic skin disorders or wounds, sores, and ulcers resulting from immobility, inability to care for one's self, or peripheral vascular disease. Additional contributing factors are general age-related changes such as decreased humoral and cellular immunity, malnutrition, and chronic medical comorbidities. These various causes of immune dysfunction may prevent elderly patients from mounting the appropriate physiologic and innate immunologic response to the bacterial endotoxins and exotoxins involved in NSTI.

Age is commonly associated with mortality and greater needs at discharge. Two groups have specifically analyzed outcomes among geriatric patients diagnosed with NSTI over the past two decades. Gebran et al. utilized the American College of Surgeons National Surgical Quality Improvement Project database to analyze the clinical course of 1460 patients over the age of 65 diagnosed with NSTI. The authors found that pre-operative liver or kidney dysfunction (as evidenced by hyperbilirubinemia, coagulopathy, or hemodialysis dependence), malnutrition (demonstrated by hypoalbuminemia), and septic shock were significant predictors of mortality, as was age above 80. In patients without these characteristics, 30-day survival was 93%. A study of Medicare claims data performed by McCarty et al. reached similar conclusions. In a sample of 1427, patients aged 65 and above with NSTI, risk factors for in-hospital mortality and worsened disposition at discharge included malignancy, liver, and kidney disease—all markers of decreased physiologic reserve. Nearly two-thirds of study patients required discharge to a facility for supplementary care.

Classification

As is the case for SSTI, several classification systems group NSTI by anatomic location or depth of infection, giving rise to a host of related monikers such as *Fournier's gangrene* (involving the genitals or perineum), *Ludwig's angina* (submandibular and sublingual spaces), or *Meleney's gangrene* (abdominal wall). The clinical utility of these methods of classification is debatable, given that the initial approach to management does not significantly differ. Of the myriad ways of describing NSTI, likely the most useful methodology is based on describing the deepest layer of tissue with necrotic involvement: whether necrotizing *cellulitis*, necrotizing *fasciitis*, or necrotizing *myositis*.

NSTI is also commonly categorized by bacterial pathogen and clinical characteristics: type I, II, or III.

- Type I is a polymicrobial infection caused by mixed aerobic and anaerobic bacteria and makes up the majority of all NSTIs. *Escherichia coli*, *Bacteroides fragilis*, and *streptococcus* are common isolates and may act synergistically to increase toxicity. These mixed infections typically affect the elderly or those with medical comorbidities, particularly diabetes. They may be associated with soft tissue gas. Necrotizing cellulitis is one variant.
- Type II is a monomicrobial infection. It may occur in healthy, immunocompetent patients and in any age group, often with no clear portal of entry. Causative agents include *Streptococcus pyogenes* and *Staphylococcus aureus* most frequently. The bacteria involved produce exotoxins, which may lead to cytokine release and inflammatory response throughout the body.
- Type III infections have been attributed to water-dwelling organisms such as *Vibrio vulnificus* or *Aeromonas hydrophila*, and Clostridium bacteria (leading to clostridial myonecrosis or gas gangrene), depending on the source.

Some authors have posited a more complex relationship between NSTI mortality, geography, and microbiology. A recently published study of microbial data at 12 centers across North America described up to 28 bacterial species involved in NSTI, with polymicrobial infections (type I) most prevalent in all regions. No geographic region or microorganism type predicted mortality though type I infection was associated with increased mortality and prolonged hospitalization. As a consequence, initial empirical antibiotic regimen should incorporate broad-spectrum agents with anti-MRSA, anti-Gram-negative, and anaerobic coverage. Clindamycin or linezolid should be included to inhibit toxin production from Gram-positive pathogens.

Presentation and Diagnosis

NSTI most commonly occurs in the extremities (lower more than upper) but can affect any region of the body, including the perineum, trunk, or head and neck. The initial presentation of the patient with NSTI may include pain out of proportion to physical findings, edema, swelling, and erythema; differentiating between cellulitis and NSTI at this point may be challenging, especially because the characteristic crepitus is not present in roughly half of cases. The "hard signs" of NSTI—advanced skin findings such as hemorrhagic bullae, ecchymosis, or visible necrosis—may develop within 1–2 days, coupled with systemic signs of sepsis (fever, tachycardia, hypotension) in intermediate or late stage of the disease. Because fascia has a relatively poor blood supply compared to muscle tissue, overlying tissue layers may initially appear unaffected while the patient experiences severe pain. Diminished pain sensation or analgesia may later develop in the involved area.

Initial misdiagnosis of NSTI is common, exceeding 70% in some studies. Commonly described pitfalls preventing prompt diagnosis include lack of vital sign abnormalities (especially fever), absence of skin findings, equivocal imaging results, and generalized symptoms attributable to other causes. Maintaining a high index of suspicion is of great importance when caring for elderly patients, who may present with atypical or subtle signs and symptoms in the setting of NSTI. Older adults may complain only of constitutional issues such as malaise, lethargy, failure to thrive, or gastrointestinal symptoms (nausea, vomiting, diarrhea) wrongly linked to other pathologies such as gastroenteritis. Fever may be masked by NSAIDs, either self-administered or prescribed for pain. Underlying cognitive impairment or functional decline can render history-taking more difficult, and age-related diminished immune system function may hinder the development of obvious vital sign or laboratory abnormalities. As such, geriatric patients may present in the advanced stages of NSTI.

Workup

NSTI is predominantly a clinical diagnosis based upon history and physical examination, yet the absence of classic physical signs should not be used to rule out presence of the disease. Laboratory testing may aid in the diagnostic process; common abnormal findings may include leukocytosis and elevated markers of acute inflammation such as C-reactive protein. In cases suspicious for NSTI, blood cultures should be drawn prior to initiation of antibiotics.

First published in 2004, the Laboratory Risk Indicator for NECrotizing Fasciitis (LRINEC) is a well-known method of stratifying suspicion for early NSTI based on six laboratory parameters: C-reactive protein, white blood cell count, hemoglobin, sodium, creatinine, and glucose. LRINEC score of 8 or higher is meant to confer a high risk of NSTI. Multiple systematic reviews and meta-analyses on the diagnostic accuracy of the LRINEC score have failed to demonstrate high sensitivity or specificity. This is of particular relevance for elderly patients, who are more likely to have abnormal laboratory values at baseline. Other NSTI scoring systems that build upon LRINEC values have been more recently developed, but none may be used in isolation of clinical suspicion.

Similarly, radiologic imaging may be a useful adjunct in the diagnostic process as long as it does not delay surgical exploration. Plain radiographs may show soft tissue gas in the affected area, but many cases of NSTI (especially those in the early stages) may not involve subcutaneous gas. In a retrospective analysis including 172 patients with surgically proven NSTI, computed tomography (CT) was diagnostic or suspicious in 97.3% of cases, while plain X-ray was significantly less sensitive. Key findings on CT scan include fat stranding, fluid and gas collections dissecting along fascial planes, and soft tissue gas. The addition of intravenous contrast may reveal thickening of the superficial and deep fascia or non-enhancing fascia, suggestive of fascial necrosis. Cross-sectional imaging can be particularly helpful when body habitus renders physical examination unreliable and also aids in surgical planning. As with X-ray, the absence of gas does not exclude NSTI.

Magnetic resonance imaging is the modality of choice for definitive identification of necrotizing fasciitis but is not recommended as first-line imaging technique, due to its low specificity and inaccessibility in the emergent setting. Some have studied the utility of bedside ultrasound in differentiating between cellulitis and NSTI, but this practice is not yet widespread. Proposed diagnostic adjuncts such as fine-needle aspiration or incisional biopsy of suspicious areas of skin are not routinely recommended.

Treatment

Management of NSTI is complex, involving multiple medical and surgical disciplines, but at its core relies upon three fundamental components: timely and adequate surgical debridement, strict microbiological surveillance, and targeted high-dose antibiotic regimens.

In any patient with an elevated suspicion of NSTI, the cornerstone of management is operative intervention. Early surgical debridement and removal of all necrotic tissue (ideally within the first 6–12 h following admission) has been overwhelmingly shown to be the most important determinant of outcome in NSTI, decreasing mortality and other complications. Recognition of this has led to the declaration by various authors that "time is fascia." Resuscitation or treatment of sepsis should not delay transport to the operating room, where NSTI may be definitively diagnosed and treatment can be initiated.

Kongkaewpaisan et al. underlined the importance of minimizing surgical delay in a recent single-center review from 2007 to 2018. Of 91 patients eventually diagnosed with NSTI, nearly a quarter of the cohort was not admitted to a general surgery service. Over half of these were misdiagnosed, and unsurprisingly, the non-surgical service patients experienced significant delays in time to surgical incision resulting in a trend towards greater mortality.

The initial surgical approach involves incising the affected area and thoroughly exploring the wound for gross findings such as absence of bleeding, loss of tissue resistance to blunt dissection (the "finger test"), and/or murky, foul-smelling, gray-brown (or "dishwater") fluid. All necrotic, infected, devitalized, and non-viable tissue in the layers of muscle, fascia, subcutaneous tissue, and skin must be removed until healthy, bleeding tissue is reached. Sharp debridement using a scalpel blade or Metzenbaum scissors for larger areas of tissue is advisable. Of note, underlying tissue necrosis may extend beyond the boundaries of skin involvement, mandating an aggressive debridement. Subcutaneous or submuscular pockets must be probed along wound margins, and irrigation with not only saline but also antiseptic solution is recommended. Intraoperative specimens should be sent for microbiological studies and histologic evaluation.

In situations where skin viability is unclear, an approach that spares as much skin as possible is recommended. Wound re-exploration will likely be necessary and viability of the remaining skin may be re-assessed at that time. The wound should be left open with coverage with saline-moistened dressings though some recommend use of dressings soaked in povidone iodine or sodium hypochlorite. For patients in need of aggressive resuscitation and correction of fluid and electrolyte abnormalities, a damage control strategy may be employed. Typically, re-exploration of the wound to determine adequacy of source control and verify lack of disease progression should take place at least within 12–24 h, or sooner depending on signs of worsening local or systemic infection. Re-exploration should continue until all necrotic tissue has been removed and the patient has clinically stabilized. Most will require multiple debridements and procedures during their hospitalization.

Fasciotomy may be required if compartment syndrome is suspected or occurs following resuscitation. In some cases of extensive extremity involvement, amputation may be necessary. In the event of Fournier's gangrene, wide debridement remains a mainstay. Diverting colostomy may be helpful to minimize bacterial load in the perineal wound. In less complex cases, fecal diversion with rectal tubes may be adequate.

Antibiotic therapy should be promptly initiated and after blood cultures are drawn. Similar to delays in surgical treatment, delays in antibiotic administration have also been linked to adverse outcomes. It is crucial to initiate a broad-spectrum regimen covering against Gram-positive, Gram-negative, and anaerobic organisms.

Patients with NSTI commonly display systemic manifestations of the inflammatory process, which require early and aggressive treatment to improve outcomes. Aside from timely initiation of empiric antimicrobial treatment, the critically ill may require hemodynamic and metabolic support in the form of generous fluid resuscitation, vasoactive medications, and other means of organ support. De-escalation of antibiotic therapy should be based on clinical improvement and microbial culture data. Principles of geriatric-focused post-operative care should be followed when determining appropriate pain management, thromboembolism prophylaxis, delirium prevention, early mobilization, and optimal enteral nutrition support.

The role of hyperbaric oxygen as adjuvant treatment following debridement remains controversial, with insufficient evidence to support its use. Based on recent evidence intravenous immunoglobulin may be considered in patients with NSTI caused by group A streptococcus but its use for other pathogens is not currently supported. Negative pressure wound therapy may facilitate wound care and improve healing following the completion of debridement. Soft tissue loss resulting from proper surgical management may be significant and require definitive closure with tissue flaps or skin grafting.

Surgical and wound care techniques commonly used in burn centers may be indicated to ensure maximal restoration of function. Though traditional teaching warns against taking reconstruction into account at the time of debridement, minimizing initial resection of uninvolved skin and subcutaneous tissue may aid in patient recovery. Tom et al. described an institutional shift in surgical approach to NSTI at their tertiary center from 2012 to 2016; in cohort of 487 patients with NSTI, the adoption of skin-sparing debridement was associated with significantly higher rates of wound closure and non-inferior rates of source control, mortality, or post-operative complications.

Outcomes

Mortality of NSTI has historically varied in the literature in the range of roughly 5–50%. Advancements in critical care and awareness of the importance of timely surgical intervention have helped reduce NSTI mortality over the past several decades. In statewide or international studies from the past two decades, predictors of increased mortality have included a range of variables such as in-patient coagulopathy, advanced age, electrolyte abnormalities, increased creatinine or need for hemodialysis, history of malignancy, and general medical comorbidities.

Nationwide analyses of geriatric patients with NSTI from recent decades have demonstrated mortality rates of 5% and 19%. Although mortality seems to have decreased in recent years, morbidity secondary to complications remains high in the elderly. Those who survive commonly suffer from functional impairment and changes in body appearance, often worsening previously limited mobility. Recently published studies have demonstrated the significant effects of NSTI on physical and psychological quality of life. A retrospective analysis by Urbina et al. found severe impairments in physical components compared to the general population among 49 patients treated for NSTI at a French tertiary center who were administered the Short-Form Health Survey at a median follow-up time of 1.5 years. In addition to physical effects, the authors noted that mental health problems were more prevalent in

NSTI survivors compared to survivors of septic shock of non-NSTI etiologies, especially in patients requiring intensive care.

References

1. Brakenridge SC, Efron PA, Stortz JA, Ozrazgat-Baslanti T, Ghita G, Wang Z, et al. The impact of age on the innate immune response and outcomes after severe sepsis/septic shock in trauma and surgical intensive care unit patients. J Trauma Acute Care Surg. 2018;85:247–55. https://doi.org/10.1097/TA.0000000000001921.
2. Gebran A, Gallastegi AD, Gaitanidis A, King D, Fagenholz P, Kaafarani HMA, et al. Necrotizing soft tissue infection in the elderly: effect of pre-operative factors on mortality and discharge disposition. Surg Infect. 2022;23:53–60. https://doi.org/10.1089/sur.2021.130.
3. McCarty AR, Villarreal ME, Tamer R, Strassels SA, Schubauer KM, Paredes AZ, et al. Analyzing outcomes among older adults with necrotizing soft-tissue infections in the United States. J Surg Res. 2021;257:107–17. https://doi.org/10.1016/j.jss.2020.06.031.
4. Moore SA, Levy BH, Prematilake C, Dissanaike S. The prediction predicament: rethinking necrotizing soft tissue infections mortality. Surg Infect. 2015;16:813–21. https://doi.org/10.1089/sur.2015.002.
5. Louis A, Savage S, Utter GH, Li S-W, Crandall M. NSTI organisms and regions: a multicenter study from the American Association for the Surgery of Trauma. J Surg Res. 2019;243:108–13. https://doi.org/10.1016/j.jss.2019.05.006.
6. Stevens DL, Bryant AE, Goldstein EJC. Necrotizing soft tissue infections. Infect Dis Clin N Am. 2020;35:135–55. https://doi.org/10.1016/j.idc.2020.10.004.
7. Fernando SM, Tran A, Cheng W, Rochwerg B, Kyeremanteng K, Seely AJE, et al. Necrotizing soft tissue infection: diagnostic accuracy of physical examination, imaging, and LRINEC score: a systematic review and meta-analysis. Ann Surg. 2019;269(1):58–65. https://doi.org/10.1097/SLA.0000000000002774.
8. Leichtle SW, Tung L, Khan M, Inaba K, Demetriades D. The role of radiologic evaluation in necrotizing soft tissue infections. J Trauma Acute Care Surg. 2016;81:921–4. https://doi.org/10.1097/TA.0000000000001244.
9. Kongkaewpaisan N, Hwabejire J, Lee JM, Narueponjirakul N, Meier K, Mendoza A, et al. Necrotizing soft tissue infection: time is crucial, and the admitting service matters. Surg Infect. 2020;21:828–33. https://doi.org/10.1089/sur.2019.262.
10. Mohanty S, Rosenthal RA, Russell MM, Neuman MD, Ko CY, Esnaola NF. Optimal perioperative management of the geriatric patient: a best practices guideline from the American College of Surgeons NSQIP and the American Geriatrics Society. J Am Coll Surg. 2016;222(5):930–47. https://doi.org/10.1016/j.jamcollsurg.2015.12.026.
11. Tom LK, Maine RG, Wang CS, Parent BA, Bulger EM, Keys KA. Comparison of traditional and skin-sparing approaches for surgical treatment of necrotizing soft-tissue infections. Surg Infect. 2020;21:363–9. https://doi.org/10.1089/sur.2019.263.
12. Eguia E, Vivirito V, Cobb AN, Janjua H, Cheung M, Kuo PC. Predictors of death in necrotizing skin and soft tissue infection. World J Surg. 2019;43:2734–9. https://doi.org/10.1007/s00268-019-05087-8.
13. Suzuki H, Muramatsu K, Kubo T, Kawasaki M, Fujitani T, Tsukamoto M, et al. Factors associated with mortality among patients with necrotizing soft tissue infections: an analysis of 4597 cases using the diagnosis procedure combination database. Int J Infect Dis. 2021;102:73–8. https://doi.org/10.1016/j.ijid.2020.10.019.
14. Urbina T, Canoui-Poitrine F, Hua C, Layese R, Alves A, Ouedraogo R, et al. Long-term quality of life in necrotizing soft-tissue infection survivors: a monocentric prospective cohort study. Ann Intensive Care. 2021;11(1):102. https://doi.org/10.1186/s13613-021-00891-9.

Perioperative Management of Geriatric Patients

39

David A. Lieb II, Dalia Alqunaibit, Srinivas Reddy, Corrado P. Marini, and John McNelis

Introduction

The percentage of the US population age 65 and older has increased from 9.2% of the population in 1960 to 16.9% in 2020. This increase translates into an increasing proportion of geriatric patients, defined as age 65 and older, among the surgical population. In addition to age-related physiological changes and frailty, these patients are more likely to have multiple medical comorbidities compared to the adult population. These can result in several challenges such as an increased risk of malnutrition, post-operative delirium, urinary retention, and pulmonary complications. All of these can result in increased morbidity and mortality if not recognized and managed appropriately. This chapter will discuss several of the unique challenges posed by geriatric patients during the pre-operative, intra-operative, and post-operative periods.

D. A. Lieb II · D. Alqunaibit · S. Reddy · C. P. Marini · J. McNelis (✉)
Department of Surgery, Albert Einstein College of Medicine, Jacobi Medical Center, Bronx, NY, USA
e-mail: John.McNelis@nychhc.org

Recommendations for the Pre-operative, Intra-operative, and Post-operative Periods

Pre-operative

The American College of Surgeons (ACS) and the American Geriatrics Society (AGS) issued joint guidelines regarding optimal perioperative management of geriatric patients. This management starts pre-operatively, which starts with a thorough discussion regarding patient treatment goals and preferences, to include any advanced health directives and designated healthcare proxies. It likewise entails a thorough pre-operative assessment to identify patients at high risk for frailty and for medical optimization.

Nutrition and Fasting

Part of this entails identifying geriatric patients at risk for malnutrition, who are at particular risk of malnutrition. This increased risk is due to several factors, namely the increased prevalence of cognitive and functional decline, socioeconomic circumstances, increased likelihood for polypharmacy and multiple medical comorbidities, and age-related changes such as diminished appetite, slower gastrointestinal transit time, and decreased oropharyngeal muscle mass that can lead to dysphagia. In fact, as many as 15% of geriatric patients overall, and around 25—60% of geriatric patients in long-term care facilities,

P. Petrone, C. E.M. Brathwaite (eds.), *Acute Care Surgery in Geriatric Patients*,
https://doi.org/10.1007/978-3-031-30651-8_39

meet criteria for malnutrition. Malnutrition is associated with several adverse outcomes and complications in surgical patients, to include impaired wound healing, increased risk of surgical site infections, increased overall length of hospital stay, and increased mortality.

Given the significant adverse effects of malnutrition and the increased risk in geriatric patients, it is important not just to identify patients at risk for malnutrition prior to surgery, but also to optimize patients' nutritional status as feasible. All patients should undergo a nutritional risk assessment to include assessment of recent oral intake, prior to surgery. While several screening tools exist, some common patient characteristics indicative for malnutrition risk include a body mass index (BMI) of less than 18.5 kg/m^2, overall weight loss of at least 10—15% within the last 6 months, pre-operative serum albumin less than 3.0 g/dL, and critical illness. Patients identified at high risk for malnutrition during assessment should undergo nutritional therapy for 7—14 days pre-operatively, even if this would require a delay in surgery. Oral nutritional supplements are preferred, and parenteral nutrition is indicated only if patients are not able to consume adequate nutrition and supplementation enterally.

Pre-operative management in geriatric patients likewise entails considerations for fasting and medical management. Traditionally, surgical patients were made strictly NPO at midnight prior to surgery to limit aspiration risks intraoperatively. However, recent evidence suggests that prolonged fasting periods are associated with worse surgical outcomes. Prolonged fasting can lead to poor nutritional status and dehydration pre-operatively, both of which are even greater risks in geriatric patients. As a result, revised ACS and American Society of Anesthesiologists (ASA) guidelines now allow for shorter preoperative fasting periods for elective procedures. These guidelines now permit consumption of clear liquids up to 2 h prior to surgery and light meals and milk up to 6 h before surgery although meals with fried food, fatty food, or meat may require more time before surgery. It is important to recognize that patients with comorbidities affecting gastric emptying (such as diabetes and hiatal hernia) may require longer times between oral intake and surgery than these guidelines specify.

Intra-operative

Anesthesia

Aging is associated with several physiological changes that become pertinent when administering general anesthesia. Several changes directly affect the ability of geriatric patients' ability to metabolize medications utilized during anesthesia. Loss of liver volume and blood flow result in decreased hepatic clearance of medications. Renal changes include decreased number of nephrons, renal blood flow, and glomerular filtration rate, which increase the risk of acute kidney injury and impair clearance of renally cleared medications and anesthetics. Additionally, geriatric patients generally have increased body fat and decreased total body water. All these changes can lead to higher plasma concentrations of medications and decreased metabolism and elimination of medications. As such, geriatric patients may take longer to emerge from anesthesia, and dosages of anesthesia should be adjusted accordingly.

In terms of cardiovascular status, geriatric patients tend to have higher systolic blood pressures due to stiffening of vascular structures, higher baseline sympathetic tone, and decreased chronotropic and inotropic responses to sympathetic stimulation. All of these can result in greater hemodynamic lability and hypotension compared to younger adult patients.

Most importantly, geriatric patients undergo pulmonary changes with age, notably reduced lung volumes, reduction in alveolar surface area, decreased chest wall compliance, reduced vital capacity and tidal volume, and reduced arterial oxygenation. These changes can result in increased work of breathing and atelectasis in response to anesthesia. Furthermore, these patients often undergo loss of pharyngeal muscle support and coughing and swallowing response, in turn increasing the risk of airway obstruction and aspiration. All the above changes and responses to anesthesia place geriatric patients at increased risk of pulmonary complications in the perioperative period.

Given these age-related changes and associated risks in geriatric patients, some providers have advocated using regional anesthesia (e.g., neuraxial blocks, epidural anesthesia) either as the primary modality or as an adjunct to general anesthesia in geriatric patients. However, definitive evidence of the benefits of regional anesthesia vs. general anesthesia is limited. For instance, a 2017 meta-analysis investigating hip fracture surgery found no significant differences in 30-day mortality or rates of post-operative delirium, pneumonia, or other complications between general anesthesia and regional anesthesia. Reducing exposure to general anesthesia may be beneficial for geriatric patients, but decisions regarding anesthesia modality should balance this against the feasibility of such methods for a given procedure.

Perioperative Analgesia

In addition to anesthetic considerations in geriatric patients, providers should also consider perioperative analgesia plans in these patients. Care should be taken to avoid certain medications in geriatric patients associated with post-operative delirium, hemodynamic impairment, or respiratory dysfunction. The Beers criteria from the AGS provide a comprehensive list of these medications that should be avoided, which include anticholinergics, barbiturates, benzodiazepines, meperidine, and muscle relaxants. Although there has been concern regarding the risk of bleeding with non-steroidal anti-inflammatory drugs (NSAIDs), such as ibuprofen, their use is likely safe in the absence of other contraindications for use. However, for geriatric patients, NSAIDs should be administered at the lowest reasonable dose for as short of a period as feasible to limit potential bleeding and gastrointestinal risks.

While opioids are explicitly among this list of medications to avoid, they should be used judiciously in geriatric patients. In addition to potentiating the sedative effects of other medications, changes associated with aging ultimately make geriatric patients more sensitive to opioids, thereby increasing the risk of delirium, respiratory depression, and possible death. As such, multimodal pain management should be utilized for geriatric patients. These approaches, particularly when utilizing NSAIDs and COX-2 inhibitors such as celecoxib, can help decrease opioid requirements and risk of pulmonary complications.

Each analgesia plan should be individualized based on individual patient characteristics, such as baseline levels of pain. However, a stepladder approach is reasonable for geriatric patients. Mild pain can be addressed with paracetamol, with or without co-administration of NSAIDs. Analgesia can be escalated to codeine or tramadol for moderated pain, with tramadol associated with fewer respiratory side effects but with an increased risk of delirium. For severe pain, opioids can be used, although doses should be started at the lowest possible and monitoring for tolerance. Additional adjuncts, such as lidocaine patches and regional anesthesia techniques, may be utilized as appropriate.

Intra-operative Management

Outside of anesthesia and analgesic considerations, it is important to consider certain intra-operative management considerations for geriatric patients. Pressure injuries are of particular concern given age-related changes in skin resulting in fragility. Advancing age, long OR cases (particularly those lasting 6 h or longer), poor nutritional status, medical comorbidities, and ASA status are all factors associated with increased pressure injury risk. Prevention of these injuries requires consideration not just for patient characteristics, but also with regard to patient positioning to identify possible sites of pressure injuries. Foam pads should be placed at potential injury sites, particularly for longer OR cases.

In addition to increased risk of pressure injuries, geriatric patients also face the risk of intra-operative pulmonary aspiration, which can cause significant morbidity and mortality. This increased risk is attributable not just to age-related changes in pulmonary and neurological function, but also the increased prevalence of oropharyngeal dysphagia due to changes in musculature and the GI system. Following pre-operative fasting recommendations can limit this risk, but intra-operative management can further limit this risk. If neuromuscular blockers are to be used, long-acting neuromuscular blockers should be avoided, and patients should have sufficient recovery neuromuscular function prior to extubation. Additionally, elevating the head of the bed prior to anesthesia induction, use of low tidal volume ventilation (i.e., 6–8 mL/kg of ideal body weight), and using laparoscopic surgical approaches when feasible can also reduce the risk of pulmonary complications.

Hypothermia

Hypothermia, defined as a core body temperature below 36 °C, is another concern for geriatric patients. Anesthetic agents impair thermoregulation, limit vasoconstriction, and lower the core temperature at which shivering occurs, all of which increase the risk of intra-operative hypothermia. This risk is further increased in geriatric patients due to age-related degeneration of thermoregulatory mechanisms. Even mild cases of intra-operative hypothermia are associated with coagulopathy and increased blood loss, wound infections, poor wound healing, and longer time to anesthesia emergence. While preventing intra-operative hypothermia is important for all surgical patients, it is particularly so for geriatric patients.

Several methods can be utilized to limit heat loss and prevent hypothermia. The most utilized include passive heating with blankets, forced air warming systems, and warmed intravenous fluids. Blankets can reduce heat loss from skin by up to 30%, which is sufficient counteract heat loss due to effects from anesthesia. However, because patients can still lose heat from exposed areas (such as the intra-operative field), blankets alone are insufficient to prevent intra-operative hypothermia. As such, active warming (typically as forced air blankets) is typically used in addition to blankets although quality evidence regarding specific benefits is limited. A 2016 Cochrane review highlighted decreased rates of surgical site infections when active warming devices were utilized, as well as lower rates of perioperative cardiovascular events in select population although insufficient evidence existed regarding other benefits.

Post-operative

Although most geriatric patients progress appropriately in the post-operative period, they are at a greater risk of complications when compared to the general population. These complications can result in persistent impairment in daily function and quality of life following discharge, or even death. Many post-surgical complications can occur across all surgical patients, but there are certain complications of concern among geriatric patients.

Nutrition in the Post-operative Period

As discussed, geriatric patients are at greater risk for malnutrition compared to the general population, and this likewise extends to the post-operative period. Given this and the associated risk of complications due to malnutrition, optimizing nutritional status postoperatively is of utmost importance in geriatric patients. In addition to pre-operative nutritional assessment, geriatric patients should also undergo nutritional assessment postoperatively to identify those at risk for malnutrition. A rule of thumb for nutritional needs postoperatively is 25–30 kcal/kg of ideal body weight and 1.5 g of protein per kg of ideal body weight.

Evidence suggests that early initiation of enteral feeding postoperatively results in improved outcomes without significantly increasing the risk of ileus or anastomotic leaks. For most patients, starting clear liquids within 24 h postoperatively and advancing diet as tolerated is reasonable. However, several patients may not be able to consume sufficient calories orally postoperatively, which can increase the risk of malnutrition postoperatively. If patients, particularly those identified as high risk for malnutrition, are not expected to be able to consume at least 50% of their caloric needs within 7 days of surgery, tube feeding should be considered. This particularly applies to patients undergoing certain surgical procedures, such as head and neck surgeries. In cases where tube feeding is indicated, feeds should ideally be started within 24 h of surgery, starting at a low rate (i.e., 10–20 mL/h) and titrated up to goal rate as tolerated. Standard whole protein formula is appropriate for most patients.

Enteral nutrition, either via tube feeding or oral intake, is preferable to parenteral nutrition due to the lower associated risk of infectious complications, shorter overall hospital stay, and lower cost. However, several patients will have conditions precluding enteral feeding, such as intestinal obstruction. Additionally, several patients may have impaired absorption within the gastrointestinal tract. Therefore, parenteral nutrition should be initiated in those patients who are not expected to tolerate oral or enteral feeds for at least 5 days following surgery, as well as those not expected to meet 50% of caloric needs for at least 7 days with both enteral and oral nutrition.

Post-operative Delirium and Cognitive Dysfunction

Post-operative delirium (POD) is one of the most well-known complications of geriatric surgical patients. The prevalence of POD in geriatric patients is around 10% although this percentage can be above 40% among patients requiring ICU admission and as high as 50% in some studies. A concurrent risk is post-operative cognitive dysfunction (POCD), in which cognitive deficits persist after surgery. Pre-operative cognitive impairment and dementia are the most significant risk factors for postoperative delirium although advanced age and pre-operative pain levels are also significant risk factors.

Given the significant increases in morbidity and mortality associated with POD, preventing POD is vital, particularly in the geriatric population. General principles in the geriatric population include environmental measures to promote natural sleep-wake cycles, as well as avoiding medications associated with delirium such as benzodiazepines. Additionally, steps can be taken at each stage of the operative period to reduce the risk of POD. Comprehensive geriatric assessment and prehabilitation prior to surgery, the use of bispectral index (BIS) and addition of dexmedetomidine to anesthesia intra-operatively, and judicious use of antipsychotics post-operatively are all associated with a lower risk of POD in geriatric patients. While reducing exposure to general anesthesia does appear to reduce post-operative delirium risk, the evidence for neuraxial anesthesia to this end is mixed. As always, any discussions regarding anesthesia in geriatric patients should be done in a multi-disciplinary manner with anesthesia, as well as other providers as appropriate.

Pulmonary Complications

Pulmonary complications are another significant source of morbidity and mortality for geriatric surgical patients. This encompasses a broad range of derangements to include pneumonia, pulmonary thromboembolism, and acute respiratory distress syndrome. Advanced age, frailty, associated infections, existing cardiopulmonary disease, hypoalbuminemia, and renal disease are all significant risk factors for pulmonary disease.

In addition to pre-operative optimization and limiting the risk of intra-operative aspiration, post-operative management should also focus on preventing aspiration and other pulmonary complications. These include early mobilization out of bed, aspiration precautions (to include elevating the head of the bed) and performing swallow evaluations for patients whose clinical or cognitive status puts them at high risk for aspiration. Multimodal pain management is also vital to reduce the need for opioid pain medications, and by extension, the risk for respiratory depressions. Additionally, regular chest physiotherapy, to include incentive spirometry and chest percussion, are associated with decreased rates of post-operative pneumonia and should be incorporated into management.

Urinary Retention

Urinary retention is a common issue in the post-operative period and is typically treated with catheterization. However, prolonged use of indwelling urinary catheters is associated with an increased risk of catheter-associated urinary tract infections (CAUTI), which is in turn associated with increased morbidity and mortality. Therefore, it is important to identify patients at high risk for urinary retention.

Geriatric patients have several risk factors for post-operative urinary retention (POUR). Aging can result in gradual degeneration of the nerves innervating the bladder, resulting in impaired sensation of bladder fullness and emptying. Male geriatric patients are at particularly increased risk of urinary retention due to the increased incidence of benign prostatic hypertrophy (BPH), which can cause obstruction and limit voiding. Additionally, geriatric patients are more likely to have neurologic comorbidities (e.g., diabetic neuropathy, stroke) associated with urinary retention. Finally, geriatric patients are more likely to be on medications that increase the risk for urinary retention, such as beta blockers and anticholinergics.

In addition to age-related risk factors, the type of surgery and anesthesia used can affect the risk of POUR as well. Urinary retention is a particular concern for inguinal hernia repair and for pelvic surgeries (e.g., anorectal cases) due to the proximity of pelvic nerves responsible for voiding. Excessive intravenous fluid administration, particularly in these cases, further increases the risk of POUR. General anesthetic agents inhibit detrusor muscle contraction, and longer cases with general anesthesia are associated with an increased risk of retention. For cases utilizing neuraxial anesthesia, large doses of anesthetic agent or use of long-acting anesthetic agents likewise increase the risk of POUR.

Management of POUR largely centers around limiting exposure to risk factors for retention. Limiting the use of IV fluids intra-operatively, as well as utilizing techniques that limit the dose and duration of neuraxial anesthesia (such as use of local anesthetic), can reduce the risk of retention. Additionally, alpha blockers can be helpful for patients at high risk of retention, especially for anorectal cases and for those with known BPH. Finally, avoiding anticholinergic medications and limiting opioid use can limit the risk of POUR.

However, even with all measures taken, patients may still develop urinary retention and require catheterization. Prior to catheterization, providers should obtain an ultrasound of bladder volume, with catheterization indicated if bladder volume exceeds 600 mL. The use of indwelling versus intermittent catheterization remains controversial, as does the recommended duration of indwelling catheter use (if utilized). Generally, for patients at lower risk for retention, indwelling catheterization can be limited to 24 h. Patients undergoing major surgery, particularly major pelvic surgery, longer indwelling catheterization may be required.

Conclusion

Perioperative management of geriatric patients follows similar principles to management for the general surgical population. However, due to age-related physiological changes and the increased rate of medical comorbidities, perioperative management should be modified accordingly. These changes include pre-operative nutritional optimization, considerations for limiting exposure to general anesthesia, multimodal pain management, and interventions to limit the risk of pulmonary complications. Interventions continue into the post-operative period with early initiation of nutrition (when feasible) to limit the risk of malnutrition, as well as prevention and optimal management of urinary retention. Post-operative delirium is of particular concern among geriatric patients, and a significant part of management entail prevention and avoiding exposures associated with delirium. All these considerations are vital for optimal outcomes in the geriatric population.

References

1. US Census Bureau 2020. Census summary file. Washington, DC: US Census Bureau; 2021.
2. Mohanty S, Rosenthal RA, Russell MM, Neuman MD, Ko CY, Esnaola NF. Optimal perioperative management of the geriatric patient: a best practices guideline from the American College of Surgeons NSQIP

and the American Geriatrics Society. J Am Coll Surg. 2016;222(5):930–47. https://doi.org/10.1016/j.jamcollsurg.2015.12.026.
3. Weimann A, Braga M, Carli F, Higashiguchi T, Hübner M, Klek S, et al. ESPEN guideline: clinical nutrition in surgery. Clin Nutr. 2017;36(3):623–50. https://doi.org/10.1016/j.clnu.2017.02.013.
4. Alvis BD, Hughes CG. Physiology considerations in geriatric patients. Anesthesiol Clin. 2015;33(3):447–56. https://doi.org/10.1016/j.anclin.2015.05.003.
5. O'Donnell CM, McLoughlin L, Patterson CC, Clarke M, McCourt KC, McBrien ME, et al. Perioperative outcomes in the context of mode of anaesthesia for patients undergoing hip fracture surgery: systematic review and meta-analysis [Corrigendum: Br J Anaesth. 2018;120(6):1442-4]. Br J Anaesth. 2018;120(1):37–50. https://doi.org/10.1016/j.bja.2017.09.002.
6. American Geriatrics Society. By the 2019 American Geriatrics Society Beers Criteria® update expert panel. American Geriatrics Society 2019 updated AGS Beers Criteria® for potentially inappropriate Medication use in older adults. J Am Geriatr Soc. 2019;67(4):674–94. https://doi.org/10.1111/jgs.15767.
7. Schofield PA. The assessment and management of peri-operative pain in older adults. Anaesthesia. 2014;69(Suppl 1):54–60. https://doi.org/10.1111/anae.12520.
8. Bulfone G, Bressan V, Morandini A, Stevanin S. Perioperative pressure injuries: a systematic literature review. Adv Skin Wound Care. 2018;31(12):556–64. https://doi.org/10.1097/01.ASW.0000544613.10878.ed.
9. Entriken C, Pritts TA. Perioperative pulmonary support of the elderly. Curr Geriatr Rep. 2021;10(4):167–74. https://doi.org/10.1007/s13670-021-00369-3.
10. Lim BG, Lee IO. Anesthetic management of geriatric patients. Korean J Anesthesiol. 2020;73(1):8–29. https://doi.org/10.4097/kja.19391.
11. Sessler DI. Perioperative thermoregulation and heat balance. Lancet. 2016;387(10038):2655–64. https://doi.org/10.1016/S0140-6736(15)00981-2.
12. Madrid E, Urrútia G, Roqué i Figuls M, Pardo-Hernandez H, Campos JM, et al. Active body surface warming systems for preventing complications caused by inadvertent perioperative hypothermia in adults. Cochrane Database Syst Rev. 2016;4(4):CD009016. https://doi.org/10.1002/14651858.CD009016.pub2.
13. Janssen TL, Alberts AR, Hoof L, Mattace-Raso FUS, Mosk CA, van der Laan L. Prevention of postoperative delirium in elderly patients planned for elective surgery: systemic review and meta-analysis. Clin Interv Aging. 2019;14:1095–17. https://doi.org/10.2147/CIA.S201323.
14. Brown CH, Edwards C, Lin C, Jones EL, Yanek LR, Esmaili M, et al. Spinal anesthesia with targeted sedation based on bispectral index values compared with general anesthesia with masked bispectral index values to reduce delirium: the SHARP randomized controlled trial. Anesthesiology. 2021;135(6):992–1003. https://doi.org/10.1097/ALN.0000000000004015.
15. Baldini G, Bagry H, Aprikian A, Carli F. Postoperative urinary retention: anesthetic and perioperative considerations. Anesthesiology. 2009;110(5):1139–57. https://doi.org/10.1097/ALN.0b013e31819f7aea.

Surgical Risk Assessment in the Elderly

40

John McNelis, David A. Lieb II, Erin R. Lewis, Dalia Alqunaibit, and Corrado P. Marini

Surgeons, like most specialists, are increasingly faced with an aging patient population. Approximately 33% of procedures in 2010 were performed in patients older than 65 years of age. The percentage is projected to double by 2030. Approximately 50% of patients over 65 years of age will undergo a surgical procedure during their twilight years. A per US Census data, the mean age of the US population has risen from 29.5 in 1960 to 38.6 in 2020. The percent of the population below the age of 18 has decreased from 35.7% in 1960 to 22.2% in 2020. Conversely, the percent of population older than 65 has risen from 9.2% of the population in 1960 to 16.9% of the population in 2020. In the elderly category, those aged 80 or greater, the percent of the population has risen from 1.4% in 1960 to 4% of the total population in 2020. Hence, surgeons are increasingly faced with operations on population often with multiple comorbid conditions. As the population ages, however, a contrast between biologic and chronologic age emerges. Surgeons will frequently encounter very vibrant 70- or even 80-year-old patients and very frail 50-year-old ones. Therefore, the need for adequate risk assessment evaluation and optimization becomes critical in determining risk of procedures and to discern the healthy elderly patients from the frail high-risk ones.

Perioperative evaluation and risk assessment of the geriatric patient is a sequential process incorporating pre-operative and perioperative decision-making and pre-operative risk assessment and risk stratification, with special attention to functional status, cognition, and frailty. In addition to traditional comprehensive evaluation, with focus on medical testing and geriatric-specific assessments followed by pre-operative optimization, several risk assessment tools can also be employed.

Risk assessment begins with surgical decision-making and an assessment of the patient's decision-making capacity. After assessment of decision-making capacity is established, discussions with the patient or surrogate to establish goals of care should be clarified at the outset. If the patient's goals and priorities are not achievable with surgery, nonoperative or palliative options should be considered. If surgery is aligned with the patient's goals and priorities, the role of surgery in achieving these goals should be thoroughly discussed including risks and benefits of surgery. It is critical at this stage to establish advanced directives including establishment of a healthcare proxy and treatment goals. Informed consent and establishment of advance directives

J. McNelis (✉) · D. A. Lieb II · E. R. Lewis · D. Alqunaibit C. P. Marini
Albert Einstein College of Medicine, Jacobi Medical Center, Bronx, NY, USA
e-mail: John.McNelis@nychhc.org; liebd@nychhc.org; lewise8@nychhc.org; alqunaid@nychhc.org; corradom@nychhc.org

P. Petrone, C. E.M. Brathwaite (eds.), *Acute Care Surgery in Geriatric Patients*,
https://doi.org/10.1007/978-3-031-30651-8_40

should be clarified early in the process. In focusing on the patients' goals and priorities it is especially important to elicit the patient's or surrogate's expectations and goals. Does the patient seek prolongation of life, independence, alleviation pain or something else? Further, all possible intra- and post-operative scenarios, including the expected quality of life post-operatively, should be clearly explained to the patient.

INCLUDEPICTURE "C:\\var\\folders\\z6\\mx5xfr8d7zq5dpx5w1p1svfm0000gp\\T\\com.microsoft.Word\\WebArchiveCopyPasteTempFiles\\page5image1970199504" * MERGEFORMAT Physiologic changes related to the aging process all organ systems: neurologic, cardiovascular, pulmonary, gastrointestinal, renal, hematologic, immunologic, endocrine, and musculoskeletal. Loss of brain mass increases with age resulting in progressive cerebral atrophy. In addition, there is decreased cerebral blood flow, peripheral neural denervation and decreased conduction velocity. Cognitive decline and behavior variability also increasingly manifests with aging. Cardiovascular effects of aging include a high incidence of a coronary artery disease and decreases in cardiac output, left ventricular compliance and baroreceptor response, as well as decreased vascular compliance which are important in mobilizing reserve and establishing homeostasis. Conduction system abnormalities leading to arrhythmias are prevalent in the elderly. Pulmonary problems of aging include decreased dynamic and static compliances, increasing VQ mismatch, decreased reserve volume, functional residual capacity and FEV_1, decreased response to hypoxia and hypercapnia and impaired ciliary function, important in clearing secretions. Elderly patients experience protein malnourishment, decrease in hepatic blood flow and impaired hepatic microsomal enzyme function, which will adversely affect the patient's ability to metabolize medications. Renal mass is decreased as is glomerular filtration, renal blood flow, with associated decrease urinary concentrating ability. The elderly also suffers from immunological dysfunction, increased insulin resistance as well as a diminished endocrine response to stress. The physiologic changes are summarized in Table 40.1.

In addition, elderly patients can also present with multiple comorbidities and polypharmacy issues, often unsure of dosing with questionable compliance compounded by poor functional and nutritional status. There are often communication comprehension issues that impede history taking and exacerbate social needs.

Collectively, these factors all diminish the elderly patient's physiologic reserve and the ability to mount an adequate stress response to surgery, which can lead to poor outcomes. It is important to note that not all elderly patients are necessarily compromised or debilitated, and

Table 40.1 Physiologic changes in the elderly

Neurologic	Loss of brain mass, <cerebral blood flow, <cerebral oxygen consumption, <neurotransmitters, cognitive decline, behavioral variability, <PNS conduction velocity, loss of peripheral neurons, denervation
Cardiovascular	CAD, <CO, <LV compliance, autonomic dysfunction, <baroreceptor response, conduction system changes, valvular disease, <vascular compliance
Pulmonary	>Parenchymal compliance, <chest wall compliance, >*V*/*Q* mismatch, <respiratory muscle mass, rapid shallow breathing, >RV and FRC, <FVC and FEV1, <central response to hypoxia and hypercapnia, <ciliary function
Gastrointestinal	Protein malnourishment, <hepatic blood flow, <hepatic microsomal enzyme function, <drug metabolism, <plasma protein concentration
Renal	<Renal mass, <renal blood flow, <GFR, <urine concentrating ability, <response to plasma hormones
Hematologic	Anemia, <blood volume, <bone marrow cellularity
Immunologic	<Immune system function
Endocrine	Insulin resistance, <hormone (free T3, GH, aldosterone) production
Musculoskeletal	Decreased muscle mass, increased fat mass, impaired thermoregulation, skin fragility

many octogenarians may still have good performance status equivalent to patients several decades younger in age. Therefore, age in itself should not exclude an elderly patient from surgery. It is more important to differentiate chronological age from biological age, a combination of the pathophysiologic processes of aging, comorbidities, and genetic factors that better predicts fitness and performance in response to physiologic challenges. As such, adequate risk assessment in the elderly population depends more on physiologic assessment than purely chronological assessment, and the need for objective risk stratification tools becomes critical.

Risk Stratification Assessments

Traditional risk stratification tools include ASA classification, basic laboratory studies, exercise tolerance, evaluation of comorbidities and the revised cardiac index scales of Eagle, Goldman, and Detsky.

The American Society of Anesthesiologists (ASA) physical status classification is the most commonly used risk assessment tool. The ASA Physical Status Classification System has been in use for over 60 years. ASA score is assigned to all patients undergoing elective and emergent procedures regardless of patient age. ASA criteria consist of six classes of increasing severity score ranging from healthy (ASA 1) to brain dead awaiting harvesting (ASA 6), with an "E" is added for emergent surgeries. The ASA model has been validated in multiple studies as a reasonable predictor of mortality. For instance, the mortality for ASA 1E is 0–6% while a high risk 5E may face a 75–100% mortality. The purpose of the system is to assess and communicate a patient's pre-anesthesia medical comorbidities. The classification system alone does not predict the perioperative risks, but when used with other factors such as type of surgery, frailty, and level of deconditioning, it can be helpful in predicting perioperative risks. The full ASA classification table is summarized in Table 40.2.

The Goldman Multifactorial Risk Index is another widely used risk assessment tool to assess mortality risk in non-cardiac patients. The Goldman Index is a scoring system that incorporates age, pre-op MI within 6 months, significant aortic stenosis, non-sinus rhythm, premature ventricular beats greater than 5 per min, S3 gallop, and jugular venous distention (Table 40.3). An adjustment factor is then added for general medical status, high-risk surgery and emergency surgery. The Modified Goldman Index, while acknowledging chronological age, weighs physiologic function more heavily. For instance, a healthy 85-year-old without any associated Goldman Criteria would have a Goldman Score of 5 (Class 1-low risk) while a 55-year-old diabetic, hypertensive, renal failure patient with a recent history of an MI and atrial fibrillation undergoing emergency surgery would be a Class 4-high-risk patient.

Detsky's Modified Mortality Risk assessment is similar to Goldman's but incorporated pulmonary edema and an angina scale (Table 40.4). Our healthy 85-year-old undergoing elective laparoscopic cholecystectomy would still be low risk

Table 40.2 ASA classification

ASA	Definition
I	healthy patient
II	mild systemic disease
III	severe systemic disease
IV	severe systemic disease that is a constant threat to life
V	A severe systemic disease that is a constant threat to life without the operation
VI	A declared brain-dead patient whose organs are being removed for donor purposes

Table 40.3 Modified Goldman Index

	POINTS
Age > 70 Years	10
MI Within 6 Months	5
S3 or JVD	11
Aortic Stenosis Critical	3
Rhythm other than Sinus with or without PACs	7
5 or greater PVCs/minute anytime before surgery	7
Poor Medical Status	3
Intra-peritoneal ,thoracic or Aortic Surgery	3
Emergency Surgery	4
Total Points	53

CLASS	Points	None/Minor Complications	Life Threatening Complications	Cardiac Death
I	0-5	99%	.7%	.2%
II	6-12	93%	5%	2%
III	13-25	86%	11%	2%
IV	>26	22%	22%	56%

Table 40.4 Detsky risk factors

A. Age older than 70 years: 5 points
B. Prior myocardial infarction
1. Last infarction within 6 months: 10 points
2. Last infarction more than 6 months ago: 5 points
C. Unstable Angina within last 6 months: 10 points
D. Angina Pectoris
1. Canadian Angina Class 3: 10 points
2. Canadian Angina Class 4: 20 points
E. Alveolar pulmonary edema
1. Pulmonary edema within 1 week: 10 points
2. Pulmonary edema at any time: 5 points
F. Suspected critical aortic stenosis: 20 points
G. Arrhythmia
1. Rhythm other than sinus or sinus with PACs: 5 points
2. More than five premature ventricular beats: 5 points
H. Emergency surgery: 10 points
I. Poor general medical status: 5 points
1. Based on Goldman Risk Index
IV. Interpretation
A. Class 1: Points 0–15 (low risk)
B. Class 2: Points 20–30 (moderate risk)
C. Class 3: Points >30 (high risk)

with a Detsky score of 5, while our previously described 55-year-old diabetic hypertensive undergoing emergent surgery would have a Detsky score of 85 (High Risk).

The Charlson Comorbidity Index (CCI) is a scoring system that incorporates a series of comorbid conditions into a risk index that also does not incorporate chronologic age. It is, however, a significant component of the various frailty indices that have been developed for risk assessment and incorporates dementia into its assessment. Again our 85-year-old scheduled for cholecystectomy would have a CCI of zero, while a chronically ill would have a CCI of 8. CCI was the first scoring system that incorporated cognitive impairment as an independent risk factor. Cognitive impairment has been associated with increased mortality in the elderly population. Gajdos and Scarborough independently examined this issue. Gajdos identified patients with impaired sensorium as having a higher rate of pneumonia, ventilator dependence, renal failure, urinary tract infection, stroke, venous thromboembolism and death Scarborough in a propensity matched NSQIP retrospective study of patients undergoing complex vascular and general surgery also reported a higher incidence of mortality, major morbidity, and re-operation.

In 2009, Robinson et al. added a new component to risk assessment, namely, frailty. Since then, multiple modifications have been developed. Robinson's Original Frailty Score (FS) evaluated five predictors: cognitive assessment, albumin less than 3.4, history of recurrent falls, hematocrit less than 35, activities of daily living <6, and CCI. These indices were reflective of cognition, function, and comorbidities. The presence of four or more predictors was associated with significantly increased mortality. This represented a significant shift from previous risk assessment tools.

Makary et al. introduced their Frailty Score (Table 40.5) from Hopkins in 2010. Frailty was identified as a predictor of surgical outcomes based on a scoring system from zero to five that included weakness, weight loss, exhaustion with low physical activity, and slowed walking speed. Scores of 0–1 were considered non-frail, 2–3 intermediately frail, and 4–5 frail. Makary demonstrated that as frailty increases, so do post-op complications, length of stay, and discharge to a rehabilitation facility.

In 2014, Kim et al. refined the frailty score to incorporate the Charlson Comorbidity Index (Table 40.6), dependence in activities of daily living, dependence in instrumental activities of daily living (ADL), independent activities of daily living (IADL), dementia (MMSE), risk of delirium and malnutrition and musculoskeletal wasting. As seen previously, high-risk patients (Frailty score >5) demonstrated higher mortality and increased length of stay.

Multiple frailty scoring systems have been developed, some expressing their value as an index (FI)—(Frailty risk factors over total factors measured). The Comprehensive Geriatric Assessment Frailty Index (CGA-FI) incorporates previously described markers of frailty and sorts them into four categories: Medical History, Functional Status, Performance Status, and Nutrition. In the CGA-FI, a total of 50 data points is described. The GFI would be dependent on how many parameters were measured. Age does not appear on the GCA-FI. Our 85-year-old could very well have an FI of 0.0 (0/50), while our 55-year-old might have an FI as high as 0.3–0.5. Multiple studies across multiple surgical specialties have demonstrated the superiority of FI and FS in predicting surgical outcomes.

Other risk assessment tools include several surgical risk calculators, the most prominent one being the NSQIP risk calculator, developed from the American College of Surgeons National Surgical Quality Improvement Database. Risk is

Table 40.5 Makary/Hopkins Frailty Score 2010

Shrinking	Unintentional weight loss ≥10 lb. in 1 year
Weakness	Grip strength measurement
Exhaustion	Questions about effort and motivation
Low activity	Questions about leisure time activity
Slowed walking speed	Time to walk 15 feet

Table 40.6 Multidimensional Frailty Score

Item	0	1	2
Malignancy	No	Yes	NA
Charlson Comorbidity Index	0	1–2	>2
Albumin (g/dL)	≥3.9	3.5–3.9	<3.5
ADLs	Independent	Partially dependent	Dependent
IADLs	Independent	Partially dependent	Dependent
MMSE	Normal	MCI	Dementia
Risk of delirium (Nu-Desc)	0–1	≥2	NA
Mini nutritional assessment	Normal	Risk of malnutrition	Malnutrition
Mid-arm circumference (cm)	≥27	24.6–27	<24.5

determined on 21 patient-related variables: multiple pre-operative, demographic and operative variables to calculate the probability of post-operative events. It has been validated in predicting cardiovascular complications, however, may be of limited value in more complex or extremely critically ill patients.

The POSSUM scale (Physiological and Operative Severity Score for the enumeration of Mortality and Morbidity) is a scoring system that is used to predict risk-adjusted mortality and morbidity rates in surgical procedures. It consists of both Physiologic and Operative Variables. Our Healthy 85-year-old would have a predicted POSSUM mortality rate of 2.7%, while our 55-year-old would be significantly higher possibly exceeding 90% predicted mortality.

	Score			
Variable	**1**	**2**	**4**	**8**
Age (years)	≤60	61–70	≥71	
Cardiac signs	No failure	Diuretic, digoxin, antianginal, or hypertensive therapy	Peripheral edema, warfarin therapy	Raised jugular venous pressure
Chest radiograph			*Borderline cardiomegaly*	*Cardiomegaly*
Respiratory history	No dyspnea	Dyspnea on exertion	Limiting dyspnea (one flight)	Dyspnea at rest (rate ≥30/min)
Chest radiograph		*Mild COPD*	*Moderate COPD*	*Fibrosis or consolidation*
Systolic BP (mmHg)	110–130	131–170 100–109	≥171 90–99	≤89
Pulse (beats/min)	50–80	81–100 40–49	101–120	≥121 ≤39
Glasgow Coma Score	15	12–14	9–11	≤8
Hemoglobin (g/dL)	13–16	11.5–12.9 16.1–17.0	10.0–11.4 17.1–18.0	≤9.9 ≥18.1
White cell count (×10¹²/L)	4–10	10.1–20.0 3.1–4.0	≥20.1 ≤3.0	
Urea (mmol/L)	≤7.5	7.6–10.0	10.1–15.0	≥15.1
Sodium (mmol/L)	≥136	131–135	126–130	≤125
Potassium (mmol/L)	3.5–5.0	3.2–3.4 5.1–5.3	2.9–3.1 5.4–5.9	≤2.8 ≥6.0
ECG (Electrocardiogram)	Normal		Atrial fibrillation (rate 60–90)	Any other abnormal rhythm ≥5 ectopics/min Q waves or ST/T changes

Pre-operative Workup and Perioperative Management

Once the decision is made to proceed with surgery, pre-operative evaluation should include testing as per the ASA practice advisory. Tests should not be ordered routinely, even in elderly patients, as routine testing has not been shown to significantly change perioperative management. Rather, tests should be but rather on a selective basis for purpose of optimizing perioperative management. Included in pre-operative optimization is a comprehensive assessment to include medical, physical, functional, psychological, and socioeconomic factors. Such comprehensive geriatric assessments have been shown to reduce mortality and increase likelihood of independent living and adequate functional status post-operatively. Such assessments may also help improve post-operative outcomes to include decreasing the rates of post-operative pneumonia, delirium, decubitus ulcers, and inappropriate catheter usage, as well as aiding pain control and early mobilization. These assessments should be multi-disciplinary and should include contributions from the operating surgeon, geriatricians, pharmacists, internists, nurse specialists, physical and occupational therapists, dietitians, and social workers.

While medical conditions can be treated and optimized, frailty in itself is difficult to treat. Interventions are better established in the community. There is limited evidence of pre-operatively administering testosterone growth hormone and vitamin D in patients who are frail, but these have not been fully established in the surgical population. In addition, orthopedic and cardiac surgeons are increasingly utilizing pre-operative rehabilitation prior to surgery, which has been shown to reduce length of hospitalization in these patients.

Conclusion

Surgeons today must contend with an increasingly elderly surgical population. In general, the combination of age-related physiological changes and medical comorbidities decreases the physiological reserve of more elderly patients. This in turn increases the risk of perioperative and post-operative adverse events. However, there is often significant heterogeneity in the geriatric population, particularly in terms of functional status and the ability to tolerate surgery. Therefore, pre-operative assessment and risk stratification should focus on factors that might impair the ability of elderly patients to tolerate surgery to include medical comorbidities, frailty, and poor functional status. Several assessment tools exist to assist with these assessments. The results of these assessments should be used not just to guide goals-of-care discussions with patients and/or their surrogates but should also be used to guide pre-operative workup and testing should the decision be made to proceed with surgery.

References

1. US Census 2020. Census summary file. Washington, DC: US Census Bureau; 2021.
2. Kim S, Brooks AK, Groban L. Preoperative assessment of the older surgical patient: homing in on geriatric syndromes. Clin Interv Aging. 2015;10:13–27. https://doi.org/10.2147/CIA.S75285.
3. Oresanya LB, Lyons WL, Finlayson E. Preoperative assessment of the older patient: a narrative review. JAMA. 2014;311(20):2110–20. https://doi.org/10.1001/jama.2014.4573.
4. American Society of Anesthesiologists. ASA Physical Status Classification System 2020. https://www.asahq.org/standards-and-guidelines/asa-physical-status-classification-system.
5. Goldman L, Caldera DL, Nussbaum SR, Southwick FS, Krogstad D, Murray B, et al. Multifactorial index of cardiac risk in noncardiac surgical procedures. N Engl J Med. 1977;297(16):845–50. https://doi.org/10.1056/NEJM197710202971601.
6. Detsky AS, Abrams HB, McLaughlin JR, Drucker DJ, Sasson Z, Johnston N, et al. Predicting cardiac complications in patients undergoing non-cardiac surgery. J Gen Intern Med. 1986;1(4):211–9. https://doi.org/10.1007/BF02596184.
7. Charlson ME, Pompei P, Ales KL, MacKenzie CR. A new method of classifying prognostic comorbidity in longitudinal studies: development and validation. J Chronic Dis. 1987;40(5):373–83. https://doi.org/10.1016/0021-9681(87)90171-8.
8. Scarborough JE, Bennett KM, Englum BR, Pappas TN, Lagoo-Deenadayalan SA. The impact of functional dependency on outcomes after complex general and vascular surgery. Ann Surg. 2015;261(3):432–7. https://doi.org/10.1097/SLA.0000000000000767.
9. Robinson TN, Eiseman B, Wallace JI, Church SD, McFann KK, Pfister SM, et al. Redefining geriatric preoperative assessment using frailty, disability and co-morbidity. Ann Surg. 2009;250(3):449–55. https://doi.org/10.1097/SLA.0b013e3181b45598.
10. Makary MA, Segev DL, Pronovost PJ, Syin D, Bandeen-Roche K, Patel P, et al. Frailty as a predictor of surgical outcomes in older patients. J Am Coll Surg. 2010;210(6):901–8. https://doi.org/10.1016/j.jamcollsurg.2010.01.028.
11. Bilimoria KY, Liu Y, Paruch JL, Zhou L, Kmiecik TE, Ko CY, Cohen ME. Development and evaluation of the universal ACS NSQIP surgical risk calculator: a decision aid and informed consent tool for patients and surgeons. J Am Coll Surg. 2013;217(5):833–42. https://doi.org/10.1016/j.jamcollsurg.2013.07.385.
12. Copeland GP. The POSSUM system of surgical audit. Arch Surg. 2002;137(1):15–9. https://doi.org/10.1001/archsurg.137.1.15.
13. Apfelbaum JL, Connis RT, Nickinovich DG, Pasternak LR, Arens JF, Caplan RA, et al. Practice advisory for preanesthesia evaluation: an updated report by the American Society of Anesthesiologists Task Force on Preanesthesia Evaluation. Anesthesiology. 2012;116(3):522–38. https://doi.org/10.1097/ALN.0b013e31823c1067.
14. Partridge JS, Harari D, Martin FC, Dhesi JK. The impact of pre-operative comprehensive geriat-

ric assessment on postoperative outcomes in older patients undergoing scheduled surgery: a systematic review. Anaesthesia. 2014;69(Suppl 1):8–16. https://doi.org/10.1111/anae.12494.

15. Kim K, Park KH, Koo KH, Han HS, Kim CH. Comprehensive geriatric assessment can predict postoperative morbidity and mortality in elderly patients undergoing elective surgery. Arch Gerontol Geriatr. 2013;56(3):507–12. https://doi.org/10.1016/j.archger.2012.09.002.

General Surgical Emergencies

41

Michael N. Jamiana, Benedict Edward P. Valdez, Halima O. Mokamad-Romancap, and Delbrynth Mitchao Smigel

Introduction

Every surgeon has to pay great respect to elderly patients coming in at the emergency room. No amount of retrospective study can perfectly predict a uniform intervention and outcome for every elderly patient. It is common knowledge that looks could be deceiving, for there are those in their 80s able to do a 5-km brisk walk, and on the other hand, some in their 60s have difficulty reaching half of the said parameter.

Nevertheless, everyone will agree that elderly people prefer a comfortable experience when asked what they would want and expect in crises such as being acutely ill with a surgical case. Commonly observed are the underestimations of the severity of illness, especially in the geriatric population, which ends in surgical ICU and affects the mortality rates.

Comorbidities certainly will be common with this age group: uncontrolled diabetes, hypertension, heart failure, COPD, liver cirrhosis, among others. These illnesses would challenge an acute surgical team in the preoperative preparation and often are the reasons for delay or avoidance of surgery. A trend of most common emergency general surgery cases in the elderly that has been occurring worldwide are colectomy, adhesiolysis, small bowel resection, repair of a perforated gastric ulcer, appendectomy, or cholecystectomy, depending on the ethnicity and demographic area.

In Southeast Asia, citing a 2018 baseline survey of the Longitudinal Study of Ageing and Health in the Philippines (LSAHP) for monitoring the Philippine Sustainable Development Goal (SDGs) commitments for older people was done and has cited Japan as an extreme example of population aging. This trend is also occurring worldwide. This demographic trend is a consequence of improvements in public health and progress in medical science, a field in which humanity has taken great strides, especially over the last 100 years. Fractures of the hip, thigh, and pelvis, digestive illnesses, and ailments of the liver or gallbladder have been prevalent in Trauma and Acute Care Surgery. Their true prevalence is likely higher because of undiagnosed cases among those with less access to healthcare.

M. N. Jamiana (✉)
Brokenshire Medical Center, Department of Trauma Surgery, Southern Philippines Medical Center, Davao City, Philippines

B. E. P. Valdez
Emergency Medicine Department, Southern Philippines Medical Centre (SPMC), Davao City, Philippines

H. O. Mokamad-Romancap
Department of Surgery, Cotabato Regional and Medical Center, Cotabato, Philippines

D. M. Smigel
Southern Philippines Medical Center, Davao City, Philippines

P. Petrone, C. E.M. Brathwaite (eds.), *Acute Care Surgery in Geriatric Patients*,
https://doi.org/10.1007/978-3-031-30651-8_41

The old and frail sometimes come at a crossroad when deciding what they want for themselves. The Frailty Index (FI) has been found in many literatures as a significant predictor of mortality. In general, elderly patients have more difficult surgeries due to their chronicity. A classic example are gallbladders in the elderly, which are often markedly thickened, difficult to dissect laparoscopically, and are reasons for conversion to open cholecystectomy.

Again, arriving at a wise judgment on what they would prefer and expect in crises is sometimes challenging, and refusing surgery is sometimes not a smart option since there are situations where giving them the simplest and quickest procedure can, in fact, significantly improve their conditions. There are concerns that elderly people sometimes have difficulty comprehending, and judgment calls are sometimes left in the hands of their children or family members.

Physiologic Changes in Geriatrics

Pertinent to understanding general surgical emergencies are physiologic changes in geriatrics that would explain their peculiarities. Homeostenosis helps one understand the vulnerability of the elderly when challenged, whether, by acute illnesses, trauma, cancer, medications, etc., those age-related changes become apparent. The concept of homeostenosis—the characteristic, progressive constriction of homeostatic reserves that occurs with aging in every organ system—was recognized by the famous physiologist Walter Cannon in the 1940s. Aging brings the individual closer to the precipice or threshold by losing physiologic reserves. The "precipice" may be defined, for example, as death or ill enough to have a cardiac arrest or hospital admission. The precipice may also present in the guise of common and protean symptoms, such as mental confusion, weight loss, sleep disorder, or weakness.

In acute care surgery, it is common to hear and read about limited physiologic reserves found in the elderly. Many studies show that body weight and body mass index (BMI) do not change significantly, but fat mass increases and muscle mass decreases. Proprioception in the elderly is markedly reduced than in young adults leading to a higher risk of trauma, wound, and falling. Cardiovagal baroreflex sensitivity decreased, which may induce several consequences, including increased levels of BP variability, higher potency of orthostatic hypotension, impaired ability to respond to acute challenges to the maintenance of BP, and increased risk of sudden cardiac death. Decreased responsiveness to β-adrenergic stimulation results in the body being unable to drive maximum heart rate or maximum cardiac output according to stimuli or stress such as exercise, infection, or shock. The skeletal muscle of breathing will gradually lose strength. The lung parenchyma loses elasticity, causing the elastic recoil to deteriorate. Cilia which function in the mucociliary clearance of sweeping mucus and dirt out of the lungs, become slower with age. The coordination of the oropharyngeal muscles and the swallowing reflex is impaired, which causes a higher risk of aspiration and leads to a higher risk of aspiration pneumonia in the elderly. In the gastrointestinal tract, the *Cajal* body decreases, which acts as a pacemaker that sends slow wave potential to the intestinal smooth muscle causing intestinal contraction. As the number of *Cajal* bodies decreases, gastric emptying and intestinal transit time are slowed. Hence, the elderly eat less, causing anorexia due to indigestion and eventually constipation which is very common. The immune response becomes altered as aging changes, called *immunosenescence*. Immunosenescence of aging reduces the ability to accumulate T-cells and decreases the output of naïve T-cells. All the changing processes make the elderly have lower immunity to infection, lower expression of inflammation, higher risk of autoimmune disease, and lower activity of vaccination. As to the skeletal system, osteoporosis is common and, along with it, are fractures year in and year out.

Approach, Clinical Assessment, and Preoperative Preparation

Nearly 27 million persons were admitted to US hospitals with a severe Emergency General Surgery (EGS) diagnosis, accounting for 7.12%

of all hospital admissions. Year by year, the number of EGS hospitalizations and the volume and rate of procedures increased. As a result, the EGS burden in the general population has risen rapidly, surpassing other major public health concerns such as diabetes, cancer, heart failure, stroke, and HIV infection. Furthermore, EGS patients have a far higher risk of morbidity and death, with 35% of patients being 70 years or older. Most of these patients have comorbidities, are on medications, and are experiencing geriatric physiological issues.

Risk and Clinical Assessment and Preoperative Preparation of EGS Cases

All geriatric surgical patients should have preoperative tests such as hemoglobin, renal function tests (creatinine, blood urea nitrogen), and serum albumin. In contrast, white blood cell count, platelet count, coagulation tests (PT, INR, PTT), electrolytes (Na, K, Cl, Ca), glucose, and urinalysis are recommended for selected geriatric surgical patients.

Preoperative optimization is critical in an older patient with acute and chronic illnesses, which might cause surgical delays. Thus, the preoperative evaluation must be goal-directed and time-limited, considering the risk of postponing life-saving surgery. In acknowledgment of the need for quality improvement in geriatric surgical treatment, the American College of Surgeons National Surgical Quality Improvement Program (ACS NSQIP) and the American Geriatrics Society (AGS) have formed a Geriatric Surgery Advisory Board to develop best practices standards. Table 41.1 shows the optimal preoperative assessment checklist for elderly patients. Surgeons must ensure a thorough preoperative evaluation and management, which is necessary for patient informed consent and optimal treatment. However, compliance with this checklist is more difficult at low-income facilities, where people and equipment are restricted to quickly handle the severely sick elderly's preoperative needs.

Frailty is characterized by reduced physiologic reserve and stress resistance, making patients more prone to adverse health outcomes such as falls, deteriorating mobility, ADL impairment, hospitalizations, and death. Comorbidity and disability are clinically separate entities. The use of the Fried Index has been recommended by both the American College of Surgeons and the American Geriatrics Society (Table 41.2). If three or more of the five characteristics (unintentional weight loss, poor walking speed, easy tiredness, history of falls, and diminished grip strength) are evident, the patient is considered frail. When combined with the American Society of Anesthesiologists' score and serum hemoglobin, unintentional weight loss and grip create a straightforward, simple risk classification system with robust prognostic information.

Table 41.1 Checklist for the optimal preoperative assessment of the geriatric surgical patient

In addition to conducting a complete history and physical examination of the patient, the following assessments are strongly recommended: • Assess the patient's cognitive ability and capacity to understand the anticipated surgery. • Screen the patient for depression. • Identify the patient's risk factors for developing postoperative delirium. • Screen for alcohol and other substance abuse/dependence. Perform a preoperative cardiac evaluation according to the American College of Cardiology/American Heart Association algorithm for noncardiac surgery patients. • Identify the patient's risk factors for postoperative pulmonary complications and implement appropriate strategies for prevention. • Document functional status and history of falls. • Determine baseline frailty score. • Assess the patient's nutritional status and consider preoperative interventions if the patient is at severe nutritional risk. • Take an accurate and detailed medication history and consider appropriate perioperative adjustments. • Monitor for polypharmacy. • Determine the patient's treatment goals and expectations in the context of the possible treatment outcomes. • Determine the patient's family and social support system. • Order appropriate preoperative diagnostic tests focused on elderly patients.

(From Optimal Preoperative Assessment of the Geriatric Surgical Patient: A Best Practices Guideline from the American College of Surgeons National Surgical Quality Improvement Program and the American Geriatrics Society.)

Table 41.2 Description of fried phenotype and clinical frailty scale

Fried phenotype	Clinical frailty scale
Weight loss: >10 lb. unintentionally in the prior year	1. Very fit people who are robust, very active, and motivated. These people commonly exercise regularly. They are among the fittest of their age.
Grip strength: Lowest 20% (by gender and body mass index)	2. Well: People who have no active disease symptoms but are less fit than those in previous category 1. Often, they exercise or are very active occasionally.
Exhaustion: Self-report	3. Managing well: People with well-controlled medical problems but rarely active beyond walking
Slowness: 15 ft. walking speed (by gender and height)	4. Vulnerable: Although not dependent on others for daily help, symptoms often limit activities. A common complaint is being "slowed up" and tired during the day.
Low activity: Kilocalories per week (men <383, women <270)	5. Mildly frail: These people often have more evident slowing and need help in high-order instrumental activities of daily living. Typically, this impairs shopping and walking outside alone, meal preparation, and housework 6. Moderately frail: People need help with outside activities and keeping house. Inside, they often have problems with stairs and need assistance with bathing and might need minimal help with dressing. 7. Severely frail: Entirely dependent on all personal care from whatever cause (physical or cognitive). Even so, they seem stable and not at high risk of dying (within approximately 6 months). 8. Very severely frail: Entirely dependent, approaching the end of life. Typically, they could not recover from even a minor illness. 9. Terminally ill: Approaching the end of life. This category applies to people with a life expectancy <6 months, which are not frail.
Frailty present if ≥3 characteristics present	Frailty present if category ≥4.

(From Fried LP, Tangen CM, Walston J, et al.; Cardiovascular Health Study Collaborative Research Group. Frailty in older adults: evidence for a phenotype. J Gerontol A Biol Sci Med Sci. 2001;56 (3):M146–56.)

Improved communication is another crucial consideration when dealing with acutely ill geriatric patients. An unanticipated operation presents a significant communication issue for the surgeon and any clinician involved in the patient's care and the patient and their family members. An advisory panel has published a prototype framework for the best communication practices at Harvard Medical School to facilitate goal-concordant care (Table 41.3). To deal with the challenges, particularly in preoperative decision-making and preferences, as well as eventual care goals, an organized approach to quality communication in the acute situation is recommended. In some cases, avoiding surgery is a better alternative than life-prolonging therapeutic procedures, which might harm the quality of life.

Table 41.3 Goals of a structured communication framework

- Place the patient's acute surgical condition in the context of the patient's underlying illness.
- Elicit the patient's goals, priorities, and what is acceptable to the patient regarding life-prolonging and comfort-focused care.
- Describe treatment options—including palliative approaches—in the context of the patient's goals and priorities.
- Direct treatment to achieve these outcomes and encourage the use of time-limited trials in circumstances of clinical uncertainty.
- Affirm continued commitment to patient's care.

(Data from Recommendations for Best Communication Practices to Facilitate Goal-concordant Care for Seriously Ill Older Patients with Emergency Surgical Conditions.)

In most cases, surgeons lack a comprehensive understanding of the current management of comorbidities and acute illnesses that their patients may develop during the postoperative period, contributing to postoperative complications. Hence, multiple specialties such as surgery, geriatrics, radiology, anesthesia, and other relevant specialties must be implicated in the patient's care to provide adequate expertise to maximize available equipment and technological advances, with possibly fewer invasive procedures and interventions.

Emergency General Surgery Cases

While the list of EGS patients is long, open small bowel resections, open large intestine resections, gastrointestinal ulcer and hemorrhage management, peritoneal adhesion lysis, and exploratory laparotomy are the most prevalent surgical emergencies. The acute abdomen might be challenging to diagnose in the elderly population. Some of the traditional signs, symptoms, and physical examinations may not be present, and some patients may be unable to communicate due to post-stroke symptoms of dementia. In this patient population, early diagnosis is critical; therefore, identifying between a surgical and nonsurgical abdomen must be done as soon as possible. Imaging modalities should be used quickly to support the working diagnosis and help the surgeon through the case treatment.

In another Swedish study, nonspecific abdominal pain (44%), appendicitis (16%), bowel obstruction (9%), diverticulitis (8%), gastrointestinal perforation (3%), gallstone disease (3%), and pancreatitis (3%) were the most common diagnoses based on computed tomography (CT); only 11 patients (0.5%) had mesenteric ischemia. Mesenteric ischemia may be a more common cause of acute abdomen in geriatric persons than previously thought; it reflects the incidence because the underlying etiology is usually atherosclerosis, atrial fibrillation, or another cardiac event, and the incidence of mesenteric ischemia was higher than the incidence of acute appendicitis in patients over the age of 75. As a result, immediate computed tomography with contrast enhancement should be performed in these patients, ideally in the arterial and venous phases. Furthermore, acute pancreatitis showed a second peak in those aged 75–85 years, which coincided with the high prevalence of gallstones in the elderly, and cholecystitis was extremely frequent in the elderly, with early mortality rates of 38%. In contrast, some individuals with minor diseases managed with conservative therapy in primary care departments (e.g., acute cholecystitis patients unsuited for surgery) may be missed.

On the other hand, diverticular illness has become increasingly common, and the full burden of the disease is likely to be underestimated. After an initial period of nonoperative management, such as a colectomy for diverticular disease, the added responsibility of care for delayed surgical operations is undertaken "semi-electively." Furthermore, the upper gastrointestinal tract has an admission rate of 16.7%, with a 31.1% operative rate and a 2% mortality rate. In comparison, the hernia has an admission rate of 3.3%, with a 72.6% operative rate and a 2% mortality rate. Colorectal conditions are the next most common, with an admission rate of 19% and a 2.2% mortality rate.

In this age group, intestinal obstruction is the most prevalent surgical emergency, and sticky intestinal obstruction is the most common cause of intestinal obstruction. It was recently found that intestinal blockage occurs in 55% of senior surgical emergency cases, with sigmoid volvulus occurring in 12.7% of patients and a 14% fatality rate. The leading causes of acute abdominal surgical emergencies appear to be an acute intestinal blockage and hollow viscus perforation. Obstructed hernia, which accounted for 14% of the causes, is usually avoidable. In senior patients, acute mesenteric ischemia and intestinal blockage due to a colonic tumor had a worse prognosis.

The Challenges

Salvageability is a complex topic to broach with elderly patients' families or any other relatives. This situation is most encountered in severe illnesses requiring immediate surgical treatment and where the prognosis is often poor. The elderly people's response is a polite decline to aggressive management, which frequently causes conflict between what patients want and what their relatives prefer. Finally, we should let our patients be our guides in the ordinary course of therapeutic practice. However, in extreme instances such as trauma and acute care surgery, elderly patients do not have the luxury of making their own decisions, and the likelihood of survival should be communicated to the next of kin. Removal of care is an ethical and end-of-life problem that will be tackled by family members and the surgical team at some point. Clinicians may be hesitant to discuss or even bring up the overall prognosis since many patients or family members may find it frightening. Hence, a poor prognosis should be made known to the family to make an informed decision. Clinicians should therefore offer to talk about the overall prognosis with very elderly patients but should respect those who decline. Underestimating clinical status in advanced age has been emphasized in numerous studies and utilizing evidence-based principles to advise emergency surgery in older people demonstrates that even using the ACS NSQIP risk calculator underestimates of surgical risk in the elderly happens. Elderly patients admitted to the ICU have a greater morbidity and mortality rate than younger patients. Severity of sickness, altered state of awareness, and infection are the most critical factors independently associated with the highest risk of death.

Intraoperative Challenges

Surgery causes physical and metabolic stress in elderly patients with a reduced cardiovascular reserve, putting them at risk for intraoperative shock and hypoperfusion. Underhydration and excessive resuscitation are toxic to these patients. As a result, goal-directed fluid therapy is a concept in perioperative fluid administration in which hemodynamic variables such as stroke volume, stroke volume variation, pulse pressure variation, and cardiac output are constantly monitored. There is mounting evidence that intraoperative hypotension is linked to heart, kidney, and brain injury, as well as an increased chance of death in high-risk patients. Intraoperative hypotension, on the other hand, is an avoidable risk factor because arterial pressure can be controlled using intravenous fluids and vasopressors.

Cardiovascular, respiratory, renal, and hepatic functions are all reduced in geriatric patients. During anesthesia and the postoperative period, the patient has a minimal functional reserve, which is a safety margin. Infectious complications, respiratory complications (hypoxia, pneumonia, need for noninvasive or invasive mechanical ventilation for respiratory failure, acute respiratory distress syndrome), neurologic complications (stroke, altered consciousness), cardiovascular complications (cardiac arrhythmia, acute heart failure, myocardial infarction), and surgical complications were all defined as occurring within 30 days after surgery (anastomotic leak, surgical site infection, reoperation). Most patients undergo abdominal surgery, which is associated with an increased risk of acute kidney injury, respiratory failure, sepsis, and death. Among patients predominantly undergoing abdominal surgery with increased postoperative risk, management targeting individualized systolic blood pressure, compared with standard management, reduced the risk of postoperative organ dysfunction.

Outcomes and Complications in the Elderly

Currently, a study predicts that by the year 2050, the percentage of the population older than 80 will double, leading to increasing demand for healthcare resources, including intensive care that requires more healthcare workers. As per study of 484 patients admitted to medical, surgical, and coronary ICUs in a big metropolitan teaching hospital, one-third of adults older than 64 who are admitted to the ICU die within 6 months of release. Independent predictors of death at 6 months were the number of days during the 30 days before the hospitalization that the patient felt their "physical health was not good" on the health-related quality of life survey [OR = 1.08; 95% CI 1.04–1.12], a higher Acute Physiology and Chronic Health Evaluation II score [OR 1.09; 95% CI 1.06–1.12], and chronic pulmonary disease as comorbidity [OR 2.22; 95% CI 1.04–4.78]. Among survivors at 6 months, health-related quality of life had significantly worsened over time in the oldest patients but improved in the youngest survivor.

Mortality in General Surgical Emergencies

In general surgical emergencies, various factors may increase the patient's risk of complications that result in morbidity and fatality. These could include the time between the beginning of symptoms and the initial consultation. The ability of the physician to diagnose and the receiving facility's ability to perform urgent surgical intervention may play a role in the management's success or failure. Surgical intervention may contribute a role in the success or failure of the treatment. The World Health Organization's (WHO) Global Health Estimates report on global disability-adjusted life years (DALYs) lost from different diseases, published in 2013, did not specifically mention general surgical emergencies but rather combined the various clinical presentations from different categories such as peptic ulcer disease, appendicitis, and digestive disease. According to McCord et al., these situations can result in DALYs being lost. This accounts for 1.5% of all DALYs in all parts of the world, with 596 per 100,000 people.

In 2020, Doglietto et al. published factors associated with surgical mortality and problems among patients with and without Coronavirus Disease 2019 (COVID-19) in Italy, which found that surgical mortality and complications were greater in patients with than without COVID-19 patients. These findings suggest that surgery in COVID-19 patients should be postponed wherever possible.

References

1. Cruz CJP, Cruz JCP, Saito Y. Ageing and health in The Philippines. Jakarta: Economic Research Institute for ASEAN and East Asia (ERIA); 2019.
2. Taffett GE. Physiology of aging. In: Geriatric medicine. New York, NY: Springer; 2003. https://doi.org/10.1007/0-387-22621-4_3.
3. Suraseranivong R. Physiologic changes in the elderly. GMSMJ. 2022;2(2):129–40.
4. Gale SC, Shafi S, Dombrovskiy VY, Arumugam D, Crystal JS. The public health burden of emergency general surgery in the United States: A 10-year analysis of the Nationwide Inpatient Sample–2001 to 2010. J Trauma Acute Care Surg. 2014;77(2):202–8. https://doi.org/10.1097/TA.0000000000000362.
5. Chow WB, Rosenthal RA, Merkow RP, Ko CY, Esnaola NF, et al. Optimal preoperative assessment of the geriatric surgical patient: a best practices guideline from the American College of Surgeons National Surgical Quality Improvement Program and the American Geriatrics Society. J Am Coll Surg. 2012;215(4):453–66. https://doi.org/10.1016/j.jamcollsurg.2012.06.017.
6. McIsaac DI, Moloo H, Bryson GL, van Walraven C. The Association of Frailty with outcomes and resource use after emergency general surgery: a population-based cohort study. Anesth Analg. 2017;124(5):1653–61. https://doi.org/10.1213/ANE.0000000000001960.
7. Cooper Z, Koritsanszky LA, Cauley CE, Frydman JL, Bernacki RE, Mosenthal AC, Gawande AA, Block SD. Recommendations for best communication practices to facilitate goal-concordant Care for Seriously ill Older Patients with Emergency Surgical Conditions. Ann Surg. 2016;263(1):1–6. https://doi.org/10.1097/SLA.0000000000001491.
8. Scott JW, Olufajo OA, Brat GA, Rose JA, Zogg CK, Haider AH, Salim A, Havens JM. Use of National Burden to define operative emergency general surgery. JAMA Surg. 2016;151(6):e160480. https://doi.org/10.1001/jamasurg.2016.0480.
9. Kärkkäinen JM, Lehtimäki TT, Manninen H, Paajanen H. Acute mesenteric ischemia is a more common cause than expected of acute abdomen in the elderly. J Gastrointest Surg. 2015;19(8):1407–14. https://doi.org/10.1007/s11605-015-2830-3.
10. Ziara Al-Hussainy A, Hawaz Al-Hawaz M, Abdulsatar AM. Acute abdominal surgical emergency in elderly patients (a prospective study). Med J Basrah Univ. 2009;27(1):34–41. https://doi.org/10.33762/mjbu.2009.49036.
11. Fried LP, Tangen CM, Walston J, Newman AB, Hirsch C, Gottdiener J, Seeman T, Tracy R, Kop WJ, Burke G, McBurnie MA. Cardiovascular health study collaborative research group. Frailty in older adults: evidence for a phenotype. J Gerontol A Biol Sci Med Sci. 2001;56(3):M146–56. https://doi.org/10.1093/gerona/56.3.m146.

12. Wrzosek A, Jakowicka-Wordliczek J, Zajaczkowska R, Serednicki WT, Jankowski M, Bala MM, Swierz MJ, Polak M, Wordliczek J. Perioperative restrictive versus goal-directed fluid therapy for adults undergoing major non-cardiac surgery. Cochrane Database Syst Rev. 2019;12(12):CD012767. https://doi.org/10.1002/14651858.CD012767.pub2.
13. Futier E, Lefrant JY, Guinot PG, Godet T, Lorne E, Cuvillon P, Bertran S, Leone M, Pastene B, Piriou V, Molliex S, Albanese J, Julia JM, Tavernier B, Imhoff E, Bazin JE, Constantin JM, Pereira B, Jaber S, INPRESS Study Group. Effect of individualized vs standard blood pressure management strategies on postoperative organ dysfunction among high-risk patients undergoing major surgery: a randomized clinical trial. JAMA. 2017;318(14):1346–57. https://doi.org/10.1001/jama.2017.14172.
14. McCord C, Ozgediz D, Beard JH, et al. Gen Surgical Emergencies. In: Debas HT, Donkor Gawande A, et al., editors. Essential surgery: ease control priorities, vol. 1. 3rd ed. Washing (DC): The International Bank for Reconstruct and Development/The World Bank; 2015. Chapter https://www.ncbi.nlm.nih.gov/books/NBK33350 https://doi.org/10.1596/978-1-4648-0346-8_ch4.
15. Doglietto F, Vezzoli M, Gheza F, Lussardi G Domenicucci M, Vecchiarelli L, Zanin L, Sarace G, Signorini L, Panciani PP, Castelli F, Maroldi Rasulo FA, Benvenuti MR, Portolani N, Bonarde S, Milano G, Casiraghi A, Calza S, Fontanel MM. Factors associated with surgical mortality ar complications among patients with and without cor navirus disease 2019 (COVID-19) in Italy. JAM Surg. 2020;155(8):691–702. https://doi.org/10.100 jamasurg.2020.2713.

Options on Conservative Treatment in Acute Surgical Emergencies

42

Leandro Stoll Coelho, Vinicius Rocha-Santos, and Joel Faintuch

Introduction

Along surgical history, decreasing tissue damage through less invasive techniques was always on the scope of the surgeons. Approaches never dreamed before like laparoscopic surgery, image-guided percutaneous procedures, angioembolizations to treat aneurisms and hemorrhage, and the cutting-edge technology of robotic-assisted surgery remarkably contributed to lessen tissue damage and consequently the immune and metabolic response to trauma, with the same safety and efficacy as conventional open surgeries. The Hippocratic motto *primum non nocere* worked like a moral compass. It probably played a major role on the mental drive of surgeons committed to good medical practice, pushing towards the use of minimally invasive techniques, in order to keep risks and complications at bay.

Can we go further and take one more step into noninvasiveness? Is there any more room for conservative treatment within contexts in which surgery would be first choice? High definition imaging devices like CT scan, MRI, advanced ultrasound, and PET scan, complemented by cutting-edge PET/MRI, laser CT scan, laser ultrasound, and endoscopic ultrasound are making it possible to access body structures with unparalleled precision and reliability, allowing the surgeon to feel more confident with periodic surveillance only. They enabled multiple conservative changes in the handling of traumatic and non-traumatic disorders of gastrointestinal, biliopancreatic, and colorectal viscera. In such circumstances, the otherwise uncontested immediate surgical indication gave place to less invasive or completely conservative options (Table 42.1).

L. S. Coelho (✉)
Regional Hospital of Registro, Sao Paulo, Brazil

Regional Hospital Dr. Leopoldo Bevilacqua, Pariquera-Acu, Sao Paulo, Brazil

V. Rocha-Santos
Liver Transplantation Unit, Gastroenterology Division, University of Sao Paulo, Sao Paulo, Brazil

J. Faintuch
Department of Gastroenterology, Sao Paulo University Medical School, Sao Paulo, Brazil
e-mail: jfaintuch@hc.fm.usp.br

P. Petrone, C. E.M. Brathwaite (eds.), *Acute Care Surgery in Geriatric Patients*,
https://doi.org/10.1007/978-3-031-30651-8_42

Table 42.1 Conservative pathways for traditional surgical emergencies

Intensive monitoring (invasive and noninvasive) • Hemodynamic, respiratory, gastrointestinal, neurological
Clinical management: • Fluid replenishment, shock management, coagulation factors, antibiotics, antacids, hormones
Interventional radiology • Drainage, embolization, stenting, clot removal
Local bleeding control • Abdominal or thoracic packing, fibrin glue, and hemostatic patches
Endoscopic maneuvers • Blood vessel sclerosis, stricture dilatation, obstruction stenting, collection drainage, visceral by-pass, fistula occluders, and sponges
Hyperbaric oxygen therapy • Refractory anaerobic infections, ischemic lesions and grafts, necrotic wounds
Other options (benign and cancerous lesions) • Radiofrequency ablation • Laser hemostasis • Cryotherapy

Gastroduodenal Problems

Complications of peptic ulcers such as perforation, bleeding or obstruction have become much less common after the advent of H2 receptor antagonists and notably proton-pump inhibitors, associated with wider employment of endoscopy and breath tests which increased *Helicobacter pylori* diagnosis and treatment. Medical and endoscopic treatment is nowadays, by far, the best option of treatment for peptic disease, even in face of complications such as partial obstruction and limited hemorrhage.

Perforated Peptic Ulcer

One should admit that acute abdomen caused by ulcer perforation, although infrequent still carries serious morbidity, mainly in those with associated health conditions including the elderly patients. Surgical repair is the best option in most cases; however, in selected patients conservative management is possible.

According to some sources, in 1870 Redwood reported a patient successfully treated without surgical intervention. It is true that at those early times surgical mortality was so prohibitive that not operating, although fraught with obvious danger, seemed rather natural. Yet even in the first half of the twentieth century with a number of advances in anesthesia, blood and fluid replacement and antibacterial sulfonamide drugs, Wangensteen defended nonsurgical treatment after spontaneous healing of a perforated ulcer. Taylor first reported a series of 28 patients receiving non-operative management in 1946 naming it the Taylor method, which consisted of nasogastric aspiration, antibiotic therapy, and intravenous fluid replacement. More recently, *Helicobacter Pylori* eradication was added to that therapeutic protocol.

The Taylor rationale is based on gastric decompression and continuous external drainage, which promotes healing. Of course, nutritional support was the weak point, in case a prolonged fasting period was required, as modern enteral and parenteral nutrition were not available in the 1940s. Nevertheless, Edward Crisp in 1843 had already noticed that inflammatory adhesions and adjacent tissues often blocked perforated ulcers after just a few days, thus preventing fluids of spreading into peritoneal cavity. A much more recent French prospective study published by Songne et al. demonstrated a 50% success rate of conservative treatment in a series of 82 consecutive patients.

Clinical phases of acute perforated ulcer

Phase 1: Chemical peritonitis caused by gastric acid. The leaked fluids have relatively scarce bacteria.

Phase 2: Occurs 6–12 h after the perforation. Pain diminishes somewhat probably due to dilution of the irritating gastric contents by the peritoneal exudates.

Phase 3: Peritoneal infection. Occurs after 12–24 h, whereas bacterial growth and sepsis are the main features.

Eligibility to Non-operative Treatment

The candidate should be within the first 12 h after symptom onset, a period in which the abdomen is still sterile or minimal bacterial contamination is present, abdominal pain is limited to the upper abdomen and hemodynamic variables are stable. Oral food and fluids should be discontinued and a decompressive gastric tube must be used to prevent additional gastric content leak. Intravenous fluids, antibiotics, and injectable proton pump inhibitors must be started. Close surveillance comprising vital signs, physical examination, and pain evaluation at least every 6 h is of vital importance.

Upon signs of hemodynamic instability, worsening of pain suggestive of generalized peritonitis or any other clinical deterioration, the patient should be taken to the operating room to be surgically treated, preferentially by the laparoscopic approach. Special attention must be given to frail or elderly individuals in whom proportionally minor cardiac, circulatory, or metabolic imbalances could be life threatening. In principle those admitted with signs of shock, tachycardia, hypotension, generalized peritonitis, fever or history of onset of symptoms longer than 12 h should not undergo conservative treatment.

Endoscopic Closure of the Perforation

Over-the-scope-clips (OTSC) are a recent attempt to close the ulcer through an endoscopic approach. It is minimally invasive and takes little time (around 10 min). The peritoneal cavity is supposed not to be infected; otherwise, surgical treatment is the best option. Further prospective randomized studies must be conducted, as current evidence is limited.

Acute Appendicitis

With a lifetime risk ranging from 7% to 8%, acute appendicitis is the most common surgical emergency and the most frequent cause of acute surgical abdomen worldwide. McBurney was the first to describe appendectomy in 1894 and the classical abdominal incision bears his name. The laparoscopic approach is related to less wound infections, less postoperative morbidity, shorter hospital stay, and better quality of life, being recommended by the Society of American Gastrointestinal and Endoscopic Surgeons (SAGES) and the European Association for Endoscopic Surgery (EAES) as the gold standard. Mortality related to appendectomy is lower than in the past however not negligible, around 0.5%.

Non-operative Management

Harrington in 1953 and Coldrey in 1959 were among the first to advocate non-operative treatment. Coldrey reported 471 patients treated with antibiotics suffering low mortality (0.2%) and low recurrence rate (14%). Such success notwithstanding, very few followed his lead.

The advantages of conservative treatment would be no wound infection, adhesions, and incisional hernias. Anesthesia-associated risks would also be excluded which could play a positive role on comorbid patients. Furthermore, it presumes shorter hospital stay, lower costs, and shorter absence from work. Failure of antibiotic therapy should not be overlooked, exposing the patient to complicated appendicitis including perforation, fecal peritonitis, and sepsis leading to greater morbidity and mortality. Moreover, without removal of the diseased organ, the lifetime risk of appendicitis would remain. Another risk for prolonged use of antibiotics during acute appendicitis would be bacterial resistance.

In the meta-analysis conducted by Prechal, 63% of patients who underwent non-operative management were successfully treated within the first year of follow-up. In the surgical (control) group, the success rate was 96%. In patients who needed secondary appendectomy for failure of antibiotic treatment, the complications were statistically the same as from primary appendectomy. There was no difference in the duration of hospital stay, and absence of work was significantly shorter in the antibiotic group. Surgery provided definitive cure; however, the conservative did not expose the patients to increased risk.

Long-term effects of nonsurgical antibiotic therapy need to be further studied. The incidence of cancer in uncomplicated appendicitis is very low; however, it still has to be taken into account as it can play a role on prognosis. Given the higher rate of failure of conservative treatment and of recurrence, the indication for conservative treatment in this setting should be tailored according to the patient's needs and expectations.

Colonoscopy Perforation

Colonoscopy is a widely performed procedure throughout the world, with over 15 million yearly interventions just in the USA. Although safe and with minimal associated morbidity, the technique is not risk-free. Iatrogenic colon perforation (ICP) is probably the most dreaded complication for patients undergoing diagnostic screening or therapy. Reported frequencies are 0.019–0.8% and 0.1–3.0% for diagnostic and therapeutic colonoscopy, respectively. This complication can lead to prolonged hospital stay, emergency surgery with or without a stoma, and sepsis. Mortality range is 5–7% and up to one third of those requiring operation get a stoma.

Therapeutic colonoscopies have a higher probability of perforation both because they may deal with an already diseased organ, and because of occasionally complex manipulations. Other aspects contributing to colon perforation include pneumatic dilatation of strictures in Crohn's disease, advanced age (over 75 years), endoscopic mucosal and submucosal dissection for colorectal neoplasia, multiple comorbidities, and female gender.

The endoscopist, promptly detects up to 60% of ICPs, such as when an intra-peritoneal structure appears on the screen during endoscopic examination. Abdominal pain (up to 95% of the cases), and deranged laboratory and radiologic tests demand urgent awareness and should be actively investigated in suspicious circumstances. Such encompass distention, rebound tenderness, fever, diffuse peritonitis, tachycardia, rectal bleeding, along with elevated white blood cell count and C-reactive protein and pneumoperitoneum. If suspicion of perforation persists, computed tomography scan should be done as it can detect not only free air, but also free fluid. Double contrast tomographic colonic imaging (intravenous and rectal) sometimes demonstrates sealed perforations, which may be eligible for non-operative treatment.

Signs of sepsis or diffuse peritonitis, immunosuppressed individuals, large perforations (such as those easily identified by the endoscopist during the primary examination), or those related to cancer almost invariably demand immediate surgery.

Conservative Treatment

Localized pain, free air but no free fluids in the abdominal cavity, hemodynamic stability and the absence of fever are usually associated with good prognosis without operation. Intravenous fluids and nutrients, bowel rest and broad-spectrum antibiotics are mandatory along with close clinical and laboratory surveillance. If the pneumoperitoneum impairs respiration, it should be percutaneously needle- or catheter-drained, a maneuver that could help closing the perforation. Initial improvement does not rule out need for subsequent surgery; therefore, the patient should be monitored for several days in the hospital. This means a longer total hospital stay than when primary operation is conducted.

Endoluminal Repair

Endoscopic treatment is a minimally invasive and effective alternative. Ideally, the damage should be recognized during the procedure and bowel preparation should be adequate. Clip closures are reported since 1997, sealing and healing perforations without surgery. Devices such as through-the-scope (TTS) clips and over-the-scope clips

(OTSC) are highly successful in closing ICP. Perforations larger than 1 cm are better treated with such modality, which includes more tissue within the clips.

Through-the-scope clips are used primarily for hemostasis; however, they are able to seal full-thickness perforations as well. Yet because of the smaller size only submucosa and mucosa tend to be reached. Nevertheless with small defects, success rates as encouraging as of 84% have been demonstrated.

If OTSC is the option, a more difficult advance of the colonoscope mounted with the OTSC system could occur in the right colon, however, not in more distal parts of the large bowel. Such barrier notwithstanding, given the overall high success rates in treating ICP, the OTSC system might become the standard approach for this lesion in the near future.

Endoscopic Band Closure

Band-ligation technique was also reported as a method of closing small perforations when the use of an endoscopic clip is difficult. Surrounding tissue and the perforation site are sucked into the banding cap and the band is deployed.

Post-endoscopy management of an ICP should include broad-spectrum antibiotics and bowel rest. A close surveillance is important to prevent clinical deterioration, and surgery must be carried out if severe abdominal pain, peritonitis, or sepsis ensues.

Acute Diverticulitis

Diverticulosis of the sigmoid colon is common in the elderly, affecting approximately 33% of persons older than 60 years of which up to 15% will proceed with an episode of diverticulitis. According to some groups, acute diverticulitis is increasing more swiftly than the expected aging of the population, as much as 26% between 1998 and 2005. Complicated diverticulitis can include abscess, fistula, stricture, and partially blocked or free perforation. For a long time, treatment of acute diverticulitis with extraluminal air has been emergent resection with or without colostomy, which is associated with high morbidity and mortality (40–44% and 4–24%, respectively). Fortunately, recurrence rates are lower compared to younger patients, those free from recurrence representing 83% of those>67 years of age.

Non-operative Treatment

Acute left colon diverticulitis (ALCD) is associated with abscess in 20% of the cases. For small collections, recommendation is broad-spectrum antibiotic therapy with close clinical monitoring. This approach has a failure rate of 19% if the median size is 4 cm. Larger abscesses are best handled by percutaneous drainage associated with antibiotics, which still carries a failure rate of 21% for abscesses with a median size of 6.1 cm. Surgery should be avoided in stable, younger patients, becoming more urgent in the elderly whenever refractory to the conservative approach, as it is associated with higher mortality.

In circumstances of distant-free intraperitoneal air and no intraperitoneal fluid, non-operative management is still a possibility if hemodynamic stability and no signs of sepsis are confirmed. The failure rate ranges from 10 to 43% and experience with the elderly is limited. With just about 2 cm of air in the absence of peritonitis or fluid effusions, 86% success rate and no mortality have been observed. If pericolic air only is detected healing could be possible, as much as 99%.

Splenic Trauma

The spleen is involved in around 32% of the events of major abdominal trauma. Over the last 40 years, splenic injuries evolved from a mainly surgical to a fundamentally non-operative management (NOM) aiming at spleen conservation in hemodynamically stable patients, thus preventing long-term risks of splenectomy which include immunological impairment and lifelong threat of severe infectious diseases. Moreover, NOM avoids anesthesia, operation, and complication costs and success rate can be as high as 97%, especially with lower injury grades. NOM is also associated with a shorter hospitalization period, thus it has become the gold standard for blunt spleen trauma in hemodynamically stable patients, in the absence of peritonitis or associated injuries requiring laparotomy.

Conservative and Minimally Invasive Treatment

It includes clinical and hemodynamic observation with or without angiography and embolization. For planning NOM, contrast-enhanced CT scan is crucial in grading lesions with sensitivity and specificity around 96–100%. NOM should only be attempted in centers capable of precise diagnosis of the severity of spleen and other injuries and around-the-clock management including close observation, with intensive care and surgery team easily available.

NOM is classically indicated for minor and moderate spleen lesions, as scored according to the World Society of Emergency Surgery (WSES) or the American Association for the Surgery of Trauma (AAST) (WSES I, AAST-II / WSES II, AAST III). If a positive blush or early aneurism is present on CT scan, angiography should be considered, as those findings are risk factors for re-bleeding. NOM failure rate ranges from 4 to 15%. Age over 55 years is a risk factor for NOM failure which is associated with a higher mortality and longer hospital stay, even though the spleen tends to shrink with aging and thus be less vascularized, within the framework of generalized atrophy of immune tissues in the elderly.

Angioembolization

If moderate lesions (WSES III / AAST IV-V) are selected for NOM, angiography/angioembolization (AG/AE) is recommended regardless of a CT blush. In AAST injury grades above IV, the failure rate of NOM may reach 54.6%. AG/AE has become a powerful ally for spleen trauma treatment enhancing success up to 86–100%. The earlier AG/AE is performed, the lower are the splenectomy odds. NOM failure in the presence of CT contrast blush ranges between 67% and 82% so AG/AE is mandatory in those cases. Nevertheless, AG/AE is not complication-free, encompassing major troubles (3.7–28.5%) such as re-bleeding, splenic infarction, splenic abscess, pseudocyst, and severe puncture-related complications, especially when conducted by non-specialized teams or in not well-equipped units. Minor morbidity occurs in 23–61% of the candidates including fever, pleural effusion, and coil migration.

Liver Trauma

Because of its large size and location in the upper part of the abdomen, the liver is one of the most affected organs by abdominal trauma, both penetrating and blunt, and its rich vascular nature makes it a source of potentially fatal hemorrhage.

Analogously to spleen injuries, NOM depends on grading of the damage by contrast-enhanced CT scan (gold standard). Hemodynamic stability is mandatory for such option as well as no other abdominal injuries requiring surgical treatment like hollow viscus perforation.

Around 80% of blunt hepatic trauma can be conservatively treated and NOM is similarly the treatment of choice for stable patients with stab and gunshot wounds. This applies to liver injuries graded as minor or moderate (WSES I–II and AAST I, II, and III), for which success rate reaches around 80% if all modalities of hepatic trauma are considered. For stab wounds more failures are to be expected (50% need for interventions if anterior lesions and 25% if posterior ones).

Clinical and hemodynamic monitoring follows the lines of splenic injuries. Special attention should be given to gunshot wounds as they carry a higher risk of associated lesions and should be conservatively treated only in specialized trauma centers.

AG/AE should be employed when a contrast blush or early aneurism is present. If NOM is selected for more severe lesions (WSES III and AAST IV-V), admission to the ICU is advised. Interventional radiology should be readily available as additional vascular damage could be present. Drops in hematocrit levels even in the absence of shock should raise the suspicion of active bleeding and immediate angiography should be considered.

As in other contexts angioembolization is occasionally followed by adverse events nominally bile leak, contained biloma, hepatic necrosis, and hepatic abscess.

Pancreatic Trauma

It occurs in less than 1% of all traumas and up to 11% of abdominal trauma. Blunt injuries are the most frequent ones. Their importance stems from the high risk of complications and death. Given the limited experience in most centers, treatment of moderate and severe pancreatic injury (PI) is still a topic of debate. Lesions graded I or II (without main duct injury) are treated conservatively. Main pancreatic duct (MPD) injury is the most important finding on the CT scan and operation is often the choice although associated with high morbidity and mortality. Pancreatic injury can be associated with other abdominal lesions rendering conservative treatment less likely, notably after penetrating trauma. Despite the dearth of solid evidence, non-operative management (NOM) is increasing in this field.

NOM in moderate and severe PI (grades III, IV, and V) has a success rate of 30% however with a high rate of subsequent pseudocysts, ranging from 65–74%. Nevertheless, these are mostly benign troubles amenable to minimally invasive interventions, particularly endoscopic drainage. After ERCP, pancreatic stent insertion could be a successful strategy for grade III PI.

Main Duct Disruption

There is still not consensus on whether NOM is a legitimate approach for MPD. However if delayed presentation with a well-walled pseudocyst is detected, MPD might benefit from minimally invasive treatment nominally endoscopic cystogastrostomy. To this aim various models of stents contribute to keep the transmural drainage open until the cyst is reabsorbed.

Pancreatic Necrosis and Abscess

Acute pancreatitis is deemed as the most common cause, after colic gallbladder, of serious upper abdominal pain in clinical practice. Although the vast majority of cases are mild and self-limited, up to 10% are associated with extensive pancreatic necrosis, which means high morbidity and prolonged hospital stay. In the relatively recent past, it could carry a mortality rate of 30%, and even 70% with associated infection.

Pancreatic necrosis may present as an acute necrotic collection (ANC), usually seen in the first 4 weeks and often extending into surrounding fat and retroperitoneal tissues, or walled-off necrosis (WON) which is a more mature, encapsulated pancreatic mass seen 4 weeks or more after the onset of pancreatitis. In both circumstances, infection of the necrotic tissue is possible, eventually encompassing anaerobic bacteria.

Early laparotomy, debridement and drainage of infected pancreatic necrosis (IPN) was the established approach during many years, yet burdened by major complications (34–95%) and death (11–39%). Recent experience demonstrates that non-operative treatment of IPN is the best alternative. In a series of 31 patients, eight were treated with antibiotics (25.8%), and the remaining ones were handled by drainage procedures (endoscopic and percutaneous). Surgical necrosectomy was necessary in only four patients (12.9%) because of treatment failure. Total mortality was 3.2% (one death).

The PANTER trial challenged open necrosectomy versus a less invasive approach named "step-up," in which minimally invasive procedures can be escalated or re-employed for draining IPN. Such encompassed percutaneous drainage, endoscopic transgastric drainage and minimally invasive retroperitoneal necrosectomy, generally employed in this sequence.

Percutaneous Drainage

Currently, this represents indeed the first line of treatment for IPN achieving 25–60% resolution of infection, with a high level of evidence (1A). Endoscopic transgastric drainage or necrosectomy and video-assisted retroperitoneal debridement are other alternatives, when required. Open surgery should be employed when those less invasive options fail as this approach relates to less new-onset organ failures although it is more aggressive and may require more interventions.

In cases of disconnected duct syndrome with walled-off necrosis, surgical transgastric necrosectomy may be also feasible, with morbidity and mortality around 38% and 2%, respectively.

Nonsurgical Pneumoperitoneum

Spontaneous non-laparoscopy-related pneumoperitoneum indicates hollow viscus perforation and conventionally demands emergent surgical exploration. However, in 5–15% of cases it is not associated to perforation and may be conservatively managed.

Common and Infrequent Conditions

Early postoperative pneumoperitoneum can of course be detected after 60% of open surgeries and 25% of laparoscopic procedures. Around two thirds of the findings will resolve within 2 days and 97% after 5 days. On CT scan, free peritoneal air may be recognized for somewhat longer, in about 50% of the cases after 6 days. A decreasing volume without worrisome clinical or peritoneal signs indicates a benign course.

Peritoneal dialysis can be associated with asymptomatic pneumoperitoneum (10–33% of the patients). Pneumatosis cystoides intestinalis is a rather rare cause of nonsurgical pneumoperitoneum. This condition is characterized by multiple intramural cysts filled with gas that may eventually rupture leading to pneumoperitoneum. Only in exceptional circumstances will intervention be required.

The lungs and thoracic structures may also be a source of nonsurgical pneumoperitoneum as occasionally occurs during prolonged mechanical ventilation with pneumothorax or pneumomediastinum. Risk factors include high airway pressures, noncompliant lungs, obstructive airway disease, and acute respiratory distress syndrome. Pneumoperitoneum in this setting, in the absence of peritoneal signs, could lead to unnecessary imaging investigation and even laparotomy.

Although unusually, air may enter the peritoneal cavity from the genital tract through the uterus and uterine tubes. Tubal insufflation during a hysterosalpingogram is an obvious mechanism; however, other local manipulations including sexual intercourse could be possible causes. Spontaneous resolution is the rule. Only in circumstances of significant pain or rebound tenderness, fever, elevated white blood cell count, or other signs of peritoneal inflammation should additional work up be provided.

Case Report

As previously alluded to, non-operative treatment of infected pancreatic necrosis is the preferred approach nowadays. Especially when percutaneous or endoscopic catheter drainage of the septic focus is feasible and material can be collected for bacteriologic profile and targeted antibiotic therapy. More than three decades ago, interventional radiology and endoscopy were not as available and effective in this condition as nowadays. Mortality with strictly conservative therapy was prohibitive; therefore, nearly all services advocated urgent open drainage. A patient seen by one of the authors was a profoundly religious man admitted to an academic hospital.

The involved microbes could not be identified as initial blood cultures were negative, and minimally invasive access to the focus was not available at that time. However, the individual was clinically septic with fever, high white blood cell count, upper abdominal distention and pain, and gas bubbles were identified during the imaging exploration of the pancreatic area, along with extensive retroperitoneal necrosis. As the case was being prepared for surgery the patient adamantly refused surgical consent. In his opinion, either his faith would save him, or otherwise he would peacefully accept that his time of dying has arrived. As he offered no alternative intravenous nutrients and high doses of antibiotics were prescribed, and the medical team crossed fingers hoping for the best. After the second week, the patient rapidly started to improve, to the point that he could be discharged home without operation. To the best of our knowledge, it was the first report of full regression with medical management only. Not surprisingly, the article was subsequently criticized, not only because of lack of bacteriologic confirmation, but because the concept of non-operative recovery after such an ominous infection was unconscionable at that time. Minimally invasive treatment started to become mainstream only about a decade after this publication, when satisfactory results were also reported.

We agree that our first plan had not been medical care either, as in the 1980s and 1990s of last century minimally invasive approaches were mostly a distant horizon, and even well-equipped surgical intensive care units (SICUs) were not easy to come by. Only today can one be confident that a critically ill subject will be well monitored when admitted to an SICU. Should conservative therapy fail and unexpected deterioration occur, the surgeon will still be able to change course and provide the required operation.

References

1. Chung KT, Shelat VG. Perforated peptic ulcer - an update. World J Gastrointest Surg. 2017;9(1):1–12. https://doi.org/10.4240/wjgs.v9.i1.1.
2. Wei JJ, Xie XP, Lian TT, Yang ZY, Pan YF, Lin ZL, Zheng GW, Zhuang ZH. Over-the-scope-clip applications for perforated peptic ulcer. Surg Endosc. 2019;33(12):4122–7. https://doi.org/10.1007/s00464-019-06717-x.
3. Salminen P, Tuominen R, Paajanen H, Rautio T, Nordström P, Aarnio M, Rantanen T, Hurme S, Mecklin JP, Sand J, Virtanen J, Jartti A, Grönroos JM. Five-year follow-up of antibiotic therapy for uncomplicated acute appendicitis in the APPAC randomized clinical trial. JAMA. 2018;320(12):1259–65. https://doi.org/10.1001/jama.2018.13201. Erratum in: JAMA 2018;320(16):1711
4. de Angelis N, Di Saverio S, Chiara O, et al. 2017 WSES guidelines for the management of iatrogenic colonoscopy perforation. World J Emerg Surg. 2018;13:5. https://doi.org/10.1186/s13017-018-0162-9.
5. Khan A, Hawkins AT. Challenging surgical dogma: controversies in diverticulitis. Surg Clin North Am. 2021;101(6):967–80. https://doi.org/10.1016/j.suc.2021.05.024.
6. Fugazzola P, Ceresoli M, Coccolini F, Gabrielli F, Puzziello A, Monzani F, Amato B, Sganga G, Sartelli M, Menichetti F, et al. The WSES/SICG/ACOI/SICUT/AcEMC/SIFIPAC guidelines for diagnosis and treatment of acute left colonic diverticulitis in the elderly. World J Emerg Surg. 2022;17(1):5. https://doi.org/10.1186/s13017-022-00408-0.
7. Cinquantini F, Simonini E, Di Saverio S, Cecchelli C, Kwan SH, Ponti F, Coniglio C, Tugnoli G, Torricelli P. Non-surgical Management of Blunt Splenic Trauma: a comparative analysis of non-operative management and splenic artery embolization-experience from a European trauma center. Cardiovasc Intervent Radiol. 2018;41(9):1324–32. https://doi.org/10.1007/s00270-018-1953-9.
8. Coccolini F, Montori G, Catena F, Kluger Y, Biffl W, Moore EE, Reva V, Bing C, Bala M, Fugazzola P, et al. Splenic trauma: WSES classification and guidelines for adult and pediatric patients. World J Emerg Surg. 2017;18(12):40. https://doi.org/10.1186/s13017-017-0151-4.
9. Pillai AS, Kumar G, Pillai AK. Hepatic trauma interventions. Semin Interv Radiol. 2021;38(1):96–104. https://doi.org/10.1055/s-0041-1724014.
10. Coccolini F, Coimbra R, Ordonez C, Kluger Y, Vega F, Moore EE, Biffl W, Peitzman A, Horer T, Abu-Zidan FM, Sartelli M, et al. WSES expert panel. Liver trauma: WSES 2020 guidelines. World J Emerg Surg. 2020;15(1):24. https://doi.org/10.1186/s13017-020-00302-7.
11. Coccolini F, Kobayashi L, Kluger Y, et al. Duodeno-pancreatic and extrahepatic biliary tree trauma: WSES-AAST guidelines. World J Emerg Surg. 2019;14:56. https://doi.org/10.1186/s13017-019-0278-6.
12. Koganti SB, Kongara R, Boddepalli S, Mohammad NS, Thumma V, Nagari B, Sastry RA. Predictors of successful non-operative management of grade III & IV blunt pancreatic trauma. Ann Med Surg (Lond). 2016;10:103–9. https://doi.org/10.1016/j.amsu.2016.08.003.
13. Leppäniemi A, Tolonen M, Tarasconi A, Segovia-Lohse H, Gamberini E, Kirkpatrick AW, Ball CG, Parry N, Sartelli M, Wolbrink D, et al. 2019 WSES guidelines for the management of severe acute pancreatitis. World J Emerg Surg. 2019;14:27. https://doi.org/10.1186/s13017-019-0247-0.
14. Mularski RA, Sippel JM, Osborne ML. Pneumoperitoneum: a review of nonsurgical causes. Crit Care Med. 2000;28(7):2638–44. https://doi.org/10.1097/00003246-200007000-00078.
15. Faintuch J, Meniconi MT, Speranzini MB, Pinotti HW, Smolentsov H. Clinical regression of infected pancreatic necrosis. Case report Int J Pancreatol. 1991;8(4):379–86. https://doi.org/10.1007/BF02952729.

Appendicitis in Elderly

43

Supparerk Prichayudh and Rattaplee Pak-art

Introduction

Appendicitis is one of the most common acute abdominal conditions in all age groups, including elderly (5–10% of patients with appendicitis). Rupture rate, morbidity, and mortality are higher in older patients due to difficulty in diagnosis and increased comorbidities. With an advance in modern medicine resulting in increased life expectancy, acute appendicitis in elderly is likely to be more common. Early diagnosis and prompt treatment are of utmost importance to achieve favorable outcomes in elderly patients with appendicitis.

Clinical Manifestations

Although migratory abdominal pain (from periumbilical area to right lower quadrant) with tenderness, anorexia, and fever are common presentations recognized in other age groups, these signs and symptoms may be less obvious in geriatric patients. Lower abdominal pain (up to 90%) and anorexia (up to 60%) are the two most common symptoms found in elderly patients with appendicitis. Furthermore, in the patients who are unable to communicate (e.g., cerebrovascular accident or dementia), presentation of acute appendicitis can be more subtle (i.e., feeding intolerance, abdominal distension, and unexplained fever/sepsis). Early diagnosis based on signs and symptoms alone can be difficult in this group of patients, resulting in higher rupture rate and mortality. Hence, high index of suspicion, laboratory tests, and imaging study are usually needed for timely diagnosis of acute appendicitis in the patients who are unable to communicate.

Pathology

Uncomplicated appendicitis is an early form of acute appendicitis, comprising acute edematous and acute suppurative appendicitis. Complicated appendicitis is usually a late form of acute appendicitis, especially the one with appendicolith leading to persistent luminal obstruction, gangrenous appendicitis, and perforation with phlegmon, abscess formation or diffused peritonitis. The elderly patients are more likely to have complicated appendicitis (60–70% in age greater than 65 years) as compared to the younger age groups (13–40%). Elderly patients who have onset of abdominal pain greater than 24 h, peritonitis, and signs of sepsis (tachycardia and tachypnea) are more likely to have complicated appendicitis.

S. Prichayudh · R. Pak-art (✉)
Department of Surgery, King Chulalongkorn Memorial Hospital, Faculty of Medicine, Chulalongkorn University, Bangkok, Thailand
e-mail: Supparerk.P@Chula.ac.th; Rattaplee.P@Chula.ac.th

P. Petrone, C. E.M. Brathwaite (eds.), *Acute Care Surgery in Geriatric Patients*,
https://doi.org/10.1007/978-3-031-30651-8_43

Diagnosis

Like other age groups, the diagnosis of acute appendicitis can be made based on symptoms (anorexia, migratory pain from periumbilical area to right lower quadrant, fever), signs (peritoneal signs, decreased bowel sound), and simple laboratory values (leukocytosis with left shift, normal urinalysis). However, these findings can be more subtle in elderly due to impaired host response to infection/inflammation and comorbidities. Several clinical scores using these simple clinical parameters have been proposed to help diagnose acute appendicitis (e.g., Alvarado score, Lintula score, and Diagnostic score). The application of these scores in elderly showed acceptable accuracy (up to 90%) with appropriate cut-off points. Nevertheless, there is no standard score dedicated specifically for elderly patients and differentiation between complicated and uncomplicated appendicitis cannot be made by these clinical scores.

Abdominal ultrasonography has been used for diagnosis of acute appendicitis especially in children and pregnancy with accuracy above 80%; however, it is operator dependent and data on elderly with appendicitis is limited. Computed tomography (CT) has been more widely used for elderly patients with acute abdominal conditions and the accuracy to diagnose appendicitis in elderly patients is great (90–100%). CT can help differentiate complicated appendicitis (the presence of appendicolith, free air, free fluid, abscess, and ileus) from uncomplicated one. Furthermore, CT can help diagnose other pathologies mimicking appendicitis in elderly (e.g., colonic diverticulitis, colon cancer, and enterocolitis).

Diagnosis of acute appendicitis in elderly can be made by detailed history, physical examination, and simple laboratory tests. Imaging study can be used when the clinical manifestation of appendicitis is not obvious, or when there are other differential diagnoses to be ruled out.

Non-operative Management

Uncomplicated Appendicitis

Non-operative management of acute uncomplicated appendicitis can be safely performed in selected patients. With two recent randomized control trials of non-operative treatment (antibiotics therapy) vs. operative treatment in uncomplicated appendicitis, majority of the non-operative treatment group underwent successful treatment with only 27–29% of the patients required subsequent appendectomy (with the follow-up time of 90 days to 1 year). A five-year follow-up study demonstrated that 39% of the patients in the non-operative group developed recurrent appendicitis and 89% of those had complicated appendicitis. Since most of the patients in these studies were young (mean age of 33–38 years) and the morbidity/mortality of appendicitis is higher in elderly, the application of non-operative treatment in elderly with appendicitis is not routinely recommended. If surgeon decides to perform non-operative management, it must be done with caution after discussing the risks and benefits with the patient and close observation with a low threshold for appendectomy (if clinical signs become worse) are mandatory.

Phlegmon and Appendiceal Abscess

In patients who present late (after 24 h of onset), perforation is more likely. Perforation can result in uncontrolled infection (peritonitis and sepsis), or a localized inflammatory mass (appendiceal phlegmon), or an appendiceal abscess. Since the morbidity of emergency appendectomy is high in patients who present with appendiceal mass (inability to identify an appendix, inadvertent injuries of bowel, and surgical site infection); they can safely undergo non-operative management with a course of broad-spectrum antibiotics, provided that there are no signs of peritonitis/sepsis. Percutaneous drainage can be added to drain an abscess demonstrated in the imaging study if the patients do not respond quickly to antibiotics. The disadvantages of the non-operative treatment included increased length of stay, increased cost of treatment, and the risk of recurrent appendicitis.

Interval appendectomy after a successful conservative treatment of an appendiceal phlegmon/abscess is controversial. Proponents suggested routine interval appendectomy at 6–8 weeks after onset due to risk of recurrence (up to 8.8%) and risk of neoplasm (1.3% in general population and up to 20% in elderly). However, observation is a viable option especially in patients who have high risk for surgery and low probability for cancer (considering the information obtained from imaging study and/or colonoscopy).

Operative Management

To date, appendectomy is still considered the standard treatment for acute appendicitis. Early surgery (less than 12 h after the onset) results in less rupture rate and less morbidity. Appendectomy can be performed in either open fashion or laparoscopic approach, depending on the surgeon's expertise and the patient's preference. While laparoscopic appendectomy has advantages of decreasing post-operative pain, hospital length of stay, and wound infection, open appendectomy carries shorter operative time and lesser intra-abdominal infection. Additionally, laparoscopy can help the surgeon explore the abdomen more thoroughly in a case with uncertain diagnosis. However, the conversion rate from laparoscopic to open appendectomy is higher in elderly patients (up to 17%). Conversion is a sign of "good judgment" when the situation cannot be handled laparoscopically (e.g., bleeding control, the need for bowel repair/resection, and suspicion of neoplasm), depending on the surgeon's expertise in laparoscopic surgery.

Negative appendectomy can be encountered up to 15% in patients undergoing appendectomy. This rate is lower in elderly (10%) due to an increasing use of preoperative imaging studies. The normal-looking appendix should be removed for a pathologic examination and for prevention of future diagnostic dilemma. Other pathologies mimicking acute appendicitis should also be sought thoroughly (e.g., Meckel's diverticulitis, ileitis, colitis, and gynecological conditions).

Post-operative morbidity for appendectomy increases in elderly (19–46%) as compared to younger patients (5–9%). The most common morbidity is surgical site infection (9–15%). Besides advanced age, the other risk factors for post-operative morbidity include higher American Society of Anesthesiologists score (ASA >3), open surgery, complicated appendicitis, and comorbidities (i.e., anemia, heart disease, and chronic renal failure).

Conclusion

Elderly patients with acute abdominal pain should be carefully evaluated. Since the signs and symptoms of acute appendicitis can be more subtle in elderly. High index of suspicion is required, and selective use of imaging study is advised to make an early diagnosis. Morbidity and mortality of appendicitis are higher in elderly patients, especially ones with complicated appendicitis. Even though the non-operative treatment for acute appendicitis is emerging, appendectomy is still considered as a standard treatment and should be done in a timely fashion to prevent perforation and other morbidities.

References

1. Lapsa S, Ozolins A, Strumfa I, Gardovskis J. Acute appendicitis in the elderly: a literature review on an increasingly frequent surgical problem. Geriatrics (Basel). 2021;6(3):93.
2. Dahdaleh FS, Heidt D, Turaga KK. The appendix. In: Brunicardi FC, Andersen DK, Billiar TR, et al., editors. Schwartz's principles of surgery. 11th ed. New York: McGraw-Hill; 2019. p. 1331–43.

3. Tantarattanapong S, Arwae N. Risk factors associated with perforated acute appendicitis in geriatric emergency patients. Open Access Emerg Med. 2018;10:129–34.
4. Alvarado A. A practical score for the early diagnosis of acute appendicitis. Ann Emerg Med. 1986;15:557–64.
5. Lintula H, Kokki H, Pulkkinen J, Kettunen R, Gröhn O, Eskelinen M. Diagnostic score in acute appendicitis. Validation of a diagnostic score (Lintula score) for adults with suspected appendicitis. Langenbecks Arch Für Chir. 2010;395:495–500.
6. Shchatsko A, Brown R, Reid T, Adams S, Alger A, Charles A. The utility of the alvarado score in the diagnosis of acute appendicitis in the elderly. Am Surg. 2017;83:793–8.
7. Eskelinen M, Meklin J, Syrjänen K, Eskelinen M. A diagnostic score (DS) is a powerful tool in diagnosis of acute appendicitis in elderly patients with acute abdominal pain. Anticancer Res. 2021;41:1459–69.
8. Ooler BD, Lawrence EM, Pickhardt PJ. MDCT for suspected appendicitis in the elderly: diagnostic performance and patient outcome. Emerg Radiol. 2012;19(1):27–33.
9. Salminen P, Paajanen H, Rautio T, et al. Antibiotic therapy vs appendectomy for treatment of uncomplicated acute appendicitis. JAMA. 2015;313(23):2340–8.
10. Salminen P, Tuominen R, Paajanen H, Rautio T, Nordström P, Aarnio M, Rantanen T, Hurme S, Mecklin JP, Sand J, et al. Five-year follow-up of antibiotic therapy for uncomplicated acute appendicitis in the APPAC randomized clinical trial. JAMA. 2018;320:1259–65.
11. CODA collaborative a randomized trial comparing antibiotics with appendectomy for appendicitis. N Engl J Med. 2020;383:1907–19. https://doi.org/10.1056/NEJMoa2014320.
12. Ahmed A, Feroz S, Dominic J, et al. Is emergency appendicectomy better than elective appendicectomy for the treatment of appendiceal phlegmon: A review. Cureus. 2020;12(12):e12045.
13. Prasertsuntarasai S, Prichayudh S. Is interval appendectomy necessary for appendiceal mass? Chula Med J. 2007;51(5):273–9.
14. Segev L, Keidar A, Schrier I, Rayman S, Wasserberg N, Sadot E. Acute appendicitis in the elderly in the twenty-first century. J Gastrointest Surg. 2015;19:730–5.
15. Renteria O, Shahid Z, Huerta S. Outcomes of appendectomy in elderly veteran patients. Surgery. 2018;164:460–5.

Management of Pancreaticobiliary Disease in the Geriatric Patient Population

44

Matthew Krell, John D. Allendorf, Matthew Morris, Amir Sohail, and Jennifer M. Whittington

Introduction

Benign biliary disease is a common diagnosis that is treated with surgery in patients worldwide. Given a multitude of healthcare advancements over the past decades, there has been a substantial increase in the geriatric population. The Institute of Medicine first formed a workforce for geriatric patients and produced a report outlining their objectives in 1978. In 2008, the Committee on the Future Health Care Workforce for Older Americans generated another report addressing the evolving geriatric patient population and how the healthcare workforce can best care for this population of patients. This committee set objectives to improve competence in delivery of care to geriatric patients on behalf of the entire healthcare workforce, increase the recruitment and retention of geriatricians, and enhance the delivery of health care. This increasing aging population creates new and unique considerations for the healthcare industry including physician and provider communication to minimize polypharmacy, ensuring safe domiciling of aging patients, and provision of optimal care for geriatric patients under the purview of Centers for Medicare and Medicaid Services (CMS). The acute care surgeon must be able to rapidly assess and care for geriatric patients to effectively determine if the patient requires emergent surgical intervention or if temporizing adjuncts such as Endoscopic Retrograde Cholangiopancreatography (ERCP) or drainage with interventional radiology are indicated prior to surgical intervention. Pancreatitis is one of the most common gastrointestinal disorders requiring acute hospitalization worldwide with an estimated incidence of 13–45 cases per 100,000 and about 270,000 cases annually in the United States. The 2012 Atlanta classification revised its outline of acute pancreatitis diagnosis to require at least two of the following three criteria: persistent abdominal pain often radiating to the back, a threefold increase in serum lipase, and/or amylase above the upper limit of normal value, and typical imaging findings of acute pancreatitis. The acute care surgeon must organize a multidisciplinary team of geriatricians, gastroenterologists, interventional radiologists, nutritionists, nursing staff, physical therapists, social workers, and supportive care to optimize perioperative and long-term postoperative care for geriatric patients treated with biliary disease. The acute care surgeon must also consider biliary malignancy as part of their

M. Krell · J. D. Allendorf · M. Morris · A. Sohail · J. M. Whittington (✉)
Department of Surgery, NYU Long Island School of Medicine, NYU Langone Hospital—Long Island, Mineola, NY, USA
e-mail: Matthew.krell@nyulangone.org; John.Allendorf@nyulangone.org; matthew.morris@nyulangone.org; Amir.Sohail@nyulangone.org; Jennifer.Whittington@nyulangone.org

P. Petrone, C. E.M. Brathwaite (eds.), *Acute Care Surgery in Geriatric Patients*,
https://doi.org/10.1007/978-3-031-30651-8_44

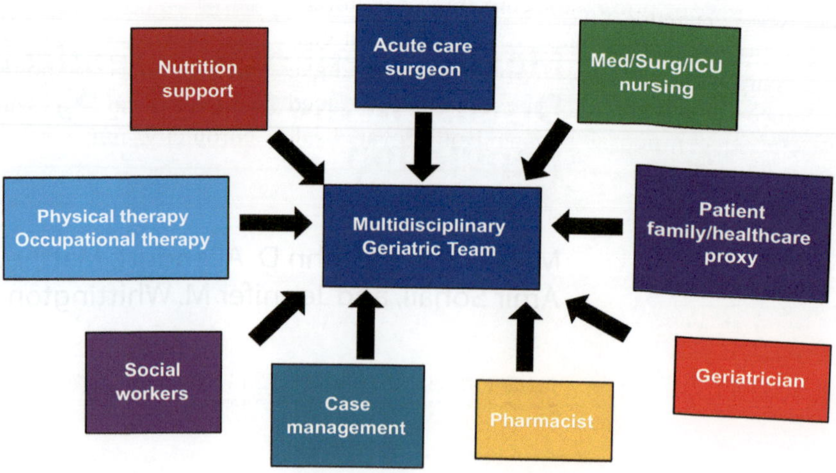

Fig. 44.1 Each member of the multidisciplinary geriatric team plays a unique and important role in delivering patient center care to geriatric patients in the acute care setting

differential diagnosis in the geriatric patient population and offer special consideration to including oncologic specialists as an integral part of the care team early in the patient's hospitalization (Fig. 44.1).

Initial Evaluation of Geriatric Biliary Pathology in Acute Care Surgery

History and Physical Examination

The acute care setting can be a particularly treacherous realm for geriatric patients presenting with biliary disease. Although benign biliary disease represents a common presentation in the acute care setting, some geriatric patients have baseline neurocognitive disorders that prevent them from effectively communicating their symptoms to the care team. If the patient is unable to clearly articulate their medical history, the acute care surgeon must obtain critical information from secondhand sources. These critical sources could include family present at time of admission, emergency service providers responsible for patient transport who may have bystander information, or nursing providers at the patient's residence if the patient is coming from an assisted living facility or nursing home (Table 44.1). Ideally, geriatric patients undergo perioperative assessment with a geriatrician with a formal frailty index prior to elective surgical intervention.

It is critical to determine if the patient has other medical comorbidities that could impact medical decision-making in the emergency setting. The acute care surgery team should make every effort to obtain records from the patient's primary care provider and any consultants. It is ideal to reach out to these consultants directly to discuss the patient's care if possible. Special considerations to review include if the patient has had a recent cardiac intervention or history of cardiac stents that may require prolonged anticoagulation in the perioperative period. Determining if the patient has any severe obstructive or restrictive lung disease that would limit their ability to liberate from the ventilator postoperatively if surgery is indicated. Assessment of metabolic status, particularly the severity of diabetes mellitus if present, as this requires careful glycemic control if the patient sustains biliary sepsis. Many geriatric patients have considered their advanced directives and prepared for medical emergencies, however many have not. It is critical for the emergency care team to have these discussions early on with the patient, directly if the patient is medically able and has decision-making capacity, or with the patient's healthcare proxy if the patient is unable to make these decisions for themselves.

In addition to determining the patient's baseline capacity for mental and physical activity, the acute care surgery team should make every attempt obtain an updated medication reconcilia-

Table 44.1 Geriatric acute care surgery patients have special considerations regarding history and physical that can impact further testing and patient management

Special considerations in Geriatric Assessment in Acute Care Surgery	
History	
	Medications, polypharmacy
	Where patient lives (nursing home, with family)
	Baseline activities of daily living
	Advance directives
	Surgical and procedural history, presence of pacemakers, prosthetics
Physical exam	
	signs of elder abuse (emaciation, wounds, reluctance to speak with family present)
	skin changes suggested with malnutrition or undiagnosed conditions (flaking, unhealing wounds)
	bruising and skin tears requiring care(patients on anticoagulants)
	presence of longstanding catheters (indwelling foley catheters)
	appreciation of more lability with abnormal vital signs (physiologic frailty)

tion from the patient or their contacts. Polypharmacy is a special consideration for geriatric patients in the acute care setting. Many geriatric patients have a reduction in lean body mass and total body water content. Therefore, they have a decreased distribution volume of hydrophilic drugs and accentuated toxic effects of medications. Their relative increase in body fat and increased distribution volume of fat-soluble drugs leads to an increased half-life and time to reach a steady-state serum concentration for certain medications. Reduced glomerular filtration rate, tubular secretion, and renal blood flow can lead to a reduction in renal drug elimination and accumulation of renally cleared drugs. Particularly before any procedural or surgical intervention, the acute care surgeon must determine if the patient is taking anticoagulants that need to be judiciously reversed. Sepsis secondary to biliary pathophysiology can exacerbate polypharmacy, and it is imperative that the acute care surgery team consider this during initial resuscitative efforts.

Physical exam findings of biliary pathology traditionally include postprandial right upper quadrant pain or nausea, fevers, and jaundice. Pain is often a discriminating feature in jaundiced patients. Jaundice secondary to malignancy is typically painless, whereas patients with jaundice and pain frequently have a benign process causing obstruction of the biliary tree. Patients with obstructive ascending cholangitis may additionally present with hypotension, tachycardia, and altered mental status. Geriatric patients presenting with biliary pathology are challenging because their symptoms may not be as pronounced as a non-geriatric patient presenting in the acute care setting. Some patients may not be able to effectively verbalize their symptoms while others may have limited pain perception due to neuropathy. Other subtle signs of biliary dysfunction can include excoriations or skin picking secondary to chronic pruritis, ecchymosis and/or petechia secondary to synthetic hepatic dysfunction, reports of biliuria or acholic stools from care providers, or loose skin from prolonged weight loss due to chronic postprandial pain. If weight loss over an acute period, i.e., 2–3 months, is noted in a geriatric patient in the setting of biliary disease, the acute care surgeon should consider malignancy as part of the differential diagnosis.

Laboratory and Radiographic Evaluation

The laboratory assessment of geriatric patients is like that of other patients with biliary disease in the acute care setting. Uncomplicated cholelithiasis, i.e., asymptomatic or biliary colic, laboratory results are frequently normal. In the acute care setting, laboratory assessment should include a complete blood chemistry (CBC) with differential to assess for leukocytosis, anemia, thrombocytosis, or thrombocytopenia. Leukocytosis suggests an inflammatory process and is frequently associated with acute cholecystitis. The differential assessment can show a left shift with respect to the neutrophil count to further support evidence of an inflammatory process or can show evidence of underlying blood dyscrasias that may warrant further evaluation prior to intervention if time permits. A geriatric patient in the acute care setting should also undergo evaluation with an arterial blood gas (ABG) to assess for correctable acid base disorders, and a basic metabolic panel (BMP) to assess for correctable electrolyte abnormalities. For patients who have coronary artery disease or cardiac electrophysiologic dysfunction, it is imperative to correct potassium, magnesium, and calcium prior to procedural or surgical intervention. It is prudent to consider testing a hemoglobin A1C (HgbA1C) as this has shown to improve perioperative and intensive care unit outcomes in the geriatric population. Additionally, endocrine function should be evaluated in geriatric patients who do not respond to initial resuscitative measures. For patients who have persistent bradycardia, decreased skin turgor, unexplained weight gain, or lethargy prior to admission, it is reasonable to assess thyroid function by testing a serum Thyroid Stimulating Hormone (TSH) as well as a T3 and free T4 measurement. For patients with persistent tachycardia not responsive to fluid TSH should be assessed to evaluate for an underlying overproduction of thyroid hormone. For patients who are being treated for sepsis not responding to fluid resuscitation with pressors, the acute care team should consider assessment of the hypothalamic-pituitary-adrenal (HPA) axis by assessing the patient's cortisol level. The most common laboratory abnormalities noted in complications associated with cholelithiasis are elevations in bilirubin. Assessment of hyperbilirubinemia should assess total, conjugated, and unconjugated forms of bilirubin. It is important to note that total and conjugated bilirubin will be elevated in jaundice associated with biliary obstruction while an increase in unconjugated bilirubin is noted in hemolysis or Gilbert's disease. Alkaline phosphatase is secreted from the lining of the bile ducts and is also associated with biliary obstruction. Measurement of aspartate transaminase (AST) and alanine transaminase (ALT) is a marker of hepatocyte function. AST is elevated 2:1 in alcoholic liver disease while ALT is raised in intrinsic hepatocyte damage. Gamma glutamyl transpeptidase (GGT) is frequently elevated in patients with alcoholic liver disease. Serum albumin is an important nutritional marker in the geriatric population. Serum albumin is often low in patients with chronic liver insufficiency and in patients with poor nutritional reserve. This can impact surgical decision-making if there is concern that the patient will not adequately heal postoperatively. Prothrombin time (PTT) is the most sensitive marker of synthetic liver function and is sometimes elevated in chronic liver insufficiency. This marker can also be elevated in prolonged biliary obstruction. Patients with acute biliary pancreatitis will typically have an elevated serum lipase level.

As with any patient, the workup begins with a thorough history and physical exam, which may be combined with appropriate laboratory testing, and imaging can help elucidate the etiology of the acute pancreatitis and guide management.

A serum lipase or amylase level three times the upper limit of normal serum in the setting of abdominal pain is diagnostic of acute pancreatitis. There does not need to be any changes in white blood cell count, but leukocytosis is commonly seen with acute pancreatitis. Elevations in total bilirubin, alkaline phosphatase, aspartate transaminase, and alanine transaminase are also often seen.

Independent risk factors for severity of acute pancreatitis include older age, obesity, hematocrit, CRP, and BUN. Elevated hematocrit >44% on admission is predictive of more severe disease as it reflects greater hemoconcentration from third space losses. Similarly, a BUN >20 at the time of admission is associated with an increased risk of death. In addition, increases in BUN on serial measurement are associated with worse outcomes. An elevated CRP >150 which rises more slowly than BUN or other acute phase reactants such as hematocrit has also been shown to correlate with severe acute pancreatitis 24–48 h after admission. The single most important lab value is often considered BUN not lipase for determining severity of acute pancreatitis. Procalcitonin is the most sensitive and strongly specific lab test for detection of pancreatic infection. Much of these values are utilized in an array of scoring systems used to evaluate severity.

When evaluating a patient with suspected acute pancreatitis, it is important to appropriately assess the severity of their disease. The severity can help with the level of care required to treat the patient and help predict morbidity and mortality. Severe acute pancreatitis is associated with persistent organ dysfunction and higher mortality. There are several scoring systems in place to help grade the severity of the disease. Some of these are the Revised Atlanta classification, Imrie classification, Ranson's criteria taken on admission and at 48 h, APACHE III score helps with prognostication and in-hospital mortality, Computed Tomography (CT) pancreatitis severity score which examines the level of edema, level of necrosis and a score of 5 or greater associated with increased hospital length of stay and 15× risk of mortality, Balthazar score stratified pancreatitis as mild (interstitial), intermediate (exudative), severe (necrotizing), BISAP score bedside index for severity in acute pancreatitis. Each score has its positives and negatives and there is not one alone that is recommended as a sole predictor of outcome. When using a severity grading score, you must take into account the ease of use and whether the score is examining qualitative data or quantitative data. The WSES (World Society Of Emergency Surgery) recommends the BISAP as one of the most accurate and applicable scoring tools for calculating severity, mortality, and organ failure along with the APACHE score, but note that there is no gold standard scoring system. The highest risk of death among acute pancreatitis patients are those who have persistent organ failure with infected pancreatic necrosis. The sooner you can evaluate the severity of the disease the sooner you can arrange a disposition for the patient, severe pancreatitis with organ failure likely requires a higher level of care such as intensive care unit compared to a mild acute pancreatitis.

Ultrasound is generally the first choice of diagnostic imaging. Ultrasound is an excellent imaging modality in that it has a high specificity and is low cost without radiation and can readily identify gallstones. Findings of pericholecystic fluid and or gallbladder wall thickening are suggestive of acute cholecystitis. While dilation of the common bile duct suggests choledocholithiasis. A sonographic Murphy's sign can often be elicited in patients with acute cholecystitis. However, ultrasound is operator dependent and can be limited by patient body habitus. Adedeji et al. demonstrated that 65% of patients presenting with acute cholecystitis have a positive Murphy's sign whereas only 48% of elderly patients exhibit this finding. Ultrasound which can identify gallstones as the potential etiology of the acute pancreatitis. CT is more expensive than ultrasound and exposes the patient to radiation but can offer additional information and is less operator dependent. The most utilized imaging modality is CT with intravenous contrast enhancement. This is optimally done as a dual phase protocol CT which includes arterial and portal venous contrast phases. The contrast aids in delineating potential etiologies in the setting of obstructive disease, as well as identifying peripancreatic fluid collections and evidence of necrosis. Typically, changes in the density of pancreatic parenchyma due to local edema and fat stranding to the surrounding retroperitoneal fat will invariably be seen. Non-enhancement of the pancreas on CT or the presence of gas is indicative of necrosis. Signs of hemorrhagic pancreatitis, include high attenuated fluid in the peripancreatic area. The optimal timing for the first CT is 72-96 h after the onset of symptoms. Other options for imaging include Magnetic Resonance Imaging (MRI) and Endoscopic Ultrasound (EUS). The timing of follow-up imaging is based on the severity of illness and the patient's clinical course.

CT imaging findings associated with biliary disease include pericholecystic fluid, cholelithiasis, gallbladder wall thickening, and common bile duct dilation/choledocholithiasis. CT imaging also provides the benefit of evaluating for separate intra-abdominal pathology that may explain the patient's symptoms. CT imaging can be utilized if the ultrasound findings are equivocal or if there is suspicion of a more insidious disease process, such as a biliary malignancy, not fully visualized with ultrasound. CT imaging should be used judiciously in the geriatric population. Many geriatric patients have underlying chronic renal disease and a contrast bolus can incite an acute kidney injury. This is particularly important because if the patient required ERCP to treat biliary obstruction, which requires contrast dye, as part of their multidisciplinary approach to treat their biliary disease, The development of an acute kidney injury could delay the implementation of a critical intervention such as imaging with contrast or utlization of certain nephrotoxic antibiotics. These types of delay in care could result in the worsening of their cholangitis and subsequent clinical decompensation. In a frail geriatric patient such a delay in care could result in failure to rescue, and ultimately create a significant morbidity, or even mortality, in this patient population.

Hepatobiliary Iminodiacetic Acid (HIDA) scan is a nuclear medicine exam that is considered the most specific/sensitive for acute cholecystitis. A stone obstructing the cystic duct, resulting in non-visualization of the gallbladder is diagnostic of acute cholecystitis. A study showing lack of tracer in the common bile duct is diagnostic for choledocholithiasis. HIDA can also be used for detection of biliary dyskinesia. The ejection fraction can be determined by administration of CCK during the exam. A biliary ejection fraction of <35% is considered abnormal. HIDA is infrequently utilized in the acute care surgery setting but is helpful in the outpatient evaluation of biliary dyskinesia and postoperative assessment of bile leak after cholecystectomy.

Further evaluation of the biliary tree can also be undertaken utilizing MRI or Magnetic Resonance Cholangiopancreatography (MRCP). This allows for excellent evaluation of soft tissue in the area, as well as good definition of the biliary tree and pancreas. It is often the best imaging for workup of choledocholithiasis and malignancy. Like HIDA scan, MRCP is also useful in the evaluation of a post cholecystectomy bile leak. In cases where choledocholithiasis or other biliary obstruction is suspected with elevated bilirubin, but the MRCP is negative, further workup may be considered with EUS to directly evaluate the biliary tree endosonographically. If EUS does identify an obstructive lesion, ERCP can then be performed at this time to clear or relieve the obstruction. Particularly in the geriatric population where there is an increased risk of malignancy, an experienced interventional gastroenterologist can be obtained biliary brushings and possibly biopsies if there is concern for an underlying malignancy.

Treatment of Geriatric Pancreaticobiliary Pathology in Acute Care Surgery

Considerations of Initial Resuscitation

The geriatric population can be particularly challenging to manage in the acute care setting for numerous reasons. Determining the patient's goals of care in a timely manner, particularly if they have not provided advance directives, is paramount. If a geriatric patient has profound biliary sepsis and has decision-making capacity but has stated that they do not want aggressive care or intervention, it would be unethical to pursue aggressive interventions to rescue the patient. If a patient is unable to make these decisions for themselves and the healthcare proxy is responsible, it is up to the multidisciplinary acute care surgery team, led by the acute care surgeon, to guide the healthcare proxy in making the decisions that the patient would make for themselves if they were there to make informed decisions. Clear and compassionate communication is a critical skillset that the acute care surgeon must embrace.

When the patient has elected to pursue intervention, or the healthcare proxy has chosen to pursue lifesaving measures on behalf of the patient, timely diagnosis, and intervention are critical for the geriatric patient's survival. Initial management should include establishing reliable IV access to administer isotonic fluids. Geriatric resuscitation in the acute care setting requires exceptional clinical vigilance since these patients often have underlying medical comorbidities and less physiologic reserve compared to younger healthier patients with biliary disease. For patients exhibiting hemodynamic lability, it is prudent to establish an arterial line to assess pulse pressure variations and utilize ABG measurements to assess end points of resuscitation including arterial pH and base deficit. Bedside point of care ultrasound (POCUS) is a useful tool to assess for bedside cardiac dynamics and resuscitation parameters including inferior vena cava fluid dynamics. Additionally, for patients with underlying cardiac disease, particularly those patients on anticoagulation, a plan for anticoagulation reversal and/or bridging must be developed based on the expediency for surgical intervention.

It is critical to start broad antibiotics in a timely manner to target organisms most commonly responsible for infections of the biliary tree. For community-acquired acute cholecystitis, single agent cefazolin, cefuroxime, or ceftriaxone are adequate. For patients with community-acquired acute cholecystitis with physiologic disturbance, advanced age or immunocompromised state, or any patient who has cholangitis of any severity, then meropenem, doripenem, piperacillin-tazobactam, or cefepime in combination with metronidazole is appropriate. Given the caveat of advanced age, most geriatric patients treated in the acute care surgery setting should be treated with this more aggressive regimen. One caveat for geriatric patients being treated with beta lactam antibiotics is that these medications lower the seizure threshold. For patients who receive atypical anti-psychotics or anti-seizure medications, this should be taken into consideration and a pharmacist should be included as part of the multidisciplinary team. Patients who will require more expeditious surgical intervention, a multidisciplinary approach including anesthesiology, cardiology, and pulmonary medicine, if indicated, is recommended.

Indications for Emergent Operative Intervention for Geriatric Biliary Pathology

Severe or chronic gallbladder inflammation or recurrent bouts of cholecystitis place patients at increased risk of more complicated pathology, especially in the elderly population. Surgical emergencies are considered in the presence of bleeding, perforation, and obstruction. Surgical emergencies that require expeditious optimization and prompt surgical intervention include emphysematous cholecystitis, gangrenous cholecystitis, gallbladder perforation, cholecystoenteric fistula, and gallstone ileus.

Emphysematous cholecystitis is more common in the elderly from an increased incidence of gas forming bacteria, particularly *Clostridium* species. Patients with diabetes are at higher risk of sepsis. Neuropathy in these patients can lead to a lessened perception of pain and later presentation in the clinical course. Aggressive glycemic control is imperative after obtaining source control, which is achieved with emergent cholecystectomy. Ideally, this is performed in a minimally invasive fashion, but considerations regarding the geriatric patient's ability to tolerate pneumoperitoneum, severity of inflammation and spread of contamination, and length of time in under anesthesia are important decision-making points in the acute care setting. If the patient cannot tolerate pneumoperitoneum or there is significant peritoneal contamination, then open cholecystectomy is the ideal approach.

Chronic cholecystitis is often caused by recurrent episodes of obstruction of the cystic duct. This leads to chronic inflammation of the gallbladder, scarring, and ultimately gallbladder dysfunction. The elderly population also suffers from vascular disease and low blood flow states that can more easily be affected by acute illness and cause ischemia. Ischemia to the gallbladder can lead to gangrenous cholecystitis, which also warrants emergent cholecystectomy and should be approached similarly to emphysematous cholecystitis. The most severe cases of gangrenous cholecystitis can result in gallbladder perforation with spillage of contents into the intra-abdominal space. Gallbladder perforation is classified into four types based on the Niemeier classification and its modification: type 1, free perforation; type 2, perforation with abscess; type 3, chronic perforation with cholecystoenteric fistula; and type 4, perforation into the biliary tree resulting in the formation of cholecystobiliary fistulae. In this setting, the geriatric patient is at particularly high risk of Mirizzi's syndrome and higher risk of bile duct injury during the index operation. Great care should be taken to delineate the critical view of safety and bail out maneuvers such as subtotal cholecystectomy should be considered as this patient population is at higher risk of failure to rescue in the setting of a perioperative technical error. The acute care surgeon should employ the assistance of hepatobiliary specialists early and often if these anatomical challenges are anticipated.

Recurrent and chronic cholecystitis also increases the risk of biliary-enteric fistula when chronic stones erode through the biliary team. This can lead to the formation of gallstone ileus. This presentation is more commonly seen in the elderly population, frequently nursing home residents, and is responsible for 25% of small bowel obstructions in this patient population. The primary focus is on relieving the bowel obstruction, which often requires an enterotomy to remove the stone and most are over 2 cm in size and cannot traverse the ileocecal valve. Cholecystectomy may or may not be performed at the index procedure. Particularly in the geriatric population, cholecystectomy should be performed with extreme caution, if at all. The fistula often creates substantial inflammation, putting the patient at increased risk of common bile duct injury. It is reasonable to leave a drain in the right upper quadrant and allow the tract to scar as this is generally better tolerated than the sequelae of a major bile duct injury requiring more substantial intervention. In the setting of bowel perforation and contamination, the acute care surgeon should weigh the risks and benefits of performing a primary anastomosis in a previously contaminated field versus offering the patient a diverting ileostomy. In general, ileostomies are often not well-tolerated in the geriatric patient population as they are associated with volume losses, dehydration, and electrolyte abnormalities. Preoperative discussion should highlight these concerns with the patient and their healthcare proxy, and if the patient does require fecal diversion, nutrition, and volume status should be optimized and ileostomy reversal should be planned within 8–12 weeks of the index procedure if possible.

In these scenarios, the acute care surgery team should discuss postoperative care including an anticipating prolonged intensive care unit stay for these patients as they are at a particularly high risk of developing postoperative abscesses and requiring subsequent drainage procedures. Challenges regarding nutrition, patient mobility, preventing other postoperative infections, and long-term placement of the patient post hospitalization should all be anticipated and reviewed daily with the multidisciplinary team.

Multidisciplinary Approaches for the Management of Non-emergent

Acute symptomatic cholelithiasis

The incidence of cholelithiasis increases with age likely having to do with a disruption in the flow of bile or stasis and the change in the composition of the bile produced. As we age, there is an increase in the activity of 3-hydroxy-3-methylglutaryl coenzyme A which is crucial in the synthesis of cholesterol and a decrease in 7$\underline{\alpha}$ hydroxylase which is the rate-limiting enzyme in the production of bile salts from cholesterol. These two changes allow for a saturation of bile with cholesterol and an increase in the ratio of secondary bile salts to primary bile salts. This alteration in ratio promotes cholesterol synthesis, increases protein in the bile, decreases nucleation time, and increases production of phospholipids that affect mucin production. Some have suggested that Virchow's triad for thrombosis (stasis, hypercoagulability, and endothelial injury) similarly can be applied to gallstone production. The last point of the triad would be endothelial injury, which could be extrapolated to chronic gallbladder inflammation from having sludge or stones for a number of years. The most common bacteria found in acute cholecystitis are *Escherichia coli*, *Klebsiella*, and *Clostridium*, which is the same as those seen in younger individuals.

Cholelithiasis is most often asymptomatic and is diagnosed incidentally through imaging. Cholelithiasis is more likely to become symptomatic in the elderly population. Ten percent of patients with asymptomatic cholelithiasis will develop signs or symptoms within 5 years. This number increases to about 25.8% by 10 years. Although cholelithiasis is frequently asymptomatic in most individuals, symptomatic cholelithiasis often warrants operative intervention. It has been reported that around 80% of the population has gallstones. Biliary colic is symptomatic cholelithiasis and is typically associated with postprandial right upper quadrant pain or nausea. It is often caused by the gallbladder contracting against a stone blocking the cystic duct transiently.

While much of the disease diagnosis and intervention is unchanged in the elderly population, the perioperative management can vary significantly due to the increased healthcare demands of geriatric patients. The diagnostic and treatment modalities are relatively unchanged as endoscopy, surgery, and percutaneous drainage are relatively safe in the geriatric population. The difference becomes apparent, and a knowledge gap remains in assessing the geriatric patient population appropriately given their reduced physiologic reserve and optimizing their multiple comorbidities that can contribute to an increase in morbidity and mortality.

For asymptomatic/incidental cholelithiasis management consists of prophylactic surgery, expectant management, or less often medical therapy. The indication for intervention on asymptomatic cholelithiasis largely depends on clinical findings, discussion with the patient about risks and benefits, and insurance authorization in the American health system.

The primary benefit of prophylactic surgical intervention in the geriatric patient population is to avoid more complicated gallbladder disease developing without the foresight of optimizing the multiple medical comorbidities that this population often have. This is also more often considered in the geriatric population due to this population being significantly more likely to develop symptomatic cholelithiasis in the future as well as an increased risk of complicated biliary pathology. A study looking at the first episode of symptomatic cholelithiasis in patients over the age of 65, who did not undergo hospitalization or elective cholecystectomy within 2.5 months of the first episode found that the 2-year emergent gallstone-related hospitalization rate was 11.1%, with associated in-hospital morbidity and mortality rates of 56.5% and 6.5%. Asymptomatic cholelithiasis have been shown to have approximately a 10% risk of developing signs or symptoms within 5 years. This number increases to about 25.8% at 10 years.

The surgical treatment of choice for cholelithiasis is cholecystectomy. Minimally invasive approaches have emerged as the gold standard with open cholecystectomy being reserved as a fall back for when the laparoscopic approach cannot be performed or during an intraoperative complication during laparoscopic cholecystectomy such as significant bleeding, damage to a neighboring structure, or patient inability to tolerate pneumoperitoneum. The geriatric patient population has a higher rate of conversion from laparoscopic to open cholecystectomy. This is likely due to the multiple medical comorbidities in this patient population, including a longer history of gallstones, more attacks of cholecystitis, and the resultant fibrosis. These combined with an increased incidence of cardiac, pulmonary, and renal disease all contribute to the increased conversion rate of laparoscopic to open cholecystectomy in geriatric patients.

Acute Cholecystitis

Biliary colic often precedes presentation of a patient who develops acute cholecystitis, where the cystic duct blockage becomes permanent. In this irreversible obstruction, there is a cessation in the flow of bile out of the gallbladder; additionally, the distension of the gallbladder can compromise blood flow to the gallbladder wall leading to ischemia, inflammation, and infection.

The treatment of acute cholecystitis includes fluid resuscitation, antibiotics, and cholecystectomy or cholecystostomy tube placement. Without surgical intervention, there is a very high rate of recurrence putting the patient at risk for more severe complications such as cholangitis, pancreatitis, emphysematous cholecystitis, gangrenous cholecystitis, gallbladder perforation, and chronic cholecystitis. The pain from acute cholecystitis should be treated, but avoidance of morphine is recommended because it causes contraction of the sphincter of Oddi. There is an extremely high rate of recurrence of acute cholecystitis for those that do not undergo cholecystectomy and recurrent episodes are associated with increased morbidity and mortality. Estimates of recurrence rate of acute cholecystitis after non-operative management with percutaneous cholecystostomy and/or antibiotics vary, but it is safe to conclude that if patient's comorbidities can be optimized, cholecystectomy should be performed (Fig. 44.2).

The decision to perform a cholecystectomy or placement of a cholecystostomy tube is often based on the severity of the inflammation, the resources of the healthcare system, patient frailty, and medical comorbidities of the patient. Hence, risk stratification becomes very important in the geriatric patient. Some patients with severe cardiac or pulmonary disease would not tolerate prolonged general anesthesia or CO_2 pneumoperitoneum and would benefit from percutaneous cholecystostomy tube placement. Nonoperative management can be considered in select patients, but a recent retrospective study from 2018 by Wiggens et al. showed a 50% readmission rate with this management. For patients who do undergo placement of cholecystostomy tube in the acute setting, timing of interval cholecystectomy is important in the geriatric patient population. For patients with ASA class IV or V, or for patients with less than 6 months life expectancy, expectant management with a cholecystostomy tube for the remainder of the patient's life is reasonable as this offers less risk of morbidity and/or mortality than undergoing definitive management with interval cholecystectomy. For patients with ASA class II or III, geriatric assessment and outpatient evaluation with necessary consultants is indicated. These patients are candidates for interval cholecystectomy as this improves morbidity and overall quality of life in this population.

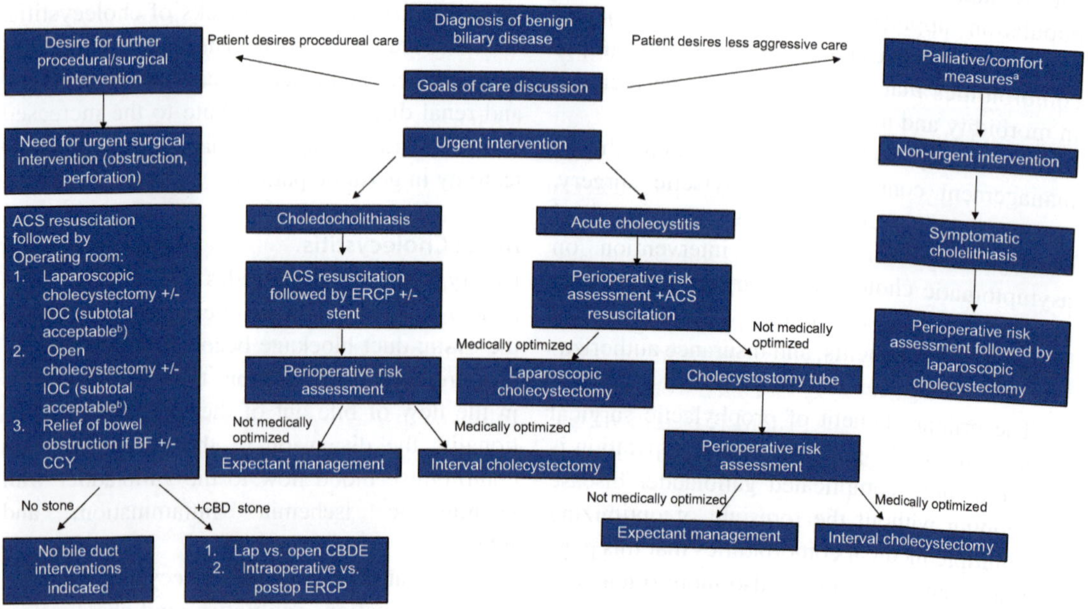

Fig. 44.2 Treatment algorithm for management of geriatric patients with benign biliary disease. (a) A detailed conversation with support care, the patient, healthcare proxy, and all members of the care team should tailor the patient's care to their goals. This could include antibiotics without plan for procedural intervention *CBDE* Common bile duct exploration, *IOC* Intraoperative cholangiogram, *ERCP* Endoscopic Retrograde Cholangiopancreatography, *BF* Biliary fistula, *CCY* Cholecystectomy, *ACS* Acute Care Surgery

A proposed 72-h period, considered the golden window, is considered standard of care for optimal timing of operative intervention on patients presenting with acute cholecystitis. Ambe et al. suggest that immediate laparoscopic cholecystectomy for acute cholecystitis within 24 h of symptom onset is not superior to surgery 25–72 h after symptoms begin. Laparoscopic cholecystectomy for acute cholecystitis therefore can be safely performed within the golden 72 h. This is particularly important for the geriatric patient population as many require perioperative risk assessment and optimization prior to surgical intervention.

Several risk stratification systems in place to help with this decision. Tokyo guidelines, American Association of Surgery of Trauma (AAST), Parkland grading scale, and the American Society of Anesthesiology (ASA). Tokyo guidelines were first put forth in 2007, revised in 2013 and again in 2018 and recommend treatments of patients with acute cholecystitis and acute cholangitis by grading the severity. This risk stratification tool rates acute cholecystitis as grade I (mild), grade II (moderate), and grade III (severe). Grade I acute cholecystitis is characterized by acute cholecystitis in a healthy patient with no organ dysfunction and mild inflammatory changes in the gallbladder, making cholecystectomy a safe and low-risk operative procedure. Grade II acute cholecystitis is associated with duration of symptoms >72 h, marked local inflammation (gangrenous cholecystitis, pericholecystic abscess, hepatic abscess, biliary peritonitis, emphysematous cholecystitis), and white blood cell count >18,000 and a palpable tenderness in the right upper quadrant. Again, pain as an exam finding may be subtle in the geriatric population due to other comorbidities like diabetes with subsequent neuropathy. Additionally, pain may exist much longer than 72 h due to neuropathy or the geriatric patient's inability to effectively communicate their symptoms. Grade III acute cholecystitis is characterized by cardiovascular dysfunction: hypotension requiring treatment with dopamine > 50 mcg/kg/min, or any dose of norepinephrine, neurological dysfunction: decreased level of consciousness, respiratory dysfunction: PaO_2/FiO_2 ratio <300, renal dysfunction: oliguria, creatinine > 2.0 mg/dL, hepatic dysfunction: PT-INR >1.5, hematological dysfunction: platelet count <100,000/mm^3. These patients require urgent resuscitative measure to reverse the sequelae of hemodynamic effects of sepsis and prevent further end organ failure. Prompt antibiotic administration in addition to guided resuscitation measures can impact early morbidity and mortality in geriatric patients who have little physiologic reserve to tolerate such hemodynamic insult.

Primary Choledocholithiasis

Primary choledocholithiasis is more often from pigmented stones than cholesterol. Pigment stones are formed by obstruction or infection of the biliary tree, or hematologic disease and are known to recur frequently. Secondary choledocholithiasis is much more common and occurs from passage of stones from the gallbladder or hepatolithiasis. Patients with choledocholithiasis, even asymptomatic choledocholithiasis, are at risk for developing cholangitis and biliary pancreatitis. Symptomatic choledocholithiasis often presents with epigastric or right upper quadrant pain, as well as signs and symptoms consistent with cholangitis. Obstruction of the biliary tree due to choledocholithiasis can cause acute cholangitis secondary to bacteria in the biliary tree and elevated intraductal pressure within the bile duct allowing for translocation of bacteria or endotoxins into the vascular system known as cholangio-venous reflux.

There is debate surrounding the management of more complicated cholecystitis such as patients with elevated liver enzymes, concern for choledocholithiasis, or proven choledocholithiasis. When there are stones within the biliary tree the patient is at greater risk of cholangitis and biliary pancreatitis. Therefore, it is important not only to remove the source, the gallbladder, but to also clear the ductal system of stones that can cause blockages. MRCP is used initially to identify patients with choledocholithiasis; however, some feel that elevated liver enzymes are enough to indicate choledocholithiasis. Definitive clearance of the biliary tree can be done endoscopically via

ERCP or intraoperatively via a common bile duct exploration that can be performed laparoscopically or open. The choice of approach is determined by the availability of resources and surgical skill set. If the acute care surgeon pursues cholecystectomy and there are intraoperative findings consistent with choledocholithiasis (i.e., enlarged common bile duct, inflammation around the infundibulum and common bile duct, concern for Mirizzi's syndrome), it is prudent to perform intraoperative cholangiogram as anatomic delineation of the hepatobiliary tree can prevent bile duct injury. Laparoscopic or open common bile duct (CBD) exploration can be performed if the acute care surgeon's laparoscopic skill set allows; however, this should be considered with caution as the area is often very inflamed and primed for iatrogenic injury. A more cautious intraoperative measure in the geriatric population would include cholecystectomy with urgent consultation of interventional gastroenterology to perform ERCP intraoperatively or urgently in the postoperative setting. Notably, geriatric patients are at higher risk of missed or forgotten stent placement; therefore, it is important to ensure that these patients are not lost to follow up and can eventually undergo stent retrieval when indicated.

MRI can be limited due to machine availability delaying testing times. ERCP must be coordinated with the gastroenterology service or a skilled endoscopic surgeon. Using a Markov model, Epelboym demonstrated that upfront cholecystectomy with routine intraoperative cholangiogram as the preferred strategy is the most cost-effective approach to the management of patients presenting with suspected choledocholithiasis. A systematic review by Dasari et al. found no difference in terms of morbidity, mortality, or success rate between the varied methods of biliary tree clearance although there was a decrease in post-ERCP pancreatitis in the group that underwent intraoperative common bile duct exploration. Additionally, open bile duct clearance was superior to ERCP in achieving CBD stone clearance.

ERCP has its own inherent risks which include pancreatitis, bleeding, perforation, and issues associated with biliary stents and gallstone treatment. A recent systematic review showed an incidence of post-ERCP pancreatitis of 3.5% and the authors noted that it is often less severe than other causes of pancreatitis. Bleeding and perforation are most often related to sphincterotomy. After clearance of the common bile duct, the acute care surgery team should consider if the geriatric patient is a candidate for laparoscopic cholecystectomy during the interval admission, or if the patient should undergo outpatient geriatric assessment and medical optimization in a multidisciplinary fashion prior to interval cholecystectomy.

Acute Pancreatitis

Pancreatitis is an inflammatory reaction to the pancreatic parenchyma due to an inappropriate activation of pancreatic enzymes and subsequent auto digestion of the surrounding tissues. The activation of trypsinogen, infiltration of inflammatory cells, and destruction of secretory cells are mediated by calcium overload, mitochondrial dysfunction, impaired autophagy, and endoplasmic reticulum stress which all play a role in the pathophysiology of acute pancreatitis.

The two most common etiologies of acute pancreatitis are gallstones and alcohol and together these etiologies account for 90–95% of cases. Less common causes of acute pancreatitis include hypertriglyceridemia, scorpion venom, trauma, congenital malformations, iatrogenic injury, cystic fibrosis, and sphincter of Oddi dysfunction.

In elderly, the differential of etiologies differs from the general population. Biliary remains the most common, but the second most common cause is idiopathic which largely differs from the general population which would be alcohol. Drugs as an etiology are increased compared to the younger population. Polypharmacy is not uncommon in the elderly population and taking 6 or more medications places them at higher risk. Many drugs can induce acute pancreatitis, but some of the more common drugs include, statins, HCTZ, furosemide, oxycodone, hydrocodone, trimethoprim/sulfamethoxazole, azathioprine, mercaptopurine, tetracyclines, macrolides, fluoroquinolones, rifampin, steroids, lisinopril, estradiol, and metformin.

There are a number of changes that take place in the pancreas in the geriatric patient population that the surgeon and radiologist should be aware of. There is decreased quantity and function of insulin secreting beta cells of the pancreas leading to insulin resistance. Calcification of the surrounding vessels, increased visceral adipose distribution, decreased muscle mass, and lower positioning of the pancreas which can present on imaging around the L3 level for the insertion of the ampulla of Vater. There are often increased calcifications and benign cysts of the pancreas, the pancreatic duct increases in size with age from 1–3 mm up to 1–2 cm without an obstruction or stricture, as does the common bile duct. Duct ectasia increases with age and can cause inter/intralobular ductules to dilate and appear as cysts. The numerous changes that geriatric patients' experience affect the way pancreatic/biliary pathologies present and can alter their management.

The International Association of Pancreatology (IAP) collaborated with the American Pancreatic Association (APA) to provide updated guidelines in 2013 for the management of acute pancreatitis. The World Society of Emergency Surgery (WSES) published its own guidelines in 2019. The IAP/APA guidelines made 38 recommendations related to 12 topics, diagnosis of acute pancreatitis and etiology, predicting severity, imaging, fluid therapy, ICU management, preventing infectious complications, nutritional support, biliary tract management, indications for intervention in necrotizing pancreatitis, timing of intervention in necrotizing pancreatitis, intervention strategies in necrotizing pancreatitis, and timing of cholecystectomy. The WSES made recommendations and offered discussion topics on severity grading, imaging, diagnostic laboratory parameters, diagnostics in idiopathic pancreatitis, risk scores, follow-up imaging, antibiotic treatment (prophylactic, infected necrosis, type of antibiotics), level of care of monitoring, fluid resuscitation, pain control, mechanical ventilation, increased intra-abdominal pressure, pharmacological treatment, enteral nutrition, operative management, indications for ERCP, indication for percutaneous/endoscopic drainage of pancreatic collections, indications for surgical intervention, timing of surgery, surgical strategy, timing of cholecystectomy, open abdomen, temporary abdominal closure, timing of dressing changes, and timing of abdominal closure. While there is a significant amount of overlap between the two society's guidelines, they both offer insight into some of the considerations that can then be tailored to fit an individual patient. Many of the statements with strong recommendations are the same and the differences mostly are with the weak recommendations such as laboratory diagnostics and surgical strategies.

The severity of pancreatitis is generally more severe in the geriatric patient population. Mortality in patients >80 years of age has been reported upwards of 25%. When pancreatitis is associated with organ failure, necrosis, pseudo cyst/peri-pancreatic fluid collection, abscess, hemorrhage can increase that number to >50% in this population. One of the most common causes of death after the first 7 days of acute pancreatitis is respiratory failure from pulmonary edema. Low threshold should be given to ICU admission given the large fluid shifts and multiple comorbidities associated with this patient population as well as the risk for rapid decompensation.

Fluid resuscitation is the mainstay of treatment of acute pancreatitis which needs careful balance in the geriatric patient population given the increased frailty and comorbidities such as heart disease. Severe pancreatitis often requires high volumes of balanced crystalloid resuscitation. The increase in pulmonary disease in this patient population also should give a lower threshold to early intubation. Another mainstay of treatment is pain control, which in the elderly population has the unfortunate risk of adding to delirium and its associated increased morbidity and discharge to places other than home. Non-narcotics should be attempted when possible, but in today's world of medicine it is important to treat patients' pain. The third major consideration during treatment is the emphasis on enteral nutrition. It was formerly commonplace to keep patients strictly nil per os (NPO) during acute pancreatitis, but now there is strong evidence for enteral nutrition unless it exacerbates the labs, imaging, or clinical exam of the patient. This can be achieved by mouth or nasogastric tube or nasojejunal feeding tube. Nasojejunal feeding should be attempted if an oral diet is not tolerated within 3–7 days of presentation and TPN should held to rare cases where enteral nutrition is not possible.

Antibiotics are not initially recommended to prevent infection as the pancreatitis is generally considered aseptic. There is a higher incidence of bacterial translocation activating the systemic inflammatory response with gallstone-induced pancreatitis. There is some debate about treatment with prophylactic antibiotic use in the geriatric patient population. These patients often present later in the disease course and are more frequently associated with gallstone etiology as well as a reduced physiologic reserve are at higher risk for acute decompensation. Early antibiotic use in geriatric patients could potentially reduce the incidence or effect of bacterial translocation and the degree of systemic inflammatory response which would decrease the morbidity and mortality in this patient population. However, general consensus still maintains recommendations against prophylactic antibiotic use in the elderly patient. There are some studies on animals suggesting an increase in bacterial infiltration in pancreatic tissues during an episode of acute pancreatitis in the older animals.

Management of Infected Pancreatic Necrosis in the Geriatric Population

Antibiotics are required with the patient develops signs, symptoms, or biopsy proven infected pancreatic necrosis. It is important to use antibiotics known to penetrate the infected pancreatic necrosis and should include both aerobic and anaerobic Gram-negative and Gram-positive coverage. Routine antifungal use is not currently recommended despite Candida species being common in patients with infected pancreatic necrosis and an indicator of high risk of mortality.

The decision on when to initiate invasive interventions is complicated. It is important to obtain cultures of infected pancreatic necrosis, but introduction of bacteria into aseptic pancreatic fluid collections can significantly worsen prognosis. The step-up approach to treatment of acute pancreatitis has been well adapted and is appropriate for the geriatric population as well as younger patients (Fig. 44.3). This aims at reducing highly morbid interventions such as open pancreatic necrosectomy. The goals are to maximize medical therapy with fluid resuscitation, antibiotics, and supportive care. If there is ongoing sepsis, percutaneous drainage and/or endoscopic drainage should be attempted. This can then be upsized and additional drains can be placed to maximize this step's utility. If there is still ongoing sepsis, endoscopic debridement should be attempted next if proximity to GI tract is safely accessible. Sometimes this is not sufficient or not accessible endoscopically and video-assisted retroperitoneal debridement surgery (VARDS) which entails utilizing the track from a large drain to laparoscopically enter the retroperitoneal space and debride the necrotic tissue. When this does not suffice and the patient continues to decompensate further, consideration of open or minimally invasive pancreatic necrosectomy should commence. Other indications for jumping to necrosectomy are hemorrhagic pancreatic necrosis with uncontrollable bleeding by less invasive measures, acute clinical decompensation that is unable to be temporized and abdominal compartment syndrome.

After treatment is initiated, consideration needs to be turned towards the etiology of the pancreatitis. If biliary/gallbladder pathology is the underlying etiology, this should be dealt with on the index hospital admission if plausible. ERCP is indicated in patients with acute gallstone pancreatitis or cholangitis with unabated common bile duct obstruction. In order to prevent additional episodes of pancreatitis, cholecystectomy should be performed prior to discharge after resolution of the acute pancreatitis because there is a high risk of readmission and recurrence of symptoms if not undertaken. In patients who are poor surgical candidates with significant risk associated with surgery, ERCP with sphincterotomy may reduce the risk of recurrent pancreati-

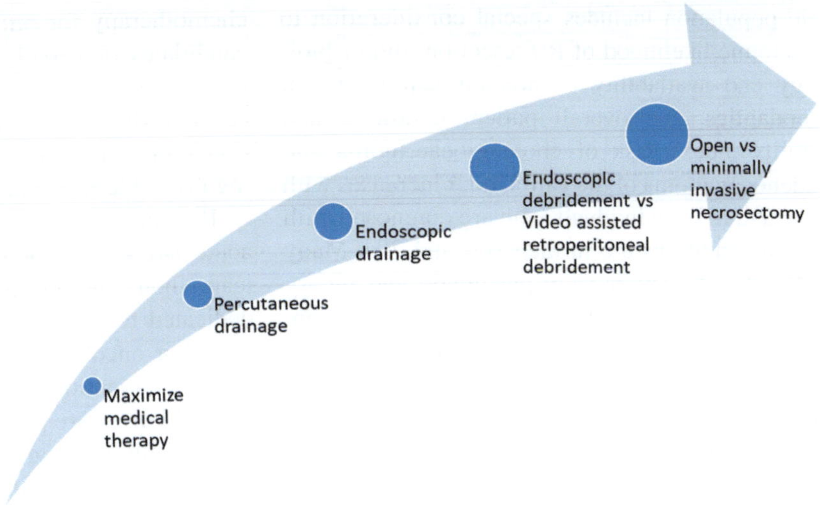

Fig. 44.3 The step-up approach treatment of acute pancreatitis has been well adapted and is appropriate for the geriatric population as well as younger patients. This aims at reducing highly morbid interventions such as open pancreatic necrosectomy

tis. A retrospective review from 2011 analyzed over 500 patients with biliary acute pancreatitis and found that ERCP with endoscopic sphincterotomy (ES) reduced the risk of recurrent disease in patients deemed too high risk for cholecystectomy. An ongoing multicenter randomized clinical trial comparing delayed cholecystectomy with endoscopic sphincterotomy in patients with biliary pancreatitis known as endoscopic sphincterotomy for delaying cholecystectomy in mild acute biliary pancreatitis (EMILY study).

In 2013, the Journal of American Medical Association (JAMA) published a study where they concluded that the risk of recurrent pancreatitis is significant in those patients who present with biliary pancreatitis and do not undergo cholecystectomy. They go on to conclude that ERCP can mitigate some of this risk when done during the initial hospitalization. They found that the risk of recurrent pancreatitis was about 17% for those undergoing no intervention on their index hospitalization, about 8% in those who underwent ERCP and approximately 5% in those who underwent cholecystectomy. The article found that both patients undergoing no intervention and those undergoing ERCP had a risk of recurrent gallstone pancreatitis but had a protective effect with ERCP. The median time from initial episode to onset of recurrence was 11 months compared to 10 months with no intervention. Kaplan-Meier estimates of recurrence for 1, 2, and 5 years in patients who underwent ERCP on index hospitalization showed a recurrence of 5.2%, 7.4%, and 11.1%. This was compared to the no intervention group yielding 11.3% for 1 year, 16.1% for 2 years, and 22.7% for 5 years and was found to be a statistically significant reduction in risk. This can be an important concept in the elderly population where surgical intervention is deemed high risk and can support the decision to avoid cholecystectomy in those cases as well as evidence that cholecystectomy at time of index admission is ideal.

Gallstone disease and pancreatitis are extremely prevalent. With the increasing size of the geriatric patient population as the "baby boomers" enter this age group, it is important to understand these pathologies to provide the best care possible. While there are not significant differences in the workup and management of these pathologies in the elderly an understanding of the changes in physiology and etiologies can help guide physicians to better outcomes and patient care.

Malignant Pancreaticobiliary Disease

The management of older patients with pancreatic and biliary tract cancers is particularly challenging owing to limited prospective data in this population. The management of malignant biliary pathology in the acute care setting for geriatric population includes special consideration to anatomic likelihood of R0 resection, tumor biology and availability of non-surgical treatment modalities, and overall patient condition and frailty index. Risk of cholangiocarcinoma and adenocarcinoma of the gallbladder increases with age and most individuals who are diagnosed with these conditions are in their 60s and 70s. Many patients who suffer from pancreatic and biliary malignancies fall within the geriatric population. Given that advanced age is common for this population, acute care surgeons who treat these conditions must be aware of physiologic changes associated with advanced age and take them into account when determining a treatment plan. The surgeon should consider the patient's age as well as associated comorbidities, functional baseline, frailty, and the patient's goals of care when developing the management plan.

Geriatric patients presenting with pancreatic cancer can present with symptoms including jaundice, weight loss, malice, pruritis, steatorrhea, and weakening of the skin, hair, and nails due to chronic nutritional deficiencies. Some patients may present with painless jaundice; however, in advanced pancreatic malignancies some patients may present with pain radiating to the back if there is tumor involvement with the celiac plexus. Initial workup for these patients should include a thorough history and physical examination, CBC, CMP, lipase, and CA 19-9. The acute care surgeon should interpret CA 19-9 with caution, as an elevated CA 19-9 in the setting of hyperbilirubinemia (total bilirubin >2.0 mg/dL) may not be accurate to assess the true value if the geriatric patient indeed has obstruction of the hepatobiliary tree secondary to a mass of the pancreatic head. Initial imaging should include a pancreas protocol dedicated triple phase CT abdomen and pelvis. The acute care surgeon should take great care the ensure the geriatric patient is appropriately intravascularly resuscitated prior to a contrast load to ensure a subsequent acute kidney injury does not develop. Such an injury could delay further diagnostic and therapeutic measures such as ERCP and stenting of the CBD. Additionally, a severe and prolonged kidney injury could potentially delay systemic chemotherapy for patients who are not surgical candidates or neoadjuvant therapy for geriatric patients with borderline resectable pancreatic cancers who are candidates for surgical intervention after treatment and restaging imaging showing favorable response to treatment.

If a pancreatic malignancy is suspected in the acute care setting, the multidisciplinary oncology team should be mobilized. It is important for a dedicated team including a surgical oncologist, radiation oncologist, medical oncologist, oncologic interventional radiologists, geriatricians, and palliative care physicians guide the management of geriatric patients with newly diagnosed malignancies. Age alone does not preclude a patient undergoing surgery, but multiple factors must be taken into account including the anatomy involved, tumor biology, and the patient's overall condition (Fig. 44.4). Surgical intervention could include a pancreatic enucleation for select neuroendocrine tumors; however, the intervention could include a pancreaticoduodenectomy, central pancreatectomy, or distal pancreatectomy and these factors should be considered carefully when determining the appropriate treatment plan for the geriatric patient. The acute care surgeon can begin the discussion regarding post-splenectomy vaccinations. Every effort to offer these vaccines 14 days prior to splenectomy as geriatric patients, particularly those who are immunocompromised due to chemotherapy, are at increased risk of overwhelming post-splenectomy infection.

Patients presenting with gallbladder adenocarcinoma can have painless jaundice, a palpable porcelain gallbladder, weight loss, or failure to

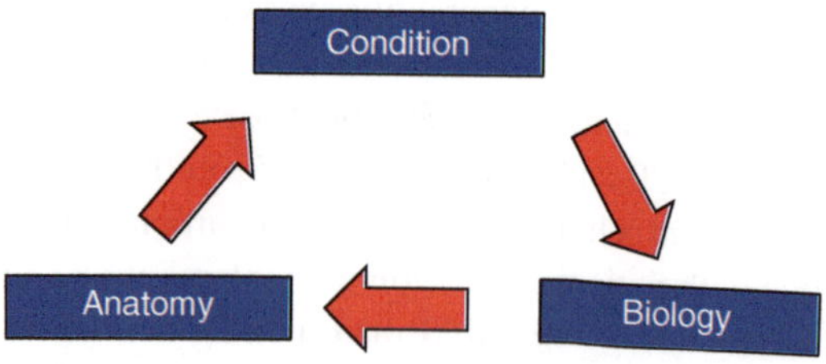

Fig. 44.4 For geriatric patients, Condition, Biology, and Anatomy, in that order, are the most important considerations for intervention in hepatopancreaticobiliary malignancies

thrive. Geriatric patients often present with locally advanced or metastatic disease due to the insidious nature of this disease and the frequently subtle of signs and symptoms in this patient population. Preoperative assessment is like that of benign biliary disease and includes laboratory analysis including liver function test, coagulation panels, and nutritional markers. Tumor markers including CA 19-9 and CEA can be assessed. The acute care surgeon should interpret CA 19-9 with caution, as an elevated CA 19-9 in the setting of hyperbilirubinemia (total bilirubin >2.0 mg/dL) can be seen in benign biliary processes. A normal CA 19-9 does not necessarily represent the lack of presence of malignancy as patients who lack the glycoprotein moiety to express CA 19-9 with serum analysis. Imaging should include ultrasound. CT and MRCP can be considered in the acute care setting to better determine the hepatobiliary anatomy. All patients being evaluated for malignancy should undergoing staging imaging with CT imaging of the chest, abdomen, and pelvis. If there is significant concern for gallbladder malignancy and the patient does not require emergent surgical intervention, the patient should be referred to a surgical oncologist for further assessment.

If the acute care surgeon has an unexpected intraoperative assessment of the gallbladder that is concerning for malignancy, it is prudent to make an intraoperative consultation to a surgical oncologist. If a surgical oncologist is not available and there is evidence of locally advanced disease (i.e., invasion into the periportal nodes or invasion into the liver), it is reasonable to obtain a biopsy for permanent pathology and refer the patient to a surgical oncologist. Do not remove the gallbladder unless it is absolutely indicated, for example, in the setting of gangrenous or emphysematous cholecystitis as this would be an operative strategy geared towards infectious source control.

Incidental gallbladder carcinoma is diagnosed in 0.3–1.5% of all cholecystectomies, but the frequency is higher in elderly patients with a rate of 9%. Acute care surgeons must follow up the pathology of all cholecystectomies. If there is evidence of dysplasia or even T1 adenocarcinoma, this should be discussed at a multidisciplinary tumor board and referred to a surgical oncologist for long-term follow-up. Elderly patients with numerous comorbidities or increased frailty index must have appropriate surgical risk stratification if formal hepatic resection is discussed with the multidisciplinary care team in the setting of gallbladder malignancy that has extended past the muscularis. For patients who are not surgical candidates, systemic chemotherapy may be considered. It is reasonable to consider a systemic chemotherapy followed by interval imaging in the setting of incidental gallbladder cancers with biliary spillage at the index operation. It is important to include any noted inflammation, anatomic abnormalities, and if there was spillage of bile during the index procedure. Up to 30% of elective cholecystectomies in the hands of board-eligible or board-certified general surgeons have spillage of biliary contents. This is important information that should be relayed to the surgical oncologist as it may change anticipated treatment sequence with regard to surgery, chemotherapy, radiation, and other regional treatment modalities.

Cholangiocarcinoma is represented by extrahepatic, hilar, and intrahepatic adenocarcinomas. Similar to other biliary tract malignancies, these malignancies often present in a delayed fashion in the geriatric population and require a multidisciplinary approach for optimal management. These patients can sometimes present with cholangitis in the acute care setting due to either extrinsic or intrinsic obstruction of the biliary tree. The acute care surgeon should include interventional gastroenterology, interventional radiology, and surgical oncology early in the management of suspected cholangiocarcinoma. It is important to carefully weigh the risks and benefits of external versus internal biliary decompression as placement of a biliary stent may increase the likelihood of the patient developing postoperative infections if they are eventually candidates for surgical resection. The management of cholangiocarcinoma, particularly intrahepatic and hilar cholangiocarcinoma are anatomically complex and often require multiple treatment considerations (i.e., staged resections, portal venous embolization, neoadjuvant chemotherapy, regional therapies) even in younger healthier patient that are outside the purview of this review. For geriatric patients, perioperative assessment becomes even more complex when taking into consideration their other comorbidities, life expectancy, and risk benefit assessment for aggressive oncologic intervention. In the acute care setting, the main objectives for these patients are expeditious physiologic resuscitation, decompression of the hepatobiliary tree, and referral to a multidisciplinary oncologic team.

Conclusion

The geriatric population can present unique challenges given the anatomic and physiologic changes that evolve with increased age. The diagnosis of both benign and malignant biliary diseases can be delayed in this patient population due to cognitive decline, communication difficulties, and decreased perception of pain. Special consideration should be given to initial history taking and physical exam for these patients. Due to delayed presentation, geriatric patients require careful resuscitation to prevent end organ failure while not compromising exacerbation of underlying cardiopulmonary comorbidities. Benign biliary disease requires a multidisciplinary approach which can include surgery after optimization, gallbladder or biliary tree decompression followed by interval cholecystectomy, or palliation with biliary decompression. Treatment of malignant biliary disease in the geriatric patient population should include early consultation of an oncologic multidisciplinary team with a focus on goals of care and quality of life. The acute care surgeon captains the team of multidisciplinary professionals in optimizing both the hospital and outpatient care of geriatric patients with biliary disease.

References

1. Institute of Medicine (US). Committee on the future health care workforce for older Americans. Retooling for an aging America: building the health care workforce. Washington (DC): National Academies Press (US); 2008.
2. Kelly KJ, Weber SM. Cholecystitis. In: Blumgart W, editor. Surgery of the liver, biliary tract and pancreas. 6th ed. Elsevier; 2017. p. 556–63.
3. Loozen CS, van Ramshorst B, van Santvoort HC, Boerma D. Early cholecystectomy for acute cholecystitis in the elderly population: a systematic review and meta-analysis. Dig Surg. 2017;34(5):371–9. https://doi.org/10.1159/000455241.
4. Adedeji OA, McAdam WA. Murphy's sign, acute cholecystitis and elderly people. J R Coll Surg Edinb. 1996;41(2):88–9.
5. Perera T, Cortijo-Brown A. Geriatric resuscitation. Emerg Med Clin North Am. 2016;34(3):453–67. https://doi.org/10.1016/j.emc.2016.04.002.
6. Hu KC, Chu CH, Wang HY, Chang WH, Lin SC, Liu CC, et al. How does aging affect presentation and management of biliary stones? Am Geriatr Soc. 2016;64(11):2330–5. https://doi.org/10.1111/jgs.14481.
7. Dimou FM, Adhikari D, Mehta HB, Riall TS. Outcomes in older patients with grade III cholecystitis and cholecystostomy tube placement: a propensity score analysis. J Am Coll Surg. 2017;224(4):502–11. https://doi.org/10.1016/j.jamcollsurg.2016.12.021.
8. Thomas M, Baltatzis M, Price A, Fox J, Pearce L, Vilches-Moraga A. The influence of frailty on outcomes for older adults admitted to hospital with benign biliary disease: a single-centre, observational cohort study. R Coll Surg Engl. 2022; https://doi.org/10.1308/rcsann.2021.0331.
9. Parmar AD, Sheffield KM, Adhikari D, Davee RA, Vargas GM, Tamirisa NP, et al. PREOP-gallstones: a prognostic nomogram for the management of symptomatic cholelithiasis in older patients. Ann Surg. 2015;261(6):1184–90. https://doi.org/10.1097/SLA.0000000000000868.
10. Wiggins T, Markar SR, Mackenzie H, Jamel S, Askari A, Faiz O, et al. Evolution in the management of acute cholecystitis in the elderly: population-based cohort study. Surg Endosc. 2018;32:4078–86. https://doi.org/10.1007/s00464-018-6092-5.
11. Ambe P, Weber SA, Christ H, Wassenberg D. Cholecystectomy for acute cholecystitis. How time-critical are the so called "golden 72 hours"? Or better "golden 24 hours" and "silver 25-72 hour"? A case control study. World J Emerg Surg. 2014;9(1):60. https://doi.org/10.1186/1749-7922-9-60.

12. van Santvoort HC, Besselink MG, Bakker OJ, Hofker HS, Boermeester MA, Dutch Pancreatitis Study Group. A step-up approach or open necrosectomy for necrotizing pancreatitis. N Engl J Med. 2010;362:1491–502. https://doi.org/10.1056/NEJMoa0908821.
13. Kucserik LP, Márta K, Vincze Á, Lázár G, Czakó L, Szentkereszty Z, et al. Endoscopic sphincterotoMy for delayIng choLecystectomy in mild acute biliarY pancreatitis (EMILY study): protocol of a multicentre randomised clinical trial. BMJ Open. 2019;9(7):e025551. https://doi.org/10.1136/bmjopen-2018-025551.
14. Epelboym I, Winner M, Allendorf JD. MRCP is not a cost-effective strategy in the management of silent common bile duct stones. J Gastrointest Surg. 2013;17(5):863–71. https://doi.org/10.1007/s11605-013-2179-4.
15. Corrigan LR, Bracken-Clarke DM, Horgan AM. The challenge of treating older patients with pancreaticobiliary malignancies. Curr Probl Cancer. 2018;42(1):59–72. https://doi.org/10.1016/j.currproblcancer.2018.01.015.

Acute Diverticulitis in the Elderly

45

Leo I. Amodu and Collin E.M. Brathwaite

Introduction

Colonic diverticular disease is a relatively common entity, which at presentation could vary in severity from mild diverticulitis amenable to outpatient treatment with or without oral antibiotics, to lower gastrointestinal bleeding (LGIB) of variable clinical significance, to acute perforation with uncontrolled intraperitoneal spillage requiring emergency surgery. The ability to appropriately diagnose and manage acute diverticulitis; the acute inflammation of colonic diverticula which could result in micro- or free perforation, is a critical requirement in surgical training and practice with significant impact on patient outcomes.

Diverticular disease has been described as a condition more commonly seen in the elderly, with some reports citing prevalence rates as high as 60% among individuals older than 65 years of age. The clinical presentation of acute diverticulitis differs in elderly patients, who present less frequently with fever and more commonly with bleeding and atypical symptoms compared to younger patients. Acute diverticulitis demonstrates a male preponderance up until the sixth decade of life, at which point it becomes more common in women. With the increasing use of flexible lower gastrointestinal endoscopy (Colonoscopy) and computed tomography (CT), it has been determined that less than 5% of patients with diverticular disease develop acute diverticulitis. While 5% seems relatively low in absolute terms, the high prevalence of diverticulosis in older adults in the western world gives rise to a significantly high rate of acute diverticulitis in this population. When emergency surgery is required for acute diverticulitis, age plays a critical role in patient outcomes, with one study citing odds ratios (OR) of 30-day mortality following the Hartmann's procedure of 2.39 and 6.28 for adults 65–79 years and ≥80 years, respectively, compared to those younger than 65 years of age. The information stated above clearly demonstrates that elderly patients have higher rates of diverticular disease including acute diverticulitis and suffer worse outcomes before and after treatment. The unfortunate combination of worse outcomes in the population mostly affected forms the basis of our work examining acute diverticulitis in the elderly.

L. I. Amodu · C. E. M. Brathwaite (✉)
Department of Surgery, New York University Langone Hospital–Long Island, Mineola, New York, USA

Department of Surgery, New York University Long Island School of Medicine, Mineola, New York, USA
e-mail: Collin.Brathwaite@nyulangone.org

P. Petrone, C. E.M. Brathwaite (eds.), *Acute Care Surgery in Geriatric Patients*,
https://doi.org/10.1007/978-3-031-30651-8_45

Immune System Changes and Physiologic Response to Infection and Sepsis in the Elderly

The task force for the third International Consensus Definitions for Sepsis and Septic Shock recommends that sepsis be defined as "life-threatening organ dysfunction caused by a dysregulated host response to infection." Acute diverticulitis as an inflammatory complication of colonic diverticulosis could result in infection, sepsis, organ dysfunction, and mortality in all patients, particularly older ones.

As individuals age, the immune system exhibits remarkable changes through a process that has been termed "immunosenescence." This is a multifactorial phenomenon that affects both natural and acquired immunity and plays a critical role in the response to acute infections, vaccinations, as well as most chronic diseases in the elderly. Immunosenescence is a dynamic process where several immune system functions are reduced, whereas others remain unchanged or increased. As immunosenescence proceeds, older people become more susceptible to infectious diseases and cancer. Unlike other causes of mortality in the very elderly, mortality due to infectious causes continues to accelerate in very late life. The human immune system is comprised of innate and acquired/adaptive branches, and both parts of the immune system are affected by aging. For instance, neutrophils play a crucial role in the innate immune system and are subject to age-related deterioration in function. This was described by Brubaker and other investigators, with age-related impairments in phagocytosis, degranulation, and production of reactive oxygen species (ROS) noted. Neutrophils, as part of their immune function produce Neutrophil Extracellular Traps (NETs), and elderly individuals have reduced ability to form NETs, which has been associated with an increased risk of sepsis and an increased susceptibility to invasive bacterial diseases.

The adaptive immune system which includes T lymphocytes (CD4+ and CD8+ subtypes) also undergoes significant changes with aging, and among these changes include (1) A decrease in naïve T cells that leads to the shrinking of the T-cell receptor (TCR) repertoire, and (2) an increase in memory T cells primed by different antigens and upregulation of pro-inflammatory molecules.

A decrease in regenerative capacity is one of the hallmarks of aging which contributes to a decline in hematopoietic cells, with a consequential effect of this decline being diminished production of adaptive immune cells. With increasing age, hematopoietic differentiation favors a myeloid line at the expense of lymphoid cells, which leads to decreased B and T lymphocyte numbers and the specific immunity they provide. While it appears that most of the changes involving the innate and acquired immune systems with age are detrimental, it is important to note that age-related changes are highly heterogeneous and variable between individuals and have been described as a determinant of development and responses to acute and chronic illness. While the intricacies of immunosenescence are well beyond the scope of this book, it is important to note how changes in innate and acquired immunity could lead to a blunted immune response in elderly individuals in the presence of bacterial infections, and how this could result in poor outcomes if diagnosis and treatment are delayed in acute diverticulitis.

Epidemiology

As mentioned in the introduction, diverticulosis and diverticulitis are seen with increasing frequency among older adults compared to younger ones, with reported rates as high as 60% in adults older than 65 years of age. Acute diverticulitis is also more common in male patients until the sixth decade of life, at which point it demonstrates a female preponderance. While the proportion of patients with diverticular disease who develop acute diverticulitis was thought to be higher in the past and stated to be approximately 10–25%, more recent studies, the increased use of CT imaging, and colonoscopic findings, have led to the determination that less than 5% of patients with diverticulosis will develop acute diverticulitis. While this chapter focuses primarily on acute diverticulitis in the elderly, it is important to note that diverticulosis and diverticulitis are being diagnosed with increasing frequency in patients younger than 50 years of age. Diet has long been thought to be the main environmental determinant of colonic diverticulosis/diverticulitis, with diets low in fiber thought to lead to generation of high intraluminal pressures necessary for the pathogenesis of colonic diverticula. This has long been considered the reason diverticular disease is more common in western countries, where diet is typically low in fiber. In geographic regions with diets high in fiber such as in Africa, earlier studies showed much lower rates of diverticular disease, with some cited prevalence rates as low as 1.85%. Even in these populations with comparatively lower prevalence rates, the incidence of diverticular disease has been found to be increasing, and occurrence is still most common in the elderly, such as in a cohort studied by Alatise et al. in a Nigerian population with a median age of 64 years. Imaeda et al. studied the burden of diverticular disease in the Japanese and other East Asian populations and reported that right colonic diverticulosis was much more common than left-sided when compared to the western population. The disease is increasing in frequency among younger patients, but still most common in the elderly. Studies of different populations arrive at similar conclusions with rising rates in both elderly and younger patients, but with older individuals most commonly affected. Imaeda cites the mean age at admission for acute diverticulitis to be 63 years of age.

Clinical Features

1. *Hinchey and modified Hinchey classification*: In 1978, Hinchey et al. wrote a landmark paper describing the management and evolution of acute colonic diverticulitis. He described acute diverticulitis as inflammation usually involving a single diverticulum with a perforation which leads to a pelvic or pericolic abscess. When the communication with the colonic lumen fails to obliterate, this results in a free perforation with persistent spillage, resulting in purulent and then fecal peritonitis if unabated. As expected, the Hinchey stage (Table 45.1) indicates clinical severity, with signs and symptoms progressing from malaise, to fever and chills, localized abdominal pain usually in the left lower quadrant (in left colonic disease) or suprapubic region, to more morbid signs and symptoms associated with generalized peritonitis (rebound tenderness and guarding), hypotension, organ failure, etc. While the Hinchey classification was widely accepted, it described only perforated disease. The use of CT imagery and the need for further refinement in clinical stratification led to the modification of Hinchey's classification, with the modification proffered by Wasvary et al. (Table 45.2) being widely adopted. The American Association for the Surgery of Trauma (AAST) developed a uniform grading system for measuring anatomic severity of disease in eight selected Emergency General Surgery (EGS) gastrointestinal conditions including acute diverticulitis (Table 45.3). The AAST grades like the Hinchey grades increase with severity of disease, and in a comparative study by Choi et al., demonstrated a correlation with severity of complications and are better at predicting the need for operative intervention when compared to the Modified Hinchey classification. What all aforementioned grading systems have in common is the correlation of grade with disease severity and the need for intervention.
2. *Distinct clinical features in elderly patients*: The clinical presentation of acute diverticulitis in elderly patients is highly variable

Table 45.1 Original Hinchey classification by Hinchey et al.

Class	Description
I	Pericolic abscess or phlegmon
II	Pelvic, intra-abdominal, or retroperitoneal abscess
III	Generalized purulent peritonitis
IV	Generalized fecal peritonitis

Table 45.2 Modified Hinchey classification by Wasvary et al.

Class	Description
0	Mild clinical diverticulitis
Ia	Confined pericolic inflammation or phlegmon
Ib	Pericolic or mesocolic abscess
II	Pelvic, distant intra-abdominal, or retroperitoneal abscess
III	Generalized purulent peritonitis
IV	Generalized fecal peritonitis

Table 45.3 AAST[a] Grading of acute diverticulitis

Grade	Description
I	Colonic inflammation
II	Colon microperforation or pericolic phlegmon without abscess
III	Localized pericolic abscess
IV	Distant abscesses
V	Free colonic perforation with generalized peritonitis

[a]American Association for the Surgery of Trauma

between individuals, and depends on baseline health status, the effects of a waning immunity described above, and the severity of disease at the time of presentation. We mentioned that in elderly patients, fever is less common and more atypical presentations may occur such as lower GI bleeding.[2] These atypical presentations have been described as "nuanced," and in a study by Lizardi-Cervera et al., only 50% of patients older than 65 years presented with abdominal pain in any lower quadrant, 17% had a fever, and 43% did not have leukocytosis. On the contrary, a higher proportion of older patients presented with diverticular bleeding. One uniquely positive feature of acute diverticulitis in the elderly that has been described by several authors are the low recurrence rates observed compared to younger patients.

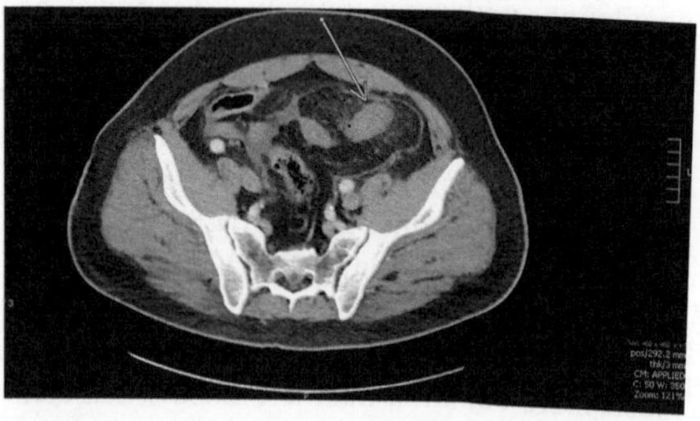

Fig. 45.1 CT scan of the abdomen and pelvis (Axial view) showing perforated diverticulitis of sigmoid colon (White arrow) with small volume scattered fluid, no drainable abscess and mild pericolic stranding

Radiological Features

The imaging modality of choice for the diagnosis of acute diverticulitis in the elderly is a CT scan of the abdomen and pelvis with intravenous contrast. CT imaging not only has the advantage of diagnosing acute diverticulitis but is also capable of distinguishing complicated from uncomplicated disease. Imaging findings on CT could include acute diverticulitis with microperforation and no abscess or phlegmon (Fig. 45.1), with associated phlegmon (Fig. 45.2), pericolic abscess (Fig. 45.3), pelvic abscess (Fig. 45.4), or significant pneumoperitoneum in patients with free perforation (Fig. 45.5). In elderly patients who cannot undergo CT scanning with IV contrast, alternative imaging modalities include CT scan without IV contrast, ultrasound (US), or magnetic resonance imaging (MRI).

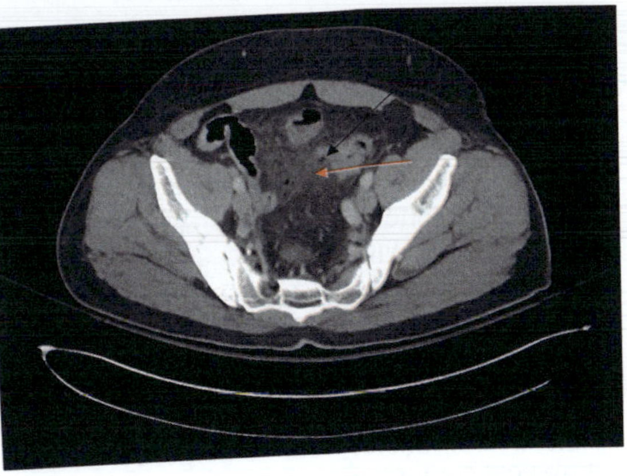

Fig. 45.2 CT scan of the abdomen and pelvis (Axial view) showing findings compatible with acute sigmoid diverticulitis, with evidence of perforation medial to the colon (Black arrow), no abscess formation, and extensive inflammatory changes in the pelvis (Orange arrow) adjacent to sigmoid colon

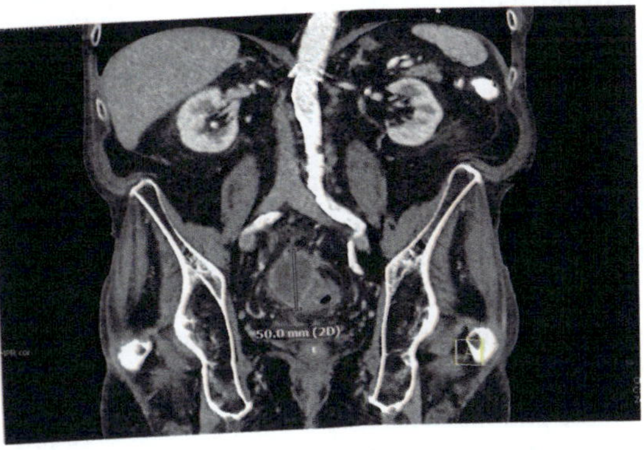

Fig. 45.3 Coronal view of a computed tomographic (CT) scan of the abdomen and pelvis showing acute sigmoid diverticulitis with a peri-sigmoid collection containing fluid and air which measures 7.0 × 5.0 × 4.0 cm, compatible with diverticular abscess/contained perforation

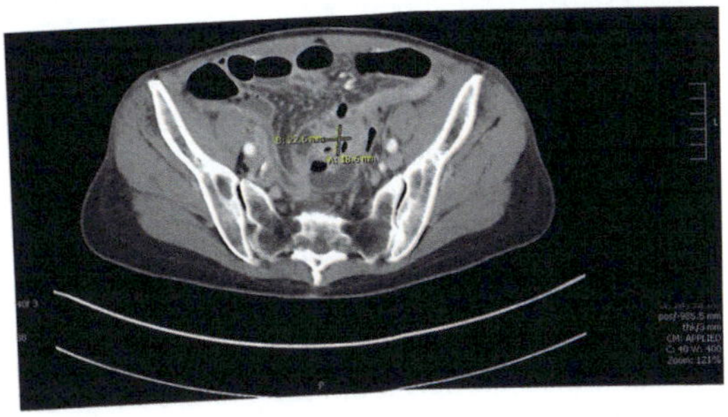

Fig. 45.4 Axial view of a Computed Tomographic (CT) scan demonstrating rectosigmoid wall thickening and adjacent inflammatory fat stranding and fluid consistent with acute diverticulitis. Descending colonic wall thickening. Adjacent pelvic ill-defined air and soft tissue density measuring 2.3 × 1.9 cm, which reflects contained perforation/phlegmon with extraluminal air, suggestive of perforation

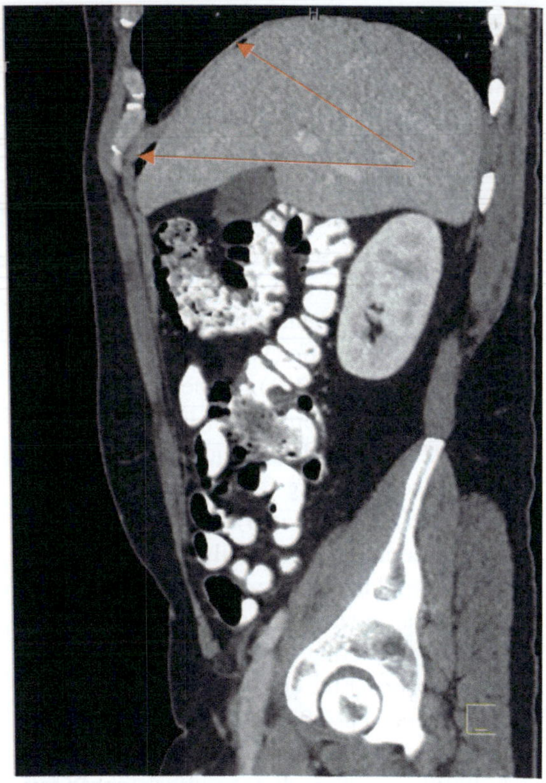

Fig. 45.5 Coronal view of a computed tomographic (CT) scan of the abdomen and pelvis demonstrating free intraperitoneal (Orange arrows) air in a patient with acute sigmoid diverticulitis and a free perforation. Patient required an urgent Hartmann's procedure

Laboratory Features

Laboratory derangements are quite often observed in acute inflammatory conditions/bacterial infections including acute diverticulitis, but care must be taken not to confirm or exclude the diagnosis based on laboratory findings alone. In the general population, leukocytosis with a neutrophil predominance is quite common, but not always the case in the elderly. Other laboratory derangements expected may include elevated pro-inflammatory markers such as C-reactive protein (CRP). Van de Wall et al. studied the diagnostic value of leukocytosis and CRP in acute diverticulitis and found that only CRP was of sufficient diagnostic value (area under the curve (AUC) of 0.715). The median CRP in patients with complicated diverticulitis was significantly higher than in patients with uncomplicated disease; (224 mg/L, range 99–284 vs 87 mg/L, range 48–151). On the basis of this, the investigators proposed a CRP cut-off value of 175 mg/L to distinguish between complicated and uncomplicated diverticulitis.

It is important to note that using this cut-off, 39% of patients with complicated diverticulitis would've been missed. Reynolds et al. in 2017 studied the diagnostic accuracy of CRP, white blood cell (WBC) count, neutrophil count, white cell to lymphocyte ratio (WLR) and neutrophil to lymphocyte ration (NLR). Values at initial presentation were compared using the Mann-Whitney U test. The diagnostic accuracy of each test was assessed using receiver operating characteristic (ROC) curve analysis. CRP, WBC, and neutrophil count, WLR and NLR all had variable accuracy in predicting complicated diverticulitis. NLR had the greatest accuracy of the five biomarkers in predicting the need for intervention, with an area under the curve of 0.79 ($p < 0.0001$), and the optimal cut-off point for NLR being 5.34 (J = 0.45). Other laboratory derangements may be indicative of severe disease, shock, organ failure, or general physiologic derangement such as lactic acidosis, hyponatremia, azotemia, and elevated creatinine.

Management

1. *Medical/Conservative management*: The decision to operate on elderly patients with acute diverticulitis depends on a number of factors including the mode of presentation, quality of life, life expectancy, initial vs. recurrent episode, presence of complications at the time of presentation, etc. In patients without a clear indication for surgery, a trial of non-operative management is a reasonable option. Recent evidence has demonstrated that in selected patients with uncomplicated diverticulitis, the routine use of antibiotics does not lead to better outcomes compared to no antibiotics. This recent development arises from the understanding that diverticulitis is primarily an inflammatory process that can result in micro-perforation, rather than a complication of micro-perforation itself. It is important to note that studies proposing the antibiotic sparing approach only included patients with uncomplicated disease (Hinchey I and Ia), and that for all other stages of disease, antibiotic use remains part of the standard of care. Antibiotic use also continues to be appropriate for high-risk patients with significant comorbidities, signs of systemic infection, or immunosuppression.
2. *Percutaneous abscess drainage*: According to the World Society for Emergency Surgery (WSES) and the American Society for Colon and Rectal Surgery (ASCRS), hemodynamically stable patients with abscesses due to colonic diverticulitis, which are amenable to percutaneous drainage (large than 3 cm for ASCRS, and 4 cm for WSES) should be offered percutaneous drainage in addition to broad-spectrum antibiotic therapy. Abscess drainage not only achieves source control, but also provides fluid samples for culture and sensitivity studies that can help guide future antibiotic therapy. Abscesses smaller than 3 cm could be treated successfully with antibiotics alone on most occasions, even in the outpatient setting.
3. *Surgical drainage*: In hemodynamically stable patients with diverticular abscesses requiring drainage without a "safe window" for a percutaneous approach, there is utility for laparoscopic drain placement without a colonic resection. The increasing use of the robotic platform in acute care surgery provides the opportunity for increased adoption of robotic-assisted abscess drainage and drain placement in the management of diverticular abscesses and should be the subject of future study.
4. *Surgical management*: The decision to operate during an acute episode of diverticulitis should be made on an individual basis. As mentioned earlier, a unique feature of diverticulitis in the elderly is the lower risk of recurrent episodes compared to younger patients. Based on this clinical peculiarity, the indication for surgery based on the number of episodes would appear to be less of a concern

in the elderly compared to younger patients. The presence of free intraperitoneal air is generally considered as a surgical indication. Free intraperitoneal air is suggestive of a free perforation with uncontrolled intra-abdominal contamination. Patients who are hemodynamically unstable or who have signs of generalized peritonitis should undergo urgent surgery, and surgery should be considered in patients who fail non-operative management evidenced by clinical deterioration with or without laboratory corroboration.

The WSES guidelines recommend elective sigmoid resection in the elderly if acute diverticulitis is associated with fistulae, stricture/stenosis, recurrent bleeding, or if symptoms are significant enough to compromise quality of life.

Resection of the diseased colon is the mainstay of surgical management of acute diverticulitis, and this was compared to laparoscopic lavage and drain placement (LLDP) in the SCANDIV trial. In this international, multicenter, randomized controlled trial, patients with perforated sigmoid diverticulitis with purulent peritonitis were randomized to either LLDP or sigmoid resection. Although there were no differences in severe complications or mortality after long-term follow-up, there was a significantly higher rate of deep surgical site infections (DSSI), and unplanned re-intervention in the LLDP group and a higher prevalence of missed malignancies compared to the resection group. Based on the SCANDIV as well as other evidence, the ASCRS does not recommend LLDP in the management of perforated sigmoid diverticulitis with peritonitis.

Where there is expertise available, a minimally invasive colectomy should be offered in preference to an open approach in acute diverticulitis, with evidence demonstrating no difference in outcomes between robotic and laparoscopic approaches. According to the WSES, the Hartmann technique is still recommended for patients with diffuse peritonitis who are critically unwell or have numerous comorbidities. Primary resection with anastomosis with or without a diverting stoma may be performed in clinically stable patients with no comorbidities, and for clinically unstable patients with peritonitis (severe sepsis or septic shock), damage control surgery (emergency laparotomy, source control, an open abdomen and abdominal vacuum-assisted closure (VAC)) may be recommended. The observation has been made in the consensus statement by the European Association for Endoscopic Surgery (EAES) and the Society of American Gastrointestinal and Endoscopic Surgeons (SAGES) that "*In Hinchey III, diverticulitis sigmoid resection with primary anastomosis with proximal diversion has similar mortality, lower morbidity and lower stoma rate at 12 months compared to Hartmann procedure with reversal.*" As such, they make the following recommendation: "*In the appropriate clinical setting, we recommend consideration of sigmoid resection with primary anastomosis and proximal diversion over HP in patients with Hinchey III/IV diverticulitis.*" The latter recommendation needs to be studied in a prospective randomized trial.

Surveillance

Following an acute episode of diverticulitis, a full endoscopic evaluation of the colon is recommended to confirm the diagnosis and to exclude malignancy. Sharma et al. demonstrated that the risk of an occult malignancy was 11% in patients with complicated diverticulitis and 0.7% in patients with uncomplicated diverticulitis. This suggests that the risk of an occult malignancy is low in patients with uncomplicated disease, and that colonoscopic evaluation may not be necessary after the acute episode. We recommend colonoscopy at least 6 weeks after an acute episode of complicated diverticulitis. In patients with acute diverticulitis who had non-operative management, there may be utility in radiologic surveillance with CT imaging. In patients with diverticulitis complicated by an abscess who underwent percutaneous drainage, it is our practice to obtain a repeat CT scan approximately after 4–6 weeks of antibiotic treatment and percutaneous drain placement to evaluate for resolution.

Conclusion

Acute diverticulitis is a relatively common condition in the elderly, which varies in severity at presentation, leading to a range of management options from non-operative treatment without antibiotics to damage control surgery. The immunologic changes that occur with aging make the presentation of acute diverticulitis more atypical and nuanced in the elderly compared to younger patients. If diagnosed and treated expeditiously, taking into account the unique complexities of the elderly patient, the management of this condition in this patient cohort will yield appreciably good outcomes.

References

1. Covino M, Rosa F, Ojetti V, Quero G, Fiorillo C, Sganga G, Gasbarrini A, Franceschi F, Alfieri S. Acute diverticulitis in elderly patients: does age really matter? Dig Dis. 2021;39(1):33–41. https://doi.org/10.1159/000509049. Epub 2020 Jun 2
2. Wheat CL, Strate LL. Trends in hospitalization for diverticulitis and diverticular bleeding in the United States from 2000 to 2010. Clin Gastroenterol Hepatol. 2016;14(1):96–103.e1. https://doi.org/10.1016/j.cgh.2015.03.030. Epub 2015 Apr 8. PMID: 25862988; PMCID: PMC4624035
3. Shahedi K, Fuller G, Bolus R, Cohen E, Vu M, Shah R, Agarwal N, Kaneshiro M, Atia M, Sheen V, Kurzbard N, van Oijen MG, Yen L, Hodgkins P, Erder MH, Spiegel B. Long-term risk of acute diverticulitis among patients with incidental diverticulosis found during colonoscopy. Clin Gastroenterol Hepatol. 2013;11(12):1609–13. https://doi.org/10.1016/j.cgh.2013.06.020.
4. Peery AF, Keku TO, Martin CF, Eluri S, Runge T, Galanko JA, Sandler RS. Distribution and characteristics of colonic diverticula in a United States screening population. Clin Gastroenterol Hepatol. 2016;14(7):980–985.e1. https://doi.org/10.1016/j.cgh.2016.01.020. Epub 2016 Feb 9. PMID: 26872402; PMCID: PMC4912930
5. Quinn S, Akram W, Hao S, Honaker MD. Emergency surgery for diverticulitis: relationship of outcomes to patient age and surgical procedure. J Am Med Dir Assoc. 2022;23(4):616–622.e1. https://doi.org/10.1016/j.jamda.2022.02.001. Epub 2022 Mar 1
6. Singer M, Deutschman CS, Seymour CW, Shankar-Hari M, Annane D, Bauer M, Bellomo R, Bernard GR, Chiche JD, Coopersmith CM, Hotchkiss RS, Levy MM, Marshall JC, Martin GS, Opal SM, Rubenfeld GD, van der Poll T, Vincent JL, Angus DC. The third international consensus definitions for sepsis and septic shock (Sepsis-3). JAMA. 2016;315(8):801–10. https://doi.org/10.1001/jama.2016.0287. PMID: 26903338; PMCID: PMC4968574
7. Seymour CW, Liu VX, Iwashyna TJ, Brunkhorst FM, Rea TD, Scherag A, Rubenfeld G, Kahn JM, Shankar-Hari M, Singer M, Deutschman CS, Escobar GJ, Angus DC. Assessment of clinical criteria for sepsis: for the third international consensus definitions for sepsis and septic shock (Sepsis-3). JAMA. 2016;315(8):762–74. https://doi.org/10.1001/jama.2016.0288. Erratum in: JAMA 2016 May 24–31;315(20):2237. PMID: 26903335; PMCID: PMC5433435
8. Santoro A, Bientinesi E, Monti D. Immunosenescence and inflammaging in the aging process: age-related diseases or longevity? Ageing Res Rev. 2021;71:101422. https://doi.org/10.1016/j.arr.2021.101422. Epub 2021 Aug 13
9. Pawelec G, Koch S, Franceschi C, Wikby A. Human immunosenescence: does it have an infectious component? Ann N Y Acad Sci. 2006;1067:56–65. https://doi.org/10.1196/annals.1354.009.
10. Brubaker AL, Rendon JL, Ramirez L, Choudhry MA, Kovacs EJ. Reduced neutrophil chemotaxis and infiltration contributes to delayed resolution of cutaneous wound infection with advanced age. J Immunol. 2013;190(4):1746–57. https://doi.org/10.4049/jimmunol.1201213. Epub 2013 Jan 14. PMID: 23319733; PMCID: PMC3563860
11. Simell B, Vuorela A, Ekström N, Palmu A, Reunanen A, Meri S, Käyhty H, Väkeväinen M. Aging reduces the functionality of anti-pneumococcal antibodies and the killing of Streptococcus pneumoniae by neutrophil phagocytosis. Vaccine. 2011;29(10):1929–34. https://doi.org/10.1016/j.vaccine.2010.12.121. Epub 2011 Jan 12
12. Hinchey EJ, Schaal PG, Richards GK. Treatment of Perforated Diverticular Disease of the Colon. Adv Surg. 1978;12:85–109. PMID: 735943.
13. Wasvary H, Turfah F, Kadro O, Beauregard W. Same Hospitalization Resection for Acute Diverticulitis. Am Surg. 1999;65(7): 632–5; Discussion 636. PMID: 10399971.
14. Shafi S, Aboutanos M, Brown CV, Ciesla D, Cohen MJ, Crandall ML, Inaba K, Miller PR, Mowery NT; American Association for the Surgery of Trauma Committee on Patient Assessment and Outcomes. Measuring anatomic severity of disease in emergency general surgery. J Trauma Acute Care

Surg. 2014;76(3):884–7. https://doi.org/10.1097/TA.0b013e3182aafdba. PMID: 24553565.

15. Francis NK, Sylla P, Abou-Khalil M, Arolfo S, BerlerD, Curtis NJ, Dolejs SC, Garfinkle R, Gorter-Stam M, Hashimoto DA, Hassinger TE, Molenaar CJL, Pucher PH, Schuermans V, Arezzo A, Agresta F, Antoniou SA, Arulampalam T, Boutros M, Bouvy N, Campbell K, Francone T, Haggerty SP, Hedrick TL, Stefanidis D, Truitt MS, Kelly J, Ket H, Dunkin BJ, Pietrabissa A. EAES and SAGES 2018 consensus conference on acute diverticulitis management: evidence-based recommendations for clinical practice. Surg Endosc. 2019 Sep;33(9): 2726–41. https://doi.org/10.1007/s00464-019-06882-z. Epub 2019 Jun 27. PMID: 31250244; PMCID: PMC6684540.

Upper Gastrointestinal Bleeding

46

Jun L. Levine

Upper Gastrointestinal Bleeding (UGIB)

Introduction

Classically, gastrointestinal bleeding is separated into upper gastrointestinal bleeding (UGIB) or lower gastrointestinal bleeding (LGIB). Bleeding can be classified as acute or chronic, with acute bleeds more sudden and apparent and chronic bleeds more insidious.

Upper GI bleeding is considered bleeding originating above the ligament of Treitz. Acute upper GI bleeding usually presents as hematemesis, coffee ground emesis or melena. However, chronic UGIB can manifest with fatigue, weakness, or syncopal episodes as a sequela to blood loss. Upper GI bleeding has a more common occurrence than lower GI bleeds. With gastrointestinal bleeding a common problem seen in the elderly, adhering to an accurate diagnostic and treatment algorithm is crucial in managing upper GI bleeds.

J. L. Levine (✉)
New York University Long Island School of Medicine, Mineola, NY, USA
e-mail: Jun.levine@nyulangone.org

Etiology/Pathophysiology

Upper gastrointestinal bleeding has a yearly incidence of 100 per 100,000 population, with a mortality risk of about 10%. Upper GI bleeding has a fourfold increase in occurrence than lower GI bleeds. The most common causes of upper GI bleeds are peptic ulcers disease (PUD) with 50% due to duodenal ulcers, followed by esophageal varices, erosive esophagitis or gastritis, Mallory-Weiss tear and seldom, gastric cancers.

Peptic Ulcer Disease (PUD)

Peptic ulcer disease accounts for 40–50% of upper GI bleeds. Gastric ulcers are usually located in the lesser curvature and prepyloric area, while the duodenal ulcers are located at the duodenal bulb. Acute ulcers have regular borders and chronic ulcers have raised borders. It is usually associated with *Helicobacter pylori* infections, long-term nonsteroidal anti-inflammatory drugs (NSAIDS) use and certain medications such as anticoagulants like aspirin and clopidogrel. There is a positive link with stress, such as acute illness or burns that instigate PUD. It is usually seen in severely ill patients in the intensive care unit with coagulopathies and multiorgan failures. Less common manifestations of PUD are due to smoking, alcohol, malignancies, or hypersecretory syndromes like Zollinger-Ellison syndrome.

P. Petrone, C. E.M. Brathwaite (eds.), *Acute Care Surgery in Geriatric Patients*,
https://doi.org/10.1007/978-3-031-30651-8_46

Signs and symptoms of PUD vary based on location. Besides association with meals that differentiate gastric versus duodenal ulcers, duodenal ulcers typically occur at night. Ulcers causing gastric outlet obstruction manifest with gastric fullness, bloating, nausea, and vomiting.

H. pylori is a Gram-negative bacillus responsible for 90% of duodenal ulcers and 70% or greater of gastric ulcers. Due to the organism's diverse virulence factors, it allows the bacterium to penetrate and then damage the gastric mucosa. *H. pylori* secretes urease to neutralize the acid and hence protect itself. The CagA/VacA toxins it produces damage to the gastric lining and causes mucosal inflammation. Additionally, the bacterium has excellent motility due to its flagella which counteracts against gastric motility and maintains it invasion in the stomach.

Nonsteroidal anti-inflammatory drugs (NSAIDS) inhibit the cyclooxygenase (COX) enzymes and thereby blocks prostaglandin synthesis. Normally, prostaglandins protect the gastric mucosa by regulating mucosal blood flow and gastric mucosal acid production by regulating mucus and bicarbonate production. This inhibition causes an imbalance of the acid-base equilibrium resulting in gastric ulcers. Hence, NSAID use is the next most common cause of PUD compared to *H. pylori* infection.

Typically, gastric ulcers are associated with pain that worsens with eating and patients with duodenal ulcers have pain that is relieved with foods. Patient with duodenal ulcers tends to gain weight versus gastric ulcer patients.

Esophageal Varices

Excluding PUD-associated upper GI bleeds, esophageal varices is the next leading culprit of UGIB. Generally, this is seen more in patient with cirrhosis with portal hypertension. In patients with cirrhosis, due to the elevated hepatic venous pressure gradient, gastroesophageal varices bleeding occurs in approximately 50% of the patients with varices. Varices have a more common occurrence in males than in females and associated with 10–20% mortality risk within 6 weeks from a bleeding episode. Common etiologies of cirrhosis are alcohol, viral hepatitis, and hepatitis B & C. Variceal bleed can be the initial presentation of undiagnosed cirrhosis. Overt acute bleeding is more common than occult, with often hematemesis, hematochezia, and melena being the initial presentation.

There are risk factors for variceal bleeding that should be determined. One is the size of the varix, with larger varices having a higher potential for bleeding. Child classification is intertwined with the risk of bleeding, with higher the Child class, the higher the risk of hemorrhage. Active alcohol consumption and endoscopic findings of varices also lead to excessive risk of rupture and bleeding.

Esophagitis

Esophagitis can be caused by multiple etiologies, inducing damage to the esophageal mucosa. The most common factor is gastroesophageal reflux leading to acid erosion of the esophagus. Abnormal reflux of gastric acid can be due to transient relaxations or decreased tone of the lower esophageal sphincter, hiatal hernias, and obesity.

Other causes of esophagitis occur in varying incidences, ranging from eosinophilic esophagitis, medication-induced, radiation, and infectious esophagitis. Eosinophilic esophagitis is noted in 0.35 per 100,000 population and associated with asthma, eczema, and food allergies. Radiation esophagitis occurs with doses of 6000 cGy causing acute injury. Infectious esophagitis is more prevalent in immunosuppressed/compromised individuals.

Medication-induced esophagitis is a direct irritation to the esophageal mucosal barrier. Damaged to the esophagus is caused by prolonged contact with medication that cause caustic injury due to acidification such as ferrous sulfate or cause tissue and vascular destruction such as potassium chloride.

Eosinophilic esophagitis pathogenesis is much more ill-defined. It is considered an allergic disorder provoked by antigen sensitization via foods or other environmental allergens. It can occur at any age and associated with patients with asthma, environmental allergens, or dermatitis. Eliminating major food or environmental allergens is the mainstay of management. Improvement is noted with acid suppression medications which indicates acid reflux playing a part.

Pathophysiology of radiation esophagitis involves cell death and DNA damage. Acute radiation injury destroys cells and impedes proliferation of cells. Chronic injury causes fibrosis which causes small vessel ischemia. This leads to strictures, ulcers, and perforation.

Infectious esophagitis is commonly caused by fungal organisms, especially *Candid albicans*. *C. albicans* initially colonizes the mucosa leading to impairments of defense mechanisms. Herpes simplex virus is the most common viral esophagitis.

Mallory-Weiss

A Mallory-Weiss tear is most often caused by forceful coughing or vomiting. It is a longitudinal mucosal laceration in the distal esophagus leading to bleeding of the submucosal arteries. Patients with substantial alcoholic use causing vomiting leads to 50% of Mallory-Weiss tears. Portal hypertension and esophageal varices are associated with more severe bleeding from Mallory-Weiss tears.

Gastric Cancer

Gastric carcinoma can be a rare cause of upper GI bleed but of a more subtle way. Because of its indolent nature, there may be no frank blood seen in emesis or in stool, except for possible fecal occult blood tests, or more likely, patient presentation of fatigue, feeling cold, weight loss, or syncope. Gastric cancer is associated with predisposing factors that include both environmental and genetic. *H. pylori* has been determined to be a major risk factor of more than 50% for gastric malignancy. *H. pylori* infection increases DNA damage and decreases the repair activities as well as initiating mutations in mitochondria and nuclear DNA and hence causing carcinogenesis. Different dietary and lifestyle factors such as alcohol consumption, smoking, high salt foods, and foods high in nitrates are implicated in gastric cancer. Dietary salt or nitrogen intake enhances *H. pylori* colonization and induced direct gastric mucosal damage. Both elevated salt and nitrogen promotes N-methyl-N′-nitro-N-nitrosoguanidine (MNNG)-induced gastric carcinomas and N-nitroso compounds (NNC) which are mutagenic compounds. Cooking practices, alcohol, smoking, and family history and different occupations have a correlation to increased risk of gastric cancer.

Gastric adenocarcinoma has the highest incidence with a two- to four-fold higher incidence in males than in females. The 5-year survival rate is 20%. Proximal gastric cancers are more predominant in developed countries with major risk factors of obesity and gastroesophageal reflux disease. Distal tumors are predominant in developing countries with *H. pylori* infection and dietary factors as causal factors.

Rare Causes

There are a wide variety of other causes of upper GI bleeds but are seldom encountered. Mostly, there are vascular lesions such as arteriovenous malformations, gastric antral vascular ectasia, aortoenteric fistula, and Dieulafoy lesions. Large arteriovenous malformations may cause significant upper GI bleeds. Gastric antral vascular ectasias are caused by liver disease manifesting as bleeding from pylorus to antrum. Aortoenteric fistulas (AEF) is an abnormal connection between the aorta and the gastrointestinal tract. Typically, there is compression between the aorta and the GI tract and a de novo tract is formed. Fistula causes are from radiation, tumor, foreign body, or transient infection. Secondary causes are resultant from a surgical intervention such as a graph adjacent to the GI tract. AEF classically presents with a herald bleed. Commonly, an episode of hematemesis or hematochezia is followed by a quiescent period with consequent substantial bleeding and cardiovascular compromise.

Evaluation

Assessment of clinical presentation should be well categorized along with a thorough history and physical. Knowledge of the description, chronicity, intensity, and onset of symptoms is crucial to understanding the severity of the bleed. Hematemesis is vomiting of fresh blood or clots. Usually, this denotes an acute upper GI bleed with rupture of blood vessels, seen in esophageal varices. Coffee-ground emesis refers to vomitus with dark old blood similar appearance to coffee grounds, signifying a bleed that has stopped and has had time to oxidize in the stomach. Melena presents as tarry stools that have a characteristic smell. This is often associated with a chronic bleed that has taken a longer pathway. Hematochezia is the passage of bright red blood per rectum. Generally, this is associated with a lower GI bleed but can be seen in a brisk upper GI bleed.

A comprehensive review of medical history, medications (NSAIDs and anticoagulant use), and social history, eliciting high risk factors such as alcohol, smoking, or substance use.

Initial vitals with attention to tachycardia, hypotension, and orthostatic hypotension needs to be addressed. Resting tachycardia is indicative of hypovolemia. Confusion and lethargy with decreased urine output are all signs of blood loss. Evidence of ascites, jaundice, or other high-risk factors for bleeding should be ascertained to evaluate for chronic live diseases. Besides a complete physical exam, attention should be placed to assess for acute abdomen, along with a digital rectal exam.

Blood work should include complete blood count, electrolyte panel, liver function tests, and coagulation profile. Serial hemoglobin levels should be obtained, as initial hemoglobin value may be falsely normal due to volume contraction and once resuscitation has begun, hemodilution may also give a false anemia. Hence, it should not be the sole predictor of bleeding severity.

Patients should be risk-stratified based on their clinical presentation. Hemodynamic instability with minimal response to resuscitation will need aggressive care and monitoring along with more invasive therapies. There are many scoring systems that have been developed to help predict rebleeding, mortality, and need for intervention, such as the Rockall or Blatchford score.

Besides fluid and blood resuscitation and hemodynamic control, endoscopy (esophagogastroduodenoscopy EGD) should be performed to identify and treat the bleeding source. Endoscopy is recommended to be performed within 12–24 h of admission, especially for patient with high-risk presentations, subsequent to optimization of hemodynamics.

Management

Acute Bleed

Acute bleeding is seen with overt bleeding, usually hematemesis, hematochezia, and melena. Majority of acute UGIB is from peptic ulcer but the often-dramatic large volume bleeding is seen in variceal bleeds, along with large arteriovenous malformations.

Two large bore intravenous peripheral access should be obtained. Intravenous fluid should be provided to maintain hemodynamic stability. Endotracheal intubations are required for patient that are unable to protect their airways such as with severe hematemesis and risk of aspirations or altered mental status.

Aggressive resuscitative efforts to achieve early hemodynamic stability with both fluid and blood products have been shown to decrease mortality. Blood transfusion initiated for hemoglobin less than 7 g/dL which may need to be adjusted for patient with unstable coronary disease or active bleeding. Halting or reversing of anticoagulants or antiplatelet therapy and assessment of risks need to be weighed when patient have underlying thromboembolic event versus active bleeding. NSAIDS should be discontinued.

Proton pump inhibitors (PPI) should be administered to patients with UGIB not due to varices. A bolus plus continuous PPI infusion versus twice daily infusion is comparable in effect.

Endoscopy should be performed within 12–24 hrs of admission in active bleeding. If a bleeding vessel is noted, therapeutic interventions, such as clipping, thermal coagulation, local epinephrine injection, or hemostatic spray should be utilized. Depending on the severity of the disease, the patient may need a combination of therapies and even endoscopic oversewing of the lesion. If a clean, non-bleeding ulcer is identified, then no intervention is required.

The Forrest classification can be used for patients with PUD. Clean ulcer base is associated with 5% rebleeding risk. Ulcers with stigmata of bleeding has a 10–43% rebleeding risk. Ulcer with active bleeding has a 55% chance of rebleeding.

Repeat endoscopy is not warranted unless there is a rebleed. Patient are placed on a 72-hr intravenous PPI twice daily and started on clear diet and advanced as tolerated. For patient with persistent bleeding despite multiple therapeutic interventions including secondary endoscopies, interventional radiology embolization, or surgical intervention may be required.

A somatostatin analog, Octreotide, may be given for suspected variceal bleeds as a bolus with continuous infusion. This can help stabilize the patient if endoscopy is delayed or is unavailable.

Use of angiography for embolization in upper GI bleeds is more challenging given collateral vessels. Given the higher complication rates associated with pseudoaneurysm, aortic dissection, bowel ischemia, and nephropathy, it is reserved for patient who cannot undergo endoscopy or have persistent GI bleeding.

Special Considerations

Aortoenteric Fistulas

Patients with aortoenteric fistulas should obtain a CT abdomen with IV contrast if hemodynamically stable. An endoscopy may be performed to exclude other sources of bleeding.

If patient is hemodynamically unstable, should proceed to surgery without further testing. However, if there is no known surgical repair, then a bedside ultrasound may be obtained.

Management is aggressive resuscitation and emergent surgical intervention in the unstable patient. Massive transfusion protocol with a 1:1:1 ratio should be performed. Operative intervention can be performed open versus endovascular aneurysm repair (EVAR). Open repair is associated with 34% mortality compared to 7% EVAR. There is difference in disease-free survival, and EVAR avoids a hostile abdomen. EVAR is preferred in the setting of no signs of infection. Even if infection is diagnosed, patients can be managed with long-term IV antibiotics and undergo a definitive repair at a more elective basis.

Varices

Patient with variceal bleeding should have their underlying comorbid condition treated. Resuscitation as above but care not to over-transfuse, as it increases portal pressure and increases rebleeding risk. Correct coagulopathy as needed, keeping in mind that fresh frozen plasma may increase rebleeding due to increased blood volume.

Erythromycin before endoscopy may promote clearance of the area, so less need for repeat endoscopy. Variceal band ligation is preferred to sclerotherapy. Ligation has lower risk of rebleeding. Failure of endoscopic therapeutic interventions may warrant self-expanding esophageal stents. If all interventions fail, liver transplantation, Portosystemic shunt/Transjugular Intrahepatic Portosystemic Shunt (TIPS) or esophageal transection in rare cases of exsanguinating bleed. There is a 70% rebleeding risk after the first episode of variceal bleeding; 30% of rebleeding episodes are fatal. Complications of variceal bleeding are multiorgan failure, encephalopathy, esophageal perforation, aspiration, and death.

Chronic Bleed

Chronic or occult bleeding presents with lightheadedness, dizziness, shortness of breath, syncope, chest pain, and fatigue. Peptic ulcer disease is responsible for the mainstay of chronic bleeding as well, along with esophagitis, NSAIDs use, inflammatory bowel disease, and gastric cancers.

PUD

Typically, patients with PUD present with epigastric abdominal pain. Gastric ulcers are associated with abdominal pain immediately after food intake, with resultant weight loss. Patient presenting with anemia, melena, or weight loss should be investigated for PUD, bleeding, perforation, or cancer. If patient is found to have gastric or duodenal ulcer likely from peptic ulcer disease, biopsies from endoscopy should be obtained and the patient should be treated with triple therapy. The gold standard with 90% sensitivity and specificity to diagnose gastric and duodenal ulcers is endoscopy. Patient with concerning symptoms or 50 years or older with dyspepsia should obtain an EGD.

Barium swallow is indicated if endoscopy cannot be performed.

H. pylori testing with serology, urea breath test, antibodies to *H. pylori*, stool antigen test or ELISA can all be performed along with endoscopic biopsy. Biopsies from 4–6 sites are necessary. Once *H. pylori* infection is ascertained, treatment consists of PPI, clarithromycin, and metronidazole or amoxicillin for 14 days. Refractory disease with ulcer greater than 5 mm not responsive to PPI therapy of 8–12 weeks may require surgical treatment. The suspicion of gastric ulcer, refractory to treatment as gastric cancer warrants a partial gastrectomy and truncal vagotomy with an emptying procedure.

Prognosis of PUD if underlying treatment is treated well is excellent. The mainstay of prevention is lifestyle modification with abstaining from at-risk factors such as smoking, alcohol, NSAIDs use, and change in dietary habits. Recurrence rates is seen in 60%.

Complications of peptic ulcer disease are upper GI bleed, gastric outlet obstruction, perforation, and gastric cancer. Treatment of underlying cause after stabilization from any active bleeding is the foundation to management of a chronic bleed.

Esophagitis

The most common presentations of esophagitis are retrosternal chest pain, heartburn, or dysphagia. Erosive esophagitis accounts for 11% of upper GI bleeds. Patients with erosive esophagitis may also experience globus sensation, regurgitation, and coughing.

Generally, erosive esophagitis is treated similarly as with PUD, with PPI or H2 blocker therapy. Lifestyle modifications of weight loss, small meals, head elevation, elimination of trigger foods like fatty foods, spicy foods, chocolate, smoking, and alcohol and not eating 2 hr before sleeping is encouraged.

If medication-induced esophagitis is at issue, patients are advised to take pills separately and remain upright for at least 30 min after taking a pill. Medication should be discontinued or switch to an alternative.

For eosinophilic esophagitis, treatment is acid suppression with PPI or H2 blocker, steroids, and removal of the food or environmental allergens.

Treatment for infectious etiology is to treat the underlying infection. Targeted therapy is provided.

Esophagitis needs to be treated by managing the underlying cause and tailoring the therapy after acute bleeding has resolved.

Complications of esophagitis are bleeding, stricture, Barrett esophagus, perforation, and aspiration pneumonitis.

Gastric Cancer

Occult bleeding is more common in gastric cancer. Once acute bleeding and resuscitative efforts are commenced, evaluation, and treatment algorithms should be maintained. Gastric cancers are 90–95% adenocarcinomas, as they originate in the epithelium. Fortunately, gastric carcinoma is declining worldwide; however, it is still responsible for 10% of deaths due to cancer worldwide especially in regions where fresh food storage is not available and water quality is poor. Gastric cancer is separated into intestinal and diffuses categories. The well-differentiated intestinal type has a better prognosis and is more common in men, and older people. The diffuse type causes thickening of the stomach wall without a discrete mass formation. Diffuse type is more common in younger patients and in women with blood group A.

More than 50–80% of gastric cancer is attributed to *H. pylori.* Gastric cancer has vague signs and symptoms. Early on, patients may feel heartburn, bloating, nausea, or decreased appetite.

Later, patients may experience abdominal pain, GI bleeding (melena), vomiting due to gastric outlet obstruction, unintentional weight loss, dysphagia, fatigue, and jaundice. Typically, patients who are symptomatic present with advanced stage of cancer. Commonly, patients have a palpable abdominal mass. Metastatic lymphatic spread is noted with Virchow's node, ascites (peritoneal carcinomatosis) or hepatomegaly (disease burden).

Patient with symptoms should undergo upper endoscopy with biopsy. Preoperative staging includes evaluations of the chest and abdomen/pelvis with computerized tomography (CT). Endoscopic ultrasound helps with staging. If negative result of malignancy is found, then positron emission tomography (PET) combined with CT will help determine resectability. Serum tumor markers of CA 125, CA 19-9, CEA, and CA 72-4 are obtained to monitor. Staging laparoscopy with peritoneal cytology is performed. Positive peritoneal cytology indicated high recurrence rate and hence surgery not recommended.

Treatment depends on preoperative staging. For limited mucosal disease, endoscopic resection can be approached. Surgical resection with lymphadenectomy is offered to patients with <T3, any N. Neoadjuvant is offered for >T2 and >T1N1 or >T3N0 is offered chemoradiation or combined with resectable lesions or palliative systemic therapy with locally advanced or metastatic disease.

Patient with localized gastric cancer have the best chance of survival. Margins of more than 4 cm is adequate. D2 lymphadenectomy is recommended for patient with resectable gastric cancer. Patients with symptomatic disease may warrant a palliative resection with positive margins due to obstruction or bleeding.

Prognosis of gastric cancer depends on stage. Early disease cases are found in 10–20% of the population with 50% cure rate. Overall survival 5-year rate is 10–15%. Due to the subtle nature of gastric cancer presentation, the cure rate is abysmally low due to advance stage of cancer at diagnosis.

Prevention strategies involve screening and treatment of *H. pylori* infection, endoscopic surveillance, restrict dietary and environmental risk factors like high salt and nitrogen consumption as well as smoking and alcohol cessation. Best health practices with good hygiene, sanitary conditions with food preparation and storage and cooking practices are considered to reduce gastric cancer risk. Several studies have demonstrated a protective effect of raw fruits and vegetable consumption against gastric cancer risk. This is also noted in people who consume antioxidants.

References

1. van Leerdam ME. Epidemiology of acute upper gastrointestinal bleeding. Best Pract Res Clin Gastroenterol. 2008;22(2):209–24. https://doi.org/10.1016/j.bpg.2007.10.011.
2. Narayanan M, Reddy KM, Marsicano E. Peptic ulcer disease and *Helicobacter pylori* infection. Mo Med. 2018;115(3):219–24.
3. Malik TF, Gnanapandithan K, Singh K. Peptic ulcer disease. In: StatPearls [Internet]. Treasure Island (FL): StatPearls Publishing; 2022. https://www.ncbi.nlm.nih.gov/books/NBK534792/.
4. Huang JQ, Sridhar S, Hunt RH. Role of helicobacter pylori infection and non-steroidal anti-inflammatory drugs in peptic-ulcer disease: a meta-analysis. Lancet. 2002;359(9300):14–22.
5. Meseeha M, Attia M. Esophageal varices. In: StatPearls [Internet]. Treasure Island (FL): StatPearls Publishing; 2022. https://www.ncbi.nlm.nih.gov/books/NBK448078/.
6. Nejat Pish-Kenari F, Qujeq D, Maghsoudi H. Some of the effective factors in the pathogenesis of gastro-oesophageal reflux disease. J Cell Mol Med. 2018;22(12):6401–4.
7. Harris JM, DiPalma JA. Clinical significance of Mallory-Weiss tears. Am J Gastroenterol. 1993;88(12):2056.
8. Velmurugan B, Mani A, Nagini S. Combination of S-allylcysteine and lycopene induces apoptosis by modulating Bcl-2, Bax, Bim and caspases during experimental gastric carcinogenesis. Eur J Cancer Prev. 2005;14:387–93.
9. Mitacek EJ, Brunnemann KD, Suttajit M, Caplan LS, Gagna CE, Bhothisuwan K, Siriamornpun S, Hummel CF, Ohshima H, Roy R, et al. Geographic distribution of liver and stomach cancers in Thailand in relation to estimated dietary intake of nitrate,

nitrite, and nitrosodimethylamine. Nutr Cancer. 2008;60:196–203.
10. Jemal A, Bray F, Center MM, Ferlay J, Ward E, Forman D. Global cancer statistics. CA Cancer J Clin. 2011;61:69–90.
11. Crew KD, Neugut AI. Epidemiology of gastric cancer. World J Gastroenterol. 2006;12:354–62.
12. Baradarian R, Ramdhaney S, Chapalamadugu R, et al. Early intensive resuscitation of patients with upper gastrointestinal bleeding decreases mortality. Am J Gastroenterol. 2004;99:619–22.
13. Serafini M, Jakszyn P, Luján-Barroso L, Agudo A, Bas Bueno-de-Mesquita H, van Duijnhoven FJ, Jenab M, Navarro C, Palli D, Boeing H, et al. Dietary total antioxidant capacity and gastric cancer risk in the European prospective investigation into cancer and nutrition study. Int J Cancer. 2012;131:e544–54.

Gastrointestinal Hemorrhage in the Elderly

47

Marlon Torres and Toyooki Sonoda

Introduction

Gastrointestinal (GI) bleeding is a significant cause of morbidity and mortality in the elderly. Bleeding from the GI tract is the most common cause of hospitalization due to gastrointestinal disease in the USA. An estimated 1% of patients over the age of 80 requires hospitalization due to GI bleeding.

Severe GI bleeding presents in multiple ways: as hematemesis (vomiting of frank blood), hematochezia (red or maroon stools), or melena (black or tarry stools). Classically, melena is associated with an upper GI source of bleeding, while hematochezia is correlated to a lower GI origin. However, massive upper GI hemorrhage can lead to hematochezia, and lower GI bleeding may present with melena. Upper GI bleeding is generally defined as bleeding proximal to the ligament of Treitz, and lower GI bleeding distal to it. These different etiologies will be considered below.

The incidence of both upper and lower GI bleeding increases with age, as conditions causing GI bleeding are more common in the elderly. Patients 80 years old or older have a three-fold increase in the rate of hospitalization from GI bleeding compared to patients aged 65–69. Additional risk factors for hospitalization include male gender, use of multiple medications, use of oral anticoagulants, presence of cardiovascular disease, difficulty with daily activities, and unmarried status. The mortality rates for both upper and lower GI bleeding have been decreasing since the early 2000s, with a current mortality of 2–3% for both entities. However, for unstable GI bleeding, the mortality is significantly higher. A National Inpatient Sample analysis of over 6 million people in the USA (years 2002–2013) demonstrated a mortality rate of 20% when patients presented with shock as opposed to 2% when shock was not present.

The management of GI bleeding is complex. Many cases require management of anticoagulation or antiplatelet therapy. Since most GI bleeding stops spontaneously, identifying the bleeding lesion *while actively bleeding* is a clinical challenge. Several diagnostic options are available, each with their own success and failure rates. Determining which test or procedure is best for each situation requires the coordinated care of a multidisciplinary team.

Key Points

- In elderly patients with GI hemorrhage, the initial focus should be on hemodynamic stabilization, including crystalloid resuscitation

M. Torres
General Surgery, NYU Langone–Long Island Hospital, Mineola, NY, USA
e-mail: Marlon.torres@nyulangone.org

T. Sonoda (✉)
Department of Surgery, NYU Langone–Long Island Hospital, Mineola, NY, USA
e-mail: toyooki.sonoda@nyulangone.org

P. Petrone, C. E.M. Brathwaite (eds.), *Acute Care Surgery in Geriatric Patients*,
https://doi.org/10.1007/978-3-031-30651-8_47

and transfusions as necessary. An effort to localize the site of bleeding should immediately follow.

- At presentation, a risk stratification should be performed. This will help to triage patients and determine which clinical services are consulted.
- For *stable* upper GI bleeding, the diagnostic procedure of choice is an upper endoscopy, performed within 24 h of presentation. Endoscopic treatment should be rendered for active bleeding. The most common cause of upper GI bleeding is peptic ulcer disease.
- For *stable* lower GI bleeding, the diagnostic procedure of choice is a colonoscopy, within 24 h of presentation. Endoscopic treatment should be rendered for active bleeding. The most common cause of lower GI bleeding is diverticulosis.
- *Unstable* bleeding warrants a multidisciplinary discussion between gastroenterology, interventional radiology, critical care, and surgery to determine the best diagnostic and therapeutic options.
- CT angiography is an excellent initial diagnostic tool for *unstable* bleeding.
  - If negative, the patient should immediately undergo upper endoscopy as the next step.
  - If positive, consider immediate transcatheter angiography and embolization as the next step.
- Surgery is necessary for patients who fail endoscopic or catheter-based therapies, or if it is deemed the best option after a multidisciplinary discussion. Every effort should be made to localize the site of bleeding prior to surgery.

Initial Evaluation

Initial patient evaluation includes a history and physical examination, with vital signs and laboratory evaluation. One should inquire about the duration, amount, and the nature/color of bleeding. Assessment for comorbid conditions is important, including cardiovascular, pulmonary, renal, and hepatic disease. A prior history of peptic ulcer disease, inflammatory bowel disease, neoplasm, or radiation is important to note. The patient's list of medications should be obtained, with attention to nonsteroidal anti-inflammatory drugs (NSAID), anticoagulants, and antiplatelet medications that may contribute to bleeding. A history of cardiac stenting or prosthetic heart valves should be noted.

Elderly patients have an increased incidence of memory loss and dementia, which can complicate the task of history-taking. Cognitive disorders impair one's decision-making abilities, and elderly patients may be unable to make rational decisions for themselves. Information should be gathered from family members and the primary care physician. The presence of advanced directives and a healthcare proxy may prove invaluable in these situations.

A focused examination should include an abdominal examination and digital rectal examination. Anoscopy should be performed as part of the initial patient examination to rule out active hemorrhoidal bleeding. Hemorrhoids contribute to up to 20% of lower GI bleeding.

Initial Treatment

Resuscitation

It is paramount to initiate immediate supportive measures in case of acute hemorrhage. Two large bore peripheral intravenous catheters are established, and patients are placed on a cardiac monitor. Supplemental oxygen is given if necessary. Patients should receive nothing by mouth (NPO).

Initial resuscitation is performed using a crystalloid intravenous infusion. Blood transfusions generally begin when the hemoglobin (Hb) is <7 g/dL (with a post-transfusion target of Hb 7–9 g/dL). Restrictive transfusion protocols, compared to more liberal protocols, demonstrate an equal or lower risk of mortality and rebleeding. In patients with underlying cardiovascular disease, transfusions should be administered with endpoint to keep Hb ≥8g/dL. A platelet transion should be given after 4 units of packed red od cells. When there is severe and unrelenting eding, blood products should be transfused th a 1:1:1 ratio between packed red blood cells, itelets, and plasma (as in trauma suscitation).

anagement of Antiplatelet nd Anticoagulant Agents

nticoagulant and antiplatelet use is common in derly patients admitted for GI bleeding. An nticoagulant such as warfarin should be stopped t initial presentation. For unstable hemorrhage, ne anticoagulant effect of warfarin is reversed vith a prothrombin complex concentrate and/or itamin K. Warfarin should be restarted in 7 days fter cessation of bleeding. Patients with high isk of thromboembolism, such as with a proshetic heart valve or recent (<3 months) venous hromboembolism, low molecular weight heparin should be started at 48 h after cessation of hemorrhage.

Aspirin for primary prevention in patients with low risk of thromboembolism should be discontinued. However, patients on aspirin for secondary prophylaxis (such as after cardiac stents) have a three-fold risk of cardiovascular or cerebrovascular events when aspirin is stopped. In these patients, low-dose aspirin (i.e., 81 g daily) should be continued.

Dual antiplatelet therapy with a P2Y12 receptor antagonist and aspirin should not be stopped without consultation with a cardiologist. Discontinuation of both medications is especially risky in patients with an acute coronary syndrome within the past 90 days or recent coronary stenting (bare metal stent placed within the preceding 6 weeks, or drug-eluting stent placed within the preceding 6–12 months). In life-threatening hemorrhage, the P2Y12 receptor antagonist should be stopped but aspirin continued. After cessation of bleeding, the P2Y12 receptor antagonist should be restarted in 5 days.

Risk Stratification

At presentation, a risk stratification should be performed for each bleeding patient. Stratification will help identify patients that are at higher risk to suffer poor outcomes. Additionally, stratification will help to triage patients (i.e., to an intensive care unit, hospital floor, or to outpatient evaluation) and assist in determining which clinical services are consulted. Risk factors for worsened outcomes include hypotension, tachycardia, ongoing GI bleeding, older age, renal dysfunction, and unstable or clinically significant coexisting conditions. Patients are categorized by acuity (low versus high, or low/medium/high) based on these criteria, with bleeding classified as either stable or unstable.

Several risk models exist to predict whether patients will need transfusions or hemostatic therapy, or whether they can safely be discharged from the emergency room. The Oakland or Strate scores are such examples. The Glasgow-Blatchford score (GBS) is helpful in identifying which patients are at risk of adverse outcomes: these include rebleeding, the need for blood transfusions, and in-hospital mortality. This tool is particularly useful in assessing the seriousness of bleeding in hospitalized patients. Our institution uses a modified Glasgow-Blatchford scoring system (Table 47.1) as part of a risk stratification strategy (Table 47.2) to determine the acuity of patients. Patients are triaged according to the risk stratification and appropriate consults are obtained.

Table 47.1 Modified Glasgow-Blatchford scale

Criteria	Value	Score
Blood urea nitrogen (BUN)	>30 mg/dL	1
Hemostasis	Hb <10 g/dL	1
	Melena	1
	Hematemesis	1
	Hematochezia	1
Shock	Any hemodynamic instability	1
	Orthostatic hypotension	1

Table 47.2 Risk stratification criteria

Low Acuity (all must be true)	**Medium Acuity** (≥ 1 criteria present)	**High Acuity** (≥ 1 criteria present)
Hemodynamic stability	Age > 50	Hemodynamic instability
Hb > 12 g/dL	BUN 20 – 30	Evidence of active bleeding: large volume hematemesis, hematochezia, or melena
BUN <20	INR 1.5 – 2	Orthostatic hypotension
Modified Glasgow-Batchford Scale (GBS) <2	GBS = 2	GBS > 2
No immediate risk criteria present	No high risk criteria present	

↓	↓	↓
Consult GI Dispo to floor or home	Consult GI Reassess in 4 hours: -To low acuity if stable -To high acuity if worsening	Consult GI and Critical Care Consult Surgery and IR as necessary Floor or ICU per Critical Care Service

Multidisciplinary Care and Treatment Algorithms

The treatment of GI hemorrhage is an interdisciplinary effort. Although different resources are available for each hospital, creation of an institutional protocol and adherence to management algorithms will standardize care and improve outcomes. A multidisciplinary team with 24/7 access to endoscopy, radiology, interventional radiology, critical care, anesthesia, and surgery is critical to the management of acute GI hemorrhage. Prompt access to endoscopic procedures and imaging is critical due to the start-and-stop nature of GI bleeding. Tables 47.3 and 47.4 are basic treatment algorithms used for upper GI and lower GI bleeding at our institution.

Table 47.3 Sample treatment algorithm for upper GI bleeding

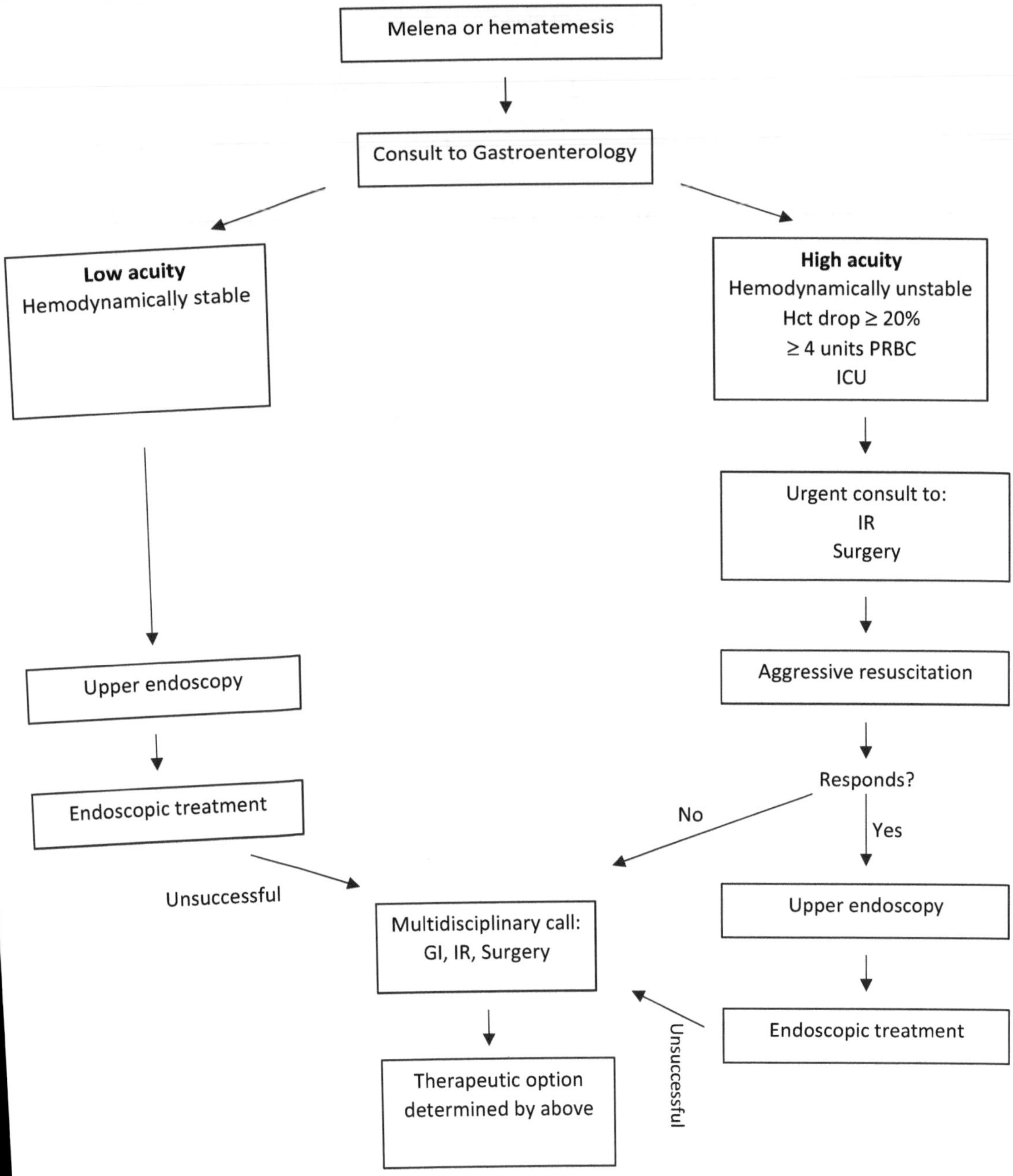

Table 47.4 Sample treatment algorithm for lower GI bleeding

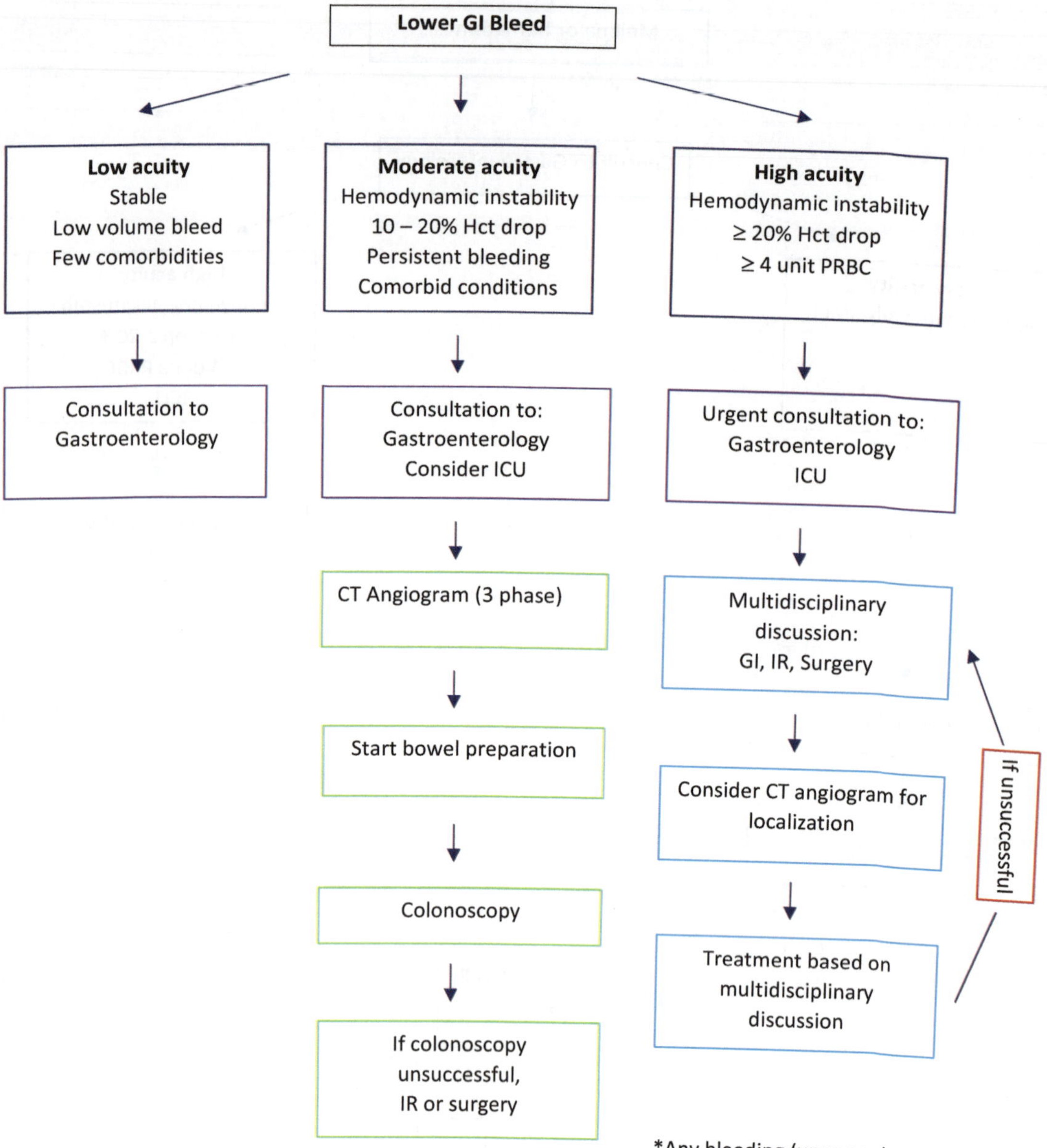

*Any bleeding (upper or lower) associated with a mass or neoplasm requires a surgical consultation

Stable or Unstable Bleeding

In patients with *stable* GI bleeding, the procedure of choice for evaluation and treatment is endoscopy. However, patients with *unstable* bleeding should undergo CT angiography after initial resuscitation. A multidetector-row helical CT can quickly establish whether active bleeding is present, and from where. CT angiography detects bleeding at a rate of 0.3–0.5 mL/min. The sensitivity and specificity of a CT angiogram are 79–95% and 95–100%, respectively, with a localization rate of near 50%. The disadvantage of CT angiography is the nephrotoxicity from the intravenous contrast; this is especially worrisome in elderly patients who have an increased incidence of chronic kidney disease. Figure. 47.1 illustrates an example of an upper GI bleed identified on CT angiography.

When CT angiography diagnoses active bleeding, the best therapeutic option should be discussed in a multidisciplinary manner. Whether to proceed with endoscopy, surgery, or percutaneous angiography is based on patient factors, volume of bleeding, and available resources. However, transcatheter mesenteric angiogram with embolization of the bleeding vessel is gaining favor as the next best step in high acuity bleeding (Fig. 47.2).

In cases of significant hemorrhage where a CT angiogram fails to localize bleeding, an upper endoscopy is immediately performed, followed by a lower GI endoscopy if this is negative.

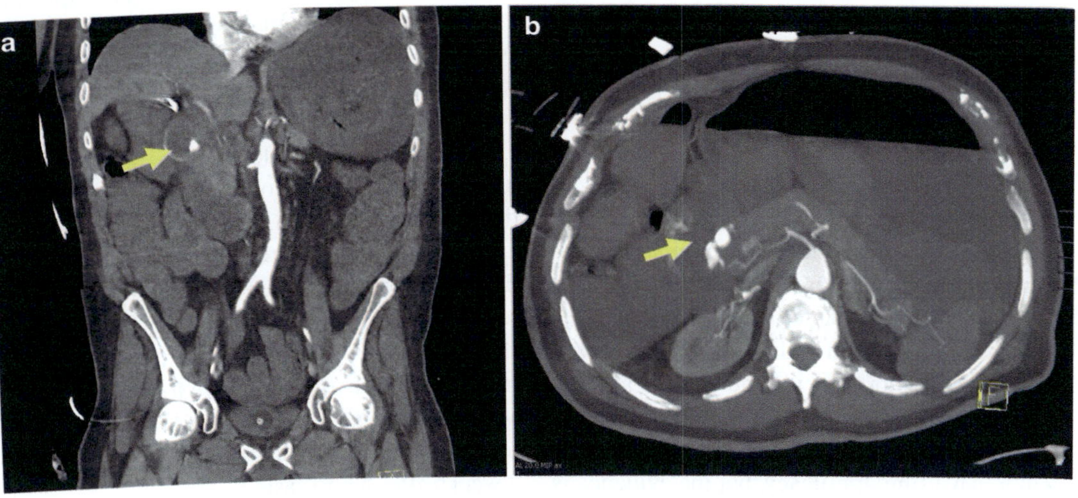

Fig. 47.1 CT angiography demonstrating extravasation of IV contrast in the duodenum (**a**) and (**b**) shows coronal and axial views of the duodenal bleeed

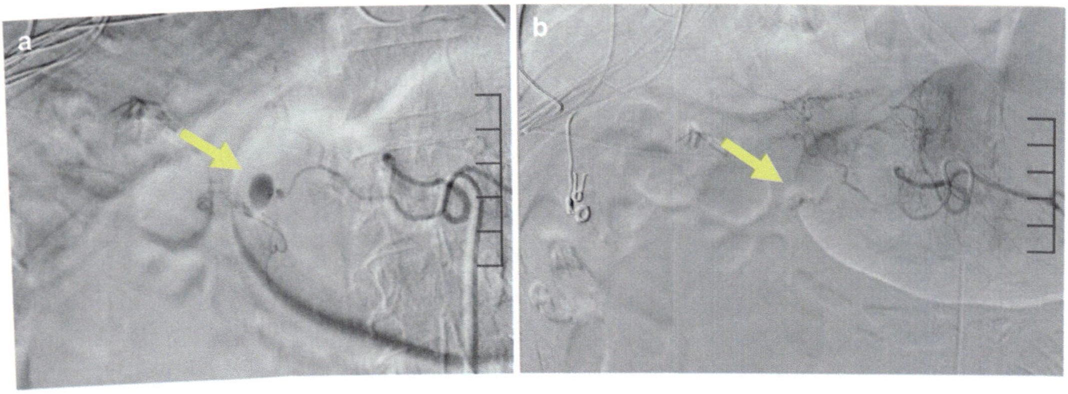

Fig. 47.2 (**a**) Mesenteric angiogram demonstrating active extravasation from the proximal gastroduodenal artery. (**b**) Superselective embolization using N butyl cyanoacrylate with complete occlusion of the bleeding artery

Upper GI Bleeding

The etiologies of upper GI bleeding are listed in Table 47.5. By far the most common cause of upper GI bleeding in the elderly is peptic ulcer disease (42–73%). This is followed by esophagitis (7–18%) and gastropathy (7–28%). Gastric and esophageal varices account for 2–11% of upper GI bleeding.

Endoscopy

For hospitalized patients with a *stable* upper GI bleed, an upper endoscopy should be performed within 24 h of presentation. A medium or high acuity bleed warrants an upper endoscopy within 12 h or sooner, based on the patient's clinical condition.

Endoscopic Management

Therapeutic endoscopic maneuvers should be performed when a bleeding site is identified. For ulcers, thermal techniques (i.e., bipolar electrocoagulation and heater probe) or an injection of a sclerosant (e.g., absolute ethanol) have been shown to be effective in both controlling bleeding and improving mortality in a number of studies. Other methods, such as clip application, argon plasma coagulation, or monopolar coagulation seem to have similar efficacy, but the evidence is not as robust. Dilute epinephrine injection (1:10,000) is helpful in stopping bleeding, but is less effective if used as the only modality. Thus, another hemostatic technology should accompany epinephrine injection.

Table 47.5 Causes of upper GI bleeding

– Peptic ulcer disease
– Esophagitis
– Gastritis and duodenitis
– Varices
– Mallory-Weiss tear
– Vascular ectasias
– Neoplasm
– Dieulafoy lesion
– Aortoenteric fistula
– Foreign body

Initial endoscopic hemostasis is successful in about 90% of bleeding peptic ulcers. The rate of rebleeding ranges from 12–25% in larger studies. More episodes of rebleeding are seen in patients with hemodynamic instability, active bleeding at initial endoscopy, large ulcer size ≥2 cm, posterior duodenal ulcers, and gastric ulcers in the lesser curve. An endoscopic clip should be placed adjacent to the site of the bleeding, which may be helpful for the interventional radiologist in case of future angiography.

Hemostatic powders have shown promise and have similar rates of efficacy as conventional therapy. It is difficult to justify hemostatic sprays as first-line therapy due to their high cost. However, this technology may be especially valuable when the application of thermal energy or clips is not technically feasible due to anatomic constraints, or when the bleeding is diffuse or massive.

After successful endoscopic hemostasis of an ulcer, high-dose proton-pump inhibitor (PPI) therapy (equivalent to omeprazole or pantoprazole ≥80 mg daily) is recommended (either continuously or intermittently) for 3 days. This reduces the rate of rebleeding significantly (RR = 0.43, 0.33–0.56). Patients at higher risk of rebleeding, such as those with a Rockall score ≥6, active bleeding, or nonbleeding but visible vessel, should be placed on twice-daily PPI for 2 weeks after hemostasis.

Patients with rebleeding after initial therapeutic endoscopy should undergo repeat endoscopy. About 75% of patients with rebleeding may achieve hemostasis this way. Two consecutive thermal modalities could increase the risk of perforation, and thus a mechanical option such as an endoscopic clip is favored. One randomized study compared repeat endoscopic treatment to surgery in patients with a recurrent upper GI bleed. Although more patients experienced rebleeding after the second endoscopic treatment compared to surgery (23% vs 7%), morbidity (15% vs 36%), and mortality rates (10% vs 18%) were significantly higher when patients underwent surgery.

For esophageal and gastric varices, pharmacologic treatment using a somatostatin analogue is initiated to reduce splanchnic circulation (e.g., octreotide 50 μg bolus, followed by a 50 μg/h infusion). Nonselective beta blockers can be effective prophylaxis for variceal bleeding as well. Both medications should be monitored for adverse cardiovascular effects. Endoscopic treatment using band ligation is the procedure of choice for varices.

Endovascular Treatment

Failure of endoscopic therapy should warrant a multidisciplinary discussion about the next optimal option. The options for patients unsuccessfully treated with upper endoscopy are either surgery or mesenteric angiography and transcatheter embolization. Embolization is performed using coils (platinum), particles (N-butyl cyanoacrylate), or liquid (polyvinyl alcohol) agents.

One systematic review and meta-analysis comparing transarterial embolization to surgery in such patients showed an increased risk of rebleeding in the endovascular treatment arm (OR = 2.44, 1.77–3.36). However, embolization had a significantly lower complication rate (OR = 0.45, 0.3–0.67) and shorter hospital stay (median 8 vs. 16 days), with similar mortality rates. Given these findings, angiography with transcatheter embolization is gaining popularity as the next step prior to surgical intervention.

Surgery for Upper GI Bleeding

Over the past few decades, improvements in endoscopic and endovascular treatment have decreased the need for surgical intervention for upper GI hemorrhage. As discussed above, even recurrent episodes of GI bleeding can be managed with repeat endoscopic procedures or percutaneous angiography. However, emergency surgery is still necessary in up to 10% of patients with bleeding ulcers, with an associated mortality rate between 2% and 36%.

Surgery for Duodenal ulcer: The most common location of a duodenal ulcer is the duodenal bulb. Thus, a longitudinal duodenotomy is made (with extension to a duodenopyloromyotomy if necessary for exposure). Ulcers located in the posterior aspect of duodenum may have erosion into the gastroduodenal artery. Thus, a suture ligation is performed of the artery proximal and distal to the ulcer, and a U-stitch is placed underneath the ulcer to control the transverse pancreatic branch. Duodenal ulcers not located posteriorly are managed by a four-quadrant suture ligation. With the widespread use of PPIs, simultaneous acid-reducing procedures have mostly become unnecessary. However, one should consider a truncal vagotomy when patients have bled while on active PPI therapy or are allergic to PPIs. Other relative indications include alcoholic patients, unreliable patients, and those who must continue NSAID use. When a truncal vagotomy is performed, closure should be in the form of a pyloroplasty. A highly selective vagotomy in an unstable patient cannot be advised.

Surgery for gastric ulcer: Bleeding gastric ulcers treated with suture ligation have a risk of rebleeding in up to 30%. Since gastric ulcers are not usually related to acid-production, acid-reducing medications are unlikely to be helpful. Thus, the treatment of choice for gastric ulcers is resection. A distal gastrectomy is recommended for ulcers in the lower half of the stomach. Ulcers in the upper stomach should be treated with a wedge resection.

Surgery for Mallory-Weiss tear: Mallory-Weiss tears are usually the result of vigorous vomiting. Non-operative treatment is successful in over 90% of cases. When necessary, surgery involves opening the cardia of the stomach with exploration of the gastroesophageal junction and direct suture ligation of the bleeding tear.

Lower GI Bleeding

The various etiologies of lower GI bleeding are listed in Table 47.6. The most common cause of lower GI bleeding is diverticulosis, accounting

Table 47.6 Causes of lower GI bleeding

– Diverticulosis
– Hemorrhoids
– Vascular ectasias
– Ischemic colitis
– Colorectal neoplasms
– Post-polypectomy bleeding
– Inflammatory bowel disease
– Stercoral ulceration
– Colorectal varices

for 30% to 65% of cases. Hemorrhoids and ischemic colitis each account for 5–20% of cases.

Colonoscopy

Colonoscopy is the procedure of choice for *stable* lower GI hemorrhage. For hospitalized patients, the procedure should be performed within the first 24 h of presentation, preceded by a mechanical bowel preparation using polyethylene glycol or similar preparation. There is no clear evidence that colonoscopy performed more urgently (<12 h) leads to any benefit in terms of diagnostic yield, transfusion requirement, hospital stay, or mortality. Colonoscopy without mechanical bowel preparation can lead to an incomplete procedure due to impaired visualization. However, one should not discount the value of an urgent flexible sigmoidoscopy (preceded by an enema preparation) if a brisk bleed is suspected from the distal left colon.

Endoscopic Management

When active bleeding is identified in the lower GI tract, there are several endoscopic options for hemostasis. As in upper GI bleeding, these include injectional therapies (e.g., dilute epinephrine solution), thermal approaches (bipolar coagulation, argon plasma coagulation, heater probe), mechanical techniques (endoscopic clips, band ligation), and hemostatic sprays. Injection using epinephrine solution (1:10,000 dilution) should be accompanied by either mechanical or thermal therapy for more definitive control of bleeding. Endoscopic treatment is successful in achieving hemostasis in over 90% of cases, but early and late rebleeding occur at a rate of 8% and 12%, respectively. Even if active bleeding is not present, a stigma of recent bleeding including a large visible vessel or adherent clot warrants endoscopic treatment. Mechanical methods are preferred over thermal techniques for diverticular bleeding, as aggressive thermal application may lead to delayed perforation.

After localization of bleeding and therapeutic maneuvers, the area of bleeding should be marked with a tattoo, both for future reference in a case of rebleeding or if surgery is required.

Endovascular Treatment

In patients with *unstable* bleeding in whom CT angiography demonstrates active bleeding, a decision should be made in a multidisciplinary manner regarding the best therapeutic option. As in upper GI bleeding, this decision should be based on patient factors, severity of bleeding, and available resources. However, a transcatheter mesenteric angiography is considered an excellent next step. If a bleeding vessel is visualized, embolization can be performed. It is yet unknown whether embolization is superior to endoscopy in lower GI bleeding as these modalities have not been directly compared. Embolization has a high technical success rate of 93–100%, with a rebleeding rate of 10–50%. However, this procedure carries a risk of bowel ischemia in up to 24%. Superselective embolization utilizes microcatheters (1.0–3.0 French) that can embolize mesenteric arteries as small as 1 mm in diameter. Superselective embolization limits the rate of bowel ischemia to a range of 1–4%, and is preferred whenever possible.

Surgery for Lower GI Bleeding

Improvements in endoscopic and transcatheter treatment have reduced the need for emergency gery in lower GI bleeding. However, surgical ervention is still necessary in 6% of all lower bleeding, and in up to 25% of cases that quire transfusions. The indications for surgery e when endoscopic and interventional radiol- y procedures fail to diagnose or stabilize tients, in cases of bowel ischemia or perfora- on, or for bleeding neoplasms. A relative dication is a blood transfusion requirement of 6 more units of packed red blood cells within 4 h. The importance of localizing the site of leeding prior to surgery cannot be stressed nough.

The options for surgical resection are either a egmental resection or total abdominal colec- omy. A segmental resection should only be per- ormed if the bleeding site has definitively been ocalized. If a hemodynamically unstable patient equires urgent surgery without clear localization of the bleeding, one should consider an intraop- erative colonoscopy and/or enteroscopy. Ultimately, in an unstable patient with a high sus- picion of a colonic bleed, a "blind" total abdomi- nal colectomy may be necessary. Rebleeding rates after this approach are higher than with seg- mental resection, as the bleeding may have occurred from a missed small bowel or anorectal source. The mortality rate for surgical interven- tion for lower GI hemorrhage is 12–17% in more recent reports.

Whether to perform an anastomosis after seg- mental or total colectomy should be based on the patient's clinical condition. Ongoing hemody- namic instability, poor nutritional state, signifi- cant comorbidities, and a massive transfusion requirement should sway the surgeon away from performing a primary anastomosis in favor of an end stoma.

A thorough exploration should be performed at the time of surgery, with examination the entire GI tract for neoplasms and potential bleeding sources, including a Meckel's diverticulum. Laparoscopic surgery has been utilized for the treatment of acute GI bleeding; however, mini- mally invasive techniques should only be consid- ered when technical expertise exists, and in a hemodynamically stable patient.

Conclusion

GI hemorrhage is a significant cause of morbidity and mortality in the elderly population. More comorbid conditions exist in the elderly, increasing the risk of poor outcomes. A multidisciplinary approach is essential for the treatment of GI hemorrhage. Institutional care protocols and treatment algorithms help to standardize care and improve outcomes. Stratification of risk based on patient stability and acuity of bleeding is important to help triage patients, determine which clinical services are consulted, and which diagnostic and therapeutic options to consider.

Upper and lower endoscopy remains the most utilized tool for diagnosis and hemostasis in patients with GI bleeding. However, in patients with high acuity hemorrhage, a multidetector-row helical CT angiography is an excellent diagnostic tool for localization of bleeding. Which hemostatic intervention is best for each patient should be a decision made in an interdisciplinary manner, considering surgical, endoscopic, and interventional radiology approaches. For active high-volume GI hemorrhage, a transcatheter mesenteric angiography with superselective embolization is gaining popularity. The acute care surgeon should be intimately involved with every patient with severe GI hemorrhage, whether surgery is ultimately required.

References

1. Kaplan RC, Heckbert SR, Koepsell TD, Furberg CD, Polak JF, Schoen RE, Psaty BM. Risk factors for hospitalized gastrointestinal bleeding among older persons. J Am Geriatr Soc. 2001;49:126–33. https://doi.org/10.1046/j.1532-5415.2001.49032.x.
2. Siddiqui NS, Paul S, Khan Z, Javaid T, Hasan SS, Khan Z, et al. Rising events and improved outcomes of gastrointestinal bleed with shock in the USA. A 12-year national analysis. J Clin Gastroenterol. 2019;53:194–201. https://doi.org/10.1097/MCG.0000000000000995.
3. Gralnek IM, Neeman Z, Strate LL. Acute lower gastrointestinal bleeding. N Engl J Med. 2017;376:1054–63. https://doi.org/10.1056/NEJMcp1603455.

4. Oakland K, Chadwick G, East JE, Guy R, Humphries A, Jairath V, et al. Diagnosis and management of acute lower gastrointestinal bleeding: guidelines from the British Society of gastroenterology. Gut. 2019;68:776–89. https://doi.org/10.1136/gutjnl-2018-317807.
5. Almaghrabi M, Gandhi M, Guizzetti L, Iansavichene A, Yan B, Wilson A, et al. Comparison of risk scores for lower gastrointestinal bleeding. A systematic review and meta-analysis. JAMA Netw Open. 2022;5(5):e2214253. https://doi.org/10.1001/jamanetworkopen.2022.14253.
6. Moss AJ, Tuffaha H, Malik A. Lower GI bleeding: a review of current management, controversies, and advances. Int J Color Dis. 2016;31:175–88. https://doi.org/10.1007/s00384-015-2400-x.
7. Yachimski P, Friedman L. Gastrointestinal bleeding in the elderly. Nature. 2007;5:80–93. https://doi.org/10.1038/ncpgasthep1034.
8. Laine L, Barkun A, Saltzman J, Martel M, Leontia GI. ACG guideline: upper gastrointestinal and ul bleeding. Am J Gastroenterol. 2021;116:899–91 https://doi.org/10.14309/ajg.0000000000001245.
9. Elmunzer BJ, Young SD, Inadomi JM, Schoenfe P, Laine L. Systematic review of the predicto of recurrent hemorrhage after endoscopic hem static therapy for bleeding peptic ulcers. Am Gastroenterol. 2008;103:2625–32. https://do org/10.1111/j.1572-0241.2008.02070.x.
10. Kazanjian KK, Hines O. Nonvariceal upper ga trointestinal bleeding: when endoscopic therap fails—a surgeon's perspective. Tech Gastrointe Endosc. 2005;7:156–9. https://doi.org/10.1016/tgie.2005.04.013.
11. Kim HS, Lee IS. Role of surgery in gastrointestina bleeding. Int J Gastrointest Interv. 2018;7:136–41 https://doi.org/10.18528/gii180029.

48 Small and Large Bowel Obstruction

Dena R. Nasir, Makenna Marty, Seija Maniskas, and Howard S. Kaufman

Small Bowel Obstruction

Introduction and General Considerations

Intestinal obstruction is an indication for emergency surgery in the elderly population. Although the incidence of small bowel obstruction (SBO) is similar across all age groups, increasing age is a predictor for increased morbidity and mortality after emergency major abdominal surgeries. Elderly patients with obstruction are more likely to have non-specific symptoms resulting in delayed diagnoses and later presentations. Although there is an increased incidence of malignancy with increasing age, adhesions and hernia continue to be the leading causes of small bowel obstruction in the elderly population.

Due to increasing frailty in patients over 65 and the increased likelihood of pre-existing malnutrition, the decision to proceed with operative management of SBO becomes a delicate balance. Aging is known to result in reduced resilience and functional performance leading to malnutrition as well as increased loss of weight and muscle mass. Specifically in the setting of bowel obstruction, where patients have often been without oral intake for multiple days, malnutrition needs to be adequately assessed.

Additional comorbidities that have increased prevalence in elderly patients, such as dementia, pulmonary disease, and kidney disease, can increase the difficulty of diagnosis in this population. Elderly patients may present with atypical symptoms or inability to vocalize their symptoms, which has also been shown to cause delay in diagnosis. With decreased oral intake and increased incidence of renal disease, the risks and benefits of obtaining a contrast radiographic study must be balanced with the increased risk of contrast-induced nephropathy. Patients with preexisting pulmonary diseases and diminished reserve may present with respiratory decompensation as a consequence of increased abdominal pressure and intra-abdominal pathology.

Clinical Presentation

Elderly patients present with small bowel obstructions later and with less profound symptoms compared to younger patients, resulting in higher incidence of misdiagnosis. Specifically, they have been shown to have less pain and are less likely to present with peritonitis even in the presence of ischemic bowel. Dehydration is a common feature of the presentation of elderly patients with SBO that has the potential to cause

D. R. Nasir · M. Marty · S. Maniskas · H. S. Kaufman (✉)
Huntington Hospital, An Affiliate of Cedars-Sinai, Pasadena, CA, USA
e-mail: howard.kaufman@huntingtonhospital.com

P. Petrone, C. E.M. Brathwaite (eds.), *Acute Care Surgery in Geriatric Patients*,
https://doi.org/10.1007/978-3-031-30651-8_48

numerous derangements including concentrated hemoglobin, hypo-or hypernatremia, hypochloremia, contraction alkalosis, metabolic acidosis, increased serum osmolality, and an increase in blood urea nitrogen to creatinine ratio. As patients age, their kidneys are less able to retain fluid in concentrating their urine and are more prone to kidney injury due to pre-renal etiologies such as dehydration.

Vital signs should be evaluated for tachycardia, hypotension, or tachypnea that can all point to a possible intra-abdominal pathology and hypovolemia from the obstructive process. In frail populations, the physiologic reserve is limited, making assessment of volume status a first priority. Foley catheter placement may be required for more accurate monitoring of fluid balance.

Presentation differs between partial and complete SBOs. Patients with partial obstructions continue with the ability to have bowel movements or pass flatus after onset of symptoms. However, differentiation between the two is important, as complete bowel obstructions have higher rates of intestinal incarceration and strangulation needing surgical intervention.

Specific consideration requiring attention in elderly patients includes evaluation for a POLST. As patients with small bowel obstructions may require immediate surgical intervention, discussion on goals of care and patient wishes should happen as early as possible. Patients with DNR (Do Not Resuscitate) status have higher risks of morbidity and mortality.

Evaluation

Evaluation should begin with a thorough history and physical examination. Care should be taken to determine last bowel movement, flatus, history of prior bowel obstructions and past abdominal and pelvic surgery, prior radiation therapy, cancer history, and dates and findings of past colonoscopies. Physical examination may be unreliable, but close evaluation for prior incisions, bloating, bulging to indicate hernias, and evaluation for tenderness is standard. Patients with ischemia, particularly those in the geriatric population, may present with atypical abdominal exams and without evidence of tenderness, so a high level of suspicion is required. In addition, medication history must be assessed for drugs that promote dysmotility, such as opioid medications and anti-psychotics.

Laboratory studies should include a complete blood count, chemistry panel, lactic acid, and lipase. Leukocytosis could indicate sepsis and increased concern for bowel ischemia, and a concentrated hemoglobin may also indicate dehydration. However, in frail elderly patients with poor nutrition or comorbidities, patients may not mount an adequate immune response in the presence of ischemia or may have a lower baseline hemoglobin. Metabolic or lactic acidosis may also indicate bowel ischemia; however, lactic acid may also be elevated in the setting of dehydration. An elevated lactic acid after volume resuscitation should raise concern for worsening visceral compromise.

Imaging studies are important tools to better characterize the etiology of obstruction. A plain abdominal series can be utilized for quick evaluation, assessing for dilated small bowel (>2.5 cm), air-fluid levels, or a large, dilated stomach. Computed tomography (CT) scan is most useful in delineating etiology of obstruction when obtained prior to nasogastric tube placement. Obstruction can be evaluated by determining transition points from dilated to decompressed small bowel. IV contrast, when not contraindicated, is important to aid in assessment for bowel ischemia or high risk for progression to bowel ischemia with bowel wall thickening, mesenteric edema, mesenteric swirling, free fluid, or in more extreme cases, pneumatosis or pneumobilia. However, absence of these findings on cross-sectional imaging does not rule out the presence of ischemia, especially in non-contrast studies. In addition, masses or hernias may be visualized. Care must be taken when giving elderly patients IV contrast as they are usually hypovolemic at the time of presentation and have higher risk of contrast-induced nephropathy.

ologies

e most common causes of SBO in the elderly pulation remain similar to the non-geriatric pulation, with adhesions, hernias, and neo-asms being the most common causes. However, cidence of diseases such as inflammatory bowel sease without a prior diagnosis is much lower the elderly population. In addition, the inci-ence of gallstone ileus and malignant bowel ostruction increases with age.

dhesive Disease

dhesive small bowel obstruction is the most ommon cause of SBO in both the general and eriatric population. History is particularly nportant, as prior abdominal and pelvic surgery s strongly predictive of adhesive small bowel lisease. A history may be difficult to elicit in an elderly patient with acute and/or chronic cogni-ive deficits, so a thorough exam evaluating for orior incisional scars is important. Although oatients typically present with a history of prior surgery, a small portion may have a virgin abdo-men. In the latter scenario, adhesions are due to past or concurrent abdominal or pelvic inflamma-tory processes. Adhesions may occur as a single band causing constriction or internal herniation of the small bowel or more commonly, matted intestines from more extensive scar tissue.

Treatment may be either nonoperative or operative depending on initial presentation. As with any other disease process, if there is evidence of bowel compromise, the patient should be appropriately resuscitated and taken for immediate surgical intervention. Such circumstances include complete or closed loop obstructions. The mainstay of medical treatment includes bowel rest with nasogastric tube decompression as well as fluid resuscitation. After decompression, imaging with water-soluble contrast can be considered, as evaluating contrast transit time into the colon can be beneficial in determining which patients are likely to resolve with nonoperative management. There is also a therapeutic benefit to water-soluble contrast due to the ability to reduce bowel wall edema and promote bowel motility. Abbas et al. suggest that contrast in the colon at 4–6 h is a reliable indicator, while others suggest that surgery was required in 96% of patients who required more than 24 h for contrast to reach the colon. Patients with water-soluble oral contrast media had an overall shorter hospital course and shorter time to resolution of their symptoms.

If symptoms do not resolve with bowel rest and decompression, surgery is typically recommended within 48 h in older populations rather than the standard 72 h. A single institution study of 144 patients demonstrated that elderly patients who underwent delayed surgery had a 14% mortality compared to 3% in the early surgery group.

Hernias

Hernias may occur in a variety of locations. Patients should be examined for prior surgical scars to evaluate for incisional hernias and other common sites of abdominal wall hernias (umbilical and Spigelian), and groin hernias, including inguinal, femoral, or obturator hernias. Prior laparoscopic and/or robotic port sites may be difficult to identify but should also be surveyed for hernias.

When bulges are noted, the overlying skin should be evaluated. With an incarcerated hernia contents are unable to be reduced back within the peritoneal cavity and strangulation indicates ischemic compromise of the hernia contents. On physical exam, skin changes, tense hernia contents, pain out of proportion of physical exam, persistent pain after reduction of hernia contents, and toxic appearance (i.e., fevers, hemodynamic instability), all indicate a strangulated hernia, requiring immediate surgical intervention. CT scans may be helpful in assessing not only the precise size and location of the hernia but the viability of the incarcerated small intestine.

Approaches may be either open, laparoscopic, or robotic depending on surgeon experience and judgment as well as institutional resources. Irrespective of the approach, the reduced bowel must be evaluated for evidence of viability and compromise. Ischemic or necrotic segments should be resected and reconstructed with primary anastomosis. The hernia defect should be closed either primarily or with the use of non-synthetic (biologic) mesh. Use of synthetic mesh is not typically recommended due to increased risk of surgical site infection.

Internal hernias caused by the passage and entrapment of viscera through congenital or acquired defects in the mesentery are not easily detected on physical examination. Diagnosis typically requires imaging with CT scan, usually assessing for mesenteric swirling or specific visualization of herniation of contents through mesenteric defects. Acquired defects usually due to prior surgical history with a Roux-en-Y reconstruction (gastric bypass, pancreaticoduodenectomy, hepaticojejunostomy). Internal hernias are closed looped bowel obstructions and necessitate surgical intervention with reduction of herniated contents, assessment and resection of irreversibly compromised intestine, and closure of mesenteric defects to prevent recurrence.

Malignancy

Primary malignant neoplasms of the small intestine are uncommon and represent approximately 2–3% of gastrointestinal cancers. While lymphoma is more commonly diagnosed in younger patients, the incidence of other tumors such as adenocarcinoma, gastrointestinal stromal tumors (GIST), and carcinoid increases with age and must be considered as an underlying cause of non-adhesive SBO. Small bowel tumors are most common in the proximal small intestine including the duodenum and jejunum, where adenocarcinoma is most common. Alternatively, carcinoid tumors more commonly occur in the ileum.

Primary abdominal and pelvic tumors not originating from the small bowel, such as gastric, pancreatic, colon, and ovarian, may result in peritoneal carcinomatosis which creates additional management challenges. Breast and other advanced extra-abdominal cancers should also be considered, especially when ascites is present on CT imaging.

Adenocarcinoma

Familial adenomatous polyposis syndrome, Lynch syndrome, celiac disease, and Crohn's disease are associated with an increased risk of developing small bowel adenocarcinoma. However, many patients develop disease sporadically.

When evaluating resectability of small bow adenocarcinoma, the surgeon must assess f superior mesenteric artery involvement as well evidence of metastatic disease of the omentu and peritoneum. If the disease is resectabl NCCN guidelines recommend that 5–8 lymp nodes adjacent to the feeding vessel should b obtained to allow for adequate staging, 5 in th duodenum and 8 elsewhere. Segmental resec tions with margins of 5–10 cm should b obtained. If the primary is located in the termina ileum, a right hemicolectomy should be per formed, and the ileocolic artery should b resected. Patients with nodal disease or T3 disease and high-risk features should be considere for adjuvant chemotherapy. NCCN reports high-risk features as: positive or close resection margins, <5 lymph nodes in duodenal or <8 lymph nodes if jejunal or ileal as well as tumor perforation.

Patients presenting with diffuse metastatic disease should be considered for palliative bypass surgery or diversion if there is evidence of obstruction and such treatment would be consistent with goals of care. Endoscopic stenting may be a feasible palliative option for obstructing duodenal adenocarcinoma and is consistent with NCCN guidelines. In this situation, chemotherapy may convert a patient with otherwise unresectable disease into a surgical candidate.

Carcinoid Tumors

Carcinoid tumor is a neuroendocrine tumor (NET) that originates from enterochromaffin cells. Carcinoids most commonly arise in the small intestine (45%), followed by rectum (20%), appendix (16%), colon (11%), and stomach (7%). Within the small bowel, they are most commonly found within the ileum 60 cm from the ileocecal valve.

Patients typically present in their 60–70s, and obstruction may be due to intussusception, intraluminal blockage, or mesenteric kinking from tumor invasion, lymphadenopathy, or desmoplastic response. Lastly, intestinal ischemia can occur in the setting of bulky disease- causing mesenteric compression or from mesenteric vascular invasion.

As all small bowel NETs have potential to etastasize regardless of size, patients without idence of metastatic disease should undergo de local excision, including resection of the volved segment of the mesentery. NETs are ultifocal in 20–55% of patients, and therefore, e entirety of the small bowel should be assessed r additional disease.

eritoneal Carcinomatosis

Ialignant bowel obstruction is most prevalent in varian cancer, followed by colorectal and gastric ancers. When peritoneal carcinomatosis results n small bowel obstruction, the burden of metatatic disease is typically high with encasement of multiple loops of intestine. When discussing urgical treatment in this patient population, a multidisciplinary meeting should be conducted aking into consideration the patient's performance status, frailty, cancer stage, estimated life expectancy, response to therapy, and goals of care.

Initially, therapy consists of nasogastric decompression and bowel rest. Total parenteral nutrition should be considered in appropriate patients. Immediate surgical management should be offered in the setting of acute bowel ischemia unless goals of care state otherwise. In addition, absolute contraindications to surgery include diffuse palpable abdominal masses, multiple levels of bowel obstruction, recurrent ascites after paracentesis, recent surgery demonstrating corrective surgery is impossible, and involvement of proximal stomach. Relative contraindications include malnutrition, low serum albumin, major renal or hepatic dysfunction, and extra-abdominal masses.

Treatment options include medical management with antisecretory drugs (e.g., octreotide), resection, bypass, ileostomy, or gastrostomy tube placement. If the tumor causing obstruction can be removed with negative margins, resection is preferred. Palliative surgery to bypass or resect obstructions may benefit patients; however, it is associated with high mortality and lengthy hospitalizations. If the bowel cannot be resected and there is healthy bowel both proximal and distal to the diseased segment, a side-to-side bypass may be created. If disease is extensive, jejunostomy or ileostomy are options if there is at least 100 cm of normal small intestine proximally. However, such a proximal stoma is associated with high output resulting in electrolyte derangements and dehydration. Lastly, a venting gastrostomy tube may be utilized.

Gallstone Ileus

While an uncommon cause of SBO in all patients, gallstone ileus has a higher incidence in the elderly. Pressure from the gallstone results in venous congestion followed by ischemia from impaired arterial inflow resulting in pressure ulcerations. This process then progresses into the development of a cholecysto-enteric fistula. Gallstones that result in fistula formation are usually over 2 cm in diameter. Obstruction most commonly occurs at the terminal ileum due to narrowing at the ileocecal valve, and the jejunum and stomach are the next most commonly affected sites.

Symptoms are typically similar to those of patients with adhesive disease. However, the mobile nature of the large gallstone may lead to more intermittent and vague symptoms. CT of the abdomen is usually diagnostic, and findings will include small bowel dilation with air fluid levels, gallbladder wall thickening, pneumobilia, and visualization of the obstructing gallstone.

At the time of initial presentation surgical intervention is recommended. A longitudinal enterotomy should be made proximal to the area of obstruction and the stone should then be milked proximally and removed. However if there is evidence of ischemia, perforation or inability to remove the gallstone at the area of obstruction, bowel resection should be considered. The entirety of the bowel should be inspected for any additional stones and the enterotomy should be closed in a transverse fashion. High-risk elderly patients with multiple comorbidities should not undergo cholecystectomy and repair of the cholecysto-enteric fistula at the time of initial intervention for the SBO. Minimally invasive surgery is an option in appropriately selected patients.

Outcomes

Defining the likelihood of adverse outcomes in elderly patients presenting with mechanical SBO is difficult due to variability in age ranges studied by various investigators. Kraus et al. compared outcomes of 80 geriatric (>65 years of age) with 136 non-geriatric patients. Both groups had similar characteristics on admission except for the presence of pre-existing cardiac disease (26.3% vs 12.5%; $p = 0.01$). There were no differences in type of treatment (medical vs surgical), time to or type of surgery, length of post-op stay, or overall complications. Cardiac complications (15% vs 0%; $p = 0.0082$) and sub-acute care facility discharge (29% vs 5%; $p < 0.001$) were more common in the geriatric cohort.

Springer and colleagues prospectively enrolled consecutive patients ≥70 years of age with SBO into an outcomes database and reported results on 104 patients; 49% managed nonoperatively; and 51% who underwent surgery. Of the nonoperative group, 86% were diagnosed with adhesive SBO; and 4% with hernias. Alternatively, within the group managed surgically, 49% were diagnosed with adhesive SBO; and 43% with hernias. The surgical group had more complications (64% v. 27%; $p = 0.002$) and longer lengths of hospital stay (10 vs 3 days; $p < 0.001$) than patients managed nonoperatively. Nonoperative management was associated with a high rate of recurrent SBO: 31% after a median follow-up of 17 months. The group of patients who required surgery after unsuccessful nonoperative management had a 14% mortality versus 3% for those who underwent immediate surgery. This difference was not significant.

Large Bowel Obstructions

Epidemiology

Large bowel obstructions (LBO) are less common than small bowel obstructions, but still account for approximately 25% of intestinal obstructions. LBO is more common in elderly patients compared to the general population, with a median age of presentation of 73, due to increased incidence of malignancy, polypharmacy, chronic constipation, and diverticulitis. The most common causes of LBO in geriatric patients include colorectal cancer (60–80%), volvulus (10–15%), and diverticulitis (10%).

LBO may be mechanical, due to intrinsic luminal obstruction or external compression, or functional. Furthermore, they can be further subdivided into partial or complete. Each of the above subtypes of large bowel obstructions can present slightly differently. There is little literature specific to these conditions in geriatric patients. Therefore, much of this discussion pertains to LBO in patients of all ages. The physiologic differences in the elderly, including cognitive factors and increased frailty discussed in the SBO section above are also relevant for LBO. Where possible, considerations specific to the elderly will be discussed.

Presentation

Acute complete LBO is a medical emergency and is associated with high morbidity and mortality if left untreated or if treatment is delayed. The onset of symptoms is typically acute but may be more indolent depending on the etiology. Most commonly, patients will present with abdominal pain, constipation or obstipation, and abdominal distention. A thorough history may help to guide investigations and treatments of underlying etiologies. As a whole, emesis is a late finding and less commonly seen in LBO compared to SBO.

While patients with LBO due to cancer may have acute onset of pain, obstipation, and distention, they may also reveal more chronic symptoms when questioned. These patients may report eeks to months of bloody stools or weight loss preceding obstructive symptoms. Diarrhea or more narrow-caliber stools are often reported prior to development of constipation, as liquid or thin, soft stool passes through a progressively narrowed lumen. Conversely, obstructions with symptoms that onset very acutely, especially pain and complete obstipation, are more typically due to volvulus.

A distal obstruction combined with a competent ileocecal valve (which occurs in most individuals) effectively creates a closed-loop obstruction, increasing the severity of symptoms and potential for complications such as perforation. Alternatively, an incompetent ileocecal valve can allow for reflux of colonic material back into the ileum and more proximal small intestine which may reduce symptom severity and decrease the risk of perforation. CT scan will differentiate between the two scenarios.

If allowed to progress, distention of the obstructed colon continues to the point of eventually compromising the blood flow to the bowel wall. Venous outflow will be obstructed first, followed later by vascular congestion and eventual obstruction of arterial inflow. Mucosal integrity is compromised with disruption of epithelial tight junctions leading to bacterial translocation and sepsis. Continued hypoperfusion from sepsis and local pressure on the colon wall leads to full-thickness colonic ischemia, which can progress to necrosis and perforation. Patients may have peritoneal findings at any point along this pathway depending on the degree of colonic compromise. Patients will appear acutely ill and distended. They are likely to appear acutely ill and exhibit tachycardia, with distension, tympany, and diffuse tenderness on exam.

Diagnosis and Radiologic Findings

While plain abdominal X-rays are most useful in the diagnosis of volvulus, CT scan is the imaging modality of choice to diagnose an LBO, identify its potential cause, identify potential complications, and guide treatment. Findings may include a dilated, stool-filled proximal colon with a decompressed distal colon, as well as identification of a transition point. Other findings such as a mass, inflammation, volvulus, or a stool filled colon with or without stercoral changes may be apparent and lead to appropriate therapy. When CT findings are equivocal, a water-soluble contrast enema may be of value in further defining the site and completeness of the LBO and may be therapeutic in cases of severe constipation and fecal impaction.

The use of intravenous contrast for abdominal and pelvic CT does not increase rates of large bowel obstruction diagnosis, but it can improve sensitivity for detecting ischemia and the presence of pneumatosis intestinalis. Therefore, intravenous fluid contrast is typically recommended if obstruction is on the differential and if its use is not contraindicated. Whether oral or rectal contrast is indicated is more controversial. Rectal contrast can be of use when there is a question of large bowel obstruction versus a functional disorder, as passage of contrast will abruptly terminate at the level of a mechanical obstruction versus its ability to flow freely to more proximal portions of colon in a functional disorder.

The diameter at which to be concerned for colonic perforation varies and is dependent on historical factors. The Law of Laplace becomes relevant when reviewing the imaging and deciding upon the urgency of intervention. Laplace's law relates the intraluminal pressure needed to stretch the wall of a hollow tube to the inverse of the radius of that tube. Therefore, the cecum, with its standard diameter being the largest of all colonic segments, is the most prone to perforation, since it requires the least amount of force to distend the walls and eventually perforate. The cecal diameter on imaging at risk for perforation ranges from 9 to 12 cm. However, the rate of distention may matter more than the actual maximal diameter found on imaging. In chronic obstruction, the colonic wall has time to gradually dilate, hypertrophy and be less likely perforate when compared with disorders that cause acute obstruction. The competence of the ileocecal valve will also affect the maximum diameter of the cecum, as luminal contents will reflux proximally into the small intestine. Colonic diameter can be trended on abdominal plain films when urgent or emergent surgery is not indicated.

Etiologies

Colorectal Cancer

Obstructing colorectal cancer remains the most common cause of LBO; however, only an estimated 7–29% of all colonic malignancies present in this fashion. The most common locations for an obstructing mass to be found are either in the sigmoid or at the splenic flexure, likely due to the relatively smaller luminal diameters.

As with the initial management of all causes of bowel obstruction, stabilization and resuscitation of the patient is paramount. Aggressive IV fluid hydration and correction of electrolyte abnormalities should be the first focus along with determination of the patient's need for emergent surgery. A nasogastric tube is of much less utility in large bowel obstruction compared to small bowel and will not be effective in decompressing the colon. Strict intake and output should be measured to guide resuscitation efforts.

Therapeutic decisions depend upon the stability of the patient, the location of the obstructing mass, and whether or not perforation is present. In an unstable patient and in those where suspected perforation, ischemia, and/or peritonitis is present, there is clear indication for immediate operative management with resection. In these situations, broad spectrum antibiotics that include coverage for Gram negative and anaerobic bacteria should be started immediately. When patients present with less severe disease, failure to improve with nonoperative management and a progressively increasing cecal diameter are also indications for urgent surgery or endoscopic stenting (when appropriate).

For left-sided obstructing masses with perforation or in an unstable patient, resection with end colostomy is the most appropriate procedure. Earlier in the course, the management becomes more controversial. Resection with primary anastomosis may be performed on unprepared obstructed colons but is associated with higher complication rates, including leak. The American Society of Colon and Rectal Surgeons (ASCRS) Clinical Practice Guideline for the Treatment of Colon Cancer addresses emergency presentations of colon cancer including obstruction. For obstructing left-sided colon cancers, management options include either stenting or resection, with treatment decisions to be individualized to the patient and expertise of the treating center. Urgent intervention to avoid perforation is paramount, as patients with free perforations have higher rates of permanent ostomy, postoperative morbidity and mortality, and peritoneal carcinomatosis with significantly lower rates of disease-free and overall survival.

A well-studied management option is placement of a self-expanding metal stent (SEMS) across the obstructing lesion. If a guidewire is able to be passed through a near-obstructing left colon or rectal mass, the immediate obstruction can be relieved to create more time for patients to be optimized for surgery prior to resection, overall allowing for better outcomes and lower complication rates. Successful SEMS placement is associated with higher chance of resection with primary anastomosis rather than a Hartmann procedure. Stenting of right colon masses has also begun to be studied, but with less robust data and likely fewer centers with the current expertise required to perform this procedure. Stenting does carry a risk of perforation with a subsequent increase in later risk of locoregional cancer recurrence and other possible risks including bleeding, stent migration, stool impaction, or tumor ingrowth. Despite the inherent risks, utilizing an SEMS as a bridge to a non-emergency surgery should be considered when feasible. Stent placement has been shown to confer lower 30- and 60-day postoperative morbidity and mortality, lower permanent ostomy rates, and similar rates of overall survival when compared to emergency colonic resection. SEMS placement is contraindicated if colonic perforation has already occurred.

When stenting is not feasible, an oncologic ;ection of involved colon following standard ınciples should be attempted. This includes ɔth proximal and distal margins of 5–7 cm and oximal ligation the primary feeding vessel(s) to ɔmplete an appropriate lymphadenectomy. In is case of synchronous right and left-sided asses, a subtotal colectomy is indicated, which ay also be required if the colon is largely chemic.

'olvulus

'olvulus occurs when an air-filled segment of owel twists around its mesentery. This condition nay reduce spontaneously or progress to luminal ›bstruction. If untreated, torsion of the mesentery :an lead to strangulation, necrosis, and perforation ɔf the bowel. The most common sites of volvulus n the large bowel are the sigmoid colon (60–75%) and cecum (20–25%). Redundancy or increased mobility of these bowel segments, whether congenital or acquired, increases the risk of torsion. Sigmoid volvulus typically presents in older adults (mean age of 70), especially those who are institutionalized or debilitated and have a history of constipation. Less common sites of colonic volvulus include the transverse colon and splenic flexure.

Presentation of volvulus can be highly variable and may range from intermittent abdominal pain to acute obstructive symptoms (nausea, vomiting, obstipation) to peritonitis with hemodynamic compromise. Symptoms for cecal volvulus tend to occur more rapidly, while sigmoid volvulus may have more of an indolent course. Management is dictated by location of the volvulus and overall status of the patient.

Sigmoid Volvulus

Unless there are obvious signs of ischemia or perforation on presentation, initial management of sigmoid volvulus is resuscitation followed by rigid or flexible endoscopic detorsion with placement of a rectal tube. Success rates range from 60–95%. If necrotic mucosa or ulceration is noted on endoscopy, this is suggestive that bowel compromise has already occurred, and the patient should be taken to the operating room.

Given a high rate of recurrence after endoscopic reduction, ASCRS recommends that elective sigmoidectomy with removal of all redundant sigmoid colon should be performed after the patient is stabilized. Stoma creation in a non-emergent setting is not usually required but may be considered for an individual patient depending on operative findings. If there is associated megacolon, a subtotal colectomy has lower recurrence rates than sigmoid colectomy with primary anastomosis.

In the setting of suspected ischemia, necrosis, or perforation, resection of the involved segment should be performed prior to detorsion of the compromised segment to reduce the chance of release of endotoxin, potassium, and bacteria into the systemic circulation. Numerous retrospective studies have reported on the choice of resection with primary anastomosis versus Hartmann procedure, and the usual patient-related factors of underlying comorbidities, current physiologic state, and stability play a role in this decision.

Other operations that do not involve resection are considered inferior to sigmoid resection due to a higher risk of recurrence. In the setting of a viable colon, detorsion alone, sigmoidoplasty (with intraperitoneal or extraperitoneal fixation), and mesosigmoidoplasty have been described with case series published. The goal of this last procedure is to tailor and broaden the base of the sigmoid mesentery to reduce the potential for repeated torsion. Elderly patients who are poor surgical candidates may be treated by percutaneous endoscopic sigmoidopexy.

Cecal Volvulus

Unlike sigmoid volvulus, the ASCRS recommends against attempts at endoscopic detorsion of cecal volvulus due to low success rates from limited series. Surgical approaches to cecal volvulus vary depending on the patient's stability and intraoperative findings. Morbidity and mortality are 3–4 times higher in patients with cecal volvulus who have nonviable or perforated bowel than those with viable bowel. Resection and anastomosis may be considered in select patients with nonviable bowel. However, resection with ileostomy (with or without mucous fistula) is appropriate in the setting of perforation or more extensive bowel necrosis.

In stable patients without bowel compromise, there are more surgical procedures from which to choose, and there is controversy as to the necessity of resecting healthy bowel. Options include detorsion alone, detorsion with cecopexy, detorsion with cecostomy, or detorsion with resection and anastomosis. Without a segmental resection, recurrent volvulus rates are higher. However, resection leads to higher rates of other postoperative complications including wound infection and anastomotic leak. Standard operations associated with the lowest volvulus recurrence rates include either ileocolic resection or right colectomy to include the volvulized segment followed by primary ileocolonic anastomosis (with or without protective loop ileostomy) if the patient is stable. However, given lack of data regarding overall superior outcomes, it is reasonable to include non-resectional procedures in management choices.

Diverticulitis

After volvulus, diverticulitis is the most common non-neoplastic cause of LBO, representing up to 10% of cases. Both acute and chronic forms of the disease can lead to obstruction. During an acute attack, partial colonic obstruction can occur from luminal narrowing caused by pericolonic inflammation or compression from a diverticular abscess. However, high-grade obstruction is more commonly associated with stricture from chronic diverticular inflammation. Diverticulitis with an associated obstruction is classified as complicated diverticulitis.

Management of diverticular LBO in the elderly differs based on the obstructive process. During an acute episode, nonoperative management may include intravenous antibiotics, rehydration, nasogastric tube decompression, and bowel rest. These modalities are usually successful to resolve the obstruction. If a pericolonic abscess is present, it may be drained percutaneously to relieve luminal compression. Surgery should be performed acutely only wi progression of disease such as in cases of perit nitis or worsening hemodynamic status, a Hartmann procedure performed in high-ri patients. The risk of malignancy is higher patients with complicated vs uncomplicat diverticulitis. Therefore, after recovery from a episode of acute complicated diverticulitis (wi or without obstruction), the colon should b evaluated endoscopically if the patient has no had a recent colonoscopy. Eventual electiv resection after an acute episode of diverticuliti with obstruction is generally recommended b ASCRS given increased risk of subsequen complicated diverticulitis episodes. Minimall invasive techniques are preferred when exper tise is available and patient factors permit thi approach.

Benign Stricture

Benign colonic stricture can be seen in Crohn's disease, patients with prior pelvic radiation, and uncommonly in those with prior surgery and anastomoses, especially if recovery was compromised by a leak. Colonoscopy is recommended to rule out a malignant stricture prior to operative management, or in the case of radiation-induced fibrosis, to determine the degree and length of stricturing. Stricturoplasty may be considered as well as segmental resection with anastomosis. Anastomotic strictures may be treated with balloon dilatation. If the degree of involved colon is extensive, especially with radiation-induced damage, a colostomy may be required if the entire involved segment cannot be resected or if there is not suitable distal large intestine for an anastomosis.

Acute Colonic Pseudo-Obstruction (Ogilvie Syndrome)

Acute colonic pseudo-obstruction (ACPO) is characterized by acute dilation of the colon in the absence of mechanical obstruction. ACPO typically presents in the setting of severe illness or after surgery or institutionalized individuals and is associated with several medications, trauma, cardiac disease, metabolic imbalances, and infection. It occurs predominantly in hospitalized patients recovering from another surgical procedure or other acute illness as well as institutionalized patients with serious comorbidities. Men over 60 years of age are most frequently affected. The precise mechanism by which Ogilvie syndrome occurs is not completely understood though it is thought to be related to a disturbance in the autonomic innervation of the distal colon. Proximal colonic dilation is seen most frequently. Occasionally, dilation extends distally to the rectum.

Initial management focuses on decompressing the colon to reduce the risks of ischemia and perforation. Ruling out mechanical causes of obstruction, correcting electrolyte abnormalities, minimizing medications, nasogastric decompression, and bowel rest are important initial steps. Supportive care may be continued for 72 h in the absence of severe pain, peritonitis, and extreme colonic distension (cecum >12 cm).

In patients who fail conservative therapy or have a cecal diameter >12 cm, intravenous neostigmine can be used and has success rates of approximately 90%. Relative contraindications to neostigmine include recent myocardial infarction, acidosis, asthma, bradycardia, peptic ulcer disease, and use of beta blockers. It should be administered with continuous cardiac monitoring with atropine at hand in the event of bradycardia. In patients who fail an initial dose of neostigmine or have a partial response, a second dose may be administered after 24 h before proceeding to colonoscopic decompression.

If neostigmine is contraindicated, colonoscopic decompression with placement of a decompression tube is the next measure. This procedure should be performed by an experienced endoscopist using minimal insufflation. After successful colonic decompression, oral polyethylene glycol should be administered daily for 7 days to prevent recurrence.

Approximately 10% of patients will not respond to supportive, pharmacologic, or endoscopic treatment. Risk factors that lead to ischemia and perforation include cecal diameter >12 cm and duration of dilatation >6 days, and surgery is indicated for these medically refractory cases. Surgical options include cecostomy, resection with anastomosis, or subtotal colectomy with ileostomy depending on the clinical status of the patient and intraoperative findings. In the pre-neostigmine era, cecal diameter >14 cm, advanced age, need for surgery, and >4 days of prolonged dilatation were associated with a higher risk of death.

Constipation

While the incidence of constipation is approximately 20% in the general population, it is more common in the elderly and approaches 50% in patients in chronic care facilities. Severe constipation is 2–3 times more frequent in females than males. The etiology in older patients is frequently multifactorial and may include both primary (slow transit, dyssynergic defecation, irritable bowel syndrome) and secondary causes (drug induced, morphologic, pelvic floor dysfunction). Chronic constipation can lead to fecal impaction and obstruction of the colon. Obstruction of this type must be addressed as it may progress to stercoral ulceration, bleeding, focal or more diffuse colonic ischemia, and perforation.

Initial management of fecal impaction, in the absence of signs of ischemia, perforation or hemorrhage, should focus on disimpaction. Manual fragmentation in combination with warm water or mineral oil enemas should be used initially to facilitate passage of a large fecal bolus. Following initial disimpaction and enemas, the colon should be thoroughly evacuated. This can be achieved with oral administration of polyethylene glycol or daily warm water enemas.

If the above measures are unsuccessful or only partially successful, manual disimpaction may need to be performed in the operating room or endoscopy suite under appropriate anesthesia, especially in the elderly or more frail individuals. Flexible or rigid sigmoidoscopy may be used to fragment and evacuate more proximal impactions and allows the endoscopist to evaluate mucosal integrity. If these interventions fail, or there is suspicion for impending perforation or ischemia, surgery is indicated.

After successful disimpaction, it is important to identify and eliminate potential causes of constipation as well as initiate a laxative regimen with the goal of producing at least one bowel movement per day. If the patient is not up to date with colonoscopy, an obstructing lesion should be ruled out after recovery from the acute obstruction and evacuation of the colon.

References

1. Cooper Z, Scott JW, Rosenthal RA, Mitchell SL. Emergency major abdominal surgical procedures in older adults: a systematic review of mortality and functional outcomes. J Am Geriatr Soc. 2015;63(12):2563–71. https://doi.org/10.1111/jgs.13818.
2. Spangler R, Van Pham T, Khoujah D, Martinez JP. Abdominal emergencies in the geriatric patient. Int J Emerg Med. 2014;7:43. https://doi.org/10.1186/s12245-014-0043-2.
3. Ozturk E, van Iersel M, Stommel MM, Schoon Y, Ten Broek RR, van Goor H. Small bowel obstruction in the elderly: a plea for comprehensive acute geriatric care. World J Emerg Surg. 2018;13:48. https://doi.org/10.1186/s13017-018-0208-z.
4. Abbas S, Bissett IP, Parry BR. Oral water soluble contrast for the management of adhesive small bowel obstruction. Cochrane Database Syst Rev. 2007;2010(3):CD004651. https://doi.org/10.1002/14651858.CD004651.pub3.
5. Ong M, Guang TY, Yang TK. Impact of surgical delay on outcomes in elderly patients undergoing emergency surgery: a single center experience. World J Gastrointest Surg. 2015;7(9):208–13. https://doi.org/10.4240/wjgs.v7.i9.208.
6. National Comprehensive Cancer Network. Small bowel adenocarcinoma (version 2.2022). Retrieved https://www.nccn.org/professionals/physician_gls/pdf/small_bowel.pdf
7. Krause WR, Webb TP. Geriatric small bowel obstruction: an analysis of treatment and outcomes compared with a younger cohort. Am J Surg. 2015;209(2):347–51. https://doi.org/10.1016/j.amjsurg.2014.04.008.
8. Springer JE, Bailey JG, Davis PJ, Johnson PM. Management and outcomes of small bowel obstruction in older adult patients: a prospective cohort study. Can J Surg. 2014;57(6):379–84. https://doi.org/10.1503/cjs.029513.
9. Cappell MS, Batke M. Mechanical obstruction of the small bowel and colon. Med Clin North Am. 2008;92(3):575–97. https://doi.org/10.1016/j.mcna.2008.01.003.
10. Vogel JD, Felder SI, Bhama AR, Hawkins AT, Langenfeld SJ, Shaffer VO, et al. The American Society of Colon and Rectal Surgeons clinical practice guidelines for the Management of Colon Cancer. Dis Colon Rectum. 2022;65(2):148–77. https://doi.org/10.1097/DCR.0000000000002323.
11. Vogel JD, Feingold DL, Stewart DB, Turner JS, Boutros M, et al. Clinical practice guidelines for colon volvulus and acute colonic pseudo-obstruction. Dis Colon Rectum. 2016;59(7):589–600. https://doi.org/10.1097/DCR.0000000000000602.
12. Hall J, Hardiman K, Lee S, Lightner A, Stocchi L, Paquette IM, et al. The American Society of Colon and Rectal Surgeons clinical practice guidelines for the treatment of left-sided colonic diverticulitis. Dis Colon Rectum. 2020;63(6):728–47. https://doi.org/10.1097/DCR.0000000000001679.
13. Naveed M, Jamil LH, Fujii-Lau LL, Al-Haddad M, Buxbaum JL, Fishman DS, et al. American Society for Gastrointestinal Endoscopy guideline on the role of endoscopy in the management of acute colonic pseudo-obstruction and colonic volvulus. Gastrointest Endosc. 2020;91(2):228–35. https://doi.org/10.1016/j.gie.2019.09.007.
14. Vazquez Roque M, Bouras EP. Epidemiology and management of chronic constipation in elderly patients. Clin Interv Aging. 2015;10:919–30. https://doi.org/10.2147/CIA.S54304.

Critical Care Management of Older Adults

49

Mira Ghneim and Thomas M. Scalea

Epidemiology and Outcomes of Critically Ill Older Adults

Age is associated with a decline of the functional reserve of multiple organ systems, progressive restriction in personal and social resources, and increasing prevalence of multiple chronic diseases. Therefore, it is not surprising that older adults utilize a disproportionate share of health care resources.

In fact, while older adults (≥65 years) represent only 17% of the US population, they account for one-half of all patients admitted to the intensive care unit (ICU) and 60% of all ICU days. Of those admitted to the ICU, the oldest-old (≥80 years) account for 25% of admissions. Furthermore, older adults represent 60–70% of ICU patients requiring invasive mechanical ventilation, and 25–30% of older adults spend their last month of life in an ICU.

Despite advances in medical and surgical care, the morbidity and mortality rate for older adults admitted to the ICU remain high. A recent meta-analysis reported an in-hospital mortality from 10% to 76%, 6-month mortality from 21 to 58%, and 1-year mortality from 33 to 72% in older adults discharged from the ICU. An equally important consideration is the quality of life experienced by older adults who survive to discharge from the ICU. This includes a significant decrease in physical function, persistent organ failure, discharge to higher level of care, and an increased risk, up to 50%, of readmission to the ICU.

Clearly, ICU utilization by older adults will increase exponentially over the next decade as this population continues to grow. Nonetheless the current critical care model and available guidelines are not geri-centric and are based on evidence from studies that often exclude older adults. Therefore, we must focus on how to best care for older adults who develop critical illness and tailor the current critical care services to better suit this vulnerable population. This chapter will review (1) the implications and influence of the changes in the central nervous cardiovascular, pulmonary, and renal systems on the management of critically ill older adults, (2) polypharmacy, (3) the need for an interdisciplinary approach to develop geriatric critical care units, and (4) ethical challenges and futility of care.

M. Ghneim · T. M. Scalea (✉)
Program in Trauma, University of Maryland School Of Medicine, R Adams Cowley Shock Trauma Center, Baltimore, MD, USA
e-mail: mira.ghneim@som.umaryland.edu; tscalea@som.umaryland.edu

P. Petrone, C. E.M. Brathwaite (eds.), *Acute Care Surgery in Geriatric Patients*,
https://doi.org/10.1007/978-3-031-30651-8_49

The Physiology of Aging and Critical Care Medicine Considerations

The Central Nervous System

The physiologic changes that the brain experiences with aging often manifest as a change in cognition due to a reduction in brain volume, a decrease in neurotransmitters and synaptic plasticity, an increase in the blood–brain barrier permeability, and a reduction in microvascular blood flow. This results in a decrease in the central nervous system's resilience, making older adults more susceptible to acute neurologic insults. Therefore, older adults experience cognitive decline in the setting of acute stressors during critical illness.

This acute brain dysfunction is manifested as hypoactive, hyperactive, or mixed delirium. Delirium is defined as a disturbance of consciousness with accompanying change in cognition. Different mechanisms have been proposed to explain the pathophysiology of delirium including, decreased cholinergic activity, increased dopaminergic activity, and abnormalities in the serotonin pathways. Hypoactive delirium is characterized by symptoms of lethargy, decreased movement, and slowed mentation. Whereas the hyperactive subtype manifests as agitation, heightened arousal, or aggression. Hypoactive delirium has been found to be the predominant subtype among critically ill older adults and is often diagnosed in a delayed fashion due to its subtle clinical presentation. In a study of older adults admitted to the ICU postoperatively after an elective surgery, patients suffering from hypoactive delirium had increased 6-month mortality (32% vs. 9%) when compared to older adults experiencing hyperactive delirium. Post-operative delirium is defined as a change in the level of consciousness that occurs 24 h after surgery and resolves within a week. Post-operative delirium is commonly seen in older adults undergoing coronary artery bypass surgery, hip fracture repairs, and in trauma patients.

Risk factors for delirium are classified into two groups: predisposing and precipitating factors. Predisposing factors include older age (≥70 years), dementia or preexisting cogniti dysfunction, history of delirium, functional di ability, sensory impairment (hearing and visi loss), comorbidities and severity of illnes depression, transient ischemic attack or strok and alcohol abuse. Precipitating factors incluc medications (anticholinergics/antihistamine benzodiazepines/opiates), surgery, trauma, ane thesia, pain, use of restraints, use of bladder catl eters, infection, acute illness, electrolyt abnormalities (Na, K, glucose), and iatrogeni events (high noise levels and constant monito alarms in the ICU). The more predisposing fac tors exist, the fewer precipitating factors ar needed to cause delirium. As a result, older adult are at much higher risk of developing deliriun compared to their younger counterparts.

The incidence of delirium in older adults has been reported to be 50–80%, with the highest incidence among critically ill patients on mechanical ventilation. Delirium has been shown extensively in the literature to be associated with worse short- and long-term clinical outcomes. These include longer duration to liberate from mechanical ventilation, increased hospital and ICU length of stay, increased hospital costs, increased risk of readmission, long-term cognitive dysfunction, and acceleration of cognitive decline in older adults with Alzheimer's disease.

Given these consequences the prevention, early detection and treatment of delirium are paramount in the management of older adults in the ICU. Proactive geriatric consultation with multicomponent interventional protocols has been shown to reduce the incidence of delirium in older adults. The Confusion Assessment Method for the Intensive Care Unit (CAM-ICU) is the most widely recognized method used to detect delirium in the ICU. The CAM-ICU has demonstrated high sensitivity and specificity for delirium in all older adults and additionally in special populations such as older adults with dementia or history of stroke. Critically ill older adults should be assessed for delirium on admission and on a daily basis post admission.

Once the diagnosis of delirium is established, reversable and modifiable risk factors must be identified and addressed. Behavioral disturbances should be managed with a non-pharmacological approach first. *Non-pharmacological interventions* include maintaining a sleep-wake cycle, frequent reorientation, minimizing noise pollution, music therapy, encouraging family to interact with the patient, early mobilization, nursing training in de-escalation techniques, using a sitter, minimizing the use of restraints and discontinuation of restraints in the intensive care unit as soon as deemed appropriate. While pain control is paramount to delirium prevention, opioid-sparing techniques using multimodal analgesia pain regimens and regional anesthesia techniques should be employed to achieve adequate pain control while minimizing opioids. *Pharmacological interventions* should be considered only after non-pharmacologic strategies have failed. This includes avoidance of opioids, benzodiazepines, and anticholinergics as the mainstay of delirium management. It should be noted that patients experiencing alcohol withdrawal should receive the standard recommended benzodiazepine therapy, and benzodiazepines should not be abruptly discontinued in older adults with benzodiazepine dependence.

The use of haloperidol to treat ICU delirium persists despite multiple randomized trials clearly demonstrating that, while haloperidol reduces agitation, it provides no benefit in terms of days spent with delirium and mortality. In fact, the current Society of Critical Care Medicine (SCCM) Guidelines recommend against the use of haloperidol routinely for the treatment of ICU delirium. On the other hand, some evidence exists to support the use of other "atypical" antipsychotics such as olanzapine, risperidone, and quetiapine to reduce the duration of delirium in adult ICU patients.

Dexmedetomidine is a highly selective α2-adrenergic receptor agonist that provides analgesia and sedation without respiratory depression. Dexmedetomidine has been shown to reduce delirium incidence and duration, mechanical ventilation days, ICU length of stay, and cost when compared with benzodiazepines and propofol. The updated SCCM sedation guidelines suggest that "in adult ICU patients with delirium unrelated to alcohol or benzodiazepine withdrawal, continuous IV infusions of dexmedetomidine rather than benzodiazepine infusions be administered for sedation to reduce the duration of delirium in these patients." As a result, dexmedetomidine is widely used as an adjunct to atypical antipsychotics in the management of delirium. Given that the SCCM guidelines are not tailored specifically to older adults, it is important to keep in mind that the antisympathetic effects of dexmedetomidine lead to the development of bradycardia and hypotension. Thus, caution should be exercised when utilizing dexmedetomidine in critically ill older adults with underlying cardiovascular disease.

Overall, current evidence does not support a single effective prevention or treatment approach in critically ill older adults. Therefore, the American Geriatric Society has recommendations for the prevention of delirium in older adults in the perioperative setting that focus on multicomponent non-pharmacologic intervention programs, optimization of pain control, avoidance of benzodiazepines and newly prescribed cholinesterase inhibitors, and use of antipsychotic medications only in patients who are agitated or of potential harm to self or others.

The Cardiovascular System

The aging cardiovascular system influences the way care is provided to older adults in the ICU in multiple ways. First, the risk of myocardial infarction, heart failure, valvular disease, and arrythmias increases with increasing age. Second, the cardiac and vascular structural and functional changes with aging have distinct implications for hemodynamic support in older adults that differ from their younger counterparts. Finally, older adults experience a decrease in cardiovascular reserve allowing for physiological stressors such as blood loss, hypoxia, sepsis, and hypovolemia to result in severe acute cardiovascular dysfunction and decompensation.

Cardiac changes with aging include increased myocardial stiffness due to myocyte apoptosis, and increased collagen deposits and fibrosis with subsequent compensatory myocyte hypertrophy. As a result, the left ventricle mass index is increased and left ventricular diastolic filling and ejection fraction are decreased. While resting cardiac output is maintained, maximal heart rate and ejection fraction decrease with aging. Ventricular relaxation, which is more energy and oxygen dependent than ventricular contraction, becomes impaired with aging as ventricular compliance decreases. As a result, diastolic dysfunction and an associated increase in pulmonary venous pressure are more common in older adults and should be taken into consideration when caring for older adults in the ICU. An important compensatory mechanism to the reduction of both left ventricular compliance and early diastolic ventricular filling is an increase in flow due to atrial contraction. The contribution of left atrial systole to left ventricular filling increases with age. Atrial fibrillation is therefore poorly handled by older adults. Therefore, new onset atrial fibrillation should be treated promptly and diligently in this patient population.

Heart failure (HF) can occur in the setting of reduced or preserved ejection fraction, although older adults mainly experience HF with preserved ejection fraction. HF presents as congestion of the pulmonary and systemic vasculature and may include evidence of end-organ hypoperfusion. Diastolic dysfunction can lead to frank HF which is further exacerbated by conditions frequently encountered in ICU patients, such as hypoxemia, volume overload, hypertension, and atrial fibrillation. Patients with diastolic dysfunction precipitated by hypervolemia should be treated with diuretics and vasodilators. Diastolic dysfunction/HF exacerbated by hypoxemia may require either noninvasive or invasive mechanical ventilation. Caution should be taken when selecting older adults for noninvasive mechanical ventilation given the increased incidence of altered mental status, inability to clear secretions, and inability to protect one's airway in this patient population.

In addition to the structural cardiac changes with aging, there is a decreased reactivity to baroreceptors and chemoreceptors, apoptosis of atrial pacemaker cells, and fibrosis of atrioventricular and bundle of his myocytes. These changes contribute to the high incidence of sick sinus sy drome, atrial arrhythmias, and bundle branc blocks experienced by older adults in the ICU.

The decrease in β-receptor stimulation ar increase in sympathetic nervous system activi occur as a result of decreased receptor affinity ar alterations in signal transduction. Therefor physiologic stressors are associated with decreased chronotropic and inotropic respons Specifically, the increased peripheral flow deman is met primarily by increasing ventricular fillin (preload) and stroke volume rather than heart rate This preload dependence renders the heart highl susceptible to volume shifts such that even mino hypovolemia can result in significant cardiac compromise. On the other hand, due to decreased ventricular compliance excessive fluid resuscitation will cause pulmonary edema. Accordingly, these changes dictate scrupulous management of volume status in older adults in the ICU. The increase in sympathetic nervous system activity with aging increases systemic vascular resistance. Clinically, these changes lead to the heightened sensitivity of older adults to sympatholytic medications. In the surgical patient, this leads to a greater likelihood of perioperative hemodynamic lability and a compromised ability to meet the metabolic demands of surgery.

There is an increased arterial stiffness with aging that manifests as an increased systolic arterial pressure, pulse pressure, and pulse wave velocity. As a result, it has been hypothesized that older adults may benefit from mean arterial pressure (MAP) goals (≥65 mmHg) in the critical care setting, especially those with chronic hypertension, to allow for adequate end-organ perfusion. Achieving these higher MAP goals is commonly accomplished with the use of vasopressors. Vasopressors, however, reduce blood flow in vasoconstricted vascular beds and are associated with negative effects on cardiac, metabolic, microbiome, and immune function in older adults with limited reserves. As a result, multiple recent pilot and multicenter trials have attempted to address whether permissive hypotension defined as a MAP of 60–65 mmHg vs. higher MAP goals affect overall mortality in critically ill older adults.

The OVATION (Optimal Vasopressor Titration) pilot study showed that increased exposure to vasopressors to achieve a MAP of 75–80 mmHg is associated with an increased 28-day mortality in older adults when compared to those experiencing lower MAP goals of 60–65 mmHg (45.8% vs 37.2%). The open label multicenter randomized controlled "65 trial" conducted in 65 ICUs in the United Kingdom randomized 2583 older adults, with vasodilatory hypotension despite fluid resuscitation and who are currently receiving vasopressors, to permissive hypotension (MAP of 60–65 mmHg) vs. MAP targets at the discretion of the ICU team (MAP 70–80 mmHg). Results from this trial showed an increased 90-day all-cause mortality control group vs. the permissive hypotension group (44% vs. 41%). Therefore, the most recent 2021 Surviving Sepsis Campaign guidelines recommend, given the lack of advantage or harm associated with higher MAP targets in older adults, targeting a MAP of 65 mmHg in the initial resuscitation of patients with septic shock who require vasopressors. Given the limited available evidence regarding the ideal MAP targets in older adults in septic shock and lack of evidence in older adults who experience a traumatic injury, MAP goals in the ICU should be main at the discretion of the intensivist until stronger evidence is available through future meta-analysis and larger randomized controlled trials.

The Respiratory System

In older adults, the declining respiratory function is the result of structural and functional changes in the chest wall, lungs, respiratory muscles, diaphragm, and small airways. With aging, there is a progressive decrease in chest wall compliance and lung volumes secondary to comorbidities such as osteoporosis, kyphosis, and decreased mobility at the rib-vertebral joints. In the lungs, elasticity is decreased leading to an increase in lung compliance. There is also a progressive decline in respiratory muscle and diaphragmatic strength resulting in a decline in maximal inspiratory and expiratory force by as much as 50%. Given that the age-related decreased chest wall compliance is proportionally larger than the increased lung compliance, the net compliance of the respiratory system is decreased. Therefore, resting work of breathing is increased and the diaphragm and abdominal muscles contribute proportionally more to the work of breathing than the thoracic muscles when compared with younger patients. These changes along with collapse of the small airways and uneven alveolar ventilation lead to a decrease in vital capacity, forced expiratory volume, and residual volume. As a result, the compensatory mechanism for increased minute ventilation during critical illness is an increase in respiratory rate. There is an increased degree of ventilation perfusion mismatching and shunting with increasing age. It is estimated that the arterial partial pressure of oxygen decreases by an average rate of 0.35 mmHg per year starting at the age of 30. The neural sensing and modulating responses by the central nervous system of the respiratory system also change with age, specifically older adults have a significantly lower ventilatory response to both hypoxia and hypercapnia. This combination of structural and physiologic changes lead to a decreased respiratory reserve in older adults such that they decompensate quicker than younger patients. Acute respiratory failure is therefore a common complication in the critically ill older adult and is due to a combination of the structural and physiological changes of the respiratory system with aging and the presence of concomitant chronic illnesses (HF and chronic obstructive pulmonary disease), acute illnesses (pulmonary embolism), major organ dysfunction, and an increased risk of acquired causes of respiratory failure (community acquired pneumonia). Accordingly, older adults represent 60–70% of ICU patients requiring invasive mechanical ventilation.

Ventilator associated pneumonia (VAP) is defined as pneumonia that occurs >48 h following endotracheal intubation. It is a common complication of mechanical ventilation and associated with an increased hospital length of stay, difficulty in weaning mechanical ventilation, and increased mortality. Given the paucity of data regarding risk factors, diagnosis, and treatment of

VAP in older patients, VAP in older adults is diagnosed and managed in a similar manner to younger patients in the ICU. VAP occurs due to inoculation of the lower respiratory tract with microorganisms from the oropharynx, subglottic area, sinuses, and gastrointestinal tract. There is some evidence that gastro-pulmonary aspiration is an important mechanism for the development of VAP in older adults. To mitigate some of the VAP risk factors, VAP prevention bundles have been developed and are often deployed in the ICU. This includes elevation of head of bed, oral care and chlorhexidine mouth care, stress ulcer prophylaxis, daily sedation assessment and spontaneous breathing trials, and early liberation from mechanical ventilation. In terms of treatment recommendations for VAP in older adults, the general Infectious Disease Society of America guidelines on VAP are usually utilized to treat older adults with VAP in the ICU and are based on facility antibiogram.

Acute respiratory distress syndrome (ARDS) is an injury to the alveolar epithelium and lung capillary endothelium resulting in acute hypoxemic respiratory failure following a known clinical insult. The Berlin criteria define ARDS as acute respiratory failure with bilateral pulmonary infiltrates not fully explained by fluid overload or heart failure, hypoxemia (PaO_2/FiO_2 ratio <300), need for mechanical ventilation, and a clinical insult within 7 days of the development of ARDS. In the United States, the overall incidence of ARDS has been reported to be 64 cases per 100,000 person-years with the incidence being 306 cases per 100,000 person-years in the 75–84 years age group. Whether age itself is a risk factor for ARDS is debatable in the current literature. Instead, the significantly increased incidence of ARDS in older adults is attributed to the higher frequency of aspiration/pneumonia, sepsis, and increased severity of illness with aging. ARDS in older adults has been shown to be associated with worse clinical outcomes, including prolonged mechanical ventilation, increased hospital length of stay, and higher mortality. The influence of age on ARDS outcomes in older adults is a function of the population studied. For example, while there is evidence in the trauma literature that age is an independent predictor of increased mortality, this is not true in other non-trauma patient populations. Additionally, while age maybe associated with an increased ARDS associated mortality, there is no significant difference between ventilator or ICU free days, length of stay in ICU or length of stay in hospital between patients <65 vs. ≥65 years of age.

In spite of the worse outcomes, no geriatric specific ARDS management guidelines exist, and the current guidelines utilized to manage ARDS are based on studies that frequently exclude older adults. This includes the ARDSnet protocol for low tidal volumes and high positive end expiratory pressure (PEEP) mechanical ventilation in addition to corticosteroid therapy, neuromuscular blocking agents, prone positioning, and in refractory cases extracorporeal membrane oxygenation (ECMO). With prone positioning being the only therapeutic modality found to be efficacious in improving outcomes in older adults.

The widely used low tidal volume/ high PEEP strategy proposed by the ARDSnet protocol is based on a patient population with an overall lower mean age and a broad array of exclusion criteria. Therefore, it is unclear whether the study is generalizable to the large population of older adults who develop ARDS. Furthermore, given that in vivo studies have shown that short-term mechanical ventilation with low tidal volumes increases pulmonary edema, lung inflammation, and decreases diaphragm function, it is unclear how the low tidal volume/high PEEP strategy utilized in the ARDSnet protocol would affect the pulmonary response in older adults. The role of corticosteroids in the treatment of ARDS has also been studied extensively. While corticosteroid use as an adjunctive therapy was associated with improved pulmonary parameters, there was an increased rate of muscle weakness and subsequent reintubations in patients receiving corticosteroid therapy, presenting a major concern regarding the risk-benefit ratio of corticosteroid use in older adults. Prone positioning, specifically placing the patient face down and continuing mechanical ventilation this position for prolonged periods of time up to 16 h, has demonstrated improved outcomes in a study population which included older adults. This includes a significant reduction in mortality and ICU length of stay. While the use of ECMO has become a valuable therapy to support recovery in ARDS, data on the use of ECMO in older adults is limited. Nonetheless, current data suggests that age is not a contraindication for ECMO, rather, its use should be decided on a case-by-case basis. Additionally, potential predictors that should be considered before initiation of ECMO support in older adults should include presence of cardiogenic shock, APACHE II, and SAPS II scores.

There are no data to suggest that one mode of mechanical ventilation is the superior mode of ventilation in older patients. Similarly, while expertise in liberation from mechanical ventilation has evolved over the past 20 years, it remains unclear specifically how the current knowledge applies to older adults. Special considerations to keep in mind when making decisions on liberation from ventilation in older adults include diminished cardio-pulmonary reserve, baseline rapid shallow breathing, a dampened response to hypoxia and hypercapnia, decreased ability to handle secretions, sarcopenia, and the duration of mechanical ventilation and its associated respiratory muscle atrophy.

Given that at baseline older adults have a respiratory exertional response that is similar to rapid shallow breathing, using this measure may be a less accurate marker of successful liberation from ventilation in older adults. Thus, physiologically, a patient may be judged to have failed a spontaneous breathing trial (SBT) when they have not. This is further complicated by the fact that older adults also have a diminished response to hypoxia and hypercapnia, and therefore an older adult patient on a SBT may be more likely to appear comfortable despite having developed significant hypoxia or hypercapnia. In the critically ill older patient, multiple factors are likely to play a role in inducing respiratory muscle atrophy including muscle inactivity, inflammation, cellular energy stress, and inadequate provision of amino acids. The diaphragm is the principal muscle of respiration. Sarcopenia in older adults' results in loss of diaphragmatic muscle mass with decreased respiratory reserve. It is therefore likely that sarcopenic patients who require mechanical ventilation have baseline diaphragmatic atrophy, which may significantly limit their respiratory reserve. Additionally, studies have shown that there is a 6% loss in diaphragm muscle thickness per day of mechanical ventilation. As a result, diaphragmatic dysfunction plays a major role in patients who fail weaning from mechanical ventilation. Many ICU patients who undergo prolonged mechanical ventilation (greater than 7 days) are not able to be weaned from mechanical ventilation, require a tracheostomy, and are frequently referred to a long-term ventilator facility. Older adults requiring mechanical ventilation have poorer short- and long-term outcomes than their younger counterparts including pneumonia, delirium, and decubitus ulcer formation.

While liberation from mechanical ventilation in older adults remains an area in which there are limited data, it is clear that intensivists should carefully consider the impact of the primary disease process and its sequelae, and the effects of aging on respiratory function when making decisions on liberation from ventilation.

The Renal System

With aging there is a decrease in renal mass, a reduction in the number of functional glomeruli associated with a compensatory glomerular hypertrophy, atherosclerosis, interstitial fibrosis, fibro-intimal hyperplasia, hyalinization, and a reduction in renal blood flow (RBF). It is estimated that RBF decreases >10% every decade of life. Consequently, in the attempt to maintain glomerular filtration rate (GFR), the compensatory glomerular hypertrophy is followed by increased filtration fraction and renal vasoconstriction. Furthermore, with aging there is an increase in the intrarenal cellular apoptosis rate, leading to a decrease in the number of functional nephrons, this coexists with the aging related reduction in cell proliferation. Overall, these senescence-related phenomena reduce the kidneys' self-renewal capacity. Thus, older adults more frequently present with baseline chronic kidney disease (CKD). Furthermore, older adults are more susceptible to develop acute kidney injury (AKI) in the setting of even the most minor hemodynamic instability and/or alterations in kidney perfusion during critical illness.

Renal tubular function also declines with advancing age. This affects the ability of the kidney to conserve sodium and excrete hydrogen ions, resulting in diminished capacity to regulate fluid and acid-base balance. The decline in function also leads to poor compensation for nonrenal losses of sodium and water and the development of hypovolemia in a preload dependent population. The tubular loss and interstitial fibrosis also contribute to a variety of salt and water syndromes in older adults that manifest as dysnatremias, hyperkalemia, and hypercalcemia which are often encountered and must be promptly addressed in the ICU setting.

AKI is a clinical syndrome that is characterized by an abrupt decrease in kidney function and is classified into three main types. (1) Pre-renal: which is due to a reduction of RBF and renal plasma perfusion and a subsequent reduction in GFR. This is the most common type of AKI in older adults and is due to the vasoconstriction of renal blood vessels with increasing age and the loss of compensatory vasodilator responses mediated by nitric oxide and angiotensin (II). (2) Renal: which is due to direct parenchymal dysfunction. This is commonly due to acute tubular necrosis of ischemic or toxic etiology (>70%), tubulointerstitial nephritis (10–20%), infections or medications, glomerulonephritis, and cortical necrosis (1–10%). (3) Post-renal: which is due to urinary tract obstruction secondary to stones, pelvic or retroperitoneal tumors, or benign prostate hypertrophy. It is the less frequent form of AKI (2–4%) in the general population but is more common in older adults (10%).

Risk factors for developing AKI in critically ill older adults include the physiological changes of the aging kidney, hypovolemia (GI losses, bleeding), comorbidities (hypertension/diabetes/heart failure/chronic kidney disease), polypharmacy (antibiotics, nonsteroidal anti-inflammatory drugs, angiotensin-converting enzyme), and other causes (contrast induced nephropathy, obstruction, sepsis, prolonged hospitalization).

In the ICU setting, the primary strategy to prevent AKI development in older adults is to recognize the specific increased vulnerability to renal injury in this cohort of patients. Given that no specific clinical or laboratory predictors of AKI development in older adults exists, management in the ICU should focus on prevention of occurrence and progression of AKI. This includes reduction of potentially nephrotoxic drugs and iodinated contrast, adequate fluid resuscitation, and prevention of hypotensive episodes especially during invasive procedures. Once AKI is established, no geriatric specific therapeutic strategies for management of AKI exist other than those suggested for the general population. Mainly, maintenance of RBF and avoidance of further renal injury are the cornerstones of supportive therapies.

Some patients who develop AKI may recover their renal function partially or completely. Others may evolve to CKD requiring dialysis. The development of CKD is due to the lack of compensatory mechanisms and adequate regeneration and microvascular damage, increased sensitivity to angiotensin II, and upregulation of genes associated with inflammation, remodeling, and fibrosis. Although variable among different studies, short-term mortality of older adults with AKI is high, ranging between 50 and 75% compared to the younger population. This is a function of severity of illness, baseline comorbidities, baseline renal function, sepsis, and multiorgan system failure.

In those who present with CKD, an accurate estimation of GFR is important for classification of CKD, patient management, and drug dosing. An important factor to keep in mind when determining GFR in older adults is that serum creatinine remains unchanged due to the concomitant decrease in lean body mass, and thus a decrease in creatinine production with increasing age. This is compounded by factors encountered during critical illness, which include medications, increased muscle breakdown due to sepsis, significant blood loss or volume infusion, trauma, protein catabolism, and immobility. This frequently leads to an overestimation of GFR and underestimation of the degree of kidney dysfunction. The current gold standard equations used to estimate GFR are the Chronic Kidney Disease Epidemiology (CKD-EPI) formula and the Modification of Diet in Renal Disease (MDRD) formula. Both formulas have been validated in older adults.

Depending on the severity of AKI and CKD in the ICU, continuous renal replacement therapy (CRRT) may be a necessity. Unlike other forms of RRT, CRRT allows for a more stable hemodynamic profile and minimizes large volume and electrolyte shifts in the setting of acute illness. Very few studies exist that have evaluated the utilization of CRRT in older adults in the ICU setting. Nonetheless indications for initiation are similar to those of the general population and include refractory volume overload, intractable metabolic acidosis, hyperkalemia, and uremia. Additionally, most of the limited available data suggest that outcomes such as renal recovery and mortality are improved if CRRT is initiated earlier. The decision to initiate CRRT in older adults is complex and should not be a function of age alone, given that the available literature does not support inferior outcomes in older adults. Instead, the decision to proceed with initiation of CRRT should consider acuity of illness, baseline medical and functional comorbidities, patient and family goals of care and wishes, short- and long-term morbidity and mortality based on the primary disease/injury process, and the likelihood of long-term renal recovery. The latter is paramount given that long-term RRT in the setting of CKD in older adults is associated with a substantial increase in mortality.

Energy Expenditure and Nutrition

Daily energy expenditure decreases with age. Resting energy expenditure falls by as much as 15% as a result of the decrease in lean muscle mass and decreased physical activity. Following acute illness or injury, the increase in oxygen consumption and energy expenditure in patients ≥65 years of age is approximately 20–25% less than their younger counterparts. These changes in energy expenditure have important implications with respect to nutritional support. Due to decreased muscle mass in the face of acute illness or even elective surgery, older adults may rapidly develop protein-energy malnutrition. Therefore, nutritional support should begin within 24 h of admission to the ICU. However, due to their decreased body mass and lower energy expenditure, overfeeding older adults with the sequelae of "stress hyperglycemia," fatty liver, and excess CO_2 production should be avoided.

Polypharmacy

There are essential changes in drug pharmacokinetics and pharmacodynamics that must be considered when managing older adults in the ICU. First, there are changes in volume of distribution, due to a decrease in total body mass, the proportion of body water, and plasma albumin, and an associated increase in total body fat. As a result, there is an increase in the concentration of hydrophilic drugs and decreased distribution of lipophilic drugs that require dose adjustments. However, any increase in lipophilic drug dosing used should be weighed against the reduced clearance and the risk of drug accumulation and adverse reactions with aging. Second, drug metabolism is altered due to reduced liver mass and blood flow, decreased CYP 450 enzyme activity, and reduced hepatic capacity. This results in accumulation of hepatically metabolized drugs in the blood. Finally, drug excretion is altered due to reduced GFR, renal tubular function and renal blood flow resulting in accumulation of renally cleared drugs. Aging is also associated with several pharmacodynamic changes that can alter the therapeutic response and lead to adverse drug reactions. These changes are due to altered receptor density, receptor affinity, signal transduction, or homeostatic mechanisms.

Polypharmacy is defined as the use of ≥5 medications. This is associated with an increased risk of inappropriate treatments due to the use of medications that are not indicated, are not effective, or constitute therapeutic duplications. Older adults have multiple chronic conditions and on average are prescribed 12 different prescription medications. This number is only increased with admission to the ICU as new therapies are initiated to treat the primary acute pathophysiology, and to manage destabilized comorbidities, anxiety, delirium, and sleep disturbances. As the number of medications administered increases, so does the potential for adverse iatrogenic events, as well as drug–drug and drug–disease interactions. It has been reported that between 50% and 85% of older adults are prescribed at least 1 potentially inappropriate medication during a hospital admission such as antipsychotics for hypoactive delirium. Similarly, medications such as opiates, benzodiazepines, and anticholinergic medications are used to alleviate symptoms but with consequences of drug-induced delirium that is associated with increased morbidity and mortality.

Therefore, it is important to recognize that the current ICU paradigm in conjunction with baseline polypharmacy in older adults is associated with an increased risk of experiencing adverse events. This is due to age-related physiological changes in drug actions; organ dysfunction affecting drug absorption, alteration in metabolism or excretion; and detrimental drug–drug and drug–disease interactions. To mitigate such events, it is essential to adopt strategies to regularly review drug therapy that are practical, systemic, and organized. This includes using lowest effective doses of "high risk" medications. Additionally, reviewing and eliminating any medications that may be causing adverse events, drug–drug interactions, or are no longer needed daily. Finally, integrating a geriatric-focused pharmacist on rounds, when possible, to optimize drug therapies.

Geriatric Critical Care: A Model for an Interdisciplinary Approach

In spite of the success of the Acute Care for Elders (ACE) model in the non-ICU setting in reducing functional disability among older adults, decreasing the risk of discharge to nursing homes, decreasing the risk of readmissions, and reducing hospitalization costs in the last two decades, this model has not yet been translated to the ICU setting. Through an interdisciplinary approach, the ACE model emphasizes maintenance of physical, cognitive, and mental health function, prevention of hospital-acquired geriatric syndromes, and transition of care planning from admission. This is achieved through (1) an interdisciplinary rounding team (2) prepared physical environment or physical environmental modifications to prevent cognitive and functional decline by fostering ambulation, functional independence, and orientation (3) improving transition of care. The focus of this section is not to introduce a new critical care model that is geriatric specific, but rather to highlight specific aspects in the current ICU care model, that could be modified based on the ACE model tenants and would therefore allow care to be tailored to the unique needs of the critically ill older adult.

The team members of an interdisciplinary geriatric critical care unit are indistinguishable from those that comprise any other highly functional critical care unit with one main exception. That is the incorporation of additional key team members, some of which possess specific expertise in geriatric medical and surgical care. This includes family members, a geriatric pharmacist, a geriatrician, and the palliative care service. Family involvement in daily rounds as members of the care team is beneficial especially when caring for older adults. This allows for the real-time discussion of active issues, progress, care plans, and goals of care between the team members and the family. In fact, these daily interactions on rounds may allow the elimination of the potential stigma associated with the "afternoon family meeting." Designating a spokesperson helps facilitate intrafamily communication as well. Due to the complexities of medication management among older adults, a geriatric-focused pharmacist is an ideal ICU team member. Pharmacists who specialize in the care of critically ill older adults, understand the renal and hepatic physiologic and pharmacologic changes that accompany aging, and assist in medication reconciliation, appropriate dosing of medication, and avoidance of harmful medications. While palliative care services have mainly been utilized for end-of-life discussions, the services that are offered by the palliative care providers extend way beyond discontinuation of life sustaining measures. This includes life circumstance adjustment (affirmation of life and emphasis on dying as a normal process of aging), help families/patients navigating the emotional, religious, and psychological implications of end-of-life decisions, and offers a support system to help families cope during a patient's illness and in their own bereavement. Finally, in certain circumstances, when there are differences of opinion, misaligned expectations, and seemingly irreconcilable differences in perspective between patients and families, among family members, and between clinicians and family or different clinical teams, the palliative care service can provide conflict resolution. Therefore, inclusion of the palliative care team early on in the ICU course is paramount.

As with all ICUs, the rooms should be arranged so that patients are easily visible from multiple vantage points within the unit to allow proper patient observation of a population that is prone to developing delirium. All rooms should have direct access to large windows with outside views and access to bright natural light. This will optimize attempts to normalize the sleep-wake cycle for these patients, in whom sleep hygiene is critical. Rooms where older adults will be managed should have larger television monitors and controls that accommodate decreased grip strength, as well as reduced digital dexterity from arthritis and related conditions, further enable comfort and communication, and reduce frustration for patients with impairments. They further provide older adults with some control over their environment at a time when they have become dependent in an unfamiliar critical care environment. Large font, high contrast signage, and large clocks and single-date calendars should be placed within rooms to facilitate reorientation. Implementation of a geriatric friendly ICU environment would also require significant subtractions from the existing environment to minimize the sensory overload, sleep disruption, and frequent use of tethering devices such as restraints and catheters that remain engrained in ICU culture. This includes maintaining a quiet environment at all times of the day. Minimizing the unwarranted noise of alarm monitors through adjustment of the monitor settings to patient's baseline status and minimizing the frequency of the alarms when deemed appropriate. Promoting wakefulness during the day through early mobilization. Discontinuation of nasogastric tubes, Foley catheters, drains, and restraints as soon as possible. Finally, assistive devices such as prescription glasses, electronic devices that speak for the patient or translate between languages, hearing aids that enable effective communication with those who may have impaired auditory or vocal capabilities should be made available in the ICU.

Modifications in how daily rounds are performed should include assessment of frailty, treatment new diagnoses of a variety of preexisting but undiagnosed conditions, continued treatment of baseline chronic conditions, daily screening, and reduction of delirium, ensuring adequate pain control, and early mobility.

Adoption of geriatric care models into the ICU is essential at this point in time. In addition to changing the built environment in the ICU to accommodate this population, integration of geriatric concepts into critical care training programs and clinical practice is vital. Critical care providers must be equipped with the skills to assess and manage geriatric syndromes, such as multimorbidity, frailty, delirium, sensory deficits, cognitive impairment, and disability. To achieve this, the current ICU workforce should be trained in foundational geriatric principles, including basic assessment tools and management strategies. This could be achieved with in-service training, quality improvement programs, interdisciplinary "geriatrics champions" to serve as peer resources, and educational programs developed by critical care societies.

Ethical Challenges: Withholding, Discontinuation of Life Sustaining Measures, and Futility

Care for older adults in the ICU presents daily opportunities for ethical dilemmas and discussions regarding goals of care, withholding life sustaining treatments (LSTs), discontinuation of LSTs, and futility of the care offered. Firstly, it is essential to define the difference between withholding and discontinuing LSTs and the dilemma of their moral differences. Withholding of LSTs refers to a decision to not start or escalate interventions. Discontinuation of LSTs refers to cessation of ongoing interventions. This includes hydration, nutrition, cardio-pulmonary resuscitation, and mechanical ventilation to name a few. Regardless of the therapy involved, dominant current ethical opinion concerning the decision to withhold or discontinue is based on the "moral equivalence" thesis. That is, if there is no moral difference between withholding and discontinuing therapy, then (all else being equal) there is no instance in which it would be allowable to withhold a treatment but not to discontinue the same treatment once it is started. Nonetheless, considerable disquiet exists among clinicians regarding the moral equivalence between withholding and discontinuing LSTs. This is compounded by the need to balance patient/family autonomy, which is often dictated by the differences in cultural and religious beliefs, with the clinical objective of ensuring beneficence (doing good) and non-maleficence (avoiding harm) with the treatments offered.

Secondly, it is difficult to determine whether withdrawing or discontinuing LSTs is appropriate without defining futility. As it is often raised as the justification for the decisions to do either. There is little, if any, disagreement among ethicists or clinicians that truly futile therapy need not be offered, should not be knowingly undertaken, and is probably actually unethical. Treatments that fail to meet a patient's goals or that maintain them in a suspended state of irrecoverable critical illness are not only costly to the healthcare system but defies the principle of non-maleficence. While this concept appears to be universally accepted, finding consensus regarding the definition of futility has proven to be problematic. Futility is often defined as a therapy that will present a patient with more burden or harm than benefit. Another commonly deployed definition of futility is that a physician must conclude that the offered therapy will succeed in fewer than 1 of 100 cases. This number appears to be extrapolated from assertions that a 1% difference in outcomes in research is usually considered statistically insignificant. Based on these definitions, the next question to be addressed is what outcomes should be used to determine futility? The truth is that no validated markers that define futility exist. In addition, using a straightforward outcome such as mortality is problematic, given that mortality is notoriously difficult for physicians to predict accurately in hospitalized patients, even with utilization of the current severity of illness scoring systems (APACHE, SAPS, CCI).

The definition of futility is not that simple and is based on an interplay between medicine, ethics, and the philosophical nature of healthcare decision-making. Clinicians often find themselves in situations where their quantitative definition of futility does not align with the qualitative definition of futility for a patient and their family. This is due to differences in values between the two entities. As a result, patients/their families and physicians often disagree about what makes a treatment futile and what benefits are worth pursuing, even if survival is unlikely. Disentangling values disagreements requires discussion, mutual respect, and negotiation.

Given the lack of consensus in the definition of futility that is useful at bedside to direct medical care, it has been proposed that a shift from determining medical/surgical "futility" to determining medical/surgical "appropriateness" is warranted. That is whether a medical or surgical treatment should be initiated or continued, regardless of whether requested or desired by the patient, the family, or the physician, should rest solely on the understanding that a treatment offered lies on the continuum of medical/surgical appropriateness where benefits outweigh the risks and harm. The determination of what treatments are appropriate will vary depending on the disease, the treatment, the anticipated outcomes, and the values of the patient, family, and physicians involved. Thus, the appropriateness of initiating or continuing a medical/surgical treatment is unique to each patient.

When caring for older adults in the ICU setting, some of the above concerns can be mitigated through (1) establishing goals of care and code status at time of admission. Ideally, this should be accomplished through direct discussion with the patient. In situations where the patient is incapacitated, efforts should be made to establish the medical power of attorney and obtain any available advanced directives early in the ICU course. In situations where the patient is unable to advocate for him or herself and has no advanced directives, it is the responsibility of the interdisciplinary care team (ICU, primary service, palliative care medicine) to counsel the family on establishing "patient-centered" goals of care that minimize prolonging patient suffering and harm; (2) involving designated family members in daily ICU rounds to provide them with real-time updates on the patient's clinical course and answer any questions that might prevent future conflicts; (3) creating an environment that is nonjudgmental with shared decision-making between the healthcare team and the family, while recognizing and honoring the fact that different people value and respond to medical data differently; (4) understanding that the decision to begin, withhold, or discontinue LSTs is as much of an ethical decision as it is a medical decision.

References

1. Akhtar S, Rosenbaum S, editors. Principles of geriatric critical care. 1st ed. Cambridge: Cambridge University Press; 2018. https://doi.org/10.1017/9781316676325.
2. Brown R, McKelvey MC, Ryan S, et al. The impact of aging in acute respiratory distress syndrome: a clinical and mechanistic overview. Front Med. 2020;7:589553. https://doi.org/10.3389/fmed.2020.589553.
3. Brummel NE, Ferrante LE. Integrating geriatric principles into critical care medicine: the time is now. Ann Am Thorac Soc. 2018;15(5):518–22. https://doi.org/10.1513/AnnalsATS.201710-793IP.
4. Damluji AA, Forman DE, van Diepen S, et al. Older adults in the cardiac intensive care unit: factoring geriatric syndromes in the management, prognosis, and process of care: a scientific statement from the American Heart Association. Circulation. 2020;141(2):e6. https://doi.org/10.1161/CIR.0000000000000741.
5. Devlin JW, Skrobik Y, Gélinas C, et al. Clinical practice guidelines for the prevention and Management of Pain, agitation/sedation, delirium, immobility, and sleep disruption in adult patients in the ICU. Crit Care Med. 2018;46(9):e825–73. https://doi.org/10.1097/CCM.0000000000003299.
6. Duprey MS, Devlin JW, van der Hoeven JG, et al. Association between incident delirium treatment with haloperidol and mortality in critically ill adults. Crit Care Med. 2021;49:1303. https://doi.org/10.1097/CCM.0000000000004976.
7. Ely EW, Inouye SK, Bernard GR, et al. Delirium in mechanically ventilated patients: validity and reliability of the confusion assessment method for the intensive care unit (CAM-ICU). JAMA. 2001;286(21):2703. https://doi.org/10.1001/jama.286.21.2703.
8. Evans L, Rhodes A, Alhazzani W, et al. Surviving sepsis campaign: international guidelines for Management of Sepsis and Septic Shock 2021. Crit Care Med. 2021;49(11):e1063–143. https://doi.org/10.1097/CCM.0000000000005337.
9. Ghneim M, Diaz JJ. Dementia and the critically ill older adult. Crit Care Clin. 2021;37(1):191–203. https://doi.org/10.1016/j.ccc.2020.08.010.
10. Kalil AC, Metersky ML, Klompas M, et al. Management of Adults with hospital-acquired and ventilator-associated pneumonia: 2016 clinical practice guidelines by the Infectious Diseases Society of America and the American Thoracic Society. Clin Infect Dis. 2016;63(5):e61–e111. https://doi.org/10.1093/cid/ciw353.
11. Lamontagne F, Richards-Belle A, Thomas K, et al. Effect of reduced exposure to vasopressors on 90-day mortality in older critically ill patients with vasodilatory hypotension: a randomized clinical trial. JAMA. 2020;323(10):938. https://doi.org/10.1001/jama.2020.0930.
12. Marik PE. Management of the critically ill geriatric patient. In: O'Donnell JM, Nácul FE, editors. Surgical intensive care medicine. Springer; 2016. p. 743–58. https://doi.org/10.1007/978-3-319-19668-8_54.
13. Medina-Liabres KRP, Kim S. Continuous renal replacement therapy in elderly with acute kidney injury. Korean J Intern Med. 2020;35(2):284–94. https://doi.org/10.3904/kjim.2019.431.
14. Palmer RM. The acute Care for Elders Unit Model of care. Geriatrics (Basel). 2018;3(3):E59. https://doi.org/10.3390/geriatrics3030059.
15. Vallet H, Schwarz GL, Flaatten H, de Lange DW, Guidet B, Dechartres A. Mortality of older patients admitted to an ICU: a systematic review. Crit Care Med. 2021;49(2):324–34. https://doi.org/10.1097/CCM.0000000000004772.

[illegible] discuss the [illegible] anticipated outcomes and the values of the patient, family, and physicians involved. Thus the appropriateness of initiating or continuing a [illegible] individualized to each patient.

When caring for older adults in the ICU [illegible] the [illegible] of the [illegible] [illegible] median [illegible] of [illegible]

[illegible]

Cardiac Hemodynamic Monitoring

50

Lili Sadri, Robert Myers, Jaleesa Akuoko,
Razvan Iorga, and Karyn Butler

ntroduction

hock is a common indication for admission to
e surgical intensive care unit (SICU). In the
lderly, as a result of pre-existing disease, organ
ystem dysfunction from shock may be present
efore the common clinical signs of shock are
pparent. Critical perfusion pressures may be
mperative to minimize cerebral, renal, and car-
diac dysfunction and the classic resuscitation
target of a mean arterial pressure (MAP) over
65 mmHg may in fact be too low to ensure ade-
quate organ perfusion in elderly patients. This
highlights the need for a patient specific resusci-
tation approach based on the physiology of
aging.

This chapter is dedicated to all the residents who give their time, their strength, their compassion, and their dedication during their rotation in the ICU.

L. Sadri · R. Myers · J. Akuoko · R. Iorga
Department of Surgery, Jefferson-Abington Health, Abington, PA, USA

K. Butler (✉)
Department of Surgery, Jefferson-Abington Health, Abington, PA, USA

Department of Surgery, Sidney Kimmel Medical College of Thomas Jefferson University, Philadelphia, USA
e-mail: Karyn.butler@jefferson.edu

Recognition of Shock

Shock is defined as inadequate oxygen delivery to meet the aerobic needs of the tissue and is typically classified into four categories; hypovolemic, cardiogenic, distributive, and obstructive. In elderly patients, multiple classes of shock may co-exist underscoring the complexity of the diagnostic and therapeutic options. The imbalance of oxygen availability and consumption results in a physiologic transition to anaerobic metabolism and subsequent metabolic lactic acidosis. Compensatory physiologic responses include tachycardia, increased systemic vascular resistance (SVR), and sodium and water retention resulting in decreased urine output. These responses serve to maintain critical perfusion to the heart and brain through augmentation of perfusion pressure and stroke volume (SV). Elderly patients may have comorbidities that alter these responses preventing the normal compensatory mechanisms from kicking in, resulting in multi-organ system dysfunction due to the delayed recognition of shock. The primary response to circulatory collapse is an increase in heart rate and an increase in SVR as a result of stimulation of systemic catecholamine's and the renin angiotensin system, respectively. These responses are blunted in the presence of agents that control heart rate and in the presence of antihypertensive therapy both commonly used by the elderly patient for management of cardiovascular dis-

P. Petrone, C. E.M. Brathwaite (eds.), *Acute Care Surgery in Geriatric Patients*,
https://doi.org/10.1007/978-3-031-30651-8_50

eases. Systemic vasodilation as a result of antihypertensive therapy may be profound and long lasting depending on the types of medications and timing of administration before the onset of the shock state.

Hard signs of shock such as MAP below 65 mmHg, tachycardia, decreased urine output, cutaneous pallor, and diaphoresis are often easy to recognize and link to a state of hypoperfusion. In the elderly, these findings may be absent or misinterpreted (e.g., diuretic induced high urine output considered "good" urine output) or may be due to pharmacologic therapy for pre-existing diseases (slow heart rate in the management of atrial fibrillation, vasodilatation for treatment of hypertension). The presence of concomitant co-morbidity underscores the need for a high index of suspicion that a shock state may be present. Moreover, information obtained from cardiac monitoring, particularly cardiac output (CO) and SVR, may facilitate early identification of hypoperfusion and clarify the shock state (Table 50.1).

Biomarkers may aid in assessing oxygen debt and monitoring organs at risk for failure. Helpful biomarkers assess metabolic acidosis as a representation of anaerobic metabolism (e.g., lactate, base deficit), assess the balance between oxygen delivery and consumption as a representation of oxygen debt ($ScVO_2$), assess changes in renal function (BUN/Cr, Cr clearance), and may suggest cardiac stress or impairment of function (troponin, brain natriuretic peptide).

Lastly, agents that impair coagulation and platelet function may indirectly affect compensatory mechanisms when shock is due to acute blood loss. Inhibition of platelet function impairs the primary hemostatic mechanism to address vascular injury with resultant ongoing blood loss and progression of shock due to intravascular blood loss.

Table 50.1 Physiologic variables and classification of shock

Classification of shock	Cardiac output	Systemic vascular resistance
Hypovolemic	↓	↑
Cardiogenic	↓↓	↑↑
Distributive	→↓	↓
Obstructive	↓	→↑

Serum lactate is a common biomarker measured in venous and arterial samples to assess the degree of hypoperfusion and help to identify when a patient is in shock. The arterial blood gas (ABG) can additionally be utilized to identify and trend the severity of acidosis and its change over time as treatment is implemented. Importantly, time to correction of the base deficit reflects the adequacy of resuscitation and correlates with survival. Moreover, the venous electrolyte panel obtained in most patients may detect a metabolic acidosis on review of the serum bicarbonate level; this may be an early indicator of anaerobic metabolism and should prompt obtaining serum lactate and/or an ABG to monitor acid-base status.

The balance of oxygen consumption (VO_2) and oxygen delivery (DO_2) is reflected by the extraction ratio ($ER = VO_2/DO_2$) and can be estimated by the measurement of central venous oxygen saturation ($ScVO_2$). Many patients who undergo resuscitation from shock have a central venous catheter in place for fluid and vasopressor support. A central venous blood gas can then easily be obtained to assess $ScVO_2$. The presence of a $ScVO_2$ less than 65% serves as an early warning that there may be an imbalance in oxygen consumption and delivery. Limitations of interpreting $ScVO_2$ include those conditions that artificially elevate $ScVO_2$ such as the presence of acidosis, arteriovenous malformations, and exposure to acid-producing toxins. In these cases, it is the $ScVO_2$ trend that is most helpful. In the absence of these conditions, a normal $ScVO_2$ may be reassuring that physiologic recovery is taking place.

Goals of Resuscitation

Goal-directed resuscitation to restore perfusion in shock states must begin with understanding the type of shock present. Classification of shock according to four categories (hypovolemic, cardiogenic, distributive, and/or obstructive) is an ential first step in developing a comprehensive tment plan. Cardiovascular, pulmonary, and al comorbidities common in elderly patients nplicate classifying the type of shock. rdiogenic, hypovolemic, and distributive ock states may co-exist and at times can be difult to differentiate without cardiac monitoring. oreover, traumatic or non-traumatic causes of structive shock may mimic hypovolemia and ust be considered based on the individual tient's history. The physiologic capability of derly patients to respond to resuscitation is lated to pre-existing co-morbidity, particularly ardiopulmonary reserve. Goal-directed therapy corporates approaches based on the patients nique physiologic reserve identified with hemoynamic monitoring and their pre-existing medial conditions.

The goals of resuscitation from shock in lderly patients are to restore and maintain organ perfusion and correct the oxygen debt so that aerobic metabolism is supported. These goals are not different from those in younger patients; it is the approach to achieving these goals that may be different. The important consideration in elderly patients is that compensatory reserves may be lost or attenuated and therefore patients may require adjunctive support such as the use of ionotropic agents, transfusion therapy, invasive or non-invasive ventilator support, and/or early renal replacement therapy.

Hemodynamic Changes with Age

Physiologic changes that occur with aging are reviewed in detail in Chap. 6. Assessment of blood pressure and understanding what "normal" is in the elderly patient is an important starting point and one that may be underappreciated particularly as traditional goals of resuscitation (MAP >65 mmHg) serve as the foundation to restore perfusion. Moreover, elderly patients may be admitted to the ICU to manage organ dysfunction unassociated with shock making it essential to determine which vascular beds, if any, have distinct needs for higher or lower perfusion pressures during the recovery from surgical disease. For example, there is significant controversy regarding optimal BP targets for elderly patients, what age breakpoints should be used to define elderly and how and where BP is measured. The new ACC/AHA hypertension guideline makes risk-stratification recommendations based on co-morbidity and characteristics for a target of systolic BP less than 130 mmHg for patients aged greater than 65 years however no diastolic target was set. Several trials, however, have shown that a BP target of 150/90 reduced mortality, stroke, and cardiac events. With these controversies in mind, care for elderly patients in the ICU must balance the risk of inadequate organ perfusion with exacerbation of cardiovascular disease emphasizing the need for an individualized approach to resuscitation guided by hemodynamic monitoring and biochemical evidence of recovery.

Cardiac and Hemodynamic Monitoring

Options for hemodynamic monitoring include devices that deliver static assessment and those that give continuous, dynamic assessment of hemodynamic parameters (Table 50.2). Each has its benefits, limitations, capabilities, and risks. Optimal and early monitoring in the elderly critically ill patient can provide clarity on the physiologic status and guide treatment during resuscitation and during recovery from critical illness. Hemodynamic parameters that assess the strength of myocardial performance (cardiac output) and cardiac responsiveness to fluid administration (SVI%) form the cornerstone of physiologic support in the ICU as patients' transition from acute illness to recovery. In particular, early identification of elderly patients who may benefit from inotropic support could improve outcomes. Although shock is a common diagnosis for admission to the ICU, not all elderly patients are in shock when their need for critical care arises. The ICU is an important resource to support recovery of organ dysfunction during treatment for surgical disease often characterized by third space fluid shifts and systemic inflammatory response syndrome (SIRS). Acute or acute-on-

Table 50.2 Hemodynamic monitoring options in shock

Clinical state	Device	Access	Measured variable
Right heart failure or pulmonary hypertension	PAC	Invasive; central venous access needed	PCWP SVR CO EDV
Assessment of acute cardiac dysfunction or intravascular volume status	TTE TEE	Non-invasive Invasive	IVC diameter, %EF Cardiac function and geometry
Assessment of cardiac output	Pulse contour analysis	Invasive; arterial catheter ± central venous access needed	CO SVI PPV
Assessment of fluid responsiveness	Bioreactance	Non-invasive	%SVI CO TPR

PAC pulmonary artery catheter, *TTE* transthoracic echocardiography, *TEE* transesophageal echocardiography, *PCWP* pulmonary capillary wedge pressure, *SVR* systemic vascular resistance, *CO* cardiac output, *EDV* end-diastolic volume, *IVC* inferior vena cava, *TPR* total peripheral resistance, *SVI* stoke volume index, *PPV* pulse pressure variation, *EF* ejection fraction

Table 50.3 Therapeutic options based on fluid responsiveness and cardiac monitoring

	Fluid responsive	Therapeutic options
↓CO ↑SVR	YES	Fluid, ± inotrope
	NO	Vasodilator, inotrope, reduce preload
↓CO ↓SVR	YES	Fluid, ± vasopressor, ± inotrope
	NO	Vasopressor, ± inotrope

CO cardiac output, *SVR* systemic vascular resistance

chronic renal events are common after surgery and management requires careful assessment of the need for intravascular volume administration balanced by the cardiac reserve to handle the fluid. A prudent approach to the use and timing of diuretic therapy and vasoactive agents to minimize cardiopulmonary dysfunction can be guided by hemodynamic monitoring to identify fluid responsiveness and cardiac reserve (Table 50.3).

Standard Monitoring

Optimizing hemodynamics in the critically ill patient restores end-organ tissue perfusion and is an important prognostic indicator for outcomes. Understanding the individual patient's physiologic response to a specific disease process can be guided with a wide range of devices to obtain hemodynamic assessments.

Adequate blood pressure (BP) control is known to prevent major adverse cardiac events in the elderly. Traditional monitoring techniques include the use of automated, non-invasive BP cuffs. Non-invasive BP monitoring has historically been a gold standard for diagnosing hypertension in all age groups given its ease of use, efficient application, and reproducibility. The accuracy of these devices may be reduced in elderly patients with decreased arterial elasticity, dysrhythmias, and/or cardiac failure. Moreover, the controversy regarding BP targets for therapeutic intervention in hypertensive elderly patients (traditionally set at ≤150 SBP) impacts BP targets selected for resuscitation endpoints. This may contribute to organ system dysfunction and impaired recovery in elderly patients that is different from their younger cohorts.

Pulse oximetry utilizes the principle of light absorption of colors at different wavelengths to determine oxygen saturation in red blood cells. A probe is placed over the front and back of a patient's distal fingertip, and different diodes of light are transmitted onto the superior aspect of the adjacent skin. The relative amount of light that is absorbed is then proportionally calculated and compared to the other side of the probe on the finger, ultimately deriving a patient's percent oxygen saturation. Pulse oximetry is advantageous in that it is an easy, non-invasive, cost-effective method for assessing a patient's percent oxygen saturation (SpO_2). Practically applied, in a patient with a normal oxygen dissociation curve, a SpO_2 >90% correlates with a PaO_2 of >60 mm. In critically ill patients, however, this association may be inaccurate. Parameters such as small vessel disease, decreased skin elasticity, and factors affecting the oxygen dissociation curve (pH, severe anemia, low core body temperature) are not well defined in the elderly. Interpretation of pulse oximetry results in elderly ICU patients should be done with caution, and confirmation with arterial sampling may be necessary.

Electrocardiography (ECG) is another standard diagnostic tool that aids the understanding of how fast and how well a heartbeat is conducted. In ischemia, timing and effectiveness of signal transduction can be detected via ECG. However, in the absence of these changes, an ECG has limited application in the acute resuscitation of patients with hemodynamic instability. For example, a common cardiac pathology presenting in the elderly is left ventricular dysfunction. As patients age, cardiac compliance decreases and comorbidities such as hypertension, coronary artery disease, and heart failure amplify this change. Cardiac contractility, compliance, and endothelial wall function decline longitudinally, and vascular and cardiac hypertrophy increases. These phenomena introduce variables that affect cardiac output and end-organ perfusion over time. The use of ECG, albeit practical and useful for detecting extremes of cardiac dysfunction, is limited in its ability to detect these important anatomic changes. Subtle findings may be identified, but confirmation with advanced imaging is often necessary and may be impractical in the acutely unstable patient.

Advanced Monitoring

Arterial Catheters, Central Venous Pressure, Pulmonary Artery Catheters

Non-invasive BP monitoring has limitations in the elderly patient due to age-specific physiologic changes. Invasive BP monitoring has emerged as the new gold standard for accurate BP monitoring in critically ill patients addressing the limitations of non-invasive BP monitoring. Arterial catheters can be used to easily obtain serial ABGs and laboratory data to monitor resuscitation and can identify hemodynamic changes quickly. Radial artery catheterization is a favored technique compared to other arterial sites secondary to decreased infection risk, ease of access due to the superficial location of the vessel, and minimal risk of distal ischemia.

Central venous pressure (CVP) monitoring via a central vein estimates right atrial pressure when the catheter tip is located at the junction of the superior vena cava and the right atrium. Compared to more advanced, invasive monitoring with a pulmonary artery catheter, CVP monitoring has fewer complications during placement and maintenance. Limitations, however, are significant and largely attributed to vascular and ventricular compliance, changes in intra-thoracic pressure, atrial dysrhythmias, valvular disease, and positioning of the patient. Despite these limitations, extreme CVP values, <6 mmHg or >15 mmHg, may be useful in guiding fluid resuscitation. Patients with little increase in CVP following a fluid bolus are more likely to be fluid responsive than patients with a large increase after fluid administration. A large increase in CVP may indicate increased right ventricular preload suggesting that additional fluid may be unnecessary and measures to reduce preload (e.g., diuretics) may be more appropriate. Due to these considerations, CVP has limited use in active resuscitation as a singular tool but may contribute aggregate information to ongoing monitoring and goal-directed therapy in select patients.

The pulmonary artery catheter (PAC) was developed by Swan-Ganz in 1970 to continuously

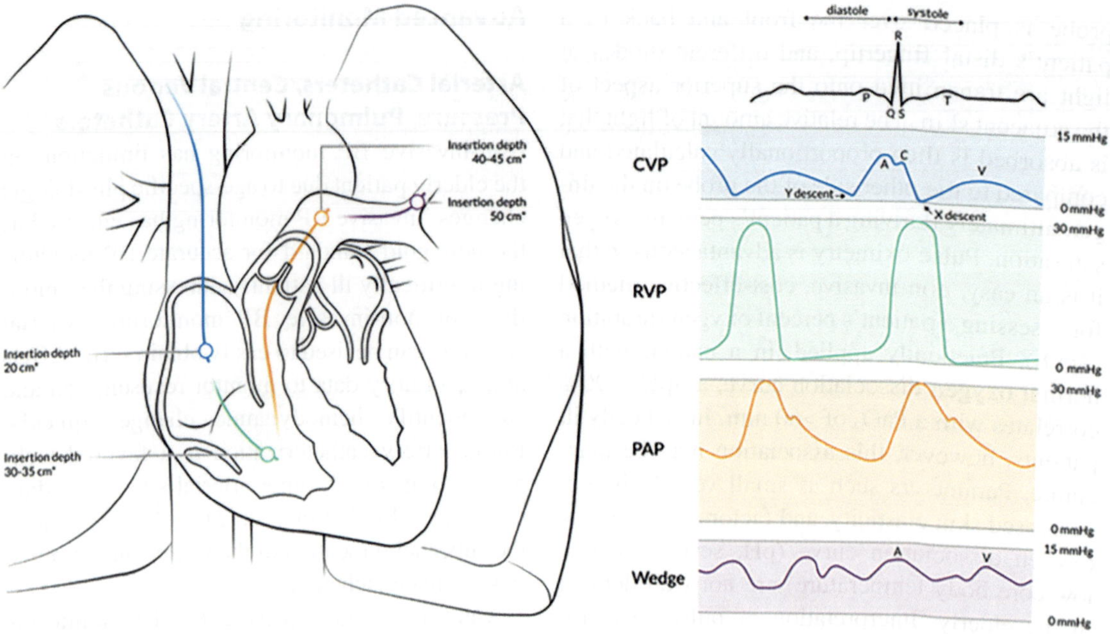

Fig. 50.1 Waveforms associated with placement of the pulmonary artery catheter. https://link.springer.com/chapter/10.1007/978-3-319-55862-2_2

Table 50.4 Normal pressure measurements

CVP	8–12 mmHg
RV	15–28 mmHg
Mean PAP	10–22 mmHg
PCWP	5–12 mmHg

CVP central venous pressure, *RV* right ventricle, *PAP* pulmonary artery pressure, *PCWP* pulmonary capillary wedge pressure

monitor cardiac performance, intravascular pressures, and oxygen delivery. The 7–8 French diameter, 110 cm long catheter has a balloon at the end and multiple ports along its length and is placed into a central vein through a large introducer. Once central venous access is obtained, the balloon is inflated and the catheter advanced while monitoring pressure changes that correlate with the anatomic location of the catheter (Fig. 50.1). The associated pressure measurements help to confirm anatomic location (Table 50.4). Upon reaching the target resting position (pulmonary capillary wedge position), the pulmonary artery waveform attenuates, the "wedge" pressure is measured at the end of expiration, and the balloon is deflated allowing the tip to rest within the pulmonary artery. This minimizes rupture of the small pulmonary vessels during balloon inflation. In the "wedged" position, the pulmonary capillary wedge pressure (PCWP) is greater than the pulmonary artery pressure and is an approximation of left atrial pressure. This can be used to assess cardiac reserve as volume resuscitation proceeds.

The most distal channel of the PAC monitors the PCWP and SvO_2. An additional lumen, 30 cm from the tip, can measure CVP and a third channel terminating in the same position can be used for infusions. The PAC permits calculation of cardiac output, using thermodilution, a technique that measures changes in blood temperature after infusion of cold fluid. Physiologic changes occurring with age make elderly patients more likely to have pulmonary hypertension and right heart failure. The early awareness of these conditions and the determination that additional fluid administration will not improve cardiac output and organ perfusion can permit consideration of pharmacologic or biomechanical support sooner for patients who remain in shock. The PAC can provide useful data in the presence of acute cardiac decompensation, however, there is little benefit for its use when primary cardiac dysfunction is not present.

Transthoracic Echocardiography

Since the 1980s, the use of echocardiography has become commonplace among critical care units, emergency rooms, and operating rooms across the country, due to its high quality, dynamic imaging, and low risk of use. Echocardiography can be performed at the bedside, can be performed serially to monitor the response to an intervention over time, and does not use ionizing radiation. It can be performed via the transthoracic (TTE) or transesophageal (TEE) routes. The transesophageal method is preferred in select patients when visibility is inadequate (e.g., obesity, edema, overlying dressings). A limitation of point-of-care ultrasonography is that the quality of results depends on the user's technical skill and interpretation. As a result, multiple organizations, including the American College of Chest Physicians and the Society of Critical Care Medicine, offer training and accreditation through simulation with guided feedback to reduce interrater variability.

Point-of-care echocardiography (POCE) is indicated for evaluation of patients with hemodynamic instability, for determination of fluid responsiveness, assessment of cardiac pathology (valvular disease, thrombi, right heart failure), and cardiac failure as a result of pulmonary embolism. In these very sick patients, assessment with TTE is risk-free. TEE on the other hand allows for unobstructed, high-definition views of the heart but requires a sedated patient. Risks of probe insertion include arrhythmias, hypotension, bleeding, and airway compromise. In the ambulatory setting, TEE has been shown to have an adverse event rate between 0.2 and 0.5%, which is slightly increased in critically ill or elderly patients. Contraindications to TEE include esophageal stricture or mass, upper gastrointestinal bleed, recent cervical spine injury, and recent esophageal or gastric surgery.

The American Heart Association recommends using POCE in "the evaluation of acute, persistent and life-threatening hemodynamic disturbances in which ventricular function and its determinants are uncertain and have not responded to treatment." Goal-directed echocardiography focuses on rapidly determining the causes of acute cardiopulmonary failure. The clinical questions to be answered include determining if shock is present and if so, what type (cardiogenic, distributive, hypovolemic, obstructive, combination) and is there a pulmonary etiology that can explain sudden clinical deterioration (pulmonary embolism). It should be noted that the goal of POC echocardiography in critical care is not to replace comprehensive echocardiography but to supplement the clinical exam and permit rapid identification of life-threatening conditions. In the acutely unstable patient, TTE can rapidly identify threat to life conditions utilizing a structured approach to assess left ventricular systolic function, right ventricular size and function, pericardial effusion, and distensibility of the IVC to evaluate volume status (Fig. 50.2).

In addition to intravascular volume status, POCE can assess fluid responsiveness. In the sedated, mechanically ventilated patient with no spontaneous breathing, ventilator-induced alterations in stroke volume and IVC diameter correlate positively with fluid responsiveness. In the spontaneously breathing patient, a change in stroke volume of 12% in response to passive leg raise, a technique which mimics the effect of a bolus of fluid to the right heart, has been shown to correlate with fluid responsiveness. A study of 220 critically ill patients by Kanji et al. demonstrated that use of fluid therapy guided by limited TTE in subacute shock resulted in lower incidence of renal failure requiring dialysis. Importantly, Khoury et al. showed that routine use of echocardiography to guide hemodynamic resuscitation resulted in changes to medical or surgical management in 60% of critically ill patients.

Pulse Contour Analysis to Measure Cardiac Output

While pulmonary artery catheters have been the gold standard for hemodynamic monitoring in critically ill patients, there is growing interest in less-invasive techniques such as pulse contour analysis. Initially characterized in the early 1900s, pulse contour analysis is based on the principle that cardiac output is proportional to

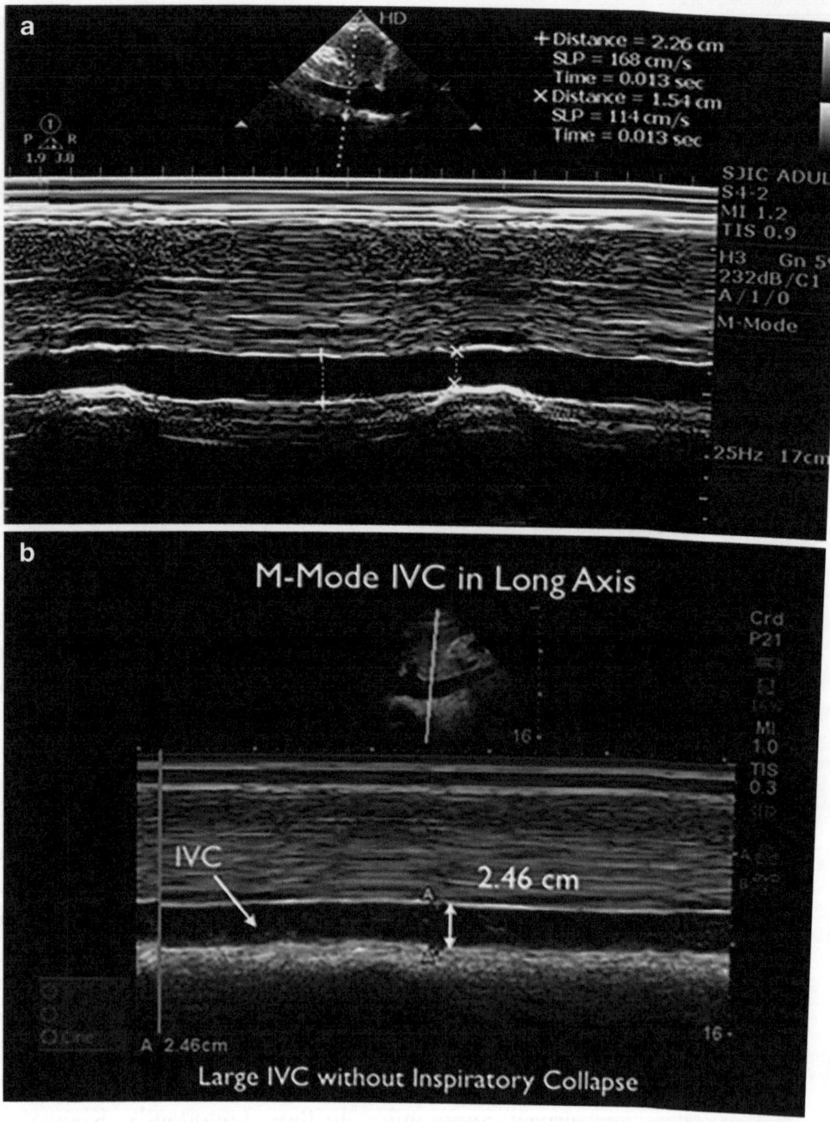

Fig. 50.2 M-mode echocardiography and IVC diameter in (**a**) hypovolemia and (**b**) euvolemia. https://onlinelibrary.wiley.com/doi/full/10.7863/jum.2012.31.12.1885. https://www.sciencedirect.com/science/article/pii/S0019483216302358

arterial pulse pressure. The arterial pressure waveform gives beat-by-beat analysis of cardiac output. Pulse contour methods are comparably less invasive than Swan-Ganz catheterization and provide accurate assessment of cardiac output in critically ill patients using arterial catheterization plus or minus central venous catheterization for calibration. Despite the need for central venous access, these methods are characterized in the literature as "less-invasive" or "semi-invasive" compared to traditional pulmonary artery catheterization, with variations in degree of invasiveness depending on the type of monitor (Table 50.5). Patients requiring intra-arterial balloon pumps, those with a history of aneurysmal disease, severe valvular disease, or prior pneumonectomy may not be candidates for this technology. In critically ill elderly patients, use of less-invasive hemodynamic monitoring reduces the risk of arrhythmias, development of heart block, thrombosis, and catheter knotting that may occur with pulmonary artery catheterization.

PiCCO

Pulse index continuous cardiac output (PiCCO, Pulsion Medical Systems; Munich, Germany)

Table 50.5 Comparison of pulse contour monitors

	PiCCO	LiDCO	VIGELEO/FloTrac	Most care PRAM
	Pulsion medical systems, Munich, Germany	LiDCO group plc, London, UK	Edwards Lifesciences corporation, Irvine, CA, USA	Vytech health, Padova, Italy
Mechanism	Sampling at 250 Hz, area under curve of the systolic portion of waveform multiplied by calibration factor	PulseCOTM algorithm, waveform independent pulse power analysis	Sampling at 100 Hz, multiplication of pulse rate with SD of arterial pressure and a conversion factor	Pressure recording analytical method, sampling at 1000 Hz, calculation from perturbations
External calibration	Yes	Yes	No – Requires input of patient demographics	No
Site of arterial signal	Femoral or brachial artery	Radial artery	Radial artery	Femoral or radial artery

(Adapted from Romagnoli et al. 2009 and Grensemann et al. 2018)

combines central venous access and large artery catheterization for cardiac output measurement. Cold saline is injected into the central venous catheter, circulates through the right heart, pulmonary system, left heart, aorta and then to systemic circulation where it is detected by an arterial transducer. Trans-cardiopulmonary thermodilution provides external calibration, whereby CO can be derived from the arterial waveform via the Stewart-Hamilton equation ($CO_{td} = (T_b\text{-}T_i)V_iK/ \int \Delta T_b dt$).

PiCCO has been compared to PAC in monitoring output and yields comparable results in perioperative patients with complex comorbid conditions, patients undergoing cardiac surgery, and in critically ill patients to guide fluid resuscitation and vasopressor support. It is not yet validated in hemodynamically unstable patients. Contraindications to PiCCO include arrhythmias, indwelling intra-aortic balloon pumps, intracardiac shunt, prior pneumonectomy, pulmonary embolism, and aortic aneurysms.

LiDCO

Similar to PiCCO monitoring, lithium dilution CO measurement (LiDCO, LiDCO Group Plc; London, UK) employs both arterial impedance measurements and venous thermodilution calibration. Instead of cold saline bolus for thermodilution calibration, a bolus of lithium chloride is instilled into a peripheral or central venous catheter.

Use of lithium chloride compared to cold saline showed improved reliability in cardiac output monitoring in critically ill patients, however in patients on long-term lithium therapy or with recent use of non-depolarizing neuromuscular blocking agents, CO measurements show decreased accuracy. Another limitation noted with this system is the requisite blood draws during calibration.

Vigileo/FloTrac

Distinct from PiCCO and LiDCO, the Vigileo/FloTrac (Edwards Lifesciences Corporation; Irvine, CA, USA) system does not require external calibration. Using an arterial waveform and the patient's age, sex, and body surface area, the system determines CO via a proprietary algorithm. As such, Vigileo/FloTrac is marketed as more user-friendly but with fewer hemodynamic parameters captured compared to PiCCO. Notably, this modality has been validated in patients with septic shock compared to transpulmonary thermodilution, demonstrating comparable assessments of CO. However, this technique reportedly overestimates CO in patients with aortic regurgitation and underestimates CO in high output vasodilatory states. Vigileo/FloTrac has not yet shown efficacy in hemodynamically unstable patients compared to invasive monitoring and has decreased utility in patients with arrhythmias, peripheral vascular disease, and aortic valvular pathology; common comorbidities in the elderly. Moreover, this technology has not been validated in mechanically ventilated patients and requires arterial catheterization.

Most Care PRAM

The Most Care/Pressure Recording Analytic Method (PRAM) system (Vytech Health; Padova, Italy) utilizes only arterial line waveforms in its analysis of hemodynamic function and requires no external calibration or patient demographic data. Compared to the other methods of pulse contour analysis, which measure the pulsatile change in the area under the curve during systole, PRAM incorporates both the pulsatile and continuous areas under the curve during systole, allowing for intrinsic assessment of systemic impedance. Using high frequency sampling, arrhythmias can be accommodated when determining CO although its use in patients with severe aortic valvular disease and dissections is limited.

Bioreactance

Non-invasive cardiac output monitoring (NICOM; Cheetah Medical; Wilmington, DE) utilizes the principles of bioreactance that result from pulsatile blood flow moving through the thorax to indirectly monitor hemodynamics. This technology does not require invasive monitoring, is portable, and is not affected by atrial dysrhythmias.

Four NICOM adhesive sensor pads placed on the patient's thorax transmit a very low current into the chest wall (Fig. 50.3). The thoracic aortic pulsatile blood flow displaces this current and transmits a voltage, a "phase shift," which correlates closely with blood volume. When this is measured over time, a value parallel to the SV is calculated and generates a Starling curve (Fig. 50.4). The same sensors can detect heart rate and calculate CO.

Starling's law, the principle that the heart changes its force of contraction as preload increases nadirs at a specific value after which

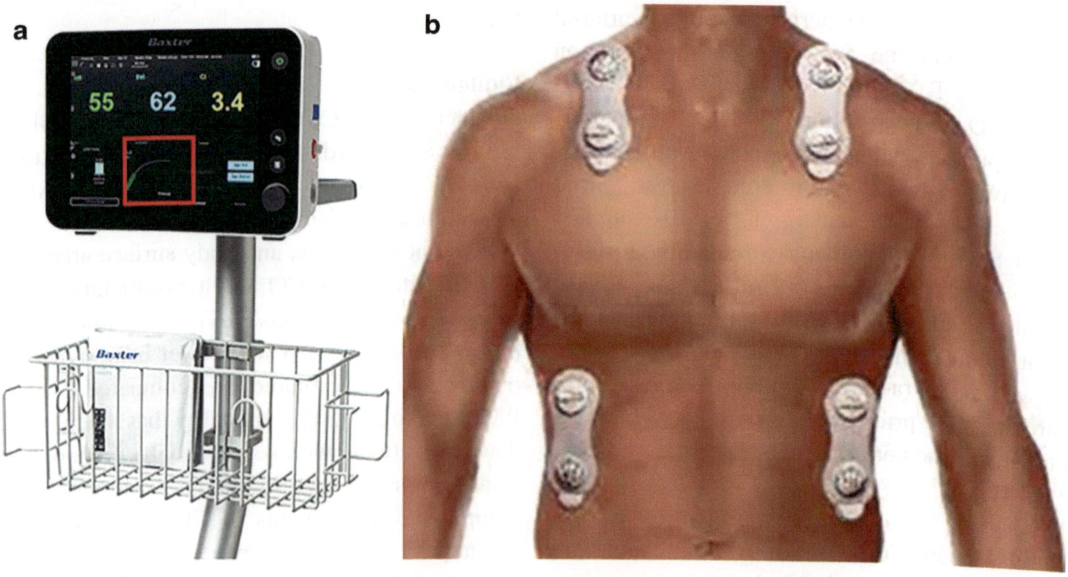

Fig. 50.3 (**a**) The NICOM monitor is a non-invasive portable device that displays cardiodynamics and generate a Frank-Starling curve (red box). (**b**) Placement of cutaneous sensors. https://usstarling.baxter.com/sites/g/files/ebysai2296/files/2020-04/Starling-Brochure.pdf

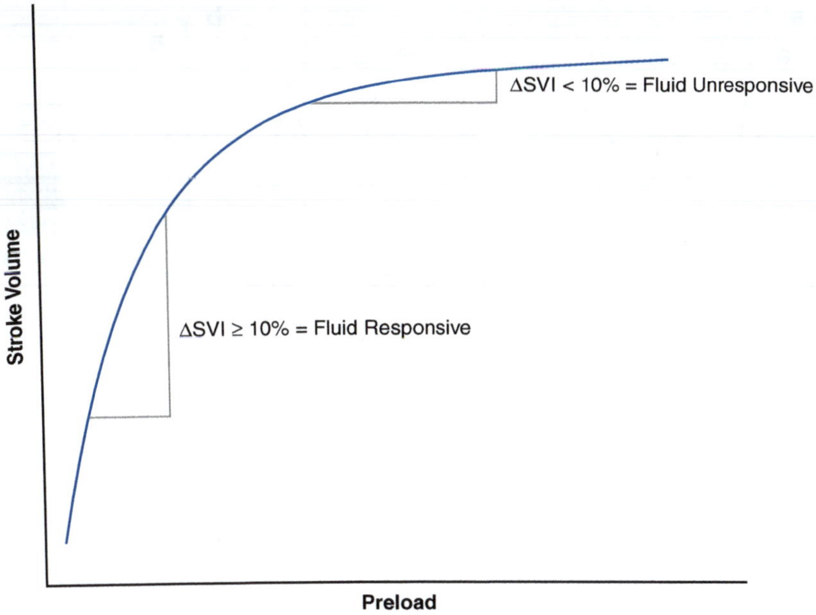

Fig. 50.4 The Frank-Starling Curve depicts changes in stroke volume as cardiac preload changes. https://www.baxter.de/de/medizinische-fachkraefte/hospital-care-stationaere-versorgung/starling-fluid-management-monitoring

further increases in preload are not beneficial. Dynamic, real-time interventions to assess the Starling curve utilizes a passive leg raise (non-invasive 250 cc fluid bolus) or a 250 mL intravenous fluid bolus (invasive bolus). The index of change in the stroke volume (%SVI) is calculated; %SVI values ≥10% are categorized as "fluid responsive." Additionally, NICOM assess total peripheral resistance and total peripheral resistance index, two values closely related to systemic vascular resistance, which can help discriminate classes of shock and guide therapy.

Limitations include improper electrode placement, inability to properly perform a fluid challenge, intra-abdominal hypertension, the presence of an open abdomen, and severe edema. These factors may reduce the accuracy of some NICOM data points. Studies have validated the accuracy of NICOM compared with the invasive PAC over a wide range of circulatory crisis. Importantly, the NICOM can be placed quickly and without risk in elderly patients where time to shock recognition and reversal is critical.

Transesophageal Doppler

Transesophageal Doppler (TED) has a role in select patients. It offers a small profile probe that can be inserted transorally or transnasally and provides continuous, reliable estimates of preload and afterload by evaluating the descending aortic waveform and calculating aortic blood flow to determine CO (Fig. 50.5). While not providing the detail of TTE or TEE, it can remain in place for up to 72 h and provides continuous hemodynamic monitoring in response to therapies such as fluid boluses. However, TED is limited by the need for sedation and airway protection in most patients. It is subject to misalignment during patient care and requires frequent repositioning to maintain a high-quality waveform. It is contraindicated in patient with local esophageal and oropharyngeal pathology or recent craniofacial trauma and may give inaccurate data in severe aortic valvular disease or in patients where surgery has altered the relationship between the aorta and the esophagus. It is advantageous in that the monitor and waveforms can be viewed without entering the patients' room. This feature is beneficial for patients on isolation, particularly during flares of COVID-19 infections.

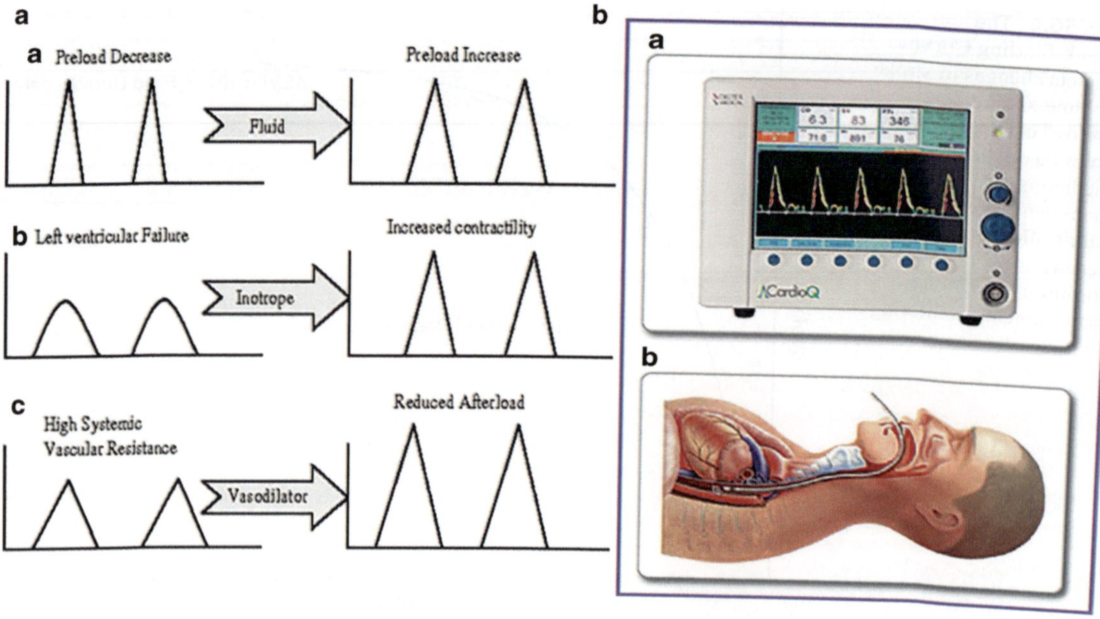

Fig. 50.5 Transesophageal Doppler showing (**a**) waveforms and compactness of monitor and (**b**) route of insertion. (D Hett, M Jonas. Non-invasive cardiac output monitoring. Intensive Crit Care Nurs. 2004;20:103–8. doi: 10.1016/j.iccn.2004.01.002)

Conclusion

The goals of resuscitation in the elderly patient who is critically ill are the same as for younger patients. That is, to restore perfusion to critical organs, correct oxygen debt to maintain aerobic metabolism and support homeostasis in the face of pre-existing comorbidities. Managing elderly patients in the ICU is challenging because of multiple comorbidities, frailty and limited physiologic reserve. These challenges demand an individualized, patient specific approach that balances obtaining valid physiologic information against the risks of intervention and erroneous data. An understanding of the patient's cardiopulmonary reserve and pre-existing disease will permit the clinician to select the best monitoring device to guide resuscitation with the goal of restorative care. Early monitoring is essential for favorable outcomes, especially in patients at the far end of the age spectrum. Age alone is an important risk factor for overall survival and the ability for recovery of pre-hospital functional status. Ultimately, outcomes with respect to performance status, return to pre-hospital living arrangements, need for ongoing medical care post-acute hospitalization, ethical considerations regarding medical futility, end of life care and cost are all impacted by the balance of providing care in the ICU to "treat acute the illness and not terminal pathology."

References

1. Weiss J, Freeman M, Low A, Fu R, Kerfoot A, Paynter R, et al. Benefits and harms of intensive blood pressure treatment in adults aged 60 years or older: a systematic review and meta-analysis. Ann Intern Med. 2017;166:419–29. https://doi.org/10.7326/M16-1754.
2. Davis JW, Shackford SR, Mackersie RC, Hoyt DB. Base deficit as a guide to volume resuscitation. J Trauma. 1988;28(10):1464–7. https://doi.org/10.1097/00005373-198810000-00010.

3. Flack JM, Bemi A. Blood pressure and the new ACC/AHA hypertension guidelines. Trends Cardiovasc Med. 2020;30(3):160–4. https://doi.org/10.1016/j.tcm.2019.05.003.
4. Benetos A, Petrovic M, Strandberg T. Hypertension management in older and frail older patients. Circ Res. 2019;124(7):1045–60. https://doi.org/10.1161/CIRCRESAHA.118.313236.
5. Zeserson E, Goodgame B, Hess JD, Schultz K, Hoon C, Lamb K, et al. Correlation of venous blood gas and pulse oximetry with arterial blood gas in the undifferentiated critically ill patient. J Intensive Care Med. 2016;33(3):176–81. https://doi.org/10.1177/0885066616652597.
6. Jentzer JC, Kashou AH, Lopez-Jimenez F, Attia ZI, Kapa S, Friedman PA, et al. Mortality risk stratification using artificial intelligence-augmented electrocardiogram in cardiac intensive care unit patients. Eur Heart J Acute Cardiovasc. 2021;10(5):532–41. https://doi.org/10.1093/ehjacc/zuaa021.
7. Richard C, Warszawski J, Anguel N, Deye N, Combes A, Barnoud D, et al. Early use of the pulmonary artery catheter and outcomes in patients with shock and acute respiratory distress syndrome: a randomized controlled trial. JAMA. 2003;290:2713–20. https://doi.org/10.1001/jama.290.20.2713.
8. Cheitlin M, Armstrong W, Aurigemma G, Beller G, Bierman F, Davis J, et al. ACC/AHA/ASE 2003 guideline update for the clinical application of echocardiography: summary article: a report of the American College of Cardiology/American Heart Association task force on practice guidelines (ACC/AHA/ASE Committee to update the 1997 guidelines for the clinical application of echocardiography). J Am Soc Echocardiogr. 2003;16(10):1091–110. https://doi.org/10.1016/S0894-7317(03)00685-0.
9. Walley PE, Walley KR, Goodgame B, Punjabi V, Sirounis D. A practical approach to goal-directed echocardiography in the critical care setting. Crit Care. 2014;18:681. https://doi.org/10.1186/s13054-014-0681-z.
10. Maizel J, Airapetian N, Lorne E, Tribouilloy C, Massy Z, Slama M. Diagnosis of central hypovolemia by using passive leg raising. Intensive Care Med. 2007;33(7):1133–8. https://doi.org/10.1007/s00134-007-0642-y.
11. Drummond KE, Murphy E. Minimally invasive cardiac output monitors. Contin Educ Anaesth Crit Care Pain. 2012;12(1):5–10. https://doi.org/10.1093/bjaceaccp/mkr044.
12. Gödje O, Höke K, Goetz AE, Felbinger TW, Reuter DA, Reichart B, et al. Reliability of a new algorithm for continuous cardiac output determination by pulse-contour analysis during hemodynamic instability. Crit Care Med. 2002;30(1):52–8. https://doi.org/10.1097/00003246-200201000-00008.
13. Mayer J, Boldt J, Poland R, Peterson A, Manecke GR Jr. Continuous arterial pressure waveform based cardiac output using the FloTrac/Vigileo: a review and meta-analysis. J Cardiothorac Vasc Anesth. 2009;23(3):401–6. https://doi.org/10.1053/j.jvca.2009.03.003.
14. Romagnoli S, Bevilacqua S, Lazzeri C, Ciappi F, Dini D, Pratesi C, et al. Most care®: a minimally invasive system for hemodynamic monitoring powered by the pressure recording analytical method (PRAM). HSR Proc Intensive Care Cardiovasc Anesth. 2009;1(2):20–7.
15. Schober P, Loer SA, Schwarte LA. Transesophageal Doppler devices: a technical review. J Clin Monit Comput. 2009;23(6):391–401. https://doi.org/10.1007/s10877-009-9204-x.

51 Nutritional Assessment and Therapy

Patrizio Petrone and Corrado P. Marini

Introduction

Malnutrition, defined as a condition where there is an imbalance between the energy derived from nutrients and the energy required to sustain cellular and tissue growth and, more importantly, normal organ function, has detrimental effects on body function and clinical outcomes. Of note, the stated imbalance may pertain to deficiencies (undernutrition) or excesses in a person's intake of nutrients. For the purpose of this chapter, we refer to malnutrition secondary to an insufficient intake of nutrients. The global prevalence of malnutrition due to insufficient intake of calories (<1000 calories per day) among elderly ranges from 23 to 46%. As people age, they eat less and tend to favor foods with lower nutritional value. The decreased food intake in the elderly, known as the "anorexia of aging," leads to a relative increase in the fat mass and a substantial decrease in muscle mass. There are many age-related physiological changes that contribute to decreased food intake, including changes in compliance of the gastric fundus, decreased stretch of the antrum, and delayed gastric emptying in response to large meals, all of which are responsible for the development of postprandial anorexia. Additional factors contributing to decreased food intake involve changes in hormonal responses, altered taste and smell, decreased appetite, and lack of pleasure when eating (dysgeusia), marital status, degree of education, and socioeconomic status. Older persons may also have inadequate food intake because of specific mechanical problems, such as the presence of tremors from Parkinson's disease, dysphagia, and senile dementia. The nine components of weight loss in the elderly, known as the 9Ds of malnutrition include: (1). Dysfunction; (2). Drugs; (3). Disease; (4). Dysphagia; (5). Diarrhea; (6). Depression; (7). Dementia; (8). Dentition; (9). Dysgeusia.

P. Petrone (✉)
Department of Surgery, NYU Long Island School of Medicine, NYU Langone Hospital—Long Island, Mineola, New York, USA
e-mail: Patrizio.Petrone@nyulangone.org

C. P. Marini
Department of Surgery, Albert Einstein College of Medicine, Jacobi Medical Center, Bronx, NY, USA

Incidence

Studies have shown that malnutrition has serious implications for recovery from disease and is associated with increased morbidity and mortality. Malnourished older adults tend to have higher rates of postoperative complications, such as wound infection, intra-abdominal abscesses, enteric fistulae, and anastomotic leakage and non-surgical sites infections (e.g., lungs, urinary tract), longer hospital stays, a higher rate of re-admission, and increased healthcare cost. It is

P. Petrone, C. E.M. Brathwaite (eds.), *Acute Care Surgery in Geriatric Patients*,
https://doi.org/10.1007/978-3-031-30651-8_51

estimated that between 24% and 51% of surgical patients are at risk of malnutrition, with the risk increasing up to 60% in the elderly. The absolute number of malnourished older people is increasing as a result of the increasing proportion of older people, and in particular, for the subset of the "very old" (age >80 years), as opposed to the "young old" (65–80 years of age). If one uses a body mass index (BMI) threshold value of 18.5 kg/m^2 to define malnutrition, then between 23% and 37% of people ≥65 years are considered to be malnourished at the time of admission to a hospital for surgical in-patient procedures. The prevalence of malnutrition depends heavily on the specific nutritional tool used to assess the nutritional status of the patient. The utility of the tool should be based on the specific patient population.

Poor nutritional status is also associated with the geriatric syndrome, which is characterized by the occurrence of health conditions affecting functionality and quality of life. Undernutrition is a cornerstone of nutritional frailty, the disability that occurs in old age due to the unintentional physiological or pathological loss of body weight and sarcopenia. Sarcopenia is the decline in muscle mass and strength that occurs with healthy aging. Studies have confirmed that malnutrition contributes to the development of delirium and pressure sores in hospitalized older patients. Additionally, malnutrition at the time of hospital admission is a major risk factor for in-hospital falls.

Diagnosis and Management

The likelihood of patients being alive and returning to their own homes after hospital discharge is an important goal in the care of hospitalized older patients. After acute hospitalization, frail older adults are more likely to be admitted to nursing facilities due to their dependency on assistance with activities of daily living (ADL). However, institutionalization often leads to a more rapid deterioration of muscle function due to the limited implementation of early physical rehabilitation aimed at mitigating the detrimental effects of protracted immobilization. Elderly surviv have long-term physical disability leading to d ficulty of ADL such as standing from a ch leading to poor health-related quality of li While the location of discharge after acute geri ric hospitalization is an important issue in old patients, studies on the association between nut tional status and discharge location are limited.

As comprehensive nutritional assessment complex and time consuming, several screenin tools are used to assess nutritional status. F instance, the Mini-Nutritional Assessme (MNA) is a validated test recommended for nutri tional screening in older populations and ha been widely used in different clinical settings The MNA is a practical, noninvasive tool tha allows rapid evaluation of the nutritional status o older adults. Various studies on the associatio between malnutrition and clinical outcomes i hospitalized older adults using the MNA have been conducted. While in some studies lower MNA scores were successful at identifying frailty in hospitalized older patients and at predicting post-discharge emergency department visits, and mortality, in another study, MNA scores at admission failed to predict long-term mortality.

Malnutrition status by the MNA is associated with adverse outcomes in older patients hospitalized in acute geriatric centers. Older inpatients with malnutrition are five times more likely to be discharged to nursing homes or long-term care hospitals and three times more likely to die within 3 months. Additionally, their chance of developing geriatric syndrome during hospitalization more than doubled.

Frailty, as a reflection of decreased physiological reserve, is closely associated with biological age, concurrent medical conditions, morbidity, and decreased survival in older adults. Malnutrition, which is included in the assessment tool of frailty, is considered a key factor in the progression of frailty. The addition of a stressor event such as pneumonia or urinary tract infection to a frail older person with impairment of balance or cognition explains the geriatric syndromes of falls and delirium, respectively, as consequences of the loss of homeostatic reserve. Unintentional weight loss, a representative criterion for the frailty phenotype model, is a major risk factor for pressure sore development.

There are various definitions for aging in place, but it generally refers to the phenomenon of older adults that remain living within their communities with some level of independence, rather than in residential care. One of the biggest threats to aging in place is that older adults become ADL dependent due to functional decline after acute disease.

The incidence of disability acquired by older patients during a hospital stay is very high and the number of hospitalized older patients is expected to continue to increase with the increasing proportion of people older than 65 years of age requiring elective and emergency surgical procedures. A recent Dutch study reported a 20% increase in functional disability in older patients at discharge after an acute hospitalization. This disability may be related to the primary reason for hospital admission, but the disease-related catabolism along with immobilization also impairs rehabilitation, even when the illness that necessitated the hospitalization was successfully treated. Currently, the interest toward functional complications after acute illness is growing, especially with the rising incidence of Long COVID and Post-Acute COVID-19 syndromes and their adverse effects on quality of life.

Functional decline may be a consequence of muscle wasting which compounds the pre-existing age-related muscle loss. Sarcopenia is defined as a reduced muscle strength combined with a reduced muscle quantity or quality. Sarcopenia due to physiological aging may be exacerbated by disease-related factors, especially inflammation. Inflammation mediates different signaling pathways in muscle cells, which leads to muscle atrophy. Hospital-associated factors such as prolonged fasting for technical or surgical reasons and protracted bed rest increase muscle wasting and muscular dysfunction. Sarcopenic patients have a three times higher risk of falls, a 50% higher risk of hospitalization, more than a twice risk of institutionalization, and a 40% higher mortality. Social isolation and depression contribute to the development of sarcopenia. Late-life depressive symptoms induce sedentary behavior, which exacerbates the vicious circle of sarcopenia. Due to the association of sarcopenia with debilitating diseases, sarcopenic patients are more likely to suffer from lower quality of life.

Massanet et al. have proposed a nutritional rehabilitation strategy to facilitate the functional recovery of patients after intensive care unit (ICU) stay. Presently, there is ongoing research aimed at improving the nutritional rehabilitation of older patients after an acute hospitalization, by identifying the specific type and duration of nutritional support targeted to the age and the disease of the patient. Given the heterogeneity of older patients, it is still not clear if there are some subgroups of patients who could benefit more from nutritional rehabilitation. In view of recent published studies, suggested approaches include dietary advice, such as energy or protein-enriched diets, anabolic agents, and essential amino acid supplementation.

Current reviews mainly focused only on malnourished older patients, mortality outcome, or muscle function. Overall, nutritional rehabilitation of any type improves functional status and muscle mass but has not been shown to change the quality of life or disposition at discharge among older acutely hospitalized patients. Identified predictors of success of nutritional rehabilitation include age, compliance, and treatment duration (at least 2 months). However, there is heterogeneity of the nutritional support provided to older patients during and following an acute illness in terms of patients' inclusion, interventions' protocol, and nutritional assessment.

Functional Status

Individualized high protein and energy dense diet combined with physical exercise improve functional status irrespective of the assessment techniques used, especially when given to "young old" patients (age 65–80) who have been admitted for acute medical conditions. It has been previously reported that aging is associated with functional decline and that younger patients recover more easily from disease-induced disability. The risk of falls is associated with aging, which may explain why patients admitted to orthopedic services tend to be older. Calcium 3-hydroxy-3-methylbutyrate monohydrate (Ca-HMB) supplementation has been shown to improve the functional status of old patients hospitalized for medical and orthopedic reasons, but not of healthy not-hospitalized old people, suggesting that the most relevant benefit of Ca-HMB appears in catabolic situations.

There is a high heterogeneity when it comes to functional status assessment across the studies. The sensitivity of the scores to assess functional status changes is heterogeneous and some scores partially assess the functional status. The findings reported by recent meta-analyses suggest a lack of benefit of nutritional interventions on the functional status of older patients. In particular, the meta-analysis of van Wijngaarden et al. focusing on older patients during geriatric rehabilitation did not show any effect of nutritional interventions on functional status. Another systematic review of Welch et al. also highlighted the lack of effectiveness of nutritional strategies on functional status of hospitalized older patients. Furthermore, Welch et al. reported that the improvement in functional status among the studies was associated with the rate of compliance, with the highest improvement rates associated with the highest rate of compliance.

The systematic review of Milne et al. published in 2009 did not corroborate an improvement in functional status from enhanced nutritional support in elderly patients. The lack of beneficial effect of nutritional support on functional outcome was in part attributed to the lack of analysis of outcomes stratified by intention to treat, the inadequate reporting of numbers of participants, and the lack of reporting reasons for losses of follow-up. Despite an improvement in the functional status of the elderly, the evidence does not show a decrease in the rate of post-discharge institutionalization. It is plausible that lack of benefit from the standpoint of discharge disposition to home instead of other institution is due to the fact that the discharge from the hospital occurs typically after a period of nutritional rehabilitation shorter than 2 months that has been shown to be beneficial from the final standpoint of disposition. Furthermore, there is a systematic exclusion of the elderly patient with several morbidities that could benefit from the nutritional rehabilitation.

Muscle Mass

Combined therapies (high protein diet + physical exercise) and Ca-HMB supplementation appeared effective to reduce the hospitalization-related loss of muscle mass. Despite a relative anabolic resistance, protein muscle synthesis is preserved even in older patients and combined therapies (nutrition + physical exercise) are the most promising to overcome the catabolic state from acute disease. Muscle mass decline may precede functional loss and it is an important treatment target as muscle wasting related to hospitalization may induce long-term disability.

Conclusion

Nutritional status evaluated using the MNA is an independent predictor of various negative outcomes among older hospitalized patients. Poor nutritional status assessed by serum albumin levels, the most widely used biochemical marker, can predict mortality, but not geriatric syndrome or discharge disposition, which might reflect the patients' functional decline. As a multidimensional tool, the MNA needs to be used more actively for the nutritional assessment of geriatric patients. Current evidence supports the use of nutritional rehabilitation for at least 2 months to mitigate the prevalence of hospital-acquired weakness and muscle mass loss, especially among patients between 65 and 80 years old. The comparative assessment of nutritional strategies would require a standard set of outcome variables, the compliance assessment, an individualized approach, and an intention-to-treat analysis. There is a need to increase the awareness of caregivers toward the nutritional component of patients' management after an acute event.

References

1. Kaiser MJ, Bauer JM, Rämsch C, Uter W, Guigoz Y, Cederholm T, et al. Frequency of malnutrition in older adults: a multinational perspective using the mini nutritional assessment. J Am Geriatr Soc. 2010;58(9):1734–8. https://doi.org/10.1111/j.1532-5415.2010.03016.x.
2. Wysokiński A, Sobów T, Kłoszewska I, Kostka T. Mechanisms of the anorexia of aging-a review. Age (Dordr). 2015;37(4):9821. https://doi.org/10.1007/s11357-015-9821-x.
3. Avelino-Silva T, Jaluul O. Malnutrition in hospitalized older patients: management strategies to improve patient care and clinical outcomes. Int J Gerontol. 2017;11:56–61. https://doi.org/10.1016/j.ijge.2016.11.002.
4. Rosted E, Prokofieva T, Sanders S, Schultz M. Serious consequences of malnutrition and delirium in frail older patients. J Nutr Gerontol Geriatr. 2018;37:105–16. https://doi.org/10.1080/21551197.2018.1470055.
5. Ishida Y, Maeda K, Nonogaki T, Shimizu A, Yamanaka Y, Matsuyama R, et al. Malnutrition at admission predicts in-hospital falls in hospitalized older adults. Nutrients. 2020;12:541. https://doi.org/10.3390/nu12020541.
6. Ellis G, Gardner M, Tsiachristas A, Langhorne P, Burke O, Harwood R, et al. Comprehensive geriatric assessment for older adults admitted to hospital. Cochrane Database Syst Rev. 2017;2017(9):Cd006211. https://doi.org/10.1002/14651858.CD006211.pub3.
7. Kang MG, Choi JY, Yoo HJ, Park SY, Kim Y, Kim JY, et al. Impact of malnutrition evaluated by the mini nutritional assessment on the prognosis of acute hospitalized older adults. Front Nutr. 2023;9:1046985. https://doi.org/10.3389/fnut.2022.1046985.
8. Yong SJ. Long COVID or post-COVID-19 syndrome: putative pathophysiology, risk factors, and treatments. Infect Dis Ther. 2021;53(10):737–54. https://doi.org/10.1080/23744235.2021.1924397.
9. Slee A, Birch D, Stokoe D. The relationship between malnutrition risk and clinical outcomes in a cohort of frail older hospital patients. Clin Nutr ESPEN. 2016;15:57–62. https://doi.org/10.1016/j.clnesp.2016.06.002.
10. van Seben R, Reichardt LA, Aarden JJ, van der Schaaf M, van der Esch M, Englebert R, et al. The course of geriatric syndromes in acutely hospitalized older adults: the hospital-ADL study. J Am Med Dir Assoc. 2019;20(2):152e8.
11. De Spiegeleer A, Kahya H, Sanchez-Rodriguez D, Piotrowicz K, Surqin M, Marco E, et al. Acute sarcopenia changes following hospitalization: influence of pre-admission care dependency level. Age Ageing. 2021;50(6):2140e6.
12. Volkert D, Beck AM, Cederholm T, Cruz-Jentoft A, Goisser S, Hooper L, et al. ESPEN guideline on clinical nutrition and hydration in geriatrics. Clin Nutr. 2019;38(1):10e47.
13. Ridley EJ, Chapple L, Chapman M. Nutrition intake in the post-ICU hospitalization period. Curr Opin Clin Nutr Metab Care. 2020;23(2):111–5. https://doi.org/10.1097/MCO.0000000000000637.
14. Ferrucci L, Cooper R, Shardell M, Simonsick E, Schrack J, Kuh D. Age-related change in mobility: perspectives from life course epidemiology and geroscience. J Genrontol A Biol Sci Med Sci. 2016;71(9):1184–94. https://doi.org/10.1093/gerona/glw043.
15. Szklarzewska S, Mottale R, Engelman E, De Breucker S, Preiser JC. Nutritional rehabilitation after acute illness among older patients: a systematic review and meta-analysis. Clin Nutr. 2023;42(3):309–36. https://doi.org/10.1016/j.clnu.2023.01.013.

Acute Kidney Injury in the Geriatric Population

52

David A. Lieb II, Corrado P. Marini, John McNelis, and Erin R. Lewis

Introduction and Epidemiology

Acute kidney injury (AKI) is an acute decrease in renal function over hours to days. Common among hospitalized patients, the number of hospitalizations specifically attributed to AKI has increased from 281,500 in 2005 to 504,600 in 2014. In that period, the total number of hospitalizations with AKI as a secondary diagnosis also increased from 1 million to over 3.2 million. AKI is of particular concern among critically ill patients (e.g., those with sepsis or severe trauma), with up to 67% of trauma ICU patients developing AKI during the course of admission.

The increasing incidence of AKI is often associated with an aging population, as elderly patients are more likely to have comorbidities such as diabetes, hypertension, and peripheral vascular disease, which may affect renal function. While these disorders are significantly associated with chronic kidney disease (CKD), their role in AKI is less clear. Factors shown to be significantly associated with development of AKI include advanced age, severity of illness/injury, use of nephrotoxic medications and antibiotics (e.g., vancomycin), use of radiocontrast agents, and hypotension. Increasing age is an established risk factor because of the associated renal changes. Several renal changes occur with advancing age including sclerosis of glomeruli, compensatory tubular hypertrophy, decreasing numbers of functional nephrons, and loss of cortical volume followed by decreased overall kidney volume. These age-related changes ultimately cause a gradual decline in renal function, thereby reducing physiologic reserve, and consequently increasing the risk of AKI following a renal insult.

Age-related changes in renal function must be viewed in the context of the heterogeneity in the overall health and functional status of elderly patients. While many geriatric patients maintain overall good health and preserved functional

D. A. Lieb II
Department of Surgery, Albert Einstein College of Medicine, Jacobi Medical Center, Bronx, NY, USA

Army Medical Department (AMEDD) Student Detachment, US Army Medical Center of Excellence, JBSA Fort Sam Houston, San Antonio, TX, USA

C. P. Marini
Department of Surgery, Albert Einstein College of Medicine, Jacobi Medical Center, Bronx, NY, USA

J. McNelis
Department of Surgery, Albert Einstein College of Medicine, Jacobi Medical Center, Bronx, NY, USA

Department of Surgery, Albert Einstein College of Medicine, Bronx, NY, USA

E. R. Lewis (✉)
Department of Surgery, Albert Einstein College of Medicine, Jacobi Medical Center, Bronx, NY, USA

Department of Population Health and Epidemiology, Albert Einstein College of Medicine, Bronx, NY, USA
e-mail: lewise8@nychhc.org

P. Petrone, C. E.M. Brathwaite (eds.), *Acute Care Surgery in Geriatric Patients*, https://doi.org/10.1007/978-3-031-30651-8_52

status, others may have significant impairments in daily function and in overall health, reflected in a concept known as frailty. Frailty, which can be determined through clinical assessments, is associated with increased morbidity and mortality among elderly patients, and it has been associated with an increased risk of AKI as well. Therefore, providers should be aware of the increased risk of AKI among older hospitalized patients, particularly among frail elderly patients.

Once AKI develops, it has significant implications in terms of morbidity and mortality. For instance, Harbrecht et al. found that among elderly trauma patients, AKI, particularly severe AKI, was associated with increased length of intensive care unit (ICU) stay, increased time on ventilator, and a more than tripled risk of mortality. These adverse outcomes are not limited to elderly patients. Approximately 27% of critically ill pediatric and young adult patients will likewise develop AKI, with development of AKI also independently associated with increased mortality in these patients. Because of these clinical implications, avoidance, prompt recognition, and appropriate management of AKI are of the utmost importance.

Definition and Staging

Several definitions for acute kidney injury exist. The Renal Injury, Failure, Loss, and End-stage renal disease (RIFLE) (Table 52.1), first developed in 2004, has 5 categories to grade AKI. The first three are based on changes in serum creatinine (S_{Cr}) and glomerular filtration rate (GFR) and/or changes in urine output (UOP), while the latter two definitions (Loss and End-stage renal disease, or ESRD) are based on duration of renal replacement therapy (RRT). These definitions progress from most sensitive for AKI to most specific for AKI.

The Acute Kidney Injury Network (AKIN) criteria (Table 52.2), published in 2007, expanded upon the RIFLE criteria. Notable differences include the exclusion of Loss and ESRD

Table 52.1 AKI Classification under the RIFLE criteria

Classification	GFR	UOP
Risk	Increase in S_{Cr} to 1.5× baseline OR ≥25% decrease in baseline GFR	<0.5 mL/kg/h for 6 h
Injury	Increase in S_{Cr} to 2× baseline OR ≥50% decrease in baseline GFR	<0.5 mL/kg/h for 12 h
Failure	Increase in S_{Cr} to 3× baseline OR ≥75% decrease in baseline GFR OR Increase in S_{Cr} to ≥4 mg/dL (with an acute increase of ≥0.5 mg/dL)	<0.3 mL/kg/h for 24 h OR Anuria for 12 h
Loss	RRT required for >4 weeks	
ESRD	RRT required for 3 months	

Table 52.2 AKIN staging system for AKI

Stage	Serum creatinine (S_{Cr})	UOP
1	Increase in S_{Cr} ≥0.3 mg/dL (≥26.4 μmol/L) OR Increase in S_{Cr} to 1.5–2× baseline	<0.5 mL/kg/h for 6 h
2	Increase in S_{Cr} to 2–3× baseline	<0.5 mL/kg/hr. for 12 h
3	Increase in S_{Cr} to ≥3× baseline OR Increase in SCr to ≥4 mg/dL (with an acute increase of ≥0.5 mg/dL)	<0.3 mL/kg/h for 24 h OR Anuria for 12 h

Table 52.3 KDIGO staging criteria for acute kidney injury

Stage	Serum creatinine level	Urine output
1	Increase to 1.5–1.9 times baseline OR ≥0.3 mg/dL (26.5 μmol/L) increase from baseline	<0.5 mL/kg/h for 6–12 h
2	Increase to 2.0–2.9 times baseline	<0.5 mL/kg/h for ≥12 h
3	Increase to ≥3.0 times baseline OR Increase to ≥4.0 mg/dL (353.6 μmol/L) OR Initiation of renal replacement therapy OR For patients <18 years, decrease in eGFR <35 mL/min/1.73m^2	<0.3 mL/kg/h for ≥24 h OR Anuria for ≥12 h

grades from RIFLE, as these were felt to be outcomes of AKI rather than measure of severity. Additionally, Stage 1 includes an absolute increase in serum creatinine of at least 0.3 mg/dL as part of its criteria to account for changes in serum creatinine associated with adverse outcomes but would otherwise be insufficient to meet RIFLE criteria.

The most recently developed staging system, the Kidney Disease: Improving Global Outcomes (KDIGO) criteria, was published in 2012 and incorporates elements of both RIFLE and AKIN (Table 52.3). AKI is defined as an increase in serum creatinine by at least 0.3 mg/dL (or 26.5 μmol/L) within 48 h, an increase in serum creatinine of at least 50% from baseline (obtained within the previous 7 days), or urine output less than 0.5 mL/kg/h for at least 6 h.

Etiology

AKI has three main etiologies: pre-renal, intrinsic, and post-renal (Table 52.4). Pre-renal AKI—also known as pre-renal azotemia—occurs due to decreased renal perfusion, in turn causing decreased glomerular filtration rate (GFR), in the setting of normal renal anatomy. Decreased perfusion can be due to decreased circulatory volume, impaired cardiac output, vasomodulation of renal blood vessels, or systemic vasodilation causing compromised perfusion.

In contrast, intrinsic AKI results from direct damage to renal structures. The most common type of intrinsic AKI, acute tubular necrosis (ATN), can result either from ischemia or nephrotoxic insults. As the causes of ischemic ATN can overlap with those of pre-renal AKI, additional testing is required to differentiate between the two. Many medications can cause nephrotoxin-mediated ATN, including multiple antibiotics such as amphotericin B, aminoglycosides, and vancomycin, contrast solutions, and immunosuppressive drugs (e.g., cyclosporine, tacrolimus). Rhabdomyolysis can also cause ATN due to the toxicity of myoglobin to tubules.

The tubules are not the only structures that can be affected in intrinsic AKI. Glomerular injury can occur due to immune complex diseases (e.g., lupus), as well as autoimmune disorders targeting glomerular structures (e.g., basement membrane disease). Tubulointerstitial injury causes include drug-induced acute interstitial nephritis (AIN), commonly associated with the use of sulfa-containing antibiotics and non-steroidal anti-inflammatory drugs (NSAIDs). Vasculature can be damaged by vasculitis disorders and other systemic conditions such as hemolytic uremic syndrome and thrombotic thrombocytopenic purpura.

Finally, post-renal AKI can result from obstruction of urine flow, either physical or functional, which creates backpressure in the tubules and—in turn—decreases GFR. While obstruction can occur at any point from the renal pelvis to the urethra, any obstructions proximal to the bladder (e.g., ureteral) must be bilateral for AKI to occur. Benign prostatic hypertrophy is one of

Table 52.4 List of types of AKI, mechanism of each type, and example causes

Type	Mechanism	Examples
Pre-renal	Decreased effective circulating volume reaching kidney	• *Hypovolemia*: Hemorrhage, burns, GI losses (vomiting or diarrhea) • *Reduced cardiac output*: Decompensated congestive heart failure, cardiogenic shock • *Renal vasomodulation*: ACEI/ARB use, NSAID use, hepatorenal syndrome, hypercalcemia, iodine-containing contrast agents • *Systemic vasodilation*: Sepsis/SIRS, anaphylaxis
Intrinsic	Damage/necrosis of nephron structures	• *Glomerular*: Post-infectious glomerulonephritis, IgA nephropathy, lupus nephritis • *Tubules*: Rhabdomyolysis, ischemia, antibiotics (e.g., aminoglycosides), contrast agents, nephrotoxins (e.g., ethylene glycol) • *Tubulointerstitial*: Acute allergic interstitial nephritis, infection • *Vasculature*: Hemolytic uremic syndrome, thrombotic thrombocytopenic purpura, vasculitis, arterial/venous thrombosis, malignant hypertension
Post-renal	Obstruction of urine flow	• *Bladder*: Benign prostatic hyperplasia, neurogenic bladder, urethral stricture, malignancy, blood clots, malignancy • *Ureter (bilateral or unilateral with one kidney)*: Nephrolithiasis, stricture, transection, retroperitoneal fibrosis, malignancy • *Pelvis*: Obstructing mass, papillary necrosis

the most common causes of post-renal AKI, particularly in men. Other causes of obstruction include neurogenic bladder, bilateral nephrolithiasis, blot clots, and malignancy.

Diagnostic Testing

Once AKI has been diagnosed efforts should be directed at determining its etiology. Workup should include a review of patient history for potentially contributory events, such as administration of nephrotoxic medications, systemic illness, and underlying medical conditions that increase the risk of AKI. Physical exam can also assist with identifying factors such as volume status and rashes. However, these alone are often insufficient to determine the specific etiology, and additional laboratory tests are usually needed.

The typical next steps include a urinalysis with urine microscopy and urine electrolytes. Urine microscopy may identify casts associated with specific AKI etiologies. For instance, ATN classically presents with "muddy brown casts" consisting of renal tubular epithelial cells and casts. Pre-renal AKI, in contrast, usually shows hyaline casts. Glomerular injury will typically present with red blood cells on microscopy, while tubulointerstitial injury often shows white blood cell casts. Acute interstitial nephritis, for instance, is classically associated with eosinophils in urine, although this finding is not sensitive. Urinalysis may also demonstrate crystals. These crystals, which can cause AKI via tubule obstruction or via inflammation and subsequently tubular necrosis, can be seen with certain medications (e.g., sulfa antibiotics, methotrexate, protease inhibitors, acyclovir, foscarnet), as well as in disorders associated with increased light-chain production (e.g., multiple myeloma).

While the above urinalysis findings can help with specific diagnoses, urine electrolytes can be more generally helpful in identifying the underlying etiology. Urine electrolytes are typically used to calculate the fractional excretion of sodium (FENa) as shown below, where U refers to urine concentration and S refers to serum concentration (both in mmol/L):

$$FENa = \frac{U_{Na} * S_{Cr}}{S_{Na} * U_{Cr}} * 100$$

Proper interpretation of FENa requires an understanding of renal physiology. Under normal circumstances, renal baroreceptors located in the juxtaglomerular apparatus detect decreases in renal perfusion and in turn trigger activation of the renal-angiotensin-aldosterone system. This system triggers increased sodium reabsorption to increase fluid retention and in turn overall circulating volume. The increase in sodium reabsorption results in decreased urinary sodium excretion. Pre-renal AKI is typically associated with a FENa of less than 1%, and a urinary sodium concentration less than 20 mmol/L.

In contrast, intrinsic AKI results in damage to kidney structures, including the tubules that affect sodium reabsorption, thereby resulting in increased urinary excretion of sodium. As such, intrinsic AKI is associated with a FENa over 1% and a urine sodium concentration greater than 40 mmol/L. The consequence of these urinary losses is also reflected in the urine osmolality. Urine osmolality will typically be over 500 mOsm/kg for pre-renal AKI, whereas intrinsic AKI will usually present with urine osmolality less than 350 mOsm/kg.

The diagnosis of post-renal AKI includes a renal ultrasound. While renal ultrasound findings may be non-specific, they can also show hydronephrosis consistent with downstream obstruction. Outside of post-renal AKI, renal ultrasound has more limited utility and will typically provide less defined findings, such as generalized atrophy in chronic kidney disease. If, after the above workup, the underlying etiology and/or diagnosis remain unclear, a renal biopsy can be performed. As this is invasive, it is usually reserved for intrinsic pathology that cannot be identified with routine workup, or those that require confirmation (e.g., autoimmune disorders) prior to initiating treatment.

Management

The goal of management for AKI is to prevent further renal injury, address any life-threatening metabolic derangements, and correct the underlying etiology. For pre-renal AKI, the objective is to ensure adequate renal perfusion. In critically ill patients, particularly those with sepsis, this typically entails a goal mean arterial pressure (MAP) of 65 mm Hg. However, since most young-old (65–80 years) and old-old elderly (>80 years) have systolic hypertension due to aging, with rates greater than 68% in the young-old and close to 85% for the old-old, the target MAP to maintain adequate renal perfusion may be much higher, particularly in elderly patients with poorly controlled hypertension. To restore intravascular volume (e.g., sepsis or GI losses), resuscitation should ideally use balanced solutions, such as Lactated Ringer's, as use of normal saline is associated with a greater rate of in-hospital mortality and renal injury.

Management of intrinsic AKI focuses on correcting the specific cause of injury and removing any offending agents/medications, if applicable. In addition to removing the offending agent, any potentially nephrotoxic medications the patient may be receiving (e.g., NSAIDs, ACE inhibitors/ARBs) should be discontinued; consideration should also include identification of alternatives to antibiotics with associated nephrotoxicity, such as vancomycin. Renally-cleared medications, particularly those with narrow therapeutic indices—such as lithium—should also have doses adjusted based on GFR to ensure appropriate therapeutic concentrations and avoid toxicity. For post-renal AKI, the obstruction to urine flow should be relieved; this may range from urinary catheter placement for urethral obstruction (e.g., benign prostatic hyperplasia) to percutaneous nephrostomy placement for proximal ureteral or renal pelvic obstruction.

For patients taking diuretics prior to admission, diuretics should be held until renal function recovers, as they can lead to further depletion of intravascular volume and worsening of renal function. Some have advocated for diuretic use in

AKI to improve urine output, which may be thought to improve outcomes, but evidence for this is limited at best. The KDIGO guidelines do not recommend routine use of diuretics, as evidence is scant regarding their overall benefit in AKI. As such, diuretic use should be limited to correcting volume overload.

Additional consideration should be given to the administration of radiological contrast, which can cause AKI in at-risk patients (e.g., pre-existing CKD) and worsen renal function with existing AKI. When possible, IV and intra-arterial contrast administration should be avoided in these patients, and alternative imaging modalities (e.g., non-contrast CT scans) should be utilized. However, for circumstances in which contrast administration cannot be avoided, several strategies can help reduce the likelihood of contrast-induced nephropathy. If contrast must be used, the lowest amount of contrast necessary should be used, and iso-osmolar or low-osmolar contrast—both of which have been shown to be less nephrotoxic—should be used. Pre-procedure/-imaging hydration can also reduce the risk of contrast-induced nephropathy. While regimens vary, IV hydration should generally take place for at least 6 h prior to contrast administration and for at least 12 h afterwards. Bicarbonate administration before administration of contrast material is also protective and has been shown to be non-inferior to peri-procedure hydration with normal saline in terms of incidence of contrast-inducted nephropathy or renal replacement therapy requirements. Either approach is appropriate per KDIGO guidelines.

Renal Replacement Therapy

If renal function remains impaired, or if life-threatening metabolic derangements arise, it may be necessary to start renal replacement therapy (RRT). Several absolute indications exist for starting renal replacement therapy (Table 52.5), often known by the mnemonic "AEIOU," which encompasses Acidosis, Electrolytes, Intoxication, Overload, and Uremia.

Beyond these absolute indications, the ideal time to initiate RRT is unclear. Some providers advocate for early initiation of RRT to avoid associated complications of severe AKI, but this approach is controversial. Many studies in the literature have found no benefit to early initiation of RRT in terms of dialysis dependence at discharge or mortality. Conversely, early initiation of RRT has associated risks, to include hypotension and infectious.

Based on this evidence, the timing of initiating RRT for patients with severe AKI should be based on a patient's overall clinical picture, rather than a specific timeframe. For severe AKI, particularly in patients with pre-existing CKD, early nephrology consultation is recommended. Nephrology can be particularly helpful in determining the appropriate timing for initiating RRT in these patients, as well as overall AKI management.

Table 52.5 Indications for initiation of emergent dialysis

Acidosis	Metabolic acidosis w/pH <7.1 and refractory to medical management
Electrolytes	Severe hyperkalemia ([K+] >6.5 mmol/L) refractory to medical management OR Hyperkalemia with associated EKG changes/arrhythmias
Intoxication	Toxicity from dialyzable compounds (e.g., salicylates, methanol, ethylene glycol, lithium, valproate)
Overload	Volume overload with pulmonary edema and refractory to diuretics
Uremia	Uremic pericarditis, uremic encephalopathy

tcomes and Follow-Up

ile AKI in many patients will resolve, renal overy is not guaranteed. Notably, Kellum et al. nd that while 58.8% of patients with KDIGO ge 2 or 3 AKI had complete renal recovery by charge, relapse of renal injury was common. tients remain at persistently elevated risk of velopment or progression of CKD, as well as pendence on renal replacement therapy, after scharge. These risks are greater in patients with vanced age, underlying cardiac disease, severe ness/sepsis during hospitalization, and pre-isting CKD. For those with incomplete renal covery or relapse of injury, short- and long-rm mortality are significantly increased.

Because of this associated morbidity and mor-lity, patients with AKI during hospitalization hould have outpatient follow-up upon discharge. ollow-up visits should entail assessments of lood pressure, weight, serum creatinine, and GFR. Urine albumin to creatinine ratio measure-nents should also be obtained, as it has been shown to correlate with progression of renal dis-ease, particularly after AKI. Nephrology referral is likewise appropriate for patients with persis-tent impairments in renal function following discharge.

Conclusion

Acute Kidney Injury is common among hospitalized patients—particularly those who are critically ill—and is associated with significant morbidity and mortality. Advancing age is a known risk factor for development of AKI, with risk further increased in frail geriatric patients. Clinicians should conduct a thorough workup and review of history to determine whether the etiology is pre-renal, intrinsic, or post-renal. Management is predominantly supportive and focused on correcting the underlying cause of injury and avoiding additional renal injury. Life-threatening metabolic abnormalities may require renal replacement therapy. Close follow-up of patients who develop AKI is warranted, as many patients will continue to have persistent impairment in renal function after discharge.

References

1. Moore BJ, Torio CM. Healthcare cost and utilization project statistical brief #231: acute renal failure hospitalizations, 2005–2014. 2017. https://www.hcup-us.ahrq.gov/reports/statbriefs/sb231-Acute-Renal-Failure-Hospitalizations.pdf. Accessed 1 Aug 2022.
2. Emigh BJ, Sahi SL, Teal LN, et al. Incidence and risk factors for acute kidney injury in severely injured patients using current kidney Disease: improving global outcomes definitions. J Am Coll Surg. 2020;231(3):326–32.
3. Harbrecht BG, Broughton-Miller K, Frisbie M, et al. Risk factors and outcome of acute kidney injury in elderly trauma patients. Am J Surg. 2019;218(3):480–3.
4. Denic A, Glassock RJ, Rule AD. Structural and functional changes with the aging kidney. Adv Chronic Kidney Dis. 2016;23(1):19–28.
5. Jiesisibieke ZL, Tung TH, Xu QY, et al. Association of acute kidney injury with frailty in elderly population: a systematic review and meta-analysis. Ren Fail. 2019;41(1):1021–7.
6. Kaddourah A, Basu RK, Bagshaw SM, et al. Epidemiology of acute kidney injury in critically ill children and young adults. N Engl J Med. 2017;376(1):11–20.
7. Bellomo R, Ronco C, Kellum JA, et al. Acute renal failure–definition, outcome measures, animal models, fluid therapy and information technology needs: the second international consensus conference of the acute dialysis quality initiative (ADQI) group. Crit Care. 2004;8(4):R204–12.
8. Mehta RL, Kellum JA, Shah SV, et al. Acute kidney injury network: report of an initiative to improve outcomes in acute kidney injury. Crit Care. 2007;11(2):R31.
9. Kidney Disease: Improving Global Outcomes (KDIGO), Acute kidney injury work group. KDIGO clinical practice guideline for acute kidney injury. Kidney Int Suppl. 2012;2(suppl 1):1–138.
10. Mercado MG, Smith DK, Guard EL. Acute kidney injury: diagnosis and management. Am Fam Physician. 2019;100(11):687–94.
11. Evans L, Rhodes A, Alhazzani W, et al. Surviving sepsis campaign: international guidelines for management of sepsis and septic shock 2021. Intensive Care Med. 2021;47:1181–247.
12. Barbar SD, Clere-Jehl R, Bourredjem A, et al. Timing of renal-replacement therapy in patients with acute kidney injury and sepsis. N Engl J Med. 2018;379(15):1431–42.

13. Kellum JA, Sileanu FE, Bihorac A, et al. Recovery after acute kidney injury. Am J Respir Crit Care Med. 2017;195(6):784–91.
14. Hickson LJ, Chaudhary S, Williams AW, et al. Predictors of outpatient kidney function recovery among patients who initiate hemodialysis in the hospital. Am J Kidney Dis. 2015;65(4):592–602.
15. Hsu CY, Chinchilli VM, Coca S, et al. Post-acute kidney injury proteinuria and subsequent kidney Disease progression: the assessment, serial evaluation, and subsequent sequelae in acute kidney injury (ASSESS-AKI) study. JAMA Intern Med. 2020;180(3):402–10.

Sepsis, Septic Shock, and Its Treatment in Geriatric Patients

53

Corrado P. Marini and David A. Lieb II

ntroduction

ngoing debates continue with regard to the chievement of a consensus about the threshold ge that should be used to identify elderly atients. An age of 65 years or greater has been reviously identified as the threshold cutoff value o identify surgical patients at risk of worse outcome. However, based on the performance data nd more recent data on life expectancy that show, as of 2020 due to a decline in mortality rates, a life expectancy of 79.0 and 84.6 years for males and females, respectively, the current threshold of 65 should be expanded from 65 to 80 years to identify "young elderly," with people older than 80 identified as "old elderly" as suggested by the World Health Organization. In fact, a recent paper regarding severe sepsis in elderly patients undergoing gastrointestinal surgery documented a mean age of 76.4 years in the group of patients requiring surgery to control intra-abdominal sepsis.

This chapter for the acute care surgeon will focus on the identification and treatment of surgical sepsis in the "young elderly" defined by an age frame of 65–80 years, and the "old elderly" defined by an age frame >80 years, with particular emphasis on the diagnosis and treatment of sepsis and septic shock in patients older than 80. From the standpoint of definitions, we will use the revised 2016 definitions of sepsis, known as Sepsis-3, because they provide higher discrimination and a more accurate prediction of sepsis-related mortality.

In 1991, sepsis was defined as systemic inflammatory response syndrome (SIRS) due to a suspected or confirmed infection with two or more of the following criteria: temperature > 38 or < 36 °C, heart rate > 90 bpm, respiratory rate > 20/min or $PaCO_2$ 32 mmHg, WBC > 12,000 or < 4000 cells/mm^3, or > 10% bands. Severe sepsis was defined as the progression of sepsis to organ dysfunction, tissue hypoperfusion, or hypotension, while septic shock necessitated the presence of hypotension and organ dysfunction that persisted despite volume resuscitation requiring vasopressor support. In 2001, the definitions were updated with the inclusions of laboratory variables, and in 2004, the Surviving Sepsis Campaign guidelines adopted the definitions to develop a protocol-driven model for the care of sepsis. In 2016, the Sepsis-3 committee introduced the new definitions: (1) Sepsis as a life-threatening condition caused by a dysregulated host response to infection resulting in organ dysfunction; (2) Septic shock as a circulatory, cellular, and metabolic abnormalities in septic patients, presenting as fluid-refractory hypotension with associated tissue hypoperfusion documented by a lactate level > 2 mmol/L requiring vasopressor

C. P. Marini (✉) · D. A. Lieb II
Jacobi Medical Center, Bronx, NY, USA
e-mail: corradom@nychhc.org

P. Petrone, C. E.M. Brathwaite (eds.), *Acute Care Surgery in Geriatric Patients*,
https://doi.org/10.1007/978-3-031-30651-8_53

therapy. Of note, the condition previously known as severe sepsis was eliminated.

There is widespread agreement that sepsis remains the leading cause of death in the intensive care units, and that unfortunately, the incidence of sepsis is increasing and will continue to rise at an approximate yearly rate of 8–11% due to a variety of reasons, including the increasing percentage of the population aged 80 years or older, the increased number of co-morbid conditions present in elderly patients, the increased use of cytotoxic and immunosuppressive drugs, and more importantly, the emergence of antibiotic resistant organisms.

Elderly have higher rates of sepsis compared with younger adults and are more likely to die from sepsis. Elderly (age ≥ 65) have a 13.1 times higher relative risk of sepsis compared to younger adults with incidence rates increasing 20.4% faster than the rates in the younger cohort. Although age has been found in some studies to be an independent predictor of mortality in patients with sepsis, other studies suggest that factors such as comorbidities and functional status contribute to mortality and not necessarily age per se. A recent study shows that early diagnosis and the early use of antimicrobials and vasopressors for the treatment of sepsis in the elderly may decrease the mortality associated with sepsis independent of age.

Aging Population and Physiological Changes Impacting the Acute Care Surgeon

The USA population is aging. Today there are more than 46 million people older than 65 living in the USA, and this number will increase to 90 million by 2050, constituting more than 25% of the total population. It is important that the acute care surgeon understand how aging changes the risk of, and more importantly, the clinical presentation of sepsis, as well as the specifics of the management of the patient with surgical sepsis as it relates to the many physiological changes that occur with aging.

Aging causes accumulating changes in every organ that ultimately lead to frailty. The definition of frailty is constantly evolving but is generally recognized as a state of compromised functional reserve characterized by impaired nutritional status, and reduced endurance, mobility, physical strength, muscle power, and cognitive function. Frailty can be identified based on the modified Frailty Index (11i-mFI), consisting of 11 variables, described in 2011 by Obeid or by the modified 5i-mFI of the National Surgical Quality Improvement Program (NSQIP) (Table 53.1).

One of the more important age-related changes pertaining to the enhanced risk of sepsis in the elderly includes immunosenescence, a functional decline in both innate and adaptive immunity that affects cell mediated and humoral immunity. The changes in innate

Table 53.1 Frailty based on the modified Frailty Index (11i-mFI) or by modified 5i-mFI of the National Surgical Quality Improvement Program (NSQIP)

NSQIP 11-mFI	NSQIP 5i-mFI	Variable
Diabetes mellitus	Diabetes mellitus	**1**
CHF within 30 days before surgery	CHF within 30 days before surgery	**2**
Hypertension requiring medication	Hypertension requiring medication	**3**
History of MI within 6 months of surgery		4
Previous PCI or angina		5
TIA or CVA with no neurological deficit		6
CVA with neurologic deficit		7
Impaired sensorium		8
History of COPD	History of COPD	**9**
Peripheral vascular disease		10
FHS before surgery—Not independent	FHS before surgery—Not independent	**11**

CHF Congestive heart failure, *MI* Myocardial infarction, *PCI* Percutaneous coronary intervention, *TIA* Transient ischemic attack, *CVA* Cerebrovascular accident, *COPD* Chronic obstructive pulmonary disease, *FHS* Functional health status

Numbers in bold indicate items included in the 5i-mFI

immunity include reduced phagocytic activity of neutrophils, macrophages, and natural killer cells in the setting of an upregulated inflammatory state characterized by an increased number of proinflammatory cytokines, including interleukin-6, C-reactive protein (CRP), tumor-necrosis factor-α, and CXC chemokine ligand-10. Characteristic of the changes in cell-mediated immunity is the reduced proportion of T-cell observed with aging as a result of the involution of the thymus. The thymus, which contributes to the adaptive cell-mediated immunity, undergoes atrophy with aging, and by age 60 causes a gradual loss of T-cell repertoire from naive CD8 T-cells and memory T-cells. The involution of the thymus causes a decrease in the production of CD4 and CD8 lymphocytes leading to a downregulated response to neoantigens exposure. The CD4/CD8 ratio can be used as a marker of both immunosenescence and immune activation. This ratio increases in the elderly due to the age-related decrease in CD8.

The altered cytokine and chemokine response in the elderly leads to the induction of proinflammatory cytokines after septic stimuli causing a protracted inflammatory state that is not adequately controlled by anti-inflammatory mechanisms, particularly by an insufficient IL-10 response. This immune dysregulation is accompanied by a more pronounced procoagulant state in older patients. Coagulation activation is a uniform finding in sepsis in the elderly. These molecular events function in concert to place elderly patients at excess risk for mortality from severe sepsis and septic shock.

Age-Related Organ-Specific Physiologic Changes Important for the Acute Care Surgeon

While all organs in the body are affected by the aging process, we will focus on the more important age-related physiological changes that impact the treatment of sepsis in the elderly, namely, the cardiovascular, renal, and hepatic systems. Of note, the changes with age occur in everyone but not at the same rate, this accounts for the difference seen in some people between chronologic and physiologic age.

Cardiovascular System

The changes in the cardiovascular system associated with aging include a decrease in elasticity and an increase in stiffness of the arterial system. Collagen and elastin provide the strength and elasticity, respectively, of the arterial wall and are normally stabilized by enzymatic cross-linking. Aging causes an increase in collagen content, collagen cross-linking, and fraying of elastin fibers which reduce arterial distensibility and increase stiffness. This results in increased afterload on the left ventricle, in isolated systolic hypertension, concentric wall thickening of the left ventricle from cellular hypertrophy, and prolonged relaxation of the left ventricle in diastole. Additionally, aging causes decreased responsiveness of adrenergic ß-receptors and decreased reactivity to baroreceptors and chemoreceptors in the setting of increased circulating catecholamines. While the left ventricular systolic function is preserved, the compromised diastolic function affects the preload recruitment of stroke volume (SV) with volume expansion and lowers the threshold for volume overload in the absence of appropriate cardiovascular monitoring. Additionally, even mild tachycardia (HR > 100 bpm) worsens the diastolic filling abnormality in the elderly (30–50% loss of early diastolic filling), which in turn causes higher left ventricular diastolic pressure that is transmitted into the lungs causing an increase in the extravascular lung water. Knowledge of the cardiovascular changes resulting from aging is necessary to optimize ventriculo-arterial coupling when treating elderly patients with sepsis and septic shock, Failure to understand how these changes affect the effects of volume expansion, inotropes, and vasopressors on the optimization of the cardiovascular function needed to enhance the overall treatment of the elderly in septic shock may lead to an unnecessary increased mortality from sepsis.

Renal System

Aging is responsible for many structural anatomic changes that cause an increase in the mesangium, obliteration of many juxtamedullary nephrons, the formation of a direct channel between the afferent and efferent arterioles, causing aglomerular circulation, and increasing zones of tubular atrophy and fibrosis in the kidney. The structural anatomic changes associated with aging lead to physiological changes in renal function. There is a decrease in the glomerular filtration rate (GFR) and the effective renal plasma flow (ERPF); the latter decreases disproportionally more than GFR—10% per decade from 600 mL/min/1.73 m^2 in youth to 300 mL/min/1.73 m^2 by the age of 80. Therefore, the filtration fraction, which is the ratio of GFR/ERPF, usually increases in the elderly. The clinical consequences of the decreased functional reserve of the kidney in the old elderly are many, including the fact that while a serum creatinine concentration of 1 mg/dL reflects a GFR of 120 mL/min in a 20-year-old person, it reflects a GFR of only 60 mL/min in an 80-year-old. Additionally, senile hypoperfusion predisposes the old elderly to CHF and kidney injury when the volume expansion needed to treat sepsis and septic shock is done with large amount of saline solutions. One important component of the bundle treatment of sepsis, namely, the dose and the dosing of antibiotics, must be adjusted to the GFR of the old elderly. Another important difference between the young elderly and the old elderly involves the laboratory findings in acute renal failure secondary to dehydration. While blood urea increases with a nearly normal creatinine in the younger with normalization after rehydration, blood urea and creatinine are both elevated in the very old, however, both altered values normalize with rehydration.

Hepatic System

The volume and blood flow of the liver gradually decrease with aging. The liver volume decreases by 25–35% in people over 65 years of age from a decrease in hepatic blood flow greater than 40%. However, despite the decrease in liver volume, the serum albumin concentration remains at almost normal levels. Of note, aging decreases the regenerative ability of the liver, which in turn delays the restoration of liver function in the setting of sepsis-induced multiple organ dysfunction syndrome (MODS). The altered functional capacity of the liver from aging has a significant effect on the pharmacokinetics and pharmacodynamics (PK/PD) of most drugs used to treat sepsis in the elderly. Reduced first pass metabolism for high hepatic extraction ratio drugs, defined by a ratio >70%, such as fentanyl and morphine sulfate causes increased bioavailability in the setting of reduced clearance. The age-related changes of the liver affect the volume of distribution and the clearance of many drugs that may require dosage adjustment in the treatment of sepsis in the elderly. In particular, the efficacy of concentration-dependent (ratio of maximum plasma concentration of unbound drug over the minimum inhibitory concentration—MIC) and time-dependent (time that the unbound drug exceeds the MIC) antibiotics and antifungal agents is affected by the changes in liver volume and hepatic blood flow.

Diagnosis

One of the more important aspects of the management of the geriatric patient with sepsis is how to establish an early diagnosis in order to provide a treatment that includes the administration of an adequate amount of fluids for volume expansion (VE), the administration of antibiotics in the first hour from diagnosis, taking into consideration the altered PK/PD due to aging, followed by early source control after the initial resuscitation phase. The changes occurring in each organ system in the old elderly patients deplete physiologic reserves and compromise the response to peritonitis. Furthermore, they limit the ability to localize, combat, and eradicate intra-abdominal infections. The early diagnosis of sepsis and septic shock as opposed to non-infectious causes of an upregulated inflammatory response is more difficult to make in the old elderly due to the downregulation of the immune system from immunosenescence. The old elderly patients with intra-abdominal sepsis present with less acute and delayed symptoms compared to the young elderly and the younger patients. Surgical patients account for more than one-third of sepsis cases in the USA. Intra-abdominal infections account for 69% of cases of surgical sepsis, with pulmonary, urinary tract, vascular access/blood stream, and wound/soft tissue infections accounting for the remaining causes of sepsis. The most common causes of intra-abdominal sepsis in the elderly include appendicitis, acute cholecystitis, cholangitis, diverticulitis, perforations on the gastrointestinal tract, intra-abdominal abscess, and more rarely, mesenteric ischemia, and infarcted colon from delayed treatment of volvulus and from colonic ischemia. Of note, one cause of sepsis that can evolve rapidly into septic shock and that can be associated with a very high mortality is severe Clostridioides difficile infection, defined by a white blood cell count greater than 15,000 cells/mL, serum albumin less than 3 g/dL, and a serum creatinine greater than 1.5 times the baseline level.

The incidence of sepsis among elderly surgical patients is the highest in patients requiring emergency surgery, with colon perforation being the predominant source of sepsis. The development of septic shock in patients after elective surgery is associated with a 30% mortality, with the mortality rate exceeding 40% in patients in septic shock requiring emergency surgery.

While the sequential organ failure assessment (SOFA) score is the score most commonly used in the ICU setting to predict the risk of mortality in septic patient, the score itself is not useful for the management of patients and is not useful for the early diagnosis of sepsis in the elderly (Table 53.2). The quick SOFA (qSOFA) score based on high respiratory rate (≥22 beats/min), low systolic blood pressure (≤100 mm Hg), or altered mentation (Glasgow Coma Scale <15) was proposed by the members of the Sepsis-3 in 2016 as a tool for the early diagnosis of sepsis in patients with suspected sepsis (Table 53.3). However, the qSOFA has a sensitivity and specificity of only 66% and 61%, respectively, for the diagnosis of sepsis, therefore, while the qSOFA may have value as a prognosticator marker for mortality and MODS in septic patients, it is not a good diagnostic marker for the detection of sepsis, particularly, in the elderly.

Table 53.2 The Sequential Organ Failure Assessment (SOFA) score

	SOFA score				
Organ system	0	1	2	3	4
Respiratory					
PaO_2/FiO_2 mmHg	≥400	<400	<300	<200	<100
Coagulation					
Platelets $10^3/mm^3$	≥150	<150	<100	<50	<20
Liver					
Bilirubin in mg/dL	<1.2	1.2–1.9	2.0–5.9	6.0–11.9	≥12
Cardiovascular	MAP ≥70 mmHg	MAP <70 mmHg	Dopa <5 Dobutamine Any dose	Dopa 5.1–15 E ≤ 0.1 N ≤ 0.1	Dopa >15 E > 0.1 NE > 0.1
CNS					
GCS	15	13–15	10–12	6–9	<6
Renal					
Creatinine mg/dL	<1.2	1.2–1.9	2.0–3.4	3.5–4.9	≥5
Urine output mL/day				<500	<200

Dopa Dopamine, *E* Epinephrine, *NE* Norepinephrine, Dobutamine; all in μg/kg/min ≥ 1 h, PaO_2 Partial pressure of oxygen, FiO_2 Fraction of inspired oxygen, *MAP* Mean arterial pressure

Table 53.3 Quick sequential organ failure assessment (qSOFA) score

qSOFA Criteria	Points
Systolic blood pressure ≤ 100 mmHg	1
Respiratory rate ≥ 22/min	1
Change in mental status (GCS <15)	1

GCS Glasgow Coma Scale

An important question regarding old elderly patients at risk of infection and/or sepsis is whether the presence of hypotension alone, defined by a systolic blood pressure less than 115 mmHg, is a sufficiently sensitive screening marker for tissue perfusion deficits to identify the transition of patients from infection/sepsis to septic shock. Many studies support the superiority of serial measurement of lactate levels over other markers, including hypotension, from the standpoint of identifying the progression of patients from sepsis to septic shock and from the standpoint of prediction of sepsis-related mortality. While anion gap and base deficits are routinely used to risk-stratify surgical patients, they are insensitive in septic patients. Normal anion gaps and base deficits have been observed in 22% and 25% of patients with mean lactate levels of 4 and 7 mmol/L, respectively. Lactate represents a useful and clinically obtainable surrogate marker of tissue hypoxia and disease severity, independent of blood pressure. Previous studies have shown that a lactate concentration >4 mmol/L in the presence of SIRS criteria significantly increases ICU admission rates and mortality rate in normotensive patients. Lactate can be measured in the ICU and in the emergency department using point-of-care devices with a turnaround time of 2 min and since peripheral venous lactate levels can be used in substitution of arterial lactate, as long as tourniquet times are short, arterial or venous lactate levels should be obtained in surgical patients who are suspected to be septic in order to initiate early therapy. The early therapy should be directed at targeting the following endpoints as soon as reasonable: (1) Volume expansion for restoration of the macro and microcirculation; (2) Administration of broad-spectrum antibiotics; (3) Normalization of lactate, venous-arterial carbon dioxide difference (Pv-aCO_2) and capillary refill time (CRT); (4) Source control with interventional procedures within 3–6 h to prevent the development of MODS.

Among the blood biomarkers available, the two that complement synergistically the clinical judgment and that appear to be more useful for the early diagnosis of sepsis and septic shock are procalcitonin (PCT) and lactate levels. These two biomarkers can be monitored to assess the response to therapy, although there is a difference between PCT and lactate with respect to tailoring therapy to the individual patient in that the former is a more sensitive biomarker of infection, useful to differentiate bacterial sepsis from a nonbacterial etiology, and to assess the response, the duration of antimicrobial treatment, including the decision to de-escalate antibiotic therapy, and the latter is a more sensitive marker of the recruitment of cellular perfusion with the administration of fluids and of the balance between oxygen delivery and consumption. Lactate level is a better predictor of ICU and in-hospital mortality. Of note, nonspecific elevations in PCT levels in the absence of a bacterial infection can occur following massive stress, such as after severe trauma and complex surgery, and in patients in cardiac shock; therefore, while it remains an efficacious biomarker of sepsis, it should be used in conjunction with other clinical parameters and the clinical judgment of the treating physician. While CRP, an acute-phase protein released by the liver, increases with tissue damage, inflammation, and with infection, in our opinion is less valuable for the diagnosis of sepsis in surgical patients.

The outcome of the elderly patients requiring emergency surgery for intra-abdominal sepsis can be predicted with an acceptable degree of accuracy by the Emergency Surgery Score (ESS) and the Predictive OpTimal Trees in Emergency Surgery Risk (POTTER) interactive calculators (Table 53.4).

Table 53.4 Predictive optimal trees in emergency surgery risk (POTTER)

Variable	Points
Demographics	
Age > 60 years	2
White	1
Transfer from outside ED	1
Transfer from acute care hospital	1
Comorbidities	
Ascites	1
BMI < 20 kg/m^2	1
Disseminated cancer	3
Dyspnea	1
Functional dependence	1
COPD	1
Hypertension	1
Steroid use	1
Ventilator requirement within 48 h of surgery	3
Weight loss >10% in the preceding 6 months	1
Laboratory values	
Albumin <3 g/dL	1
Alkaline phosphatase >125 U/L	1
BUN >40 mg/dL	1
Creatinine >1.2 mg/dL	2
INR > 1.5	1
Platelets <150,000/μL	1
SGOT >40 U/L	1
Sodium >145 mEq/L	1
WBC × 10^3 μL	
<4.5	1
16–24	1
≥25	2
Maximum score	29

BMI Body Mass Index, *COPD* Chronic Obstructive Pulmonary Disease, *BUN* Blood Urea Nitrogen, *INR* International Normalized Ratio, *SGOT* Serum Glutamic Oxaloacetic Transaminase, *WBC* While Blood Cell Count

Treatment

Source Control and Antibiotics

The choice and dosing of antimicrobials should be based on the understanding the emergence of multi-drug-resistant organisms (MDROs) and on the age-related differences in PD/PK parameters such as decrements in renal function including glomerular filtration rate, tubular secretion, and renal blood flow, reduced lean body mass and increased body fat, and shock-induced reduction in hepatic blood flow. Novel, higher generation antibiotic agents that have been developed for resistant Enterococcus faecium, Staphylococcus aureus, Klebsiella pneumoniae, Acinetobacter baumannii, Pseudomonas aeruginosa, and Enterobacter (ESKCAPE) species organisms should be preferred over the more conventional ones (Table 53.5).

While there is an increased incidence of antimicrobial-related adverse effects in the elderly, the principle of initial bolus dose and overall aggressive dosing to achieve maximal therapeutic dose should not be sacrificed to avoid potential adverse effects. Source control of infection and early appropriate antimicrobials remain the two vital components of the management bundle of surviving sepsis guidelines. The source of infection should be identified without delay when possible, and appropriate source control measures like removal of infected foreign bodies (intravascular catheters), drainage of abscesses or other infected fluid collections, or definitive surgical management of intra-abdominal sepsis should be undertaken early whenever possible.

The early institution of antimicrobial therapy has been found to significantly decrease mortality in elderly sepsis patients. Broad-spectrum empirical antibiotic therapy should be initiated within 1 h of the recognition of sepsis, after samples of blood and other suspected sites of infection have been obtained for culture, in conjunction with adequate volume expansion resuscitation to optimize the PD/PK on the selected antimicrobials.

One important aspect of the treatment of the elderly is the target systolic and mean blood pressure needed to optimize macro and microperfusion. This is especially a problem for old elderly patients as they need higher systolic blood pressures for adequate perfusion due to arterial stiffening. Moreover, because of their blunted heart rate response, their cardiac output mainly

Table 53.5 Higher generation antibiotic agents

Antibiotic	Activity against the type of bacteria
Ceftaroline (fifth-generation cephalosporin)	MRSA
Ceftolozane-tazobactam (beta-lactam-beta lactamase inhibitor) (beta lactam inhibitor—BLI)	Pseudomonas aeruginosa MDR
Meropenem-vaborbactam (carbapenem—BLI)	MDROs
Eravacycline (tetracycline of the fluorocycline group)	MRSA, VRE, Enterobacteriaceae with ESBL gram negative
Ceftazidime-avibactam	ESBL gram negative
Ceftazidime-avibactam + metronidazole	ESBL gram negative + anaerobes (CREs, cIAI)

MRSA Methicillin-resistant Staphylococcus aureus, *MDR* Multi-drug resistant, *MDROs* Multi-drug-resistant orga isms, *VRE* Vancomycin-resistant enterococcus, *ESBL* Extended spectrum beta-lactamase, *CREs* Carbapenem-resista Enterobacteriaceae, *cIAI* Complex intra-abdominal infections

depends on cardiac filling pressures with adequate preload. Old elderly patients may therefore require different targets for fluid resuscitation. In clinical practice however, clinicians often withhold a large amount of fluids in old elderly patients because of a fear of overloading the heart. In addition, in most sepsis guidelines, the threshold for hypotension is typically set at systolic blood pressure (SBP) < 90–100 mmHg, while old elderly patients are probably already in shock with higher SBPs. In the old elderly ED patients with suspected infection, a SBP < 140 mmHg is linearly associated with a higher mortality. The same has been suggested in older patients with trauma or surgical sepsis. Therefore, the old elderly patients may receive insufficient fluid volumes for adequate perfusion, which may affect outcome.

Volume Expansion

The initial management of the septic elderly patient focuses on cardiovascular stabilization, early administration of broad-spectrum antibiotics, and source control. The four determinants of cardiac output (CO) are HR, preload, afterload, and contractility (Fig. 53.1). The sequential approach to the optimization of CO involves control of the HR, increase in preload, assessment of the impact of the afterload on contractility, load-independent improvement in contractility, and optimization of ventriculo-arterial coupling (VAC). Volume expansion with the administration of a balanced salt solution is the initial ste toward the optimization of the cardiovascular sta tus of the patient in fluid-responsive patient because it decreases tachycardia and increase preload, two of the four determinants of CO.

The choice between an isotonic solution suc as normal saline (NS 0.9%) and a slightly hypo tonic solution such as Lactate Ringer's solutio (LR) as the solution of choice for the resuscitation of the septic elderly patient depends on the effects of the tonicity and of the specific ions o each solution on the restoration of the intravascular volume and on the potential side effects of each solution. With 154 mmol/L each of sodium and chloride, NS is isotonic to the extracellular fluid but contains a chloride concentration significantly higher than plasma. In contrast, LR, a more balanced solution, is slightly hypotonic to extracellular fluid but provides anions that more closely approximate plasma pH. The administration of large amount of NS (≥3 L) causes hyperchloremic metabolic acidosis in critically ill patients. The increased concentration of chloride in NS decreases the strong ion difference and induces a non-anion gap metabolic acidosis. Additionally, since the delivery of chloride to the macula densa drives mesangial contraction and the consequent decrease in glomerular filtration rate, the hyperchloremia caused by the administration of NS predisposes the patient to the development of acute kidney injury (AKI). We prefer the use of LR, as the balanced salt solution of choice for the resuscitation of the septic elderly patient based on a meta-analysis that

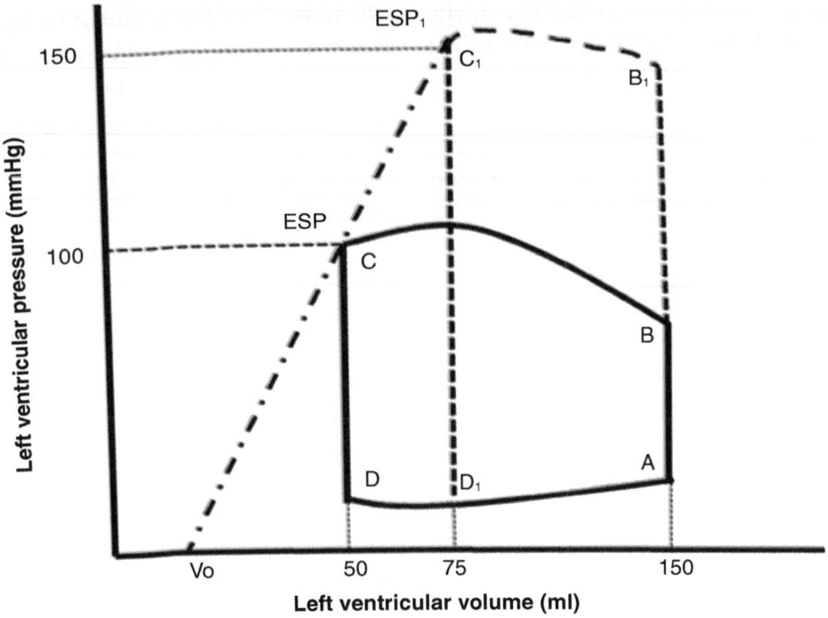

Fig. 53.1 Illustrated above is the PV relation for the left ventricle over an entire cardiac cycle. The area ABCD represents the energy added to the aortic root by the ventricular contraction. The heat dissipated in the ventricular wall during isovolumic relaxation is represented by the area contained within the triangle C, V_0, D. The end-systolic volume is 50 mL at the end-systolic pressure of 100 mmHg. Of note, no work is done on the aortic root during isovolumic contraction from point A to B because the volume of the ventricle is unchanged. Work, however, is done on the aortic root from the opening of the aortic valve to end-systole, from point B to C. The stroke volume of 100 mL, the difference between the end-diastolic volume of 150 mL minus the end-systolic volume of 50 mL is generating an aortic root end-systolic pressure of 100 mmHg. Therefore, the effective elastance of the aortic root, namely, the end-systolic pressure divided by the stroke volume, is 1.0 mmHg/ml, a value approaching the optimal ventricular-arterial coupling with optimal efficiency value of 0.5. The value of 0.5 implies that the afterload related to the maximum efficiency for a given SW is lower than Ees (Ea = 1/2 Ees). Following the administration of a vasopressor, such as norepinephrine and/or phenylephrine, there is an increase in the afterload (impedance) facing the left ventricle. The pressure has increased from the ESP to ESP_1; however, the result is more energy wasted as heat dissipation during isovolumic relaxation as depicted by the C_1, V_0, D_1 triangle and decreased efficiency of ventricular-arterial coupling as shown by an end-systolic pressure 150 mmHg divided by a stroke volume of 75 mL, yielding a 2 mmHg/1 mL ratio. VA uncoupling occurs when Ea exceeds the value of Ees (Ea/Ees >1). Described in terms of ventricular efficiency, defined as stroke work/pressure volume area (SW/PVA), the increased ESP to ESP_1 has yielded a decreased SW in relation to the PVA, therefore, a reduced ventricular efficiency

suggests improved mortality among patients with sepsis.

To understand the effects of VE on MAP, we must remember that MAP = CO (SV × HR) × SVR. Volume expansion will increase the mean BP in septic patients with increased vascular tone (high SVR) by increasing CO through increased preload. However, VE will not be effective in raising mean BP in patients with decreased vascular tone because the increased CO will be offset by a further decrease in SVR caused by the activation of NO and vascular recruitment from the increased blood flow. Therefore, the issue surrounding the role and the amount of VE in the septic patient depends on the existing hemodynamic profile of the patient at the early stage of sepsis. At the earliest stage of sepsis, the patient could be hypotensive from a preload independent compromised CO or less likely from decreased SVR in the setting of normal cardiac function. The preload dependent patient has a higher sympathetic tone as evidenced by higher dynamic arterial elastance (Ea_{dyn}), defined as the ratio of PPV to SVV, higher SVR, and lower total arterial compliance (Ca = SV/arterial PP). An initial fluid challenge (250 mL/15–30 min) or the passive leg raising test can be used to assess whether the patient will benefit from VE. A fluid responder can be identified by a 10–15% increase in SV and by a 10% increase in SV or pulse pressure after an FC and a PLR test, respectively.

A key to optimize cardiovascular function is understanding VAC, particularly in the old elderly. Ventriculo-arterial coupling is defined as the ratio between arterial elastance (Ea), an index of left ventricular (LV) afterload, and end-systolic elastance (Ees), a load-independent index of myocardial contractility (VAC = Ea/Ees). Ea = ESP/SV mmHg mL^{-1} and Ees = (0.9 × ESP)/[ESV−V_0] mmHg mL^{-1}. LV efficiency (LV_{ef}) is the ratio between the pressure-volume loop (SW) and the stroke work plus the potential energy (SW + PE). An increase in Ea with minimal or no increase in Ees will increase PE, therefore, decreasing LV_{ef} (Fig. 53.1). We could view it as thermodynamic waste since the increased pressure does not yield an increase in SV.

The old elderly has an already relatively compromised LV_{ef} even in the absence of cardiac hypertrophy because of the arterial stiffening from aging that causes an increase in Ea, and because of the maximal ventricular systolic stiffening, as measured by the end-systolic elastance (Ees). With aging, the arterial stiffening and a reduction in peripheral vasomotor regulation affect VAC by imposing far greater pulsatile and late-systolic loads on the heart. This is accompanied by tandem increases in left ventricular end-systolic stiffness and reduced diastolic compliance. These changes cause a greater systolic pressure lability with LV preload changes that in turn may affect macro and microvascular perfusion in the old elderly.

The cardiovascular management of the old elderly with sepsis must take into consideration that, at baseline, these patients will have already a mild to moderate degree of ventriculo-arterial uncoupling, which could be exacerbated by the additional uncoupling seen in septic patients with elevated lactate at baseline, before resuscitation, which has been documented in septic patients by Guarracino et al. The old elderly may require VE with a much lower volume than the 30 mL/kg suggested by the recent sepsis guidelines because of the age-related changes in VAC and more importantly, because he/she may respond with further VA uncoupling when treated with the infusion of norepinephrine (NE). Evidence shows that the infusion of NE is associated with a deterioration in LV_{ef} from uncoupling of VAC from the increase in Ea with negligible rise in Ees in septic patients. In the old elderly, the infusion of dobutamine or modulation of Ea with vasodilators may optimize VAC by increasing Ees while causing a relative minor decrease in Ea. It is important to understand the issues surrounding VAC in the old elderly to avoid the indiscriminate use of NE to increase systemic BP in view of its effect on Ea and LV_{ef}, and because of the potential detrimental effect on the microcirculation. Ideally, in view of the significant relationship between Ea_{dyn}, VAC, LV_{ef}, and the present ability to obtain PPV and SVV at the bedside, the cardiovascular treatment of the septic old elderly patient should be guided by monitoring VAC through serial measurement of Ea_{dyn}.

We suggest the following time-sensitive approach to the treatment of old elderly septic patients with a lactate level > 4 mmol/L after instrumentation that includes placement of a radial arterial line with stroke volume variation (SVV) and/or pulse pressure variation (PPV), monitoring capabilities, an oximetric central venous line to monitor superior vena cava pressure and oxygen saturation, a disposable transesophageal probe, and a Foley catheter to monitor urine output. The initial step within the first hour should be VE with the administration of Lactated Ringer's bolus at a rate of 10–15 mL/kg and the administration of a broad-spectrum antibiotic. In 2/3 of patients, VE alone may restore MAP to >80–85 mmHg while simultaneously increasing CO, LV end-systolic elastance (Ees) and simultaneously decreasing arterial elastance (Ea), hence improving VAC.

Once the patient becomes unresponsive to additional VE from the standpoint of improvement of SVV and increased CO and the achievement of a MAP>80–85 mmHg with decreasing lactate levels, then the infusion of norepinephrine titrated between 0.01 and 1.0 μg kg^{-1} min^{-1} is initiated as long as there is no evidence of uncoupling of the VAC. To limit the detrimental effect of the increased LV afterload caused by the infusion of NE, we suggest the addition of the infusion of dobutamine at a dose of 7.5–15 μg kg^{-1} min^{-1}, if there is persistent biochemical evidence of hypoperfusion by lactate levels, $ScvO_2$, CRT, and ΔPCO_2. If available, the simultaneous measurement of PPV and SVV provides us with the ability to assess dynamic arterial elastance (Ea_{dyn}) which predicts the response of blood pressure to changes in CO and to increasing or decreasing doses of NE infusion. While a MAP pressure ≥ 65 mmHg appears a reasonable blood pressure target in non-hypertensive patients up to age 65 to normalize lactate level and CRT, it is probably too low for the young and old elderly patients with systolic hypertension and decreased diastolic pressure who may benefit from a MAP between 80–85 mmHg to reach the same endpoints.

Resuscitation of the Microcirculation

The microcirculation consists of microvessels, namely arterioles, capillaries, post- capillary venules, and their cellular components with diameters <20 μm. It is the most distal site for the oxygen transfer from the RBCs to the parenchymal cells to maintain their functional activity via two mechanisms: (1) RBCs flow (convection of oxygen-carrying RBCs); and (2) Diffusion of oxygen from the RBCs to tissues cells (diffusional component quantified by functional capillary density). The autoregulation of the microcirculatory flow is implemented through myogenic, metabolic, and neurohumoral mechanisms. NO is considered a key component in the maintenance and autoregulation of the homeostasis and patency of the microcirculation.

In normal conditions, there is hemodynamic coherence between the macro and microcirculation in that an improvement in macrocirculatory flow from optimization of its variables will result in a parallel improvement of the microcirculation, which in turn will improve tissue oxygenation to match the specific oxygen demand heterogeneity of the organs' parenchymal cells. However, hemodynamic coherence is lost in septic shock. The tissues can remain hypoperfused from lack of recruitment of microcirculatory flow despite successful resuscitation of the macrocirculation with administration of fluid and vasoactive drugs. Of note, loss of coherence can occur between the different compartments of a single organ and even between groups of cells. The septic old elderly has an heterogenous microcirculation with the presence of obstructed capillaries next to capillaries with normal, fast, and slow flowing RBCs.

The gold standard to assess tissue perfusion through the evaluation of the functional status of the microcirculation is the use of hand-held vital microscopy (HVM). Of note, the finding of an initial low microcirculatory flow independent of systemic hemodynamics predicts the responsiveness of the microcirculation to VE as opposed to the absence of fluid-responsiveness in the setting of normal microcirculatory flow by HVM. The most commonly monitored site of the microcirculation assessed with HVM is the sublingual microcirculation.

Indices of microcirculation include total vessel density (TVD mm/mm^3), perfused vessel density (PVD n/mm^2), proportion of perfused vessels (PPV %), heterogeneity index (HI %), and microvascular flow index (MFI). Two scores are used in clinical practice, the De Backer score and the MFI [47–48]. The De Backer score is based on the principle that density of the vessels is proportional to the number of vessels crossing arbitrary lines. The MFI score is based on the determination of the predominant type of flow in four quadrants with the assignment of 0 = absent flow; 1 = intermittent flow; 2 = sluggish flow; 3 = normal flow. The values of the four quadrants are averaged.

Despite the support for the use of HVM by the second consensus on the assessment of sublingual microcirculation in critically ill patients and the resulting set of guidelines on microcirculatory imaging with the use HVM, the use of HVM remains subject to the interpretation of the microcirculatory images for the verification of the recruitment of the microcirculation and to the issue of the dissociation between the sublingual and intestinal microcirculation in postoperative patients with abdominal sepsis. Therefore, based on these limitations, we believe that the use of HVM limited to the monitoring of the sublingual microcirculation is not generalizable at this time. Consequently, we suggest the use of the following surrogates to monitor microcirculatory organ perfusion and anaerobic metabolism, namely, lactate, lactate/pyruvate ratio, CRT, peripheral temperature, $P(v\text{-}a)CO_2$ (ΔPCO_2), and the ratio between the $P(v\text{-}a)CO_2$ and arterio-venous oxygen content difference ($\Delta PCO_2/C(a\text{-}v)O_2$). We believe that, at this time, taking into consideration all limitations of each parameter combined monitoring of serial lactate, $ScvO_2$, CRT, ΔPCO_2, and $\Delta PCO_2/C(a\text{-}v)O_2$ during the early phases of resuscitation and optimization of septic shock reflects the adequacy of microvascular blood flow and should be used to guide the early therapy of sepsis and septic shock.

Of note, since $ScvO_2$ during anesthesia tends to be higher because of the decreased O_2ER, it is important to monitor also the ΔPCO_2 taking into consideration that an $ScvO_2 > 70\%$ with a $\Delta PCO_2 > 8$ mmHg and a $\Delta PCO_2/C(a\text{-}v)O_2 \geq 1.4$ indicate suboptimal microcirculatory perfusion. Following the control of the source of intra-abdominal sepsis, the patient should undergo ongoing stabilization for 1–2 days in the ICU settings, with therapy targeted to normalization of all perfusion and hypoxia-related parameters pertaining to the macro and microcirculation, and maintenance of a steady state, making efforts to avoid excessive volume overload (> 10%) by day 3. Volume overload is defined as the cumulative fluid balance in liters divided by the patient's baseline weight times 100. By the end of day 3, we should focus on the fourth phase of treatment, namely, the mobilization/evacuation/recovery or what others call the de-escalation phase (flow phase).

Conclusions

The incidence of sepsis and septic shock con[t]ues to rise due to a variety of reasons and mortality associated with it, while decreasi[ng] remains high ranging from 20% to 30%, a[nd] reaching 80% when complicated by the develo[p]ment of MODS. The best approach to decreasi[ng] the mortality is to implement a time-sensiti[ve] approach comparable to that employed to tre[at] stroke, myocardial infarction, and traum[a] patients. Therefore, early diagnosis, prompt in[i]tiation of antimicrobial therapy, source contro[l] and an early goal-directed approach targeted [to] normalization of the macro and microcirculatio[n] should be implemented as soon as possible. Th[e] treatment should be aimed at optimization of car[]diovascular function with initial VE and manipu[]lation of the physiological determinants o[f] cardiac function to provide adequate oxyge[n] delivery to meet the oxygen demand at the leve[l] of the microcirculation to prevent the progressio[n] of patients from sepsis and septic shock to MODS in order to improve the overall mortality.

References

1. World Health Organization (WHO). Definition of an older or elderly person. 2011. http://www.who.int/healthinfo/survey/ageingdefnolder/en/index.htmlrr.
2. Ukkonen M, Karlsson S, Laukkkarinen J, Rantanen T, Paajanen H, Finnespsi Study Group. Severe sepsis in elderly patients undergoing gastrointestinal surgery–a prospective multicenter follow-up study of the Finnish intensive care units. J Gastrointest Surg. 2016;20(5):1028–33. https://doi.org/10.1007/s11605-016-3076-4.
3. Obeid NM, Azuh O, Reddy S. Predictors of critical care-related complications in colectomy patients using the National Surgical Quality Improvement Program: exploring frailty and aggressive laparoscopic approaches. J Trauma Acute Care Surg. 2012;72:878–83.
4. Bone RC, Balk RA, Cerra FB, et al. Definitions for sepsis and organ failure and guidelines for the use of innovative therapies in sepsis. The ACCP/SCCM consensus conference committee. American College of Chest Physicians/Society of Critical Care Medicine. Chest. 1992;101(6):1644–55. https://doi.org/10.1378/chest.101.6.1644.

5. Levy MM, Fink MP, Marshall JC, et al. 2001 SCCM/ESICM/ACCP/ATS/SIS international sepsis definitions conference. Crit Care Med. 2003;31(4):1250–6. https://doi.org/10.1097/01.CCM.0000050454.01978.3B.
6. Fleischmann C, Scherag A, Adhikari NKJ, Hartog CS, Tsaganos T, Schlattmann P, et al. Assessment of global incidence and mortality of hospital-treated sepsis. Current estimates and limitations. Am J Respir Crit Care Med. 2016;193(3):259–72.
7. Martin GS, Mannino DM, Moss M. The effect of age on the development and outcome of adult sepsis. Crit Care Med. 2006;34:15–21. https://doi.org/10.1097/01.CCM.0000194535.82812.BA.
8. Collerton J, Martin-Ruiz C, Davies K, et al. Frailty and the role of inflammation, immunosenescenceand cellular ageing in the very old: cross-sectional findings. Mech Ageing Dev. 2012;133(6):456–66.
9. Guarracino F, Bertini P, Pinsky MR. Cardiovascular determinants of resuscitation from sepsis and septic shock. Crit Care. 2019;23:118. https://doi.org/10.1186/s13054-019-2414.
10. Bakker J, Gris P, Coffernils M, et al. Serial blood lactate levels can predict the development of multiple organ failure following septic shock. Am J Surg. 1996;171:221–6.
11. Suistomma M, Ruokonen E, Kari A, et al. Time-pattern of lactate and lactate to pyruvate ratio in the first 24 hours of intensive care emergency admissions. Shock. 2000;14:8–12.
12. Meregalli A, Oliveira RP, Friedman G. Occult hypoperfusion is associated with increased mortality in hemodynamically stable, high-risk, surgical patients. Crit Care. 2004;8:R60–5.
13. McNelis J, Marini CP, Jurkiewicz A, et al. Prolonged lactate clearance is associated with increased mortality in the surgical intensive care unit. Am J Surg. 2001;182:481–5.
14. Hernandez G, Bruhn A, Ince C. Microcirculation in sepsis: new perspectives. Curr Vasc Pharmacol. 2013;11:161–9.
15. Ince C. Hemodynamic coherence and the rational for monitoring the microcirculation. Crit Care. 2015;19:S8.

Elder Abuse

54

Nancy Lopez, Arman Alberto Sorin Shadaloey, and D'Andrea K. Joseph

Introduction

The global population is rapidly aging, but limited information on healthy aging is available. In 2017, globally there were an estimated 962 million people aged 60 or above, comprising 13% of the global population. Demographic projections demonstrate that the proportion of the aged population will continue to grow and by 2050, all regions of the world with the exception of Africa will have a quarter or more of their population of age 60 and above. Studies have shown that increasing economic development has served, supported a greater proportion of the population advancing into older age during adulthood. There will be an increasing likelihood that people will die at adult ages, comparable to high-income countries. The first world report on aging and health, jointly issued by the WHO's Department of Ageing and Life Course and the NIA, provides a platform of discussion with the intention to uncover knowledge gaps, which when filled would assist in creating public health measures addressing the future needs of an aging population. The WHO reports that 1 in 6 people aged 60 or older has experienced some sort of abuse in the past year. In 2021, the National Council on Aging reported that 1 in 10 Americans had experienced some form of elder abuse.

In the setting of a rapidly aging population, it is instrumental to investigate the causes of stagnating progress in advanced age healthcare, part of which elderly abuse is a fundamental contributing factor. As the advanced age population increases in proportion to the total population, elder abuse is expected to become exponentially an even more pressing problem. Ultimately, the abuse of older people has serious repercussions on physical and mental health with financial and social consequences, including, but not limited to, physical injuries, avoidable mortality, depression, cognitive decline, and overall loss of healthy years.

Definition of Elder Abuse

In 2003, the US National Academy of Sciences proposed a widely accepted scientific definition of elder abuse described as "(a) intentional actions that cause harm or create a serious risk of harm (whether or not harm is intended) to a vulnerable elder by a caregiver or other person who stands in a trust relationship, or (b) failure

N. Lopez · A. A. S. Shadaloey
Department of Surgery, NYU Langone Hospital — Long Island, Mineola, NY, USA
e-mail: nancylopez@nyulangone.org; Arman.Shadaloey@nyulangone.org

D. K. Joseph (✉)
NYU Long Island School of Medicine, NYU Langone Hospital—Long Island, Mineola, NY, USA
e-mail: d'andrea.joseph@nyulangone.org

P. Petrone, C. E.M. Brathwaite (eds.), *Acute Care Surgery in Geriatric Patients*, https://doi.org/10.1007/978-3-031-30651-8_54

by a caregiver to satisfy the elder's basic needs or to protect the elder from harm." According to the Centers for Disease Control and Prevention, "elder abuse is an intentional act or failure to act that causes or creates a risk of harm to an older adult." The abuse is commonly at the hands of a person who is assigned as caregiver but can also occur at the hands of others. Like other populations, elder abuse occurs across all forms of ethnic, social, and gender groups. However, the data in some groups remain less well defined and may be a function of cultural differences. The response to abuse is also different in different ethnic populations with one study touting trans-generational factors as playing a key role in response to abuse in the African-American population. A study by Burnes et al. showed that neglect of the elder population was lower in people of Hispanic ethnicity. Members of the LGBTQ community have higher rates of isolation and are at higher risks for abuse as compared to other groups, suggesting that older people who identify as such are at an even higher risk. Ultimately, this definition describes an elder individual that suffered injury or deprivation by another individual responsible for their wellbeing.

Incidence and Prevalence

It is important to note that how institutions, communities, and culture define elder abuse may differ, therefore data can have an inherited bias, thus prevalence and incidence may be underreported. The population tends to be subdivided into community and institutionally living older adult populations due to the lack of reliable prevalence studies in institutional settings such as long-term care or nursing facilities. However, numerous large-scale population surveys of community-dwelling individuals in a number of countries have been conducted. The results have ranged widely with self-reported data far outpacing that of individuals living at home. It is well understood that reports of abuse are often underreported due to a myriad of factors that include dependence or cognitive impairment.

The prevalence of elder abuse in the USA is estimated to be between 10% and 16%. Overall, studies reported an aggregated elder abuse prevalence ranging from 2.2% to 36.2%, with a mean of 14.3%. Emotional abuse appears to be the most common type of abuse at 11.6% in one study, with financial abuse occurring at about 6.8%. Sexual abuse was reported ranged from 0.9% to 6% depending on the study. The highest aggregated prevalence was reported in China (36.2%) and Nigeria (30.0%), followed by Israel (18.4%), India (14.0%), Europe (10.8%), Mexico (10.3%), the USA (9.5%), and Canada (4.0%).

Physical abuse encompasses acts carried out with the intention to cause physical harm or injury. Psychological or emotional abuse refers to acts carried out with the intention of causing emotional damage or injury. Sexual assault is sexual behavior or a sexual act forced upon an individual without their consent. Material exploitation involves the misappropriation of the elder's money or property. Neglect is the failure of a designated caregiver to meet the needs of a dependent older person. In the USA, the definition of elder abuse is state dependent, making the true incidence of abuse difficult to ascertain. However, some data exist with respect to the types of abuse as previously described.

Physical Abuse

In a systematic review of global population studies, in 1-year, physical abuse prevalence rates across studies ranged from 0.2% to 4.9% with a mean of 2.8%. Worldwide, Canada (0.5%) and the USA (1.4%) reported the lowest prevalence rates of elder physical abuse, followed by Europe (1.67%). Two studies from Asia reported somewhat higher physical abuse rates (India: 4.3%, China: 4.9%), whereas a single study from Nigeria found by far the highest rate (14.6%). The typical presentation of an elderly patient suffering physical abuse ranges from serious physical injury such as broken bones, traumatic brain injuries to bruises and lacerations. The patient may also exhibit signs of emotional distress and withdrawal, which could also be signs of emotional abuse.

Sexual Abuse

It is not uncommon for the victim of sexual abuse to also present with bruises and lacerations, or with signs of emotional distress. The location of these bruises could help guide the clinician as these injuries will also be present in areas around the genitalia. The presence of unexplained sexually transmitted diseases also serves as an indication of sexual abuse. A 1 year study on the incidence of sexual abuse across countries found that while Nigeria had a higher prevalence of physical abuse, they had the lowest prevalence of sexual abuse at lowest 0.04%.

Financial Abuse

The decrease in functionality that can occur with physiological aging is a risk factor for financial abuse. Patients may be unable or chose not to report their abuser as this may commonly be a family member. In one study, family members were the perpetrator about 54% of the time, while healthcare workers and partners were 31% and 13%, respectively. The review of 1-year prevalence of financial abuse ranged from 1.0% to 9.2% with a mean of 4.7%. Studies from Nigeria and Israel reported the highest prevalence of financial abuse at 13.1% and 6.4%, respectively. Mexico had the lowest prevalence of financial abuse (2.6%), whereas mean rates across Europe (3.8%) and the USA (4.5%) fell in the middle. Financial abuse can range from stealing of funds to neglect, where the victim's bills will go unpaid. It may also include using the individual's assets for the perpetrator's own benefit.

Psychological Abuse

Studies using substantive threshold criteria typically defined emotional/psychological abuse cases as 10 or more events in the past year, and some studies added a criterion that the mistreatment be perceived as somewhat or very serious by the older adult. Patients can experience emotional distress with any of the aforementioned abuses and with psychological abuse independently. Frequently, the abuser is a partner or a spouse, but abuse can also be experienced at the hands of others such as a caretaker. The victim can present with physical decline, decreased self esteem, and feelings of shame and guilt and may also present with post-traumatic stress disorder. Among studies that used substantive threshold criteria, 1-year emotional/psychological abuse prevalence ranged from 0.7% to 6.3%, with a mean of 3.3%. Studies that did not use substantive threshold criteria reported 1-year emotional abuse prevalence ranging from 4.6% to 27.3%, with a mean of 13.6%. The variant definitions of psychological abuse may be oversensitive reporting, such as single insult between 60-year-old spouses in the last year. Among studies that used the higher threshold criteria, India reported relatively high emotional abuse prevalence (10.8%), whereas Canada, the USA, and Europe had lower mean rates of 1.4%, 1.5%, and 2.9%, respectively.

Neglect

One of the most prevalent of elder abuse, neglect is often at the hands of persons known to the victims. Perpetrators of neglect are most commonly the offspring of the victim. Patients will present with signs of neglect that include poor hygiene, starvation, dehydration, and poor overall health. Studies show that neglect constitutes 60–70% of all types of elder abuse. Many standardized tools exist to screen for elderly neglect, however prevalence studies either defined neglect cases as one or more events within a given time period or according to substantive threshold criteria based on event frequency and elder self-perceived seriousness. Studies using substantive thresholds typically defined neglect as 10 or more events in the past year, compared to some studies, which included the criterion that the events be perceived as somewhat or very serious by the elder. The difference in 1-year neglect prevalence between studies that used threshold criteria and those that did not was not significant. Among studies that incorporated threshold criteria, Canada reported the lowest rate of elder neglect (0.4%), followed by Europe (0.5%) and the USA (1.1%), whereas India reported the highest neglect prevalence (4.3%).

Impact of COVID-19

The COVID-19 pandemic and the resulting stay-at-home orders in order to prevent transmission demonstrated a concomitant increase in IPV across countries. Prior to the COVID-19 pandemic, elder abuse affected one in ten older Americans annually, however, post pandemic data report now that one in five are affected (21.3%), an 83.6% increase. The surge in elder abuse is multifactorial. A multivariate logistic regression analysis examined elder abuse in a diverse sample of 897 older persons from April to May 2020, when all states had implemented stay-at-home orders. In the final models, sense of community emerged as a persistent protective factor against elder abuse. At the relational level, physical distancing was associated with a reduced risk for elder abuse. At the individual level, financial strain was associated with increased risk of abuse.

Signs of Abuse

It is important that the clinician be alert to signs of abuse when evaluating patients. With the increasing age of the population, there is a greater need to investigate elder abuse. Victims may conceal their abuse for fear of retaliation or may be unable to articulate secondary to cognitive impairments. Additionally chronic illness in the elderly may create false findings of abuse, such as ecchymosis.

Multiple screening forms have been developed to identify elder abuse, however, a gold standard that would assess elder abuse is difficult to determine due to the various legal definitions, a variety of clinical experiences and situations, signs of abuse having great overlap with markers of disease, and other standards in different regions. For example, The QualCare Scale is a direct observational scale that was originally developed as a measure of the quality of caregiving provided by family caregivers including the dimensions of physical care, psychological care, medical care maintenance, environmental care, human rights violations, and financial care.

The EARAE tool was developed for community-based caseworkers working with older adults. The tool is used to capture information from elder abuse cases in order to determine changes in the level of risk for primary and secondary types of abuse and abuse outcomes to identify and determine changes in contributing risk factors and track interventions and outcomes; however, the tool needs to be validated. Additionally, the FAMOASQ is also a questionnaire that is answered verbally and is culturally and socially tailored to Mexican older adults. More validity testing of the current assessment tools is needed; however, a multi-systemic approach rather than a single tool needs to be used to screen for elder abuse.

At this time, the US Preventive Services Task Force does not recommend screening for elder abuse or neglect, which is of particular concern. However, risk factors for abuse are well known and should prompt further investigation if this exists. These include being female, cognitive decline, limited social support and isolation, mental health problems, functional impairment and dependence, and lower socioeconomic status. Factors such as financial dependence and substance abuse in the perpetrator as well as high stress and poor coping mechanisms are risks for elder abuse. As such, the presence of notable risk factors and clinical judgment in the presence of one the following findings should warrant additional evaluation:

- Physical abuse—abrasions, lacerations, ecchymosis, fractures, burns, depression, delirium with or without worsening of dementia or dementia-related behavior problems.
- Psychological abuse—direct observation of verbal abuse, subtle signs of intimidations such as deferring questions to a caregiver, evidence

of isolation of victim from trusted friends and family members, depression, anxiety.

- Sexual abuse—bruising, abrasions, lacerations in the anogenital area or abdomen, newly acquired sexually transmitted diseases, urinary tract infections.
- Financial abuse—inability to pay for medicine, medical care, food, rent, or other necessities, failure to renew prescriptions or keep medical appointments, unexplained worsening chronic medical problems that were previously controlled, nonadherence to medication regimen or other treatment, malnutrition, weight loss, or both, without an obvious medical cause, depression, anxiety, evidence of poor financial decision making provided by the patient, firing of home care or other service providers by abuser, unpaid utility bills leading to loss of service, initiation of eviction proceedings.
- Neglect—decubitus ulcers, malnutrition, dehydration, poor hygiene, nonadherence to medication regimen.

Risk Factors for Elder Abuse

There are multiple risk factors that place the elderly population at risk for abuse. Below, Pillemer et al. describe risk factors in the setting of validated evidence for which there are three levels of evidence: Strong risk factors have validated by substantial evidence that have unanimous or near unanimous support from several studies; potential risk factors evidence is mixed or limited; and contested risk factors for which there has been a hypothesis concerning increased risk, but for which there is a lack of clear evidence.

Strong Risk Factors

- Functional dependence or disability
- Poor physical health
- Cognitive impairment/dementia
- Poor mental health
- Low income/SES
- Mental illness
- Substance misuse
- Abuser dependency

Potential Risk factors

- Gender
  - Women are more likely than men to experience elder abuse, specifically, emotional and financial abuse.
- *Age*
  - In the USA, younger age has been consistently associated with greater risk of elder abuse, including emotional, physical, financial abuse, and neglect. However, studies from Mexico and Europe report that older individuals are at heightened risk.
- *Financial dependence*
  - Lack of resources and lower socioeconomic status are associated with increased risk of elder abuse.
- *Race/ethnicity*
  - Compared with Caucasians, African-American older adults may be at increased risk of financial abuse and psychological abuse and aboriginal older adults have demonstrated higher risk of physical and sexual abuse, whereas Hispanic older adults have shown lower risk of emotional abuse, financial abuse, and neglect.
- *Relationship type*
  - Varies according to mistreatment type and culture.
  - In the USA, Israel, and Europe, the most common perpetrator of elder emotional and physical abuse is a spouse/partner, whereas the most common perpetrators of these mistreatment types in Asian countries are children and children-in-law.
- *Marital status*
  - Mixed data from the USA, Canada, and Europe indicate that being married is associated with aggregated elder abuse, emotional and physical abuse. However, other studies found that being single, separated/divorced, or widowed is associated with higher odds of aggregated elder abuse.
- *Geographic location*
  - Individuals living in urban areas may be at greater risk for elder abuse as well as specific countries.
  - A prevalence study of seven European countries found that residing in Greece was

associated with increased risk of sexual abuse, whereas residing in Portugal was associated with increased risk of financial abuse.

Less apparent are the following risk factors

- *Ageism.*
- *Older individuals may be perceived as fragile, dependent, or burdensome, making it more permissible for younger generations to mistreat them.*
- *Social and cultural norms.*

Prevention Strategies

Although great strides have been made to improve the knowledge gap regarding elderly abuse, preventative intervention studies are much scarcer. Approximately 10 intervention studies have been conducted with the results of most of these efforts being negative or equivocal and no international comparative studies of prevention programs have been conducted. Fortunately, taking on a multidisciplinary approach to targeting the five types of abuse is an acceptable initial step.

There is preliminary evidence of several prevention options, however. The most promising programs include MDT, helplines for potential victims, financial management for elders at risk of financial exploitation, caregiver support interventions, and emergency shelter for victims.

Multidisciplinary Teams

Multidisciplinary teams are likely to be an effective response to coordinating care and reducing fragmentation, leveraging resources, increasing professional knowledge, and improving. A possible limitation is that MDTs are more available in higher-income nations where multiple resources can be allocated. In lower-income countries, a higher priority is likely to be the establishment of basic elder abuse services, with later attention to coordination.

Helplines

Helplines provide an anonymous platform for elder patients to seek help about their abusive situation. Examples of hotlines exist in multiple countries such as "Helpline for Abused Older People" in Milan, Italy, which counsels abuse. The most extensive helpline system is a national network of helpline centers created by ALMA France that provides both immediate counseling and longer-term follow-up.

Money Management

Money management programs targeted to groups at high risk for financial exploitation and in particular individuals with some degree of cognitive impairment and who are socially isolated. These programs provide money management assistance, such as help with paying bills, making bank deposits, negotiating with creditors, and paying home care personnel.

Caregiver Support

Caregiver interventions provide services to relieve the burden of caregiving, such as housekeeping and meal preparation, care, education, support groups, and day care. There is suggestive evidence that these interventions, when directed specifically to abusive caregivers, may help prevent revictimization. Additionally, there is some indication that the potential for the onset of abuse may be reduced by caregiver support interventions.

Shelter

Emergency shelter currently exists for women and children, however underutilized by older women. Additionally, battered women's shelters typically are not designed to accommodate older women with physical health problems or dementia, and they do not offer services to abused men. However, specialized shelter programs for elder abuse victims have been developed and provide a safe medically appropriate environment. Descriptive studies of shelter programs suggest positive results.

Reporting and Documenting Elder Abuse

In the USA, all states have some form of mandated elder abuse reporting law; however, each state law has variations. Variations include the circumstance required to mandate a report, the action that can be taken if the victim has capacity, and how the reports are filed. Additionally, each state has its own definition of what is considered elder abuse and has different laws to prosecute those who committed the abuse. Depending on the laws in any given state, mandated reports may include doctors, nurses, home health care providers, and nursing home staff members, and few states also required any person who suspects elder abuse to report it.

Mandated reports must contact the state's Adult Protection Services (APS) or similar agency. Abuse reports may also be made to local law enforcement agency if additional criminal acts are involved.

When a report is made, several services are provided. The elder or dependent adult will be given options to keep him/her safe from harm. The unaware family members and friends can be alerted to step in to help. In some cases, the abuse perpetrator can be prosecuted, lessening the harm to others.

As an example of a guideline in reporting elder abuse, the Western Australia Elder Abuse Protocol describes the following five steps:

- Identify whether abuse is taking place
  - Gain more information about the elder person's situation.
  - Gather information from other sources as well.
- Provide emotional support
  - Give them your full attenuation.
  - Reassure them that it is okay to talk about the situation.
  - Do not confront the perpetrator.
- Assess risk and plan safety
  - Determine the level of urgency.

    An emergency describes a situation where there is an immediate threat to life or serious risk of injury or property damage.

    An urgent situation describes threats to the safety of the older person, others, or damage or loss of property or finances.

    A non-urgent situation involves no immediate threat to safety.
  - Take steps to safeguard the elder person and others in any response to the abuse.
- Contact the appropriate service according to the level of risk
  - Seek consent if it is not an emergency.
  - To note, capacity should be evaluated for ability to consent in the elderly person. Capacity is the ability to make and communicate a decision. If capacity is uncertain, a clinician will need to formally assess capacity.
  - If they refuse assistance, safely provide contact information.
- Maintain documentation of concerns and actions taken.

Conclusion

Part of the challenge with elder abuse is how it is defined. It is well accepted that IPV exists in that population, but in that group, the terminology used is usually "elder neglect," negating the other aspects of IPV that the population experiences. IPV includes neglect, emotional and psychological abuse, financial abuse, and of course can include sexual abuse. Data suggest that recognizing patients at risk and implementing forms of social support can work toward decreasing the incidence of elder abuse. Adoption of social interventions could have far-reaching implications, which can translate into improved quality of life and better outcomes with illness.

References

1. Burston GR. Letter: granny-battering. Br Med J. 1975;3:592. https://doi.org/10.1136/bmj.3.5983.592-a.
2. Van Royen K, Van Royen P, De Donder L, Gobbens RJ. Elder abuse assessment tools and interventions for use in the home environment: a scoping review. Clin Interv Aging. 2020;15:1793–807. https://doi.org/10.2147/CIA.S261877.
3. Beard JR, Officer A, de Carvalho IA, Sadana R, Pot AM, Michel JP, et al. The world report on ageing and health: a policy framework for healthy ageing. Lancet. 2016;387(10033):2145–54. https://doi.org/10.1016/S0140-6736(15)00516-4.
4. Pillemer K, Burnes D, Riffin C, Lachs MS. Elder abuse: global situation, risk factors, and prevention strategies. Gerontologist. 2016;56(Suppl 2):S194–205. https://doi.org/10.1093/geront/gnw004.
5. Chang ES, Levy BR. High prevalence of elder abuse during the COVID-19 pandemic: risk and resilience factors. Am J Geriatr Psychiatry. 2021;29(11):1152–9. https://doi.org/10.1016/j.jagp.2021.01.007.
6. Lachs MS, Pillemer KA. Elder abuse. N Engl J Med. 2015;373(20):1947–56. https://doi.org/10.1056/NEJMra1404688.
7. Blundell B. Elder abuse protocol: guidelines for action. 2017. https://www.researchgate.net/publication/333842899_Elder_Abuse_Protocol_Guidelinesfor_Action.
8. Mikton C, Campo-Tena L, Yon Y, Beaulieu M, Shawar YR. Factors shaping the global political priority of addressing elder abuse: a qualitative policy analysis. Lancet Healthy Longev. 2022;3(8):e31–e539. https://doi.org/10.1016/S2666-7568(22)00143-X.
9. Burnes D, Pillemer K, Caccamise P, Mason A, Henderson CR, Berman J, et al. Prevalence of and risk factors for elder abuse and neglect in the community: a population-based study. J Am Geriatr Soc. 2015;63(9):1906–12. https://doi.org/10.1111/jgs.13601.
10. Ayalon L. Reports of elder neglect by older adults, their family caregivers, and their home care workers: a test of measurement invariance. J Gerontol B Psychol Sci Soc Sci. 2015;70(3):432–42. https://doi.org/10.1093/geronb/gbu051.
11. Elman A, Rosselli S, Burnes D, Clark S, Stern ME, LoFaso VM, et al. Developing the emergency department elder mistreatment assessment tool for social workers using a modified Delphi technique. Health Soc Work. 2020;45(2):110–21. https://doi.org/10.1093/hsw/hlz040.
12. Li M, Chen R, Dong X. Elder mistreatment across diverse cultures. Generations. 2020;44(1):20–5.
13. Joseph J, Gonzalez A. Elder abuse in communities of color in the United States: a literature review. In: Kratcoski PC, Edelbacher M. Perspectives on elderly crime and victimization; pp 125–139 Springer: New York; 2018.

55 Post-Operative Care in Skilled Nursing and Long-Term Care

Donna Seminara, John Maese, Lorri Senk, Anita Szerszen, and Annarose Taylor

Overview

After surgical services in an acute care environment have stabilized postoperatively, there are patients for whom discharge to home is not feasible. This is usually because the discharge is clearly unsafe or there are ongoing clinical needs that overwhelm the ability for care at home.

Determination of safety for discharge is a complex analysis best served by a multidisciplinary team. Team leaders in this arena are usually represented by the social services department. Once medical necessity for Skilled Nursing Facility (SNF) is determined, then the social services team will communicate with family and analyze the home environment and available financial resources. Economic and social disparities in health are significant contributors leading to SNF after acute hospitalization. The social services team leads the effort in coordinating a post-acute care transfer to SNF for Restorative Rehabilitation (RR) and ongoing medical care.

Interestingly, acute surgical needs may uncover patients who are "on the brink of collapse" of independent living. For instance, a fall leading to hip fracture may uncover the patient with chronic sarcopenia and multiple falls who can no longer be safely at home without supervision or is in need of nursing home placement. Chronic psychological impairments from personality disorders complicated by cognitive impairment or complexities of hoarding may make returns to home environments unsafe. Unmasked poverty may bring a case to the attention of social workers for Medicaid applications. Evidence of abuse may be uncovered warranting Adult Protective Services consultation.

Patients who stay in acute care hospitals for inpatient rehabilitation must meet clinical criteria. Most importantly, they must be able to interact with some form of therapy twice a day for a

D. Seminara (✉)
Division of Geriatrics, Staten Island University Hospital, Northwell Health, Staten Island, NY, USA

Eger Health Care and Rehabilitation Center, Staten Island, NY, USA

J. Maese
Division of Geriatrics, Staten Island University Hospital, Northwell Health, Staten Island, NY, USA

L. Senk
Eger Health Care and Rehabilitation Center, Staten Island, NY, USA
e-mail: lsenk@eger.org

A. Szerszen
Inpatient Geriatrics and Research, Staten Island University Hospital, Northwell Health, Staten Island, NY, USA
e-mail: aszerszen@northwell.edu

A. Taylor
Lafayette College, Easton, PA, USA

P. Petrone, C. E.M. Brathwaite (eds.), *Acute Care Surgery in Geriatric Patients*,
https://doi.org/10.1007/978-3-031-30651-8_55

total of 3 hours of therapy daily. Limitations to such care may include:

(a) Overwhelming comorbidities such as brittle heart disease, infectious complications requiring isolation such as Clostridium difficile colitis, COVID pneumonia, or intensive wound care.
(b) Mental status challenges that inhibit a patient's ability to meaningfully interact, such as cognitive impairments secondary to dementia, delirium, chronic psychiatric illness, or traumatic brain injury.

Patients who are limited in their ability to perform the rigors of a program described above may then be appropriate for ongoing care and rehabilitation in an SNF. Social service needs such as a lack of home supervision, comorbid medical illnesses such as heart failure and complex geriatric syndromes such as protein/calorie malnutrition and sarcopenia may be additional factors that lead to the decision to have disposition to a SNF.

The application process to a skilled nursing facility for postoperative restorative rehabilitation varies from state to state. Most will utilize an admission tool. The state of Florida utilizes the AHCA 5000–3008 form which assesses medical certification for Medicaid Long-Term Care Services and Patient Transfers. In New York, the tool used is a Hospital and Community (H/C) Patient Review Instrument or PRI. The PRI provides a collection of basic information including demographics, diagnoses, prognoses, behaviors, therapy needs, treatments, and scoring of a patient's ability to perform activities of daily living (ADLs). ADL functions include bathing and personal hygiene, dressing and undressing oneself, using the toilet, mobility/transferring, and eating. For complex post-op patients who have had an extensive LOS in a hospital, the actual completion of the PRI may be a further barrier to timely discharge.

Once it is decided that a nursing facility is required for ongoing post-operative care the next issue is to coordinate payment for such services. Payor sources include Medicare, Medicaid, third-party private insurance, specialty combination programs such as Managed Long-Term Care (MLTC), and private pay resources. If a patient is Medicaid eligible, but is not acutely covered, there are processes that accelerate Medicaid enrollment.

Another important factor in preparation for care in post-acute nursing facilities is the clear determination of the goals of care for the individual patient. This is where nuanced choices between specific skilled nursing facilities may determine where the optimal rehabilitation plan can be devised for a patient. This will vary quite a bit on a case-by-case basis. Some patients may require a mechanical ventilation unit with pulmonary stepdown whereas others would benefit from on-site hemodialysis. Furthermore, recognition of ultimate patient disposition may be a factor in choosing a particular facility. For instance, for an 85-year-old cognitively intact post ORIF of right hip, an eventual plan to return to home after restorative rehabilitation may be a clear goal. For another patient with post stroke cognitive impairments and a dense right-sided hemiparesis, multiple issues will impact ultimate disposition. Options may range from returning to home to long-term care enrollment in a skilled nursing facility based upon the degree of success of rehab as well as social issues such as financial resources and family/community support.

From day one of admission to a nursing facility, their Case Management and Social Service departments will be intimately involved in assuring payment for services and ongoing payment to support the post discharge from SNF needs of the patient. The economic reality of the individual patient will often define their post discharge options. Additionally, the relationship of the individual with their family and the strength of those bonds also plays a significant role in final disposition determinations. Socially isolated, economically challenged, and undocumented populations have a higher rate of failure to sustain independent and safe living in the community. These cases are especially challenging for skilled nursing facilities.

This chapter seeks to educate on the nuances of choosing the right facility for the right patient and to inform medical personnel on the resources and services provided in skilled nursing environments for post-operative care.

Understanding Skilled Nursing Facility Admission Categories

Through advances of technology, developments in the scientific practice of medicine and improvements in living conditions patients are living longer. Moreover, increasing percentages of older patients are living (and expecting) a higher functional quality of life than previous generations. Yet, all patients do not age in the same way. There are persons 60 years of age who are physiologically 90 and those 90 years of age who play pickleball. The patient that needs a skilled nursing home likely has multiple risk factors contributing to that decision which should be less dependent upon age but more upon the fragility of the patient, their home situation, and the available number of caregivers they will have. In a population where the average life span is increasing and the number of children being born is decreasing, skilled nursing homes will continue to be an essential option in geriatric health care.

The goals of restorative rehabilitation in a SNF are directly linked to successful outcomes of post-surgical care: optimizing the ability of the individual to return to their pre-surgical home with their pre-surgical level of function.

Admission categories to SNFs include Short-Term Rehab (STR), Long-Term Care (LTC), Hospice, and Respite Care.

SNFs appropriate for post-op care of geriatric patients are health care facilities capable of a wide range of medical services including:

1. Individualized treatment plans led by a physician and a multidisciplinary team including nurses, social workers, rehabilitation specialists, dietitians, and recreational team members.
2. RR including physical, occupational, and speech therapy teams.
3. Consultant services such as psychiatry, dentistry, and podiatry.
4. Ability to credential consultants to staff from every medically appropriate specialty including general surgery, orthopedics, wound care, cardiology, pulmonary, urology, GI, etc.
5. Administration of scheduled medications.
6. Administration of IV antibiotics.
7. Administration of IV fluids.
8. Nebulizer administration of medications.
9. Wound management.
10. Plain film radiographs.
11. Ultrasound capabilities (for example, duplex US of lower extremity to rule out DVT).
12. Laboratory services to process phlebotomy, urine, and sputum collections.

During STR stays care will be supervised by a medical team to manage acute and chronic medical needs of the patient. During the course of rehabilitation these needs may fluctuate considerably especially with respect to geriatric specific conditions (sarcopenia, delirium), hypercoagulable states (DVT/PE), fluid imbalance (edema, CHF), and infectious diseases (COVID, C. diff, cellulitis, pneumonia, and wound infection). Additionally, a physiatrist will lead the PT/OT team in directing care with an end-goal of safe physical discharge. An ongoing coordination with the surgical team cannot be over emphasized. Medical and Rehabilitation trained physicians are not equipped with the nuanced insights that the surgical team will have to assure post-operative success. A patient that required daily rounds by a surgical team should not be acutely left without that input for a month after acute hospital discharge. With consideration from that perspective, it is advisable to have a scheduled follow-up visit made at the time of discharge so the patient can be evaluated by the surgeon within a reasonable time frame, usually within one week. When a patient does not have an appointment pre-scheduled, there are multiple barriers to timely follow-up. These include:

1. Patient or family barriers linked to the patient feeling fatigued or overwhelmed by the hospitalization and a vague desire to wait "until feeling stronger."

2. Insurance barriers where authorizations are required for specialty appointments; in general, managed care facilitators in the SNF are not as savvy as those in the hospital in obtaining needed authorizations as they usually multitask and perform multiple SNF roles/ functions. It is rarely a dedicated individual with only authorization responsibilities, as the SNF volume for this activity does not demand it.
3. Medical barriers such as acute complications which make it more difficult to transport the patient such as sepsis and delirium.
4. Financial barriers such as ambulette transport costs to medical offices, which are not covered by insurance. When a patient is in a SNF; the patient or family must agree to pay for transportation, and this cost often runs into several hundreds of dollars.

In addition to Short-Term Rehabilitation admissions, Long-Term Care admissions are the cornerstone of care provided in traditional skilled nursing facilities. These units are inhabited by patients who are living in the nursing home and who are not expected to ever leave the facility for another residence. There may be intense nursing time involved in the care of residents who qualify for skilled nursing homes. Such care includes wound care for pressure injury, enteral feedings via G-Tube, ostomy and Foley care, or administration of IM, SQ, or nebulizer medications. When these residents are acutely ill, management may be more intense with administration of IV fluids and IV medications, and maintainence of flow charts to document vital signs and input–output measurements. This level of skill assures actionable coordination with consultant surgical teams to provide data and directed care needed by surgeons to further assist in the recovery of their post-op patients who reside in LTC units.

Within long-term care there may be specific units or programs designed for hospice patients. Usually, hospice patients are not involved in acute surgeries, but a small percentage of patients may proceed from post-op care to hospice care. Ongoing coordination for surgical and wound care must be coordinated with the hospice team. Another SNF admission category is for Respite Care and these cases are rarely involved in surgical interventions. Respite patients have their stay paid for by the Medicaid system or by private pay for up to two weeks of care in a SNF; during this time, caregiving family members are given a respite from patient care duties for time needed for personal issues (may be a medical need or even time for vacation with family).

Payor Sources and their Influence on Length of Stay (Los)

For most geriatric patient populations, the primary payor is the Center for Medicare and Medicaid Services.

In traditional Medicare Part A, acute hospitalizations are covered as well as care at inpatient rehabilitation facilities and hospitals, so long as a physician certifies the medical need for such care. A Medicare Benefit Period (MBP) starts on the first day of the hospitalization and will continue through the time in a skilled nursing facility and extend for 60 days post discharge. Patient responsibilities for deductibles and copayments will vary over the course of care. Only one deductible will need to be paid per MBP (starting with hospital, not repeated at SNF if one is directly transferred from acute hospital or is within 60 days of acute hospital discharge). In the hospital for days 1–60 of the MBP the deductible is $1600 (as of 1/1/2023). On days 61–90 there is $400 coinsurance each day; from days 91 and beyond there is $800 coinsurance for each "lifetime reserve day." There are a maximum of 60 reserve days over the course of one's lifetime.

Once in an SNF, 2023 Medicare out-of-pocket costs are as follows: Days 1–20 there is $0 coinsurance, days 21–100 the daily coinsurance is $200 and beyond day 100 the patient is responsible for all costs. Thus, there are financial incentives by the patient to resolve rehabilitation needs within 20 days. When ongoing care is overwhelming and needed, most patients are financially motivated to work to resolve their needs by day 100.

Medicare covers the costs at an inpatient rehabilitation facility for the following:

1. Rehab services including physical therapy, occupational therapy, and speech-language pathology
2. A semi-private room
3. Meals
4. Nursing services
5. Prescription drugs
6. Medical supplies

Medicare does not cover private duty nursing, phones or TVs, personal items, or a private room unless they are medically necessary. Medicare Part B covers the cost of physician services.

In addition to traditional Medicare where copays and other costs may be covered by fee-for-service coinsurances, Medicare also offers a private plan option known as Medicare Advantage (Part C). They combine Medicare parts A and B with other benefits. Each private insurance company that sponsors such a plan has different deductible and copay structures. Enrollments in these plans have risen rapidly; in April 2022, enrollments were estimated at 29 million individuals, representing 46% of all Medicare beneficiaries. It is estimated that by 2025 this program will be the dominant source of Medicare coverage. Note that with Medicare's quality reporting system for Medicare Advantage, these regulations apply to plans as entities rather than to individual subunits such as hospitals, physicians, and nursing homes. So, quality data reported from these plans is in the aggregate and is not as useful as data collected on individual SNFs under traditional Medicare. If comparisons on quality measures are a driving force in choice of SNF, the data from Advantage plans can be misleading.

Medicaid coverage of care in a nursing facility (NF) is available only for SNFs and NFs that are licensed and certified by its state survey agency as a Medicaid Nursing Facility. The need for nursing facility services is defined by each state with their own criteria. A covered individual's plan of care must by oriented to that unique resident's needs for services in order to reach the highest practicable level of wellbeing. Coverage by federal law must include all nursing related services, specialized rehab services, medically related social services, pharmaceutical services, dietary services, professionally directed activity programs, emergency dental and routine dental services, room and bed maintenance, and routine personal hygiene items.

Most older persons who require post-operative ongoing care in a SNF will be covered by either Medicare or Medicaid plans. There will be some, however, who are only covered by third party plans—private insurance usually obtained by continuing to work after age 65. Their coverage for SNF services may be quite variable. Another option for a smaller group could be private pay where the entire bill is satisfied by the individual patient or their family outside of insurance coverage. There may be options specific to individual homes where additional services are offered for out-of-pocket payment such as access to private rooms.

Another subset program of CMS are the dual-eligible programs; dual eligibility refers to being enrolled in both Medicare and Medicaid. One such regional program is Managed Long-Term Care (MLTC). In New York, MLTC is mandatory for those who are dual eligible, over the age of 21, and in need of community-based long-term care services for more than 120 days. Many such programs, in addition to supporting services in nursing homes, will also provide home care, adult day health care, home delivered meals, medical equipment, and services such as podiatry, audiology, PT/OT/ST, etc.

SNF Care for Post-Operative Patients

The first medical matter to be addressed when a patient is being admitted to a SNF for post-operative care is to determine specific goals of care for the individual. If a patient is recovering from an ORIF of a hip fracture, a reasonable goal would be to ensure ambulation with an assistive device that allows for a patient living alone to function independently in their home. The number of steps that a patient needs to navigate will vary based upon the home environment and this understanding will allow for the design of a safeplan tailored to the individual. A patient with a Stage IV pressure injury to the sacrum with an exudative wound may need enough time to assure that use of a wound-vac and high-tech nursing is in place for training the family on how to manage equipment. A patient post debridement of bone may require high-tech nursing for PICC line maintenance at home. The short game in a SNF resolves around knowing what the long-range plan is for ongoing care.

An essential component of a SNF treatment plan is a successful transition of care (TOC) from an acute care facility. The treatments in acute care must be clearly understood with direct input from the acute medical management team on what needs to be done next. Successful transition to SNF requires good communication with the facility as well as a thoughtful discharge plan. For example, lower cost once daily antibiotics helps the SNF fiscally manage the case. A direct line of communication between inpatient acute care teams and SNF medical and nursing teams will avoid pitfalls of poorly described treatment goals. Follow-up labs and imaging studies should be clearly defined with target dates for these studies along with parameters for interpretation to decrease risk of early readmission back to an acute care facility. For example, in the case of post-surgical debridement of osteomyelitis, target dates for completion of antibiotics, frequency of lab checks of sedimentation rates, and specific time intervals for surgical follow-up care (in person or via telehealth) should be clearly written and sent to the receiving SNF. Clear discharge plans will improve chances for a successful post-operative recovery.

Some post-op patients will need to follow up directly with a medical specialist as well. A common need is for cardiology follow-up, especially if there were cardiac complications during acute care of the patient. Did the acute care team leave information for the SNF staff in setting parameters for care? For example, titration with diuretics may be focused upon maintenance of a specific weight or urine output. If that is being maintained but at the cost of worsening renal function, how does the medical team at the SNF relay that information to the acute care cardiologist? How do patients with compromised post-operative wounds follow up with their treating surgeon? If there are clear expectations made at the outset, then it is likely that complicated medical matters will benefit from direct communication with acute care teams.

CMS has incentivized enhanced communication between acute care and rehab facilities in that both hospitals and skilled nursing facilities will be economically penalized for early readmission back to the hospital within 30 days of discharge from acute care. Financial clawbacks from future payments are one way that adverse clinical outcomes (readmission to acute care) have a significant economic impact on both hospitals and SNFs. The reasoning from the payor (CMS) is that a bi-directional coordinated team will work closely on care and avoid pitfalls that precipitate readmission. Medical setbacks most commonly involve complications of sepsis, delirium, exacerbations of congestive heart failure, brittle chronic obstructive pulmonary disease, and acute gastrointestinal bleeds. Any of these can derail the best-laid plans of post-operative care.

In recent years, sepsis protocols have been established in many SNFs to optimize early intervention in cases of potential sepsis. This has mirrored the work done in acute care facilities to combat the devastation of sepsis with timely intervention of antibiotics and vasoactive agents. Quality NFs should be able to identify patients at risk by vigilance for changes in vital signs and clinical scenarios consistent with sepsis. IVF and IV AB should be initiated immediately along with samples being taken for blood cultures, urine cultures, sputum culture if indicated, CXR and baseline labs with CBC and CMP. These measures should be initiated 24/7 when indicated and if ongoing IV access is necessary most facilities have relationships with services for placement of a mid-line to support ongoing IVF or IV AB. Usually after evaluation by medical personal within 24 h, ongoing treatment may be modified. Consultation with the primary surgical team may be critical within the first hours of identifying sepsis in a post-op patient.

Delirium is another medical problem that extends the LOS and complication rate of post-op patients. Delirium affects 37–46% of the general surgical population and in the ICU has been reported in up to 87% of patients. Consequences of delirium include not only functional decline but also increases in rates of all-cause mortality. Delirium is a medical emergency and as such recognition and early intervention are key. As increasing numbers of surgical patients are discharged quickly post operatively, the risk of delirium can be exacerbated by changes of location contributing to disorganized interpretation of surroundings. It is not uncommon for a patient with an acute hip fracture to be in an Emergency Department, temporary holding unit, operating room, recovery room, stepdown unit, general surgery floor and then out of acute care to SNF all within 72 h. Furthermore, individual types of surgical interventions carry higher delirium risks; other generalized surgically related delirium risks include time under anesthesia, use of analgesics, and inadequate pain control. It is imperative that the surgical team monitor for delirium risks in the acute setting and that they communicate these concerns to the SNF. No assumptions about changes in mental status should be presumed to be a routine response of older persons to the "stress of hospitalization." Patients with underlying cognitive impairments are at increased risk for delirium. This includes not only the overtly demented patient but also those with mild cognitive impairments. Additionally, delirium as an initial presentation of cognitive impairment in an individual may be a marker of dementia in the near future.

Hyperactive (hypermanic) delirium (approximately 25% of cases) is more easily recognizable for its overt symptomatology. Patients may be restless and agitated with symptoms of hallucinations and delusions. New cases of sundowning or insomnia in a SNF may represent symptoms of delirium. Hypoactive (hypomanic) delirium may be more subtle with patients being described as calm, and unusually quiet with decreased speech. These patients are often misrecognized as depressed. Appropriate recognition of the underlying delirium should launch a search for precipitant factors. All such factors must be addressed in a timely fashion. Enhancing a patient's sensory input by having them wear glasses, hearing aids, and dentures can significantly help in maintaining organized thinking in older persons. Evidence continues to support use of the Confusion Assessment Method (CAM) in screening patients for delirium.

Vascular complications are also increased in post-op patients who require SNF for RR. The incidence of Deep Vein Thrombosis in general surgical patients has been reported in Western studies to vary from 33–35%. A CDC study found the rate to be 1% for a life-threatening blood clot. Virchow's triad of intravascular vessel wall damage, stasis of flow, and the presence of a hypercoagulable state may be further exaggerated in SNF patients who have greater mobility challenges and age-related vascular disease complications. Vigilance in monitoring patients for DVT is essential in SNF rehab care.

Several options exist to facilitate follow-up by surgical teams at NFs:

1. If there is a brisk consultative business at a specific SNF, surgical teams may benefit from having a team member have consultative privileges at that SNF. This way direct visits can assist with postoperative surgical follow-up, even if by a junior team member who can report back to team leaders.
2. Emergency privileges are easy to obtain for specific individual cases where hands-on surgical care is necessary.
3. Telehealth has expanded the reach of surgical teams into SNFs. With fine resolution available on cameras, wounds may be easily evaluated. Peripherals such as a stethoscope can allow for good evaluations of breath sounds and fair evaluations of cardiac examinations. See below re telehealth and its influence in this arena.

The surgical team needs to also be made aware of the patient's ultimate discharge destination. It may be directly to the patient's home or the patient may be moving in with a family member while continuing their recuperation. This change of address and contact phone information should be shared with the surgical team. In addition to advanced cases sometimes converting within a SNF from Restorative Rehab to LTC, other patients may find themselves in new residential communities such as assisted living. The assisted living staff may need to assist the patient in coordinating ongoing surgical care and so again, the sharing of information about all medical and surgical teams of the patient is vital. Another potential discharge may be to a NY PACE program. These Programs for All-Inclusive Care for the Elderly (PACE) are a long-term care delivery and financing plan. The goal is to prevent unnecessary use of hospital and nursing home care; the program provides all care services for patients in the place where they live and in general, there is significant social service support to assist in scheduling appointments for transitions of care, medical and surgical visits. In Pennsylvania, PACE is known as Living Independence for the Elderly (LIFE).

Specific Post-Operative Specialty Considerations

Orthopedic Surgery

For a case of ORIF of a femoral neck fracture the American College of Surgeons National Surgical Quality Improvement Program Surgical Risk Calculator estimates the risk of discharge to a SNF for an overweight patient 75–84 years of age whose case is emergent with underlying oral medications for diabetes and hypertension to be 70.2%. This is a significant risk for a broad geriatric population of patients with these specifically listed common risk factors. In the post COVID era there has been a push to "rehabilitate at home" after orthopedic procedures but this is an approach best utilized for younger geriatric patients (under 75) with elective procedures (such as total joint replacements) who are highly motivated to do the work of rehab at home.

Orthopedic rehabilitation is a subset of SNF post-operative care with the greatest success in getting patients eventually back to their pre-surgical environment; there may be a transitional period of stay either with supervising family or with use of a home health aide (HHA) to continue to assist patients upon discharge. Community Health Agencies (CHA) such as Visiting Nurse Services will often continue in the role of supervision at home with ongoing PT/OT services.

Quality RR programs will incorporate clearly defined benchmarks for success at home. This may include training for ambulation on stairs, practicing getting into and out of a motor vehicle, and training in the functional use of the bathroom and kitchen. Patients will have needed durable medical equipment (DME) such as hospital beds or wheelchairs delivered home before the patient arrives there.

Most importantly for orthopedic cases, there should be a strong affiliation in place between the surgical team, physiatry and the SNF. Specifically, follow-up radiographs can be obtained at the SNF and reviewed by the operative team. Often well-entrenched orthopedic groups will have a consultative presence in the SNF to assist in supervising the specialty care of the patient. This is usually a high-volume service for SNFs and as such these relationships are longitudinal. Embedded orthopedic groups will also have a close relationship with the physiatrist orchestrating the rehab of the patient. This model is widely reproduced across the country.

Cardiac Surgery

Most noncomplicated Coronary Artery Bypass Graft patients go directly home postoperatively. There is a subset of patients with wound complications (usually in diabetics) who may require skilled nursing for frequent dressing changes and ongoing IV ABs.

Older geriatric patients may have symptomatic aortic stenosis requiring either SAVR or TAVR. More SAVR patients are discharged to SNF than TAVR, but TAVR patients are still at risk. One regional analysis of patients after TAVR found that 2.7% were discharged to an SNF. Independent predictors of this risk included age over 75, being female, a 5 meter walk test of over 7 seconds and not using oxygen at home prior to surgery. Patients that have complications of heart failure associated with their CAD and/or valvular heart disease are at increased risk to be discharged to SNF. Increased risk is associated with a longer LOS, female sex, advanced age, hypotension, and higher ejection fractions.

Congestive heart failure SNF programs will include tight measurements of fluid intake, urine output, and daily weights. The clearer the discharge instructions are regarding management targets for CHF, then the better the outcome. This is usually an area where performance can be enhanced. For instance, treatment adjustments for specific parameters (i.e., if weight gain of 3 lbs., then administer 40 mg extra of Lasix for one day) can enhance immediate responses to subtle clinical changes. When subspecialists are not going into SNFs to see patients, the use of telehealth services, especially by surgical cardiothoracic and medical cardiology teams, can be quite helpful in the management of this at-risk vulnerable population.

Urologic Surgery

The high numbers of patients receiving cystectomies, radical and partial nephrectomy, nephroureterectomy, and prostatectomy amplify the risk for geriatric patients to experience complications. These risks are increased by comorbid obesity, prolonged operative times, diabetes, steroid use, history of bleeding, use of ASA or NSAIDs, smoking, and hx of CHF and COPD. According to one review of readmissions after urologic surgery, it found high rates of the following diagnoses being associated with readmission: infection, sepsis, wound complications, UTI, VTE, and bleeding. An appropriate discharge plan from acute care should include specific recommendations to avoid and screen for these complications.

Another urologic complication at the SNF is the patient discharged to SNF after any surgery who has had post-operative urinary retention. They are often sent to rehab facilities with a Foley catheter and no specific orders for follow-up. Recommendations on how long to continue the Foley, when to try clamping, and whether or not it is expected for the patient to recover healthy bladder control should be documented. If specific forms of urologic therapy or follow-up are to be followed, then it should be clearly stated and defined.

Surgical Management of Wounds

The complexity of wound care is often underestimated. Wounds that do not heal are usually a result of infection, poor nutrition, or decreased vascular supply. As any surgeon knows keeping a wound clean and well debrided is important to successful healing. However, this is easier said than done. The Skilled Nursing Facility often has the right resources to engineer successful wound healing. Most common wounds managed in SNFs include pressure injury, vascular ulcers, post-operative wounds, burns, and exudative sequelae of advanced peripheral vascular disease. There is no one perfect therapy. Success is based upon using the right treatment for the right patient. Approaches vary in different facilities but having a specialized nurse evaluating each wound on a regular basis provides for stability in screening, evaluating, and administering care. When the same person is taking accountability for wound management, there is generally a more active and coordinated wound management program in that facility. The wound care coordinator can also work directly with surgical consultants to optimize care and assure that patients are being seen when they need to for interventions. Measurements and photographs are essential to sharing information with the surgical team and evaluating progress. Coordination with the surgical team is critical for success. Negative wound pressure devices and hyperbaric oxygen can present challenges for the homebound patient. These devices are effective in situations where the vascular supply may be compromised, and oxygenation of the tissue is limited. A wound specialist can work with the surgical team on optimizing treatments that the patient can go home with based on the patient's willingness, education, fragility, and skill level in taking care of the wound. There are sophisticated vascular teams that will visit SNFs on a business model where they provide diagnostic and treatment services in this area of wound care.

Vascular Surgery

Skilled Nursing facilities are in a unique position to provide care to the patient that suffers vascular injury. After initial surgery, about 3% of these patients require skilled nursing care. They are medically complex or their home is not safe for their discharge. These patients are frail and suffer from comorbid conditions like diabetes, which slows the healing process and increases recovery time. Frailty as an independent risk for the postoperative vascular patient has been well studied. High impact frailty domains such as mobility, nutrition, cognition, and psycho/social conditions increase risk for discharge into SNF after vascular surgery. The team approach for the patient is critical. The internist, physiatry, and surgeon playing important roles in the care of the patient. The access to behavioral health services is also essential because very often the member has a distorted body image that requires treatment. These services, often limited in the community and difficult to obtain, are more readily available in a SNF environment. Appropriately identified pre-surgical patients with frailty syndromes should be appropriately counseled of the potential for discharge to SNF.

Trauma

The Trauma patient may present with complex challenges because of multi-organ damage from the trauma, long recovery times, and complexities of medical management. The patient having survived the initial trauma in the hospital may need ongoing care before transitioning to home. An adequately staffed Skilled Nursing Facility can provide that transition of care. One challenge to this transition may be financial. Nursing homes get a fixed reimbursement for the care they provide, and medication costs are borne by the SNF. Thus, they may be reluctant to take on high-cost patients. There needs to be creative solutions for payment of expensive antibiotics and TPN. This can be accomplished by negotiations between the insurance company and the acute care hospital partnering with the SNF. The SNF partnering with the hospital is critical because ongoing care of the patient does not stop when the patient leaves the hospital. The SNF needs to be considered an extension of the hospital with appropriately shared financial risks, access to specialty supplies, and appropriate ongoing communication between acute care and SNF medical teams. The advent of telehealth has been a useful tool facilitating multiple consultations with the patient without the cost and hardship of transferring the patient to the acute care facility. Telehealth also leverages the limited availability in some locations of subspecialty care. Studies have demonstrated that the majority of high-cost trauma patients survive and that over 50% return to productivity. This return to productivity may be enhanced by utilizing skilled services to transition to home and by incorporating input by trauma teams on optimal products and therapeutic schedules in caring for this subset of patients. For instance, less expensive wound care dressings may increase costs in the long run by prolonging time to heal wounds and injury. By integrating further in the rehabilitative journey of their patients, trauma teams can continue to evolve their influence in the full recovery of their patients.

How to Compare Skilled Nursing Facilities

SNFs are categorized as either for-profit or not-for-profit. In the for-profit sector some SNFs are singly owned private corporations administered by families or small investment groups. Larger networks may own several local or regional chains of significant numbers of facilities, and they benefit from streamlined central business practices (i.e., centralized billing, case management, use of vendors for electronic records, laboratory services, etc.). Not-for-profits may be funded from government or private sources. For instance, in NYC the NYC Health + Hospitals is an integrated health care system which is publicly funded and includes five long-term care facilities. Other facilities may have been established with donated funds and are subsequently managed by not-for-profit entities such as religious institutions.

Comparisons between different nursing homes may be accomplished with resources that evaluate different state and federal benchmarks of care. www.Medicare.gov is a resource that will directly compare nursing home quality measures including health inspections, nursing home staffing, and quality of resident care parameters. Survey findings can be reviewed for individual facilities under their CMS Form 2567; each SNF is required to have this available for review upon request. Nursing home quality can also be investigated by contacting the Long-Term Care Ombudsman; this office addresses individual resident complaints and also advocates for changes at local, state, and national levels to improve resident care and quality of life.

State health departments and licensing agencies also track quality of care delivery at SNFs. Copies of full surveys of an individual SNF may be requested as well as complaint investigation reports. In New York State the Department of Health has a link on its website for NYS Health Profiles. This site provides information about every nursing home in NYS and examines the following parameters: quality of care received, quality of life achieved, safety of residents, preventive care practices, inspections, and complaint information. The Nursing Home Profiles quality data for all NYS SNFs can be downloaded from the Health Data NY website. Direct comparisons between different SNFs can be viewed such as comparative data on quality measures such as successful discharge to the community, occurrence of pressure Injury to skin, and use of psychotropic medications. Also, on the NYS DOH website is information to download for consumers on alternatives to LTC and average regional costs of SNF care.

When choosing an appropriate SNF for post-operative care, consideration of the individual's other comorbid conditions may direct a disposition choice because of other pressing medical needs. Specialty services may be pursued at specially designed and certified units that excel in their care for specific needs. Specifically licensed units may be optimal for End Stage Renal Disease on dialysis (both hemodialysis and peritoneal dialysis), Traumatic Brain Injury, Dementia Units, Mechanical Ventilation Units with respiratory support and infectious disease programs for HIV. Furthermore, other specially designed programs may benefit specific patient populations such as for those with neurologic impairments post CVA or Congestive Heart Failure programs. Palliative care programs exist but are not usually uniform when compared facility to facility. Some may have consultants in palliative care that focus on pain management while others specialize in assisting families with advanced directives and other medical orders for life sustaining treatments (MOLST). Other programs may not have specialty input but do address end-of-life issues and work with families to determine revised goals of care as a resident's global condition declines.

Telehealth in Skilled Nursing Facility Care

Technologic advances and the COVID-19 pandemic have been a breath of fresh air supporting the use of telehealth. In varied forms telehealth has been in limited use for decades but the technology was clinically disappointing and reimbursement for services was minimal. The COVID-19 pandemic aligned perfectly with meaningful advances in software, hardware, internet access, and streaming bandwidth. Telehealth during COVID-19 provided the ideal push for a newly supported political will to guarantee payment to providers. Telehealth utilization now allows for provision of care in locations unthinkable a decade ago. The number of Medicare Fee-For-Service beneficiary telehealth encounters increased 63-fold in 2020, from approximately 840,000 in 2019 to nearly 52.7 million in 2020. A Michigan study demonstrated that during the COVID-19 pandemic telehealth encounters were logged by 2588 of 4405 active surgeons (58.8%). Surgeons have clearly embraced the concept of Telehealth.

Skilled Nursing facilities can extend the reach of subspecialty care in a cost effective and beneficial manner using telehealth. The benefits are well documented. This technology is of great value to the healthcare system where the focus becomes more patient-centric. Care is directed by the surgical consultant while problematic issues are avoided. For example, patient comfort is maintained by avoiding an often uncomfortable ambulette ride. Potentially needed serial visits are more easily facilitated via Telehealth. Fiscal barriers such as the costs of transport (the ambulette paid for by the patient and the cost of an accompanying staff member to travel with the patient being borne by the SNF) are avoided. SNF patients traveling on stretchers by ambulette with accompanying staff members are often disruptive to the flow of surgical clinics.

Furthermore, visualization of the patient and their post op wounds brings more to an evaluation than review of labs and data alone. A picture can be worth more than a thousand words. It should be noted that the cameras on newer technology are excellent and allow for meaningful evaluations under magnification and have built-in capabilities for exact measurements of wounds and lesions. Camera-enhanced telehealth is not a simple Zoom experience with a patient. Meaningful data is obtained with this technology. The ability to visualize, interview, and remotely examine the patient adds immeasurable value to surgical remote follow-up. A study in the Journal of Surgery supports this in that they found only a 2.6% readmission rate and positive patient satisfaction when Telehealth was utilized.

Of course, there are limitations. Technology can malfunction, staff may have anxiety using a new forum, poor IT support when emergent troubleshooting is needed can waste valuable time and disoriented patients may still be disruptive. We have found that preparation for Telehealth is invaluable in assuring success. The SNF must use technology, which can be easily accessed by the surgical consultant. A SNF clinical staff member must facilitate their side of the consultation including downloading pertinent clinical changes and data. They also must be there to direct the exam and be a trusting team member for the patient to feel comfortable. SNFs may find that they need to enhance their WiFi capabilities. Financial investment will be needed on the SNF side to support enhanced WiFi and purchase hardware and software programs. Based upon the size of the SNF, portable technology may be beneficial or multiple units may be necessary to support larger facilities.

Most cloud-based programs can allow for remote linkages but on the surgical side someone should practice receipt and retrieval of needed links. Rarely software is shared by SNFs already embedded in hospital networks. Most importantly one person at the SNF and another on the surgical team must be responsible for coordinating and assisting in the visit—this includes scheduling and testing of WiFi bandwidth and ease of use/training on the telehealth software. Some programs may allow for notes to be shared on each side of the telehealth communication, but many do not. Furthermore, if telehealth is new to the surgical team, then education on billing telehealth services is essential to having an engaged surgical post-acute care team. CMS must continue to be lobbied for policies of pay parity for telehealth visits. As quality visits evolve, clinical benefits will continue to support of this valuable practice.

Conclusions

In summary, a working knowledge on how patients get admitted to nursing facilities, on the economic driving forces in these centers, on what care SNFs may provide and on the benefits of a highly integrated acute care and SNF team will improve chances for enhanced post-operative care in the subacute setting. The initial decision where to specifically send the patient is integral to success. Specific clinical problems need to be managed at centers with the greatest experience in that area. A working knowledge of nuanced differences in local SNFs will enhance suitable discharge decisions. Team building between acute surgical care and skilled nursing facility practitioners aids in the success of postoperative outcomes.

References

1. https://elderaffairs.org/wp-content/uploads/instructions-for-completing-the-medical-certification.pdf or ahca.myflorida.com/medicaid/review/Forms
2. www.nyconnects.ny.gov/services.pri
3. www.medicare.gov
4. Jacobson GA, Blumenthal D. Medicare advantage enrollment growth: implications for the US health care system. JAMA. 2022;327(24):2393–4. https://doi.org/10.1001/jama.2022.8288.
5. www.medicaid.gov
6. www.sccm.org
7. Whitlock EL, Vannucci A, Avidan MS. Postoperative delirium. Minerva Anestesiol. 2011;77(4):448–56.
8. Wei LA, Fearing MA, Sternberg EJ, Inouye SK. The confusion assessment method: a systematic review of current usage. J Am Geriatr Soc. 2008;56(5):823–30. https://doi.org/10.1111/j.1532-5415.2008.01674.x.
9. Goltz DE, Baumgartner BT, Politzer CS, DiLallo M, Bolognesi MP, Seyler TM. The American College of Surgeons National Surgical Quality Improvement Program Surgical Risk Calculator has a role in predicting discharge to post-acute care in total joint arthroplasty. J Arthroplast. 2018;33(1):25–9. https://doi.org/10.1016/j.arth.2017.08.008.
10. Horne CE, Goda TS, Nifong LW, Kypson AP, O'Neal WT, Kindell LC, et al. Factors associated with discharge to a skilled nursing facility after transcatheter aortic valve replacement surgery. Int J Environ Res Public Health. 2018;16(1):73. https://doi.org/10.3390/ijerph16010073.
11. Baack Kukreja J, Kamat AM. Strategies to minimize readmission rates following major urologic surgery. Ther Adv Urol. 2017;9(5):111–9. https://doi.org/10.1177/1756287217701699.
12. Arya S, Long CA, Brahmbhatt R, Shafii S, Brewster LP, Veeraswamy R, et al. Preoperative frailty increases risk of nonhome discharge after elective vascular surgery in home-dwelling patients. Ann Vasc Surg. 2016;35:19–29. https://doi.org/10.1016/j.avsg.2016.01.052.
13. Morris JA Jr, Sanchez AA, Bass SM, MacKenzie EJ. Trauma patients return to productivity. J Trauma. 1991;31(6):827–34. https://doi.org/10.1097/00005373-199106000-00014.
14. Maese JR, Seminara D, Shah Z, Szerszen A. Perspective: what a difference a disaster makes: the telehealth revolution in the age of COVID-19 pandemic. Am J Med Qual. 2020;35(5):429–31. https://doi.org/10.1177/1062860620933587.
15. Groom LL, McCarthy MM, Stimpfel AW, Brody AA. Telemedicine and telehealth in nursing homes: an integrative review. J Am Med Dir Assoc. 2021;22(9):1784–1801.e7. https://doi.org/10.1016/j.jamda.2021.02.037.

Nursing Considerations in Management of Geriatric Patients

56

Barbara M. Brathwaite

troduction

evelopments in surgical techniques and sophis-cated monitoring are factors that have contrib-ed to the increased number of older adults ndergoing surgery. These developments have inimized, but not eliminated the risks, as many lder adults have multiple comorbid conditions, n addition to limited functional reserve, which nay affect recovery and lead to incapacity and leath. A postoperative complication is much nore serious and may lead to other complica-ions, and failure of one bodily system is more ikely to lead to failure of other systems. Diseases associated with older age including diabetes, hypertension, osteopenia and osteoporosis, peripheral neuropathy, and peripheral vascular disease can cause bodily systems to deteriorate over time. The older adult is vulnerable and less tolerant of harm.

According to estimates, half of older adults in the USA will undergo surgery at age 65 or older. Current guidelines focus on the patient's age when considering surgical hardiness in the older adult. Age in years versus physiological age varies from one patient to another. Functional status and functional reserve must be considered and may be more important than the older adult's given age.

To ensure optimal health outcomes for older adults, nurses in all settings should be familiar with geriatric health problems and demonstrate expertise in delivering care. Providing appropriate geriatric health assessments and nursing care can help reduce hospitalization rates, prevent complications, and enhance quality of life and independence. In caring for the older adult, it is imperative that nurses understand the pathophysiologic changes of the aging process and use critical thinking skills in assessing and treating the hospitalized older adult.

Physical and Physiological Changes in the Older Adult

More than one-third of all surgical procedures in the USA are now performed on adults aged 65 and over. The concern and the challenge is that the structural and physiological changes associated with aging, in addition to the presence of multiple comorbidities, place them at greater risk for postoperative complications and worse outcomes.

Age-associated physiological changes occur in all organ systems. Changes noted in the cardiovascular system include a decrease in cardiac output, increase in blood pressure, and development of arteriosclerosis. Lungs exhibit

B. M. Brathwaite (✉)
Stony Brook University School of Nursing, Stony Brook, New York, USA
e-mail: barbara.brathwaite@stonybrook.edu

P. Petrone, C. E.M. Brathwaite (eds.), *Acute Care Surgery in Geriatric Patients*,
https://doi.org/10.1007/978-3-031-30651-8_56

diminished gas exchange, slower flow rates upon expiration, and a reduction in vital capacity. Aging can have significant effects on the digestive system including decreased appetite, an alteration in smell and taste, a decrease or slowing of function and motility, and an increased risk of digestive tract disorders. Changes in pharyngeal and esophageal function and motility may lead to reflux and dysphagia. Progressive elevation of blood glucose, altered hepatic drug metabolism, and osteopenia and osteoporosis are frequently noted. A loss of skin integrity, tone, and elasticity is caused by changes in collagen and elastin, and the biological aging of the cells. Age-related muscle loss causes a decrease in lean body mass. Joint degeneration combined with the loss of muscle mass can severely affect mobility. In addition, the alterations in metabolism affect responses to commonly used medications and as a result, different medications and decreased dosages may be necessary.

These changes have important implications for nursing management of the geriatric patient. The gradual but steady physical impairment and functional disability results in increased dependency. A focus on a healthy lifestyle including nutrition, dietary supplements, hydration, stress reduction, smoking cessation, and exercise may help to delay some of these changes.

Geriatric Syndromes

Geriatric syndromes refer to a group of health conditions in older adults that do not fit into discrete disease categories. The term is used extensively to highlight the unique features of common health conditions which include frailty, functional limitation, falls, cognitive impairment, delirium, depression, polypharmacy, malnutrition, incontinence, and pressure ulcers. Reduction in functional reserve puts hospitalized older adults at high risk for development of these geriatric syndromes and often leads to functional decline and dependence.

Geriatric Assessment

A comprehensive geriatric assessment includes an assessment of health status and social support of the older adult, spirituality needs, risk factors, medication list, differentiation of normal aging from the disease process, signs of aging syndromes and diseases of old age, complications and treatments, and interpretation of laboratory results and diagnostic tests.

Functional Decline

Approximately one-third of hospitalized patients older than 70 years will suffer a hospital-associated disability affecting their activities of daily living or their ability to live independently. Half of these patients will not recover enough to function at their previous levels over the long term. Functional decline can be categorized into three areas: prehospitalization, hospitalization, and posthospitalization. Prehospitalization factors include advanced age, decreased mobility, impaired cognitive function, symptoms of geriatric syndrome including falls and incontinence, limited social functioning, and presence of depression and anxiety. Hospitalization factors include restricted mobility, inadequate nutrition, enforced dependence resulting in lack of independence and self-care, and polypharmacy. Posthospitalization factors include environmental and financial resources, family and community support, and quality of discharge planning.

The treatment of functional decline is complex, must be individualized, and holistic. Many of the treatments to prevent functional decline are associated with the above factors previously discussed, such as falls prevention, avoidance of sensory issues and delirium, and enhancing nutrition. Functional ability is clearly associated with one's social well-being and social involvement, mental status, and sense of family and community. Regaining lost functional capacity is challenging, and the best treatment occurs from collaboration with multidisciplinary teams specializing in the care of older adults. There are programs to help prevent or regain the lost function, but these can be labor-intensive and very costly. However, this is worth the cost of increased complications and loss of quality of life and independence.

Patient Safety

The Institute of Medicine has defined patient safety as preventing harm to patients. Patient safety is an essential part of nursing care that aims to prevent avoidable errors and patient harm. Evidence-based nursing interventions are necessary to ensure high quality of care and safety in the geriatric patient. Hospitalization safety risks included delirium, malnutrition, pressure ulcers, urinary incontinence, depression and anxiety, falls, restraint use, infection, functional decline, adverse drug effects, and death.

Elder Abuse

Recognizing and reporting symptoms of elder abuse are responsibilities of the nurse and can include physical, emotional, or psychological abuse, neglect, abandonment, sexual abuse, and financial abuse. Signs and symptoms to watch for include signs of depression, withdrawal, or confusion; isolation from family and friends; unexplained bruises, burns, or scars; wounds and bed sores; a dirty, dehydrated, underfed, or overmedicated appearance; and recent changes in banking or expenditure patterns. The nurse must be a patient advocate and make the appropriate referral to prevent further harm to the older adult.

Medications

Polypharmacy is characterized as the regular use of five or more medications which include prescription and over the counter vitamins, and herbal or dietary supplements, and includes the presence of the possibility of at least one serious drug interaction. It is a widespread problem in older adults as half of this population takes one or more medication that are unnecessary. Studies reveal a relationship between the presence of multiple medications and serious, negative outcomes. Adverse outcomes include the probability of a drug–drug interaction and the occurrence of drug–disease interactions.

Aging is associated with numerous physiological changes that affect drug absorption, distribution, metabolism, and excretion and therefore are important to consider. Perioperative analgesics, including opioids, should be carefully administered and monitored. The lowest necessary doses should be prescribed. Opioids can lead to adverse effects such as changes in cognition or delirium and increase the risk of respiratory and hemodynamic complications.

Nursing Evaluation of the Geriatric Patient

Health History, Physical Exam, and Assessment

Information obtained from an accurate assessment serves as the foundation for appropriate nursing care. A complete health history, physical exam, and assessment have a significant impact on the management and outcomes of older patients undergoing surgery. It is vital that nurses identify the potential for certain risks and complications and recommend and develop evidence-based treatment plans that minimize the risks.

A thorough health history includes past and present medical history and history of smoking, previous surgical and anesthesia history, and current medications. The patient's medication list should be carefully reviewed and assessed for inappropriate and unnecessary medications, and for potential harmful drug effects and/or interactions. It is important to determine if the patient has a history of cardiovascular, pulmonary, renal, or neurologic disorders, diabetes mellitus, cancer, injuries, or falls. Ascertaining if the patient has any sensory impairments, if they use glasses or a hearing aid, and if there are any language or learning obstacles can help determine if there are barriers to the patient understanding their medical care.

Upon admission, note and document which family members or significant others are accompanying the patient. If the older adult is having outpatient surgery, it is critical they have a responsible caregiver to provide home care and that they have postoperative transportation. Establishing and verifying a mutually agreed upon date and time for the postoperative phone call increases the likelihood that follow-up communication will take place. The preoperative nursing assessment should confirm all preadmission information. Patient identification and correct site surgery are vital and recognized as standard patient safety goal priorities of care.

Advance Directive

Assessment should include whether the patient has a written statement of their wishes regarding medical treatment. The focus of care for many older adults is to maintain the quality of their lives and to make the most of their remaining years. This may go against the beliefs of others. Family members or caregivers who might have to make life-and-death decisions for an older loved one may be unaware of the patient's views and preferences. The patient and caregiver's goals for treatment should be discussed, mutually agreed upon, and documented. It is vital the patient have an advance directive documented to ensure they will receive care in accordance with their wishes in the event that they become unable to communicate.

Communication and Trust

Communicating with the patient by speaking slowly and calmly in a reassuring manner helps to establish a therapeutic environment of mutual trust and respect. Questions should be presented gently in a nonthreatening, nonjudgmental manner. Asking the patient to repeat what they have just heard ensures comprehension and prevents miscommunication. Before implementing procedures, blood work, and tests, explain the reasons which helps ensure understanding and cooperation An important thing to remember is that age-related changes in cognition and anxiety can result in short-term memory impairment. Be patient and understanding when interacting with the geriatric patient.

Communication Cues

- Be attentive to the patient.
- Speak slowly and clearly.
- Be prepared to repeat questions and instructions as needed.
- Assess body language.
- Actively listen.
- Provide sensory aids such as glasses, hearing aids, and communication tools, such as dentures, or paper and pencil.
- Respond to the patient's calls in a timely manner.
- Ask the patient to repeat back instructions for confirmation of their understanding.
- Avoid overstimulation, reduce background noise and lighting.
- Provide comfort, pain relief.
- Create an environment of peace, independence, and safety.

Patient and Family Centered Care

The presence of family caregivers in the hospital is one of the main factors in providing mental and emotional support to the patient. Family members play important roles in the treatment of patients such as assisting the healthcare team in providing care, improving patient safety and quality, contributing to decision-making, and assisting in discharge, follow-up and home care. In fact, research shows that when patients and families are engaged in their health care, it can lead to increased adherence, improved communication and patient satisfaction, reduction in length of hospitalization and medical errors, and lowered costs in addition to measurable improvements in safety and quality.

Culture/Health Belief Assessment

Culture, ethnicity, and social norms may influence the older adult's response to different aspects of their hospitalization, such as trust in health care providers, acceptance of medical treatments, response to pain, and compliance with self-care activities. Understanding the health beliefs of different cultures and how healthcare is viewed aids in development of questions and treatment plans for patients. Being sensitive to general differences can strengthen the relationship between nurse and patient. Many patients retain their traditional health practices as links to their heritage in an effort to maintain their identity. Respect for alternative healing methods and traditional health practices should be maintained. The use of alternative medicines, herbal treatments, and traditional remedies is common in many cultures. Be sure to ask if the patient takes any of these.

Variations in the cultural structure and hierarchy of the family unit contribute to differences in the size of extended families and the roles of different members among cultures. Many factors affect family dynamics including personalities, communication styles, religion, cultural, educational, and legal aspects, in addition to beliefs regarding family involvement in patient care. Extended families with diverse backgrounds and education may present a challenge to healthcare providers in terms of communication and family involvement and may lead to disagreements and dissatisfaction among staff and the patient and family.

Nurses play a vital role in including family members in patient care as they are often the first point of contact for patients' families and are a consistent presence at the bedside. Understanding family members' knowledge, educational levels, coping skills, emotional states, stress levels and needs, combined with direct, open communication is necessary to assist in conflict resolution and to keep the focus on the patient's needs and wishes. Goals for treatment should be discussed with the patient and family and documented in the medical record.

When working with patients who do not speak English as a first language, be sure to ask which language they prefer to speak and if they can read English. They may need a medical interpreter. Federal policies require healthcare providers who receive Federal funds, such as Medicare payments, to make interpretive services available to people with limited English. Many rely on patients' family members or on staff members to interpret, but the use of trained medical interpreters should be applied. Although a patient may choose to have a family member translate, the patient should be offered access to a professional interpreter.

General Nursing Considerations in the Care of the Geriatric Patient

Nursing care of the geriatric patient consists of the development, implementation, and evaluation of plans of care regarding management of cognitive disorders, pain, sleep disorders, common urinary and intestinal disorders, and prevention of medication adverse reactions, falls and injuries, hospital-acquired infections, nutritional and fluid disorders, and eliminating or minimizing the use of restrictive measures, and meeting the spiritual needs of the older adult.

Encouraging patients to participate in their care as much as possible contributes to their independence and empowerment.

Skin Assessment and Care

Due to possible vascular and neurological conditions, and the loss of elasticity and skin turgor with aging, special attention should be given to skin, bony prominences, and wound healing.

Pressure Ulcers

The patient should be assessed for the presence of pressure ulcers, especially on the trochanters, sacrum, and heels. Risk factors for pressure ulcers are numerous and can include advanced age, friable skin, abnormal positioning in patients with diseases involving spasticity or contractures, edema, incontinence, infection, limited mobility, loss of sensation, shearing forces, prolonged moisture, and unrelieved pressure. All patients at risk should be frequently assessed and provided care.

Prevention is the primary goal regarding skin breakdown with the focus on decreasing insult to the skin and improving nutrition. Nursing care should include proper positioning and padding of bony prominences in patients undergoing surgery, and postoperatively, to preserve skin integrity and reduce pressure on peripheral nerves. If the patient is on bed rest and unable to turn themselves, ensure they are turned and positioned frequently, avoid sliding patients which increases shear force, and use specialized mattresses or beds that shift pressure points. It is vital to promote mobilization and assist the patient in getting in and out of bed when they are able. (Always make sure bed rails are in the up position and bed in low position.)

Nutritional care includes assessing and charting intake and output and ensuring the patient receives adequate nutrition. If necessary, this should be supplemented with vitamins, minerals, meal supplements, and tube feedings.

However, even the best preventative measures can fail, requiring wound care and tissue debridement. Dressing changes may be necessary, be sure to keep wounds and the surrounding areas clean and dry. In certain cases, diversion of urinary or fecal output via catheters and/or colostomies can help keep ulcers free of infection and expedite healing.

Cardiovascular Assessment and Care

The presence of cardiac comorbidities increases with age, and this highlights the importance of focusing on appropriate cardiac care. Multiple indices have been developed over the years to identify high-risk individuals prior to surgery. One of the most widely used is the Revised Cardiac Risk Index. This tool identifies six independent risk factors that have been correlated with increased cardiac risk. These are: high risk type of surgery, history of ischemic heart disease, heart failure, cerebrovascular disease, diabetes requiring treatment with insulin, and preoperative serum creatinine over 2 mg per dL. Age has not consistently been found to be the sole predictor of cardiac risk. However, intraoperative or perioperative mortality is higher in geriatric as compared with younger patients in the event of an acute myocardial infarction.

Hypertension

Hypertension is extremely common among the older adult and is associated with increased incidence of coronary artery disease and other comorbidities such as cerebrovascular and renal disease. During the preoperative period, the presence of hypertension and whether the patient is taking antihypertensive medications should be assessed. Every effort should be made to control hypertension preoperatively, and it is also important to avoid abrupt discontinuation of antihypertensive medications.

Venous Thrombus

Thrombosis in the venous system such as deep venous thrombosis (DVT) or pulmonary embolism (PE) is a serious complication. The thrombus can cause partial or complete blockage of circulation in the vein, which in the lower extremity (DVT) can lead to pain, swelling, tenderness, discoloration, or redness of the affected area, and skin that is warm to the touch. While a DVT can affect anyone of any age, adults over the age of 60 have a higher risk of developing this condition. A PE occurs when a portion of the thrombus breaks loose and travels in the bloodstream, first to the heart and then to the lungs, where it can partially or completely block one of the pulmonary arteries or one of its branches. A PE is a serious, life-threatening complication with symptoms that include shortness of breath, rapid heartbeat, sweating, and/or sharp chest pain (especially during deep breathing). Some patients may have hemoptysis while others may develop severe hypotension and resultant syncope. Pulmonary embolism frequently causes sudden death particularly when one or more of the vessels that supply the lungs are completely blocked.

The incidence of venous thrombosis increases significantly with age and is associated with other risk factors such as immobility, acute infection, falls, presence of comorbidities such as congestive heart failure, (CHF), COPD, diabetes, obesity, malignancies, hormone replacement therapy, genetic factors. Vulnerable older adults need to be identified in order to employ risk stratification and target preventive measures such as prophylactic treatment with anticoagulants, thrombolytics, and insertion of a vena cava filter. However, major bleeding is one of the life-threatening side effects of anticoagulants and thrombolytics.

Nursing interventions include educating the patient on these risk factors, being alert to the signs and symptoms of a venous thrombus, encouraging ambulation and mobility, hydration, and the use of intermittent pneumatic compression (IPC) devices, and application of compression stockings while in bed.

Medications

Many older adults are on some type of statin drug to reduce lipid levels, decrease vascular inflammation, and stabilize atherosclerotic plaques. Abrupt discontinuation of statins has been associated with increased risk of myocardial infarction and death. Continuing statin therapy in the perioperative period is recommended.

Thermoregulation

Perioperative hypothermia has been shown to be a significant cause of postoperative adverse events including susceptibility to infections, poor wound healing, shivering, discomfort, and increased cardiovascular complications. Several age-related physiological changes predispose the older patient to the development of hypothermia which include impaired temperature regulation, altered shivering threshold, impaired vasoconstriction, and reduced metabolic activity.

Anemia

The blood pressure and pulse should be assessed frequently after surgery. Many older adults have some degree of preoperative anemia and may need a blood transfusion. Evaluate hemoglobin and hematocrit levels and coagulation factors pre- and post-operatively. Assess for bleeding.

Dehydration

Because the patient may have been fasting, the nurse should ensure that they receive adequate IV supplementation to prevent symptoms of dehydration and decrease in blood pressure and urine output. Temperature control is necessary for older patients, and they may require more active warming than younger patients.

Pulmonary Assessment and Care

An older adult undergoing a surgical procedure and general anesthesia, combined with the age-associated reduction in lung elasticity, decrease in chest wall compliance, and respiratory muscle strength, significantly contributes to development of postoperative pulmonary complications. Additional procedure-related risks include emergency surgery, surgical time over 3 h, and multiple transfusions. Upper abdominal surgery close to the diaphragm is a risk factor for aspiration and inadequate lung expansion resulting in atelectasis. As with most other postoperative complications, pulmonary complications lead to increased morbidity, length of stay, and mortality. Although the presence of comorbidities predisposes patients to postoperative complications, age remains a significant risk.

Aspiration

Aging is associated with a decline in the usual protective reflexes in the oropharynx contributing to aspiration. Patients with swallowing disorders and neurological syndromes have a particularly elevated risk. In cases where the airway is unprotected and in the postoperative period, administration of pain medication and sedation should be carefully monitored and strict NPO restrictions adhered to even for minor surgical procedures.

Hypoventilation and Atelectasis

As advanced age is associated with a continuing decrease in chest wall compliance and decreased respiratory muscle strength, any reduction in strength may lead to hypoventilation and pulmonary complications. Postoperative pain, aspiration, drowsiness, immobilization, and bed rest can lead to shallow breathing, and the potential development of atelectasis resulting in hypoxemia, pneumonia, bronchospasm, acute respiratory failure, exacerbation of previous lung disease, and pulmonary problems due to accumulated secretions. These complications increase the risk for negative outcomes.

In addition to interventions which optimize pulmonary status during the pre- and perioperative periods, post-operative strategies can prevent pulmonary complications in the older patient. Lung expansion treatments increase functional residual capacity and expand partially or completely collapsed alveoli. Postoperatively, it is essential to closely monitor the patient's status, blood pressure, pulse, oximetry, and the presence of dyspnea and/or shortness of breath. Make sure the patient is able to clear their airway. Aspiration risk is increased in the older adult and requires attentive care. Postoperative mobilization and ambulation should be done as soon as possible. This helps prevent deep vein thrombosis (DVT) and allows for chest expansion and clearance of secretions.

Preventative measures include:

- Monitor patient's condition closely.
- Institute inspiratory muscle exercises using incentive spirometry.
- Start chest physical therapy.
- Assist with coughing and deep breathing exercises.
- Mobilize and ambulate patient as early as possible.
- Elevate head of bed while eating, and during turning and repositioning.
- Assist patient, when possible, in getting out of bed for all meals and for toileting needs.
- Evaluate for signs of dysphagia that can lead to aspiration pneumonia.
- Reduce opioid and analgesia medications.
- Educate—explain to the patient before and after surgery, the important reasons for these preventative measures.

Musculoskeletal Assessment and Care

Investigate for abnormalities suggested by the health history, such as loss of balance, gait disorders, mobility issues, or inability to transfer from a chair to a standing position. Does the patient use a cane or walker to ambulate? Assess the patient's functional status. Is the patient able to perform activities of daily living (ADLs), including bathing or showering, getting in and out of bed or a chair, walking, using the toilet, and eating? Does the patient have a history of osteoporosis which can increase risk of falling?

Fall Risk

Postoperatively, older adults experience physiologic and cognitive changes that increase the risk of falling. Hospital-based falls are believed to account for about 40% of all accidental injuries of hospitalized patients and are the most common adverse safety events in healthcare facilities. Risk factors can include change in cognition and mental status, sensory impairments, dehydration, medications, functional decline and muscle weakness, frequent trips to the bathroom, past history of falls, and coordination and balance issues.

Universal fall precautions aim to reduce the factors that lead to falls as well as offer practical solutions. Nursing interventions include familiarizing patients with the environment, keeping areas clean, dry, well lit, uncluttered, and ensuring there are sturdy handles on walls in patient bathrooms and in hallways. Beds and wheelchairs should be locked with bed heights low when the patient is at rest and adjusted to aid in transferring. Using night lights or supplemental lighting helps to prevent falls from tripping over objects. The patient should have their sensory devices, glasses, hearing aids, and other personal belongings within reach, understand how to call for help, and wear appropriate footwear (well-fitting, comfortable, non-slip shoes). Patients should be toileted every 2 h, if possible, or offered the bedpan, which will help prevent the patient from getting out of bed to use the bathroom.

Avoid at all costs frequent use of restraints to prevent falls and injuries, or unnecessary insertion of a urinary catheter which can affect patients' dignity and create potential complications for the geriatric patient.

Evaluate the patient's fall risk. Evidence-based strength training interventions such as physical therapy, being mindful of fall safety hazards, and use of assistive devices have been found to significantly reduce the rate of falls. Falls may lead to increased morbidity, decreased function, injuries, fractures, and mortality.

Frailty

Frailty may be a more significant factor than age when assessing postoperative risk in surgical management. Frailty assessment in elderly patients is recommended due to the associated irreversible alterations that may result in disability. The frail older adult is at higher risk for complications, longer hospital stays, and has a much lower rate of return to baseline function after surgery. There is a decrease in their ability to correct physiological stressors. Perioperative management must include strategies to minimize the disruption to physiologic function as well as maximize the return of function as efficiently as possible. Surgery can be a major physiologic stressor and the lack of having a physiologic reserve or ability to correct a physiologic stressor is what needs to be anticipated and ameliorated.

Neurological Assessment and Care

Cognitive Impairment/Delirium

Neurologic complications are the most common complications in the hospitalized older adult and postoperative delirium is one of the most serious with an incidence range from 15–53%, depending on the surgical procedure.

Delirium

Delirium is a serious age-related postoperative complication. The most significant risk factors are advanced age, cognitive impairment and dementia, visual and hearing impairment, sleep deprivation, sensory overload, fluid and electrolyte imbalances, and immobility. A majority of studies identify contributing factors such as certain medications, infections, organ failure, pain, fecal impaction, urinary retention, and the surgery itself. Alcohol use, abuse, and withdrawal have been implicated in postoperative delirium and cognitive decline; therefore, it is important to obtain an accurate history regarding alcohol use during the preoperative admission process.

The serious disturbance and acute decline in cognitive function may result in confusion, agitation, inattention, disorientation, changes in consciousness, hallucinations, delusions, and disorganized thinking. Symptoms of delirium may begin over a few hours and often fluctuate throughout the day, with an increase in symptoms at night. If delirium occurs, it will usually present within hours or the first 3 days after surgery. Acute delirium is often preventable and temporary if recognized and treated promptly. Treatment focuses on the causes and symptoms.

It is important to assess for the possibility of dementia which will identify patients at high risk for postoperative delirium. Dementia and delirium may be particularly difficult to distinguish as they have similar symptoms, such as confusion, agitation, and delusions, but it is essential to be aware of the difference. Delirium is an acute process with symptoms that start suddenly. Dementia is the gradual, progressive decline of cognitive function that does not readily respond to medical or pharmacologic treatment. The most common cause of dementia is Alzheimer's disease. Identifying vulnerable patients will allow for the possibility of instituting delirium prevention protocols or prophylactic drug administration. Nurses must care for patients with understanding, patience, and compassion.

Treatment includes management of the symptoms:

- Adjust the environment by ensuring the room is well-lit and quiet with decreased stimulation.
- Orient the patient with the presence of a clock, watch, calendar.

- Reorient the patient frequently to their surroundings.
- Reassure the patient that they are safe.
- Surround patient with presence of loved ones and familiar objects, if possible.
- Ensure the presence of the same healthcare workers when possible.
- Decrease sensory deprivation by making sure the patient has their glasses and/or hearing aid.
- Facilitate communication by ensuring the patient has their dentures or partial plates and provide paper and pencil or tablet computers.
- Speak clearly and slowly, repeat information as needed.
- Refrain from restraint use.
- Remove potentially dangerous items from the room.
- Manage pain with medications, use the smallest doses possible.
- Treat symptoms with non-pharmacologic interventions, if possible.
- Control anxiety and agitation with medications only if the patient poses risk of harm to themselves or others.
- Promote rest and relaxation and institute sleep hygiene measures.

Control of postoperative pain and anxiety is important. Studies indicate that higher pain scores during the first three postoperative days are associated with delirium in patients undergoing surgery. Opioids and sedative medications may induce delirium and older adults have an increased cerebral reaction to opioids. To avoid these effects, non-opioid analgesics are increasingly used as part of a multimodal pain management treatment. Use of low dose haloperidol for delirium prophylaxis in high-risk older patients may be considered.

Remember, surgery is a psychological and physiological stressor, intervene as needed to prevent delirium. Delirium is related to poor surgical outcomes, physiological and functional decline, longer hospitalizations, increase in rates of institutionalization, increase in mortality, and higher healthcare costs.

Gastrointestinal/Genitourinary Assessment and Care

Nutrition and Fluids

Limiting the time patients are NPO, particularly in older adults that have pre-existing nutritional issues or diabetes, is important. Postoperatively, practical issues such as ensuring the patient has fluids at the bedside, and access to their dentures to encourage eating, is important. Accurate fluid intake and output documentation to carefully titrate fluid requirements should also be considered.

Urinary Tract Infections

Urinary tract infections (UTIs) are one of the most common nosocomial infections, of which older adults are at increased risk. Many times, UTIs are linked to the use of urinary catheters, therefore, determining if a urinary catheter is necessary, using proper hygienic techniques to insert and maintain catheters and discontinuing catheters as quickly as possible, is extremely important. Other strategies to reduce UTIs include educating staff about proper insertion and maintenance techniques of catheters, and frequent toileting of the patient.

Nursing Care and Management in the Perioperative and Postoperative Periods

Preoperative Management

Preoperative nursing care includes perioperative teaching and thorough assessment of the patient's preoperative data, such as the history and physical examination, EKG, laboratory testing, clearances, and other pertinent information. Orders for preoperative medications, antibiotics, venous thromboembolism prophylaxis, and fasting recommendations should be written and reviewed.

Considerations for factors related to pulmonary complications should be reviewed. Smoking history, presence of pre-existing respiratory illnesses, type of anesthetic, control of nausea and vomiting, pain control (especially if increased pain during breathing is anticipated), and the use of intraoperative muscle relaxants and other medications all may contribute to pulmonary issues postoperatively. As complications in the older adult are associated with greater mortality, nursing care initiatives should focus on risks and the prevention of complications.

Preoperative teaching begins in the surgeon's office and continues during the preadmission period to prepare the older adult for surgery and extends through to discharge for follow-up care. Each period of teaching should reinforce successive perioperative teaching and appropriate geriatric educational strategies should be used. The older adult requires extra time to comprehend information when being prepared for elective and emergency surgery. Nurses must exhibit patience and use active listening communication skills to reduce anxiety and promote positive surgical outcomes.

Intraoperative Management

Intraoperative assessment involves validating patient information obtained in the preoperative unit or in the operating room (OR) holding area. The OR nurse must be attentive to every detail to ensure all surgical care issues are addressed and documented. Consent for surgery must be signed and witnessed. Surgical site must be marked and verified in the medical record and on the surgical schedule.

In addition, other vital information, such as patient's fasting status, the presence of dentures or partial plates, or sensory aids such as hearing aids or glasses must be documented. It is vital to note skin condition or skin breakdown, especially at the surgical site, before positioning the patient on the operating table. Preparing the older adult by explaining the operating room process helps decrease anxiety. After the preoperative assessment and teaching have been completed and documented, the OR nurse collaborates with the anesthesiologist. Once the patient is transferred to the OR, it is important that the OR nurse remains in visual contact with the alert patient. If possible, allow the patient to keep sensory aids or dentures. Keep noise to a minimum. Provide blankets if possible. Ensure correct positioning and pad skin pressure areas to prevent pressure ulcers.

It is the responsibility of the team to implement the safety standards which ensure the right patient, right procedure, right site. The Joint Commission, a not-for-profit group in the USA that accredits hospitals and other healthcare organizations, provides guidance regarding patient safety initiatives. The Joint Commission standard, The Universal Protocol, consists of three crucial steps: conducting a pre-procedure verification process, marking the procedure site, and performing a pre-procedure time-out with the attending surgeon, anesthesiologist, or nurse anesthetist, and circulating nurse.

Post Anesthesia Management

The post anesthesia care unit (PACU) nurse must be attentive in providing care to patients in various stages from one who is still anesthetized to one who is awake and alert. The PACU nurse employs critical thinking and assessment skills in managing the older adult recovering from anesthesia and surgery. Assessment includes airway, circulation, vital signs, mental status, and fluid and pain levels. Once stable, patient then is prepared for transfer to an inpatient unit or home.

Postoperative Management

Older adults, especially those with frailty and limited functional capacity, experience an increased complication rate in the postoperative period. The need for surgery and anesthesia creates a sentinel event for these patients and can result in negative outcomes. Outcome studies reveal that morbidity and mortality are increased following surgery in the older as compared to the younger patient.

Postoperative nursing care should include prevention and treatment of complications more frequently noted in the older adult, including postoperative cognitive impairment, confusion and delirium, pulmonary complications, pain, falls and injury, functional decline, urinary tract infections, pressure ulcers, and discharge needs. Specific concerns for the older surgical patient are hydration, nutrition, skin integrity, pain management, and promotion of safety, relaxation, sleep, and comfort.

Two critical issues upon which the nurse should focus on are the impressive effects of early mobilization and patient education. Early mobilization can bypass many postoperative complications including pulmonary complications, skin breakdown, and functional decline. Mobilization can improve appetite, reduce urinary tract infections as patients are able to toilet themselves and avoid catheter insertions, help preserve muscle strength, and prevent postoperative delirium.

Patient and family education is vital. The patient and family should have preoperatively already been given some information regarding the post-operative phase of care and what to expect. However, postoperatively, this begins with the surgeon discussing the surgical findings and the prognosis with the patient. It should also include a reiteration of the events that will occur, the expectations, and with whom the patient will interact postoperatively. This may require a reassessment of patient wishes and goals, advanced directives, and the patient's expectations for their care. Discussing the issues that patients may encounter allows the patient to take charge of their care. A patient who has been educated about the problems with immobility and pulmonary complications may be self-motivated to ambulate more frequently after surgery and/or may be more apt to practice deep breathing exercises to help avoid complications and aid in their recovery.

Pain Control

One of the goals of pain control is to provide relief while minimizing the dose of analgesics in order to decrease the dose-related risks, particularly with opioids. Opioids are typically the pain medication of choice immediately after surgery. However, the side effects can limit a patient's ability to mobilize postoperatively and participate in their care. The administration of non-opioids such as planned dosing of acetaminophen, the use of nerve blocks, or the use of different classes of drugs to minimize the dose of each drug, should be considered. Avoiding sedatives, hypnotics, tranquilizers, narcotic analgesics, muscle relaxants, and non-steroidal anti-inflammatories can be helpful.

Discharge

Discharge planning before the day of surgery is the key to positive surgical outcomes.

Discharging the same-day surgery older adult requires that the PACU nurse ensures that the patient and the family or caregiver are prepared to care for the patient in the home environment properly. Written discharge instructions should be reviewed with the patient and family carefully and thoroughly. The patient should repeat the discharge instructions back to the nurse. Demonstrations for procedures or wound care should be given with the patient or caregiver giving a return performance. Emergency telephone numbers should be listed on the discharge instruction forms. Signs and symptoms of infections are important for the patient and family to recognize and report to their healthcare provider. The home should be prepared for the older adult who is recovering to prevent falls or injuries.

Older adults are at increased risk for morbidity and mortality after injury or surgery in both the inpatient and post-discharge settings. The importance of comprehensive discharge planning is increasingly recognized as a determinant of long-term survival. Multidisciplinary communication sets the foundation for effective discharge planning and transitions of care. The older adult face several psychosocial, functional, and financial difficulties that pose significant challenges to successful transitions of care.

It is important to assess the level of readiness and the knowledge, skills, and needs of the patient and their families in discharge planning. Be sure they comprehend instructions by asking them to repeat the information, and then provide corrective feedback. Involving the patient and their family in the discharge plan and providing education increases their empowerment and participation. Discharge plans should include medication and treatment plans, palliative and rehabilitative care, post-discharge follow-up, and available financial and community resources.

Considering the age-related changes, it is essential to pay increased attention to the special needs and abilities of older adults. Rehabilitation and physical activity should be considered while keeping in mind the patient's general health condition. In addition, maintaining autonomy is the highest priority, so the patient can be released from the acute inpatient stay strengthened for follow-up care or their home environment.

Conclusion

To ensure the best possible health outcomes for the geriatric patient, nurses in surgical settings should be familiar with the risks and challenges and demonstrate proficiency in assessment and the provision of care. Appropriately assessing the health needs of the geriatric patient can reduce the length of their hospitalization and provide positive outcomes.

To become adept in geriatric assessment, there needs to be an understanding of the physiologic changes unique to the older adult, as well as the differences between normal age-related changes and changes caused by illness, disease, and other factors. Assisting the older adult in maintaining their independence as long as possible enhances their quality of life. This is an essential principle of nursing.

References

1. Boss GR, Seegmiller JE. Age-related physiological changes and their clinical significance. West J Med. 1981;135(6):434–40.
2. Cary M, Lyder C. Geriatric assessment: essential skills for nurses. American Nurse. 2011. https://www.myamericannurse.com/geriatric-assessment-essential-skills-for-nurses/.
3. Collier R. Hospital-induced delirium hits hard. CMAJ. 2012;184(1):23–4. https://doi.org/10.1503/cmaj.109-4069.
4. Korc-Grodzicki B, Downey R, Shahrokni A, Kingham TP, Patel SG, Audisio R. Surgical considerations in older adults with cancer. J Clin Oncol. 2014;32(24):2647–53. https://doi.org/10.1200/JCO.2014.55.0962.
5. Gjorgjievski M, Ristevski B. Postoperative management considerations of the elderly patient undergoing orthopaedic surgery. Injury. 2020;51(Suppl 2):S23–7. https://doi.org/10.1016/j.injury.2019.12.027.
6. Gupta S, Perry JA, Kozar R. Transitions of care in geriatric medicine. Clin Geriatr Med. 2019;35(1):45–52. https://doi.org/10.1016/j.cger.2018.08.005.
7. Jazieh AR, Volker S, Taher S. Involving the family in patient care: a culturally tailored communication model. Glob J Qual Saf Healthc. 2018;1(2):33–7. https://doi.org/10.4103/JQSH.JQSH_3_18.
8. Kretschmer R, Trögner J, Schindlbeck M, Schmitz P. Postoperative multiprofessional comprehensive treatment. Orthopade. 2022;51:98–105. https://doi.org/10.1007/s00132-021-04208-3.
9. Mamaril ME. Nursing considerations in the geriatric surgical patient: the perioperative continuum of care. Nurs Clin North Am. 2006;41(2):313–28. https://doi.org/10.1016/j.cnur.2006.01.001.
10. National Institute on Aging. NIH Spotting the signs of elder abuse. 2019. https://www.nia.nih.gov/health/infographics/spotting-signs-elder-abusec.
11. Sieber FE, Barnett SR. Preventing postoperative complications in the elderly. Anesthesiol Clin. 2011;29(1):83–97. https://doi.org/10.1016/j.anclin.2010.11.011.
12. Uchmanowicz I, Jankowska-Polańska B, Wleklik M, Lisiak M, Gobbens R. Frailty syndrome: nursing interventions. SAGE Open Nurs. 2018;4:2377960818759449. https://doi.org/10.1177/2377960818759449.
13. Wirtz D, Kohlhof H. The geriatric patient: special aspects of peri-operative management. EFORT Open Rev. 2019;4(6):240–7. https://doi.org/10.1302/2058-5241.4.180087.
14. Woolcott JC, Richardson KJ, Wiens MO, Patel B, Marin J, Khan KM, Marra CA. Meta-analysis of the impact of 9 medication classes on falls in elderly persons. Arch Intern Med. 2009;169(21):1952–60. https://doi.org/10.1001/archinternmed.2009.357. Erratum in: Arch Intern Med. 2010 Mar 8; 170(5): 477.

it is important to assess the level of readiness and the knowledge, skills, and needs of the patient and their families in discharge planning. Be sure they comprehend instructions by asking them to repeat the information, and then provide corrective feedback. Involving the patient and their family in the discharge plan and providing [illegible] their empowerment and par- [illegible]ipation. Discharge pieces should include medication and treatment plans, palliative and [illegible] available financial and community resources.

Considering the age-related changes, it is essential to pay increased attention to the [illegible] ment and [illegible]

References

1. Boss GR, Seegmiller JE. Age-related physiological changes and their clinical significance. West J Med. 1981;135(6):434–40.
2. Carr[illegible] M, [illegible] C, [illegible] essential skills for nurses. American Nurse. 2011. [illegible]
3. [illegible] Hospital-acquired malnutrition [illegible] AMA [illegible] https://doi.org/10.[illegible]
4. Kitchen[illegible] D, [illegible] SR [illegible] (2002).

57 Emergency Nursing Considerations

Robert Asselta, Zoila Nolasco, and Tisha D. Thompson

Background

Older US adults make up more than 22 million Emergency Department (ED) visits annually. Of those, 30% are related to injuries and the remainder are evaluated with surgical or medical emergencies. According to current statistics, there is a high likelihood that the older adult with an acute surgical emergency will present to the ED. According to the American College of Emergency Physicians, approximately 20% of all ED patients are admitted to the hospital. In contrast, 37% of adults age 65 and older that are seen in the ED are hospitalized. This statistic implies the higher acuity of illness or injury of the older adult patient evaluated in the ED.

Many older adults present to the ED with multiple comorbidities, polypharmacy, and functional and cognitive impairments. They also demonstrate subtle signs and symptoms as well as atypical clinical presentations. For these reasons, accurately identifying a potential life-threatening condition in the ED setting can be a challenging endeavor. Emergency nurses understand these challenges when providing accurate and expeditious care for this vulnerable population. It is imperative that the older adults get the specialized care they deserve when being evaluated in the ED. Early recognition of high-risk presentations with the appropriate interventions can influence outcomes in a positive way. It is the emergency nurse that will assess and implement the plan of care for the acutely ill or injured older adult. There are a number of circumstances where the older adult will require an ED evaluation. The most common indication for emergent evaluation will be for acute injury or illness. These patients can present out of their own concern or they can be referred by their primary care provider or surgeon for further diagnostic workup or hospital admission.

R. Asselta · Z. Nolasco · T. D. Thompson (✉)
NYU Langone Hospital - Long Island, Mineola, NY, USA
e-mail: robert.asselta@nyulangone.org; zoila.nolasco@nyulangone.org; tisha.thompson@nyulangone.org

Patient Evaluation

The ultimate goal for all ED clinicians is to provide high quality emergency care. This includes stabilization, symptom management, diagnostics, and transfer of the patient to the next appropriate level of care. In order to meet these goals, the emergency nurse, as well as the ED providers, needs to institute a systematic approach when assessing and reevaluating a patient's emergency care plan. An organized assessment process will reduce the probability of failing to identify a critical clinical cue, especially for the older adults where atypical presenting symptoms are

P. Petrone, C. E.M. Brathwaite (eds.), *Acute Care Surgery in Geriatric Patients*,
https://doi.org/10.1007/978-3-031-30651-8_57

common. The ED is a dynamic environment with unpredictable patient volume and acuities therefore a focused and organized assessment is key during nursing and provider evaluations.

Triage

Emergency care begins at ED triage. The triage area is usually in close proximity to the ED entrance. Patients will arrive via private conveyance or by ambulance. In the emergency department "triage" refers to the methods used to assess patients' severity of injury or illness within a short time after their arrival, assign priorities, and move each patient to the appropriate place for treatment. The triage nurse performs a brief assessment by first establishing the chief complaint. Based upon the reason for the ED visit, the nurse will ascertain a history of present illness or injury through an interview with the patient, family, accompanying companions, or Emergency Medical Services (EMS). A focused physical exam may be done, along with collecting a past medical/surgical history, medications taken at home, allergies, and vital signs. The triage nurse can also initiate stabilizing measures during that initial encounter such as wound care, splinting of potential fractures, cervical collar application, and pain management. Pain control may be administered via pharmacological measure with an order by a provider or by non-pharmacological measures which can be implemented independently by a nurse. To safely administer medications for pain or otherwise, the nurse must first assess medications being taken at home for potential interactions.

The triage nurse is trained to identify immediate life-threatening situations by noticing the patient's general appearance, work of breathing, and perfusion status. This "across the room assessment" will identify clinical "red flags" such as an altered mental status, accessory muscle use in breathing, pallor, or active bleeding. When utilizing a systematic approach in the assessment process, time sensitive findings or other concerning clinical signs may be identified. Once identified a multidisciplinary team response may be necessary. A few high-risk findings are acute stroke symptoms, sepsis, STEMI, and acute injuries requiring a trauma team. At times the triage assessment, including vital signs, will be deferred and the patient will be immediately brought to a treatment area where comprehensive emergency care will begin. All of the previously mentioned specialty notifications are activated by the triage nurse. Triage is typically a brief encounter with an emergency nurse. Due to the ED's fluctuating and unpredictable volume, it is recommended by the Emergency Nurses Association (ENA), as well as the American College of Emergency Physicians (ACEP) to complete the triage assessment in less than 5 min. Therefore, an accurate, focused nursing assessment is critical in the identification of high-risk medical or surgical emergencies that need to be managed in the appropriate treatment area within the ED.

Initial Nursing Assessment

Depending on the triage acuity level, the patient may be evaluated in specific locations throughout the ED. In many EDs, locations are assigned according to anticipated resources. Some areas may be fashioned as a treat and release section or perhaps configured for resuscitations. The emergency nurse will evaluate the patient and perform a more comprehensive assessment. The initial assessment is frequently completed prior to the patient being seen by the emergency physician. Again, the importance of a systematic approach to the patient assessment is key in identifying a crucial piece of data, either subjective or objective, that need to be urgently escalated to the ED physician.

Primary Assessment

The emergency nurse begins their assessment by carrying out the primary survey. This is an evaluation of one's airway, breathing, circulation, and disability status. This assessment is done to quickly assess, identify, and to begin treatment for immediate life-threatening conditions. For example, blood in the airway as a result of facial trauma after a fall. Or perhaps absent peripheral pulses and pallor due to hemorrhagic shock from a GI bleed. The primary assessment performed by the nurse in less than 2 min along with the appropriate interventions can affect the patient's outcome. Some of these interventions, besides provider notification, may be patient positioning, airway clearance, applying supplemental oxygen, and providing direct pressure to an actively bleeding wound or establishing venous access. The primary assessment, done by the emergency nurse is an essential piece of the initial assessment of the older adult.

Secondary Assessment

If the primary survey is negative, the ED nurse will conduct the secondary assessment, obtaining subjective and objective data with the goal of identifying acute illnesses or injuries and anticipating the plan of care. The secondary assessment includes interviewing the patient and verifying signs and symptoms of the presenting complaint. A focused physical assessment will be performed that includes inspection, palpation, and auscultation when indicated. Other elements of the secondary assessment include collecting information related to a past medical/surgical history, medication reconciliation, allergies, and vital signs. The emergency nurse may identify acute physiological risks at any point during the assessment and will escalate their findings to the emergency provider.

In addition to collecting data related to the patient's chief complaint, all patients in the ED are screened for suicide risk and abuse which could be physical, financial, and other forms of neglect. The emergency nurse will anticipate the needs of the patient and initiate interventions such as cardiac monitoring, supplemental oxygen application, venous access, wound care, and non-pharmacological pain management to name a few. The older adult poses many challenges for the ED clinicians in accurately assessing and diagnosing emergent syndromes. For instance, there may be communication barriers due to sensory deficits or cognitive disorders that may inhibit ascertaining accurate subjective data. In addition, medications or polypharmacy may alter vital signs, masking a sympathetic response to hypovolemia or pain, for example.

The ED Workup

The patient will be seen and examined by the ED provider. Based upon the history of presenting symptoms and physical examination, a plan of care will be established. Hemodynamic stability and symptom management are prioritized. This plan may also include diagnostics including lab work, imaging studies as well as specialty consultation. Based upon the results of the workup, an appropriate disposition will be rendered. By 2040, the demographic shift of the older adult population will encompass approximately 24% of the world's population which adds a fast-growing need to the surgical population. It is estimated that half of this population will be requiring operative procedures.

Older Adult Common Presentations

Abdominal pain is the most common chief complaint among patients over 65 presenting to the ED, representing 1.4 million visits in 2017. Abdominal pain accounts for 7% of all ED visits for older adults, or 7.5 million ED visits per year. Older adults that present to EDs with abdominal pain are at extremely high risk. Abdominal pain in younger patients is considered urgent, however stable vital signs and no red flag physical signs (pallor, diaphoresis, pain on palpation) the patient may wait to be evaluated by an ED provider. That is not the case with the older adult. The older adult with abdominal pain is triaged and assigned a higher acuity level. They are prioritized and are brought to a treatment area as soon as possible. Multiple factors such as underlying conditions (e.g., cardiopulmonary, diabetes, malignancy, etc.), decreased physiologic reserve, and delays in seeking medical care all contribute to a high incidence of complications. The emergency nurses receive the complaint of abdominal pain with a sense of urgency in the older adult. Some causes of abdominal pain in the elderly that may be life threatening are bowel obstruction, biliary disease, abdominal aortic aneurysm, gastrointestinal perforation, or hemorrhage just to name a few. Emergency nurses are aware of high-risk signs and symptoms in the older adult with abdominal pain. Abdominal distention, pain on palpation, nausea, vomiting, anorexia, fever, tachycardia, tachypnea, and hypotension are some symptoms highly suspicious for a serious underlying problem.

It is imperative for ED nurses to utilize a systematic approach in assessing the older adult with abdominal pain. It is also a priority to advocate for symptom management. Early treatment with anti-emetics and/or pain medications is essential in providing comfort for these patients. The patient's diagnostic workup may be more easily tolerated, especially when moved for imaging studies or during surgical consultation. Ongoing reassessments that include vital sign measurements are necessary in order to evaluate therapeutic interventions as well as in recognizing warning signs of decompensation or deterioration. Accurate patient assessment, timely treatment, effective communication, teamwork with providers, and effective symptom management are crucial in promoting a positive outcome.

The incidence of traumatic injuries in the older adult increases as they advance in age. According to the Center for Diseases Control and Prevention, falls have been identified as the primary cause of death among adults aged 65 and greater, resulting in millions of emergency department visits and accruing billions in cost. A range of injuries can be sustained from falls as a consequence of slowed responses, decreased perception, and alteration in balance. Depending upon the frailty of the aging adult vulnerability ensues and can be accompanied by alteration of normal physiological systems. For the older adult many traumatic events have the potential to lead to surgery, permanent disability, and death.

Emergency department nurses must evaluate potential risks and outcomes for the older adult when preparing their patients for surgery. As physiological changes ensue emergency nursing considerations must be tailored to meet those needs. This holds true not only for the physical but psychosocial factors need to be considered as well. The older adult is at a higher risk for surgical related complications and age-specific care must be provided to minimize adverse outcomes and even morbidity. Careful nursing considerations are indispensable and will positively affect surgical outcomes.

Due to the nature of surgery for the older adult, the precision in planning and execution is vital. The nurse must consider care plans, advance directives, pain management, education and various other consideration of lifetime age-related changes prior to surgery. The ability to expedite the accurate collection of key information in an abbreviated amount of time also factors into patient outcomes. The care plan will be designed and individualized to the type of surgery, risk factors, comorbidities and include education regarding recovery and can enhance postsurgical compliance. The patient and their designated support person must be educated and informed of any expected outcomes referenced in the care plan. Identifying and involving of a support person will ensure that there is a reliable and effective support system in place. Support in the recovery process allows nursing to work collaboratively to set expectations for the postoperative phase. The nurse should inform the patient and their support person what will be expected if they go to surgery, remain in the hospital or are released home. A comprehensive handoff is key during this transition. The nurse should always include transition of care in their discussions. The priority here is the nurse being able to identify immediate risks and anticipate the needs of the patient.

Wishes of each patient should be made known through advanced directives with special consideration being given to wishes surrounding resuscitation. A comprehensive cognitive assessment should be performed to validate that the patient has the capacity to understand and consent to treatment. The competent patient will be able to understand benefits, risks, and verbalize their concerns and understanding. The patient's emotional state should be considered at all time throughout treatment. They should be included in decision-making and nursing care should always be delivered with compassion and demonstrating respect for this vulnerable patient population. Spiritual support should also be considered and encompasses the identity of a large portion of patients. Spirituality can also be connected to how one perceives wellness.

Disposition

The disposition for many older adults will be inpatient admission to a unit that provides the appropriate level of care or perhaps due to a surgical emergency, they may be taken to the operating room initially. In addition to high admission rates and the need for emergency surgery, the older adult demonstrates a mortality rate approaching 10%. Avoiding hospital admission can also avert many complications associated with inpatient care and the older adult such as a functional status decline. Some of the complications of hospital admission may be an onset of delirium, hospital-acquired infections, and psychological and physiological effects of immobility. The older adult will usually prefer to recover in a familiar place among family, friends, and companions. In the event of an inpatient admission after surgery, the ultimate goal is to discharge the patient symptom free and returned to their optimal level of wellness with close follow-up. Coordinating follow-up care with the patient and support person ensuring that all aftercare instructions are clear will reduce hospital readmissions.

Discharge of the older adult should be well planned, conducted with a team approach and carried out with the intent that the patient will be able to manage their care with the appropriate resources in place. The older adult requires a holistic, precise approach to treatment that will allow them to maintain their dignity as they go through the aging process.

References

1. Center for Disease Control and Prevention. Emergency department visit rates by selected characteristics: United States, 2019. 2022. https://www.cdc.gov/nchs/data/databriefs/db434.pdf.
2. Yancey C, O'Rourke M. Emergency department triage. Treasure Island: Stat Pearls; 2021.
3. Gilboy N, Tanabe P, Travers D, Rosenau A, Eitel D. Emergency severity index, version 4: implementation handbook. AHRQ publication no. 05–0046-2. Rockville, MD: Agency for Healthcare Research and Quality; 2005. https://www.sgnor.ch/fileadmin/user_upload/Dokumente/Downloads/Esi_Handbook.pdf.
4. Akyuz E, Unlu H, Cevik B. Nursing care perceptions of older individuals undergoing surgery. J Educ Res Nurs. 2021;18(3):290–5. https://doi.org/10.5152/jern.2021.04875.
5. Center for Disease Control and Prevention. National Hospital Ambulatory Medical Care Survey. 2019.
6. Friedman A, Chen A, Wu R, Coe N, Halpern S, Hwang U, et al. Evaluation and disposition of older adults presenting to the emergency department with abdominal pain. J Am Geriatr Soc. 2022;70(2):501–11. https://doi.org/10.1111/jgs.17503.
7. Center for Disease Control and Prevention. Older adult fall prevention. 2021. https://www.cdc.gov/falls/index.html.
8. Johnson JA. Perioperative considerations for the older adult population. Urol Nurs. 2021;41(5):284–90. https://doi.org/10.7257/1053-816X.2021.41.5.284.
9. Proehl JA. Resuscitative decisions in the emergency care setting. J Emerg Nurs. 2021;47(6):933–7. https://doi.org/10.1016/j.jen.2021.08.004.
10. Bryan ED, Brenner BE. Abdominal pain in the elderly persons. Medscape. 2018. https://emedicine.medscape.com/article/776663-overview.

Perioperative Nursing Considerations

58

Theresa Criscitelli

Introduction

The year 2030 marks a demographic turning point for the USA in that one in every five Americans will be older than 65 years of age and by 2034, these older adults will outnumber children for the first time in American history. These aging Americans greatly influence the delivery of healthcare and perioperative leadership must understand these challenges and increased risks associated with the geriatric population preoperatively, intraoperatively, as well as postoperatively, in order to deliver high quality and safe surgical care.

Perioperative care within this vulnerable population is complicated and requires a multidisciplinary approach. A team-based approach is optimum that includes allied health professionals, social work, and nursing alongside medicine to be able to manage the comorbidities with outcomes that can yield fewer complications. The multidisciplinary team must appreciate the epidemiological and pathophysiological changes that occur with aging and be able to accurately assess and clinically manage these patients across the perioperative continuum. This chapter will address the preoperative, intraoperative, and postoperative nursing considerations that the perioperative nurse must be proficient to meet the needs of this patient population in order to provide safe care and proffer positive patient outcomes.

T. Criscitelli (✉)
NYU Langone Hospital—Long Island, Mineola, NY, USA
e-mail: theresa.criscitelli@nyulangone.org

Preoperative Considerations

The preoperative period is considered the time prior to surgery that is focused on preparing and optimizing the patient physically and mentally for the surgical procedure. Optimization of the geriatric patient should not begin the day of surgery, but should begin in the surgeon's office months before the surgery, so that the patient is in the best clinical condition to avoid adverse outcomes after surgery.

The preoperative time on the day of surgery provides opportunity to gather necessary information to identify risk factors and develop a perioperative plan of care that should include a physical assessment, psychological assessment, medication review, and establishment of safety measures for the perioperative setting. Ample time should be allotted and the use of collateral history from a caregiver or family member can provide additional information and clarity.

P. Petrone, C. E.M. Brathwaite (eds.), *Acute Care Surgery in Geriatric Patients*,
https://doi.org/10.1007/978-3-031-30651-8_58

Physical Assessment

When conducting the physical assessment the preoperative nurse should be cognizant of the physiologic functioning that is unique to this patient population. Table 58.1 highlights e body system and relevant potential changes this patient population that could affect the c of the surgical patient.

Table 58.1 Body system and relevant potential changes

Body system	Potential changes
Cardiovascular	– Valves thicken and become rigid – Arterial wall thickens and stiffens – Increase in peripheral resistance – Increase risk of arrhythmias – Potential for induced hypotension and syncope – Decrease in cardiac reserve
Pulmonary	– Decrease in lung capacity – Reduced pulmonary functional reserve – Loss of pharyngeal support – Increase risk for pulmonary infection and bronchospasm – Decrease response to hypoxia and hypercapnia
Gastrointestinal	– Increase chance for periodontal disease and gum recession – Impaired dentition – Decreased saliva production – Decrease muscle strength to chew, taste, and thirst perception – Increase risk of aspiration – Decrease peristalsis – Impairment of nutrient absorption and chance of indigestion/constipation – Decreased hepatic reserve and decrease metabolism of medications
Renal	– Decreased renal functional reserve and increase risk for renal complications – Decreased kidney size – Increased risk for nephrotoxic injury and adverse drug reaction – Reduced bladder elasticity, muscle tone, and capacity – Increased prostate size – Increase risk of urinary urgency, incontinence, infection, nocturnal polyuria
Musculoskeletal	– Increase weakness and decreased exercise tolerance because of decreased muscle mass – Decreased ligament and tendon strength, intervertebral disk degeneration, articular cartilage erosion that can lead to kyphosis and reduced height – Increase risk of osteoporosis, osteopenia leading to risk of fractures – Tissue elasticity and mobility decrease
Nervous and sensory	– Decrease in nerve cells, central blood flow and metabolism – Altered vision, hearing, taste, smell, and touch – Impairment of deep tendon reflexes and nerve conduction velocity causing slower motor skills and imbalance/coordination – Increased risk of delirium
Endocrine and immune	– Decrease thyroid activity – Altered release of insulin – Depress of immune response – Increase risk for infections
Integumentary	– Compromised thermoregulation – Decrease in temperature sensitivity – Decrease in subcutaneous tissue with thinner, drier, fragile tissue – Altered response to environmental temperature extremes – Decrease in shivering response – Slower metabolic rate – Decrease vasoconstrictor response – Diminished sweating – Desynchronization of circadian rhythm – Decreased heat/cold perception

Psychological Assessment

The preoperative nurse should assess the geriatric patient's cognitive and sensory function, by determining whether the patient can follow directions and perform tasks, as well as assess if a family member or caregiver has the ability to assist. This can be assessed by way of observation and continued conversation throughout the preoperative visit. It is best that the nurse face the patient, speaking clearly, slowly, and with an elevated volume, if necessary, as well as limiting background noise. Assistive devices such as hearing aids and glasses should be available as long as feasible before and after surgery.

Dementia should be evaluated preoperatively using a cognitive assessment tool by either the preoperative nurse or possibly a geriatric consultation can assist in the cognitive assessment. Understanding the preoperative status of the patient can assist in strategies for prevention postoperatively for delirium and ultimately decrease postoperative mortality.

Depression screening, using a pre-established and validated tool such as the Patient Health Questionnaire-9, is important to assess prior to surgery, since depression can have implications on surgical outcomes and has been shown to be associated with increased infections, delayed wound healing, and a decreased postoperative emotional and functional status.

Nutritional Status

Nutritional status should be assessed prior to surgery, using a validated tool such as the Mini-Nutritional Assessment or the Nutritional Risk Screening, since malnutrition can be associated with an increased rate of complications and delirium postoperatively. Unnecessary perioperative fasting should be avoided, and providing clear fluids permitted up to 2 h prior to surgery to prevent dehydration. The use of carbohydrate-containing drinks and perioperative nutritional therapy should be considered preoperatively for geriatric patients with malnutrition, since excessive fasting increases discomfort, can lead to agitation, and promotes the onset of postoperative delirium.

Medication Review

The geriatric surgical patients can be at a risk for polypharmacy due to their multiple medical conditions, multiple physicians, and number of prescriptions. Polypharmacy is a risk factor in this population and is associated with poor postoperative outcomes. This patient population may also be hoarding medications and self-medicating with over-the-counter products to supplement their prescriptions; therefore, a complete medication reconciliation must be performed. Any nonessential medications, as well as non-prescription medications, should be discontinued prior to surgery in effort to avoid any medication interactions. Usually, long-term cardiac medications, such as beta blockers, are continued in order to prevent rebound phenomena, and pain medications should be continued, especially opioids. The use of opioid medications for multi-modal pain management should be examined and when possible, an opioid alternative should be considered when discussing with the multidisciplinary care team.

Safety Measures

Safety measures should be taken to assess the complex geriatric patient that presents to the perioperative setting. The gold standard for caring for these patients is to use a Comprehensive Geriatric Assessment, as well as receiving recommendations from the primary care provider, cardiologist, anesthesia provider, and ideally a geriatric specialist.

Geriatric patients are at an increased risk of deep vein thrombosis. Therefore, prophylaxis should be accomplished by use of medication, application of sequential compression devices or anti-embolism stockings, and range of motion exercises to prevent the pooling of blood in the extremities.

Fragility screening is recommended by the American College of Surgeons and the.

American Geriatrics Society to assess older patients using the FRAIL Scale, Edmonton Frail Scale, Risk Analysis Index, Modified Frailty Index, or Clinical Frail Scale. Screening for frailty can help identify risks, determine interventions that can prevent complications, and ensure the best possible outcome for the patient. Optimization of these patients include rehabilitation programs, nutritional supplements, and co-management of care with a geriatric specialist. This can prevent patient injury and falls, as well as comprise part of the handoff of care.

Fall risk assessment must be completed on the geriatric surgical patient the day of surgery, since the risk of falling increases in high-risk patients following surgical procedures, due to frailty, diminished muscle strength, and decreased mobility. Prehabilitation can assist in functional improvement when optimizing patients prior to surgery.

Functional status of the geriatric patient should be assessed based upon the patient's activities of daily living, such as ability to use the bathroom and bathing, and instrumental activities of daily living, such as medication management, cooking, and cleaning. Functional capacity can be measured by using a validated scale, such as Duke Activity Status Index or Timed Up and Go Test. These scales can provide an accurate picture of the patient's abilities prior to surgery and can assist in creating attainable patient goals postoperatively.

Environmental factors and sensory triggers can precipitate postoperative delirium. Therefore, the nurse should create an environment throughout the perioperative setting that is a comfortable temperature and calming with as little commotion as possible. Patients should be encouraged to use their corrective devices, such as hearing aids, corrective lenses, and dentures for as long as possible prior to surgery and they should be kept safe and returned during the postoperative phase, as soon as feasible. The nurse should also speak slowly and clearly while leaning into the patient closely, as well as providing simple and brief instructions and information that is easy to comprehend. The nurse may have to reorient the patient frequently if it is observed that the patient is exhibiting sensory deprivation symptoms.

Intraoperative Considerations

The intraoperative phase comprises the time immediately prior to the surgical procedure, the induction and maintenance of anesthesia, the surgical procedure, and the emergence from anesthesia. The geriatric patient should be approached through the lens of critically thinking about the customized care that will meet the need of the specific patient based upon the physiological and psychological attributes, which are based upon assessment of risk factors and mitigating risk through preventative measures.

Anesthesia Induction

The choice of anesthesia for this patient population is dependent upon the patient's physiologic status, the length of the procedure, and the preference of the anesthesia provider and surgeon. If possible, regional anesthesia may be a viable option over general anesthesia, but it is important to assess the patient's flexibility and arthritis prior to attempting the positioning required for administration of this type of anesthesia.

Geriatric patients commonly have a decrease in the function of their systems, such as reduced liver and kidney function, altered body composition, decreased albumin level, and decreased cardiac output, as well as having an altered anti-inflammatory and pharmacokinetic response to medications. Therefore, it is more difficult to gauge the response to anesthetics and a lower dose may be required to reach a therapeutic level.

Positioning of the Geriatric Patient

Positioning of the geriatric patient is vital in effort to prevent patient injury. This patient population has a loss of subcutaneous fat, poor skin turgor, and fragile tissue, as well as a decrease in range of motion and skeletal changes from chronic pain and comorbidities. Care must be taken to pad any boney prominences with foam or gel padding and at times have the patients position themselves prior to the induction of anesthesia, especially if there are limitations that would go unnoticed once anesthetized.

The supine position, although common for many surgical procedures, can be restrictive for air flow in the geriatric patient; therefore, the head and chest may need to be elevated slightly to reduce any respiratory issue, as well as it is vital to properly align the body on the operating room bed to help prevent the compromise of blood flow. The length of surgery should be considered to reduce the risk of skin damage and pressure, so careful positioning with padding and supportive devices can be helpful.

Due to skin integrity concerns, it is important to avoid the use of tape on the geriatric patient's skin and caution should be taken when removing EKG leads and return electrode pads that can damage delicate skin. Pooling of fluids such as skin preparation should be avoided to prevent skin damage, such as irritation or chemical burn.

Thermoregulation

Geriatric patients exhibit the increased risk of hypothermia due to a decrease in muscle tissue, reduced subcutaneous fat, and diminished peripheral circulation. These attributes coupled with the cold temperatures and fluids in the operating room create an environment that can easily lead to hypothermia. Hypothermia can lead to postoperative myocardial ischemia, ventricular tachycardia, agitation, confusion, and delirium.

Thermoregulation should begin with preoperative warming of the patient using active and passive warming methods for minimum 15 min prior to surgery and then continue these methods throughout the intraoperative and postoperative phases of care in order to maintain the patient's core body temperature. Additional warming of anesthesia gases, IV fluids, irrigation solutions, insufflation gases, and ambient room temperatures can also serve as an adjunction to the forced hot air device. It is important to keep a subtle balance between how much heat is gained and how much heat is lost during the perioperative phase of care. The temperature of the geriatric patient should be carefully monitored during all phases of perioperative care.

Safety Measures

It is the responsibility of the entire surgical team to keep the geriatric patient safe during the perioperative phases of care. Changes in fluid volume, deficit or excess, are common in this patient population and can lead to impaired respiratory function, swelling of the extremities, and potentially heart failure. Therefore, the surgical team must clearly communicate blood loss during the procedure, irrigation usage, urine output, fluid intake, sponge saturation, and amount of fluid collected in suction canisters. Keeping track of input and output will help adjust for variability and assist in maintaining homeostasis.

Postoperative Considerations

The postoperative phase is considered the time the geriatric patient is received in the Post Anesthesia Care Unit and through the duration in this unit. The geriatric patient should be transferred after a verbal handoff of pertinent patient information is conveyed that will affect postoperative outcomes. It is important to discuss any events that may have occurred preoperatively or intraoperatively that could potentially affect the postoperative outcomes. The assessment and management will be governed by the type and length of the procedure that was performed. After electronic record review and physical assessment, the nurse can render the appropriate treatments, solicit necessary interventions, and determine the necessary interprofessional team members.

Pain Management

Literature supports that geriatric patients communicate pain less than younger patients, resulting in the under treatment of pain. This situation coupled with renal and neurological sensitivities to pain medications yields the need for less opioids after surgery. The postoperative nurse must assess pain by using the appropriate pain scale, but must also discuss the use of both medications and therapeutic alternatives, such as complementary approaches including relaxation techniques, distraction techniques, and hot/cold therapy. Managing postoperative pain is a precipitating risk factor for delirium, so adequate management with appropriate analgesia is vital, as well as comparing to the baseline and reviewing prior pain assessments.

Postoperative Delirium

Postoperative delirium (POD) is a complication of surgery amongst the geriatric patient population that should be accurately assessed and intervened quickly when early symptoms are noted. POD can cause delayed recovery, extended hospitalization, and increased medical cost to treat these patients. Contributing factors that can lead to POD include advanced age, cognitive impairment, comorbidities, and a previous history of delirium or cognitive impairment. POD presents beyond the initial emergence of anesthesia and can reoccur during a later postoperative phase of care. POD initially presents as agitation/hyperexcitability or somnolence/confusion and can be exhibited in behaviors such as a lack of focus or awareness, altered cognition and mental status, disinhibition, crying, or restlessness. Risk factors such as polypharmacy and frailty, as well as dementia, depression, and cognitive impairment contribute to POD.

A baseline assessment or screening questionnaire to assess cognitive function prior to anesthesia can be helpful for early postoperative identification of POD. Also, reorienting the patient to place and time, returning assistive devices such as hearing aids and glasses, avoiding relocating the patient to different rooms, and having a family member, photos, or favorite music can assist in minimizing POD. Avoiding medications that exacerbate POD, such as anticholinergic medications, sedative-hypnotics, corticosteroids, and meperidine can be helpful in minimization of POD.

Infection

Postoperative infection amongst the geriatric patient can be higher than in other patient populations. The most common sites for postoperative infection include the surgical site, urinary tract, and respiratory tract. It is imperative to watch the patient vigilantly and antimicrobial prophylaxis should be considered 1 h prior to surgery and continued at minimum for 24 h after surgery, if warranted. Additionally, the nurse should be cognizant of vital sign changes, promotion of removal of indwelling urinary catheter, use of incentive spirometer/deep breathing/ambulation, and the need for sterile dressing changes.

Safety Measures

Frequent turning and repositioning of the postoperative geriatric patient can help improve respiratory function, along with encouraging deep breathing, coughing, and incentive spirometry to maintain adequate lung function. It is necessary to provide oral hygiene to patients on mechanical ventilation to decrease the microflora load to prevent ventilator-associated pneumonia. This can be accomplished with a small-headed toothbrush or a suction toothbrush, along with the use of dry mouth gel that can be applied to the mouth and lips, when needed.

Geriatric patients should resume fluid intake as soon as possible during the postoperative phase of care, since oral or enteral diets reduce the risk of infection and can reduce the length of stay in the hospital setting. It is important to encourage consumption of fluids often to reduce the risk of dehydration and to encourage the intake of food, enteral supplements, and parenteral supplements when needed.

Beginning early ambulation and rehabilitation can facilitate postoperative recovery and prevent nerve damage, immobility, and atrophy of the muscles. These patients present a fall risk and can have apprehension when ambulating, so solicitation of additional staff to assist and encourage the patient is necessary.

Future of Perioperative Care of the Geriatric Nurse

Hospitals around the world have implemented many strategies to care for the geriatric patient. In 2017, specialists in both the USA and Canada launched the Geriatric 5 Ms that include Mind, Mobility, Medications, Multi-complexity, and Matters most, which are individual health outcome goals and care. These are five of the most important aspects of care that should be managed daily by the healthcare professional within an Age-Friendly health system. This can lead to collaborative care and potential consultations that may have been overlooked if absent such a care guide.

In an effort to prepare for the increase in this patient population, the American College of Surgeons has launched the Geriatric Surgery Verification program that will enable hospitals to create centers for geriatric surgery that can promote safe and effective care that are rooted in evidence-based standards. This can create a road-map to care for the geriatric patient inter-professionally and create an environment to share resources, as well as metrics.

Conclusion

This fast growing segment of population will continue to increase and as a whole perioperative nurses will be caring for these complex patients that will require specialized perioperative care to ensure optimum clinical outcomes and safe care to this patient population. Understanding and implementing the appropriate care within the preoperative, intraoperative, and postoperative settings will help prevent readmissions and reduced functional decline that can lead to a lower quality of life. It is also imperative that hospitals create comprehensive organizational structures that are tailored to this population of patients.

References

1. AORN. AORN eGuidelines+. Practice Point, 2020 Edition: Practice point: postoperative delirium. 2020. https://aornguidelines.org/books/content?sectionid=245920322#245920322.
2. AORN. Guidelines for perioperative practice: positioning the patient. 2022. https://aornguidelines.org/guidelines?bookid=2260.
3. Cooper L, Abbett SK, Feng A, Bernacki RE, Cooper Z, Urman RD, et al. Launching a geriatric surgery center: recommendations from the Society for Perioperative Assessment and Quality Improvement. J Am Geriatr Soc. 2020;68(9):1941–6. https://doi.org/10.1111/jgs.16681.
4. Croke L. Preoperative management of frailty in older patients undergoing elective surgery. AORN J. 2020;111(1):P8–P10. https://doi.org/10.1002/aorn.12936.
5. Ellis G, Sevdalis N. Understanding and improving multidisciplinary team working in geriatric medicine. Age Ageing. 2019;48(4):498–505. https://doi.org/10.1093/ageing/afz021.
6. Janssen TL, Alberts AR, Hooft L, Mattace-Raso FUS, Mosk CA, van der Laan L. Prevention of postoperative delirium in elderly patients planned for elective surgery: systematic review and meta-analysis. Clin Interv Aging. 2019;14:1095–117. https://doi.org/10.2147/CIA.S201323.
7. Little MO, McDonald S, Schlientz D, Kim YH. Perioperative medical assessment of older adults. In: Sinclair AJ, Morley JE, Vellas B, Cesari M, Munshi M, editors. Pathy's Principles and Practice of Geriatric Medicine, vol. 2; 2022. p. 1407–20. https://doi.org/10.1002/9781119484288.ch112.
8. Molnar F, Frank CC. Optimizing geriatric care with the geriatric 5Ms. Can Fam Physician. 2019;65(1):39.
9. Olotu C, Weimann A, Bahrs C, Schwenk W, Scherer M, Kiefmann R. The perioperative care of older patients: time for a new, interdisciplinary approach. Dtsch Arztebl Int. 2019;116(5):63–9. https://doi.org/10.3238/arztebl.2019.0063.
10. Oster KA, Oster CA. Special needs population: care of the geriatric patient population in the perioperative setting. AORN J. 2015;101(4):443–59. https://doi.org/10.1016/j.aorn.2014.10.022.
11. Putnam K. Strategies to improve postoperative brain health in geriatric patients. AORN J. 2017;105(1)
12. Rothrock JC. Alexander's care of the patient in surgery-E-book. Amsterdam: Elsevier; 2018.

13. Vespa J, Armstrong DM, Medina L. Demographic turning points for the United States: population projections for 2020 to 2060. Washington, DC: US Department of Commerce, Economics and Statistics Administration, US Census Bureau; 2018.
14. Wainer C. The importance of oral hygiene for patients on mechanical ventilation. Br J Nurs. 2020;29(15):862–3. https://doi.org/10.12968/bjon.2020.29.15.862.
15. Wolfe JD, Wolfe NK, Rich MW. Perioperative care of the geriatric patient for noncardiac surgery. Clin Cardiol. 2020;43(2):127–36. https://doi.org/10.1002/clc.23302.

59 Implementing Nursing Care Plans

Nicole Mascellaro

The Nursing Care Plan

The nursing care plan (NCP) is a plan of action. It is the written expression of the nursing process individualized to a patient. The NCP is an instrument meant to enable nurses to document a hospital course as well as provide consistent goal-directed care and collaborate with the healthcare team. Nurses use this instrument to document information relevant to specific patients' care in one place as part of a structured centralized document.

Main Reasons to Write a Nursing Care Plan

NCPs play a critical role in the delivery of patient care. NCPs are individualized, holistic, and patient centered. Additionally, consideration is taken to actual and potential patient problems. As such, NCPs provide guidelines for nursing and treatment outlining what the nurse is responsible for and how to do it. Communication between nurses and other health care providers is also facilitated by the NCP. Using this approach, the healthcare team can effectively work together to achieve common objectives.

N. Mascellaro (✉)
Adjunct Professor of Nursing, Hofstra Northwell School of Nursing and Physician Assistant Studies, Hempstead, NY, USA

Introduction to the Nursing Process

Nursing care plays a vital role in positive patient expereinces as well as in achieving favorable outcomes from admission and especially for the geriatric patinet, beyond the immediate discharge period. To assist with the care of patient, and collection and transmission of information, a problem-solving approach to facilitate nursing care was created. Developed in the 1950s, this concept consisted of three steps: (1) assessment, (2) planning, and (3) evaluation. Over time and through study and use, this process has evolved into five sequential steps: (1) assessment, (2) diagnosis, (3) planning, (4) implementation, and (5) evaluation. In any clinical setting, these five steps are essential to guide action and provide high-quality, individualized patient care. As a problem solving instrument the nursing care plan provides a framework to allow comprehensive care taking into account multiple patient factors.

Components of a Nursing Care Plan

As part of a hospital admission nurses are repsonsible for developing a plan of care based on the needs and goals of each patient. The NCP is a

P. Petrone, C. E.M. Brathwaite (eds.), *Acute Care Surgery in Geriatric Patients*,
https://doi.org/10.1007/978-3-031-30651-8_59

structures process, serving as a guide, to facilitate nurses' action and as a means to assess patient outcomes. Each step of the nursing process is interconnected and associated with specific nurisng actions. The process is continous throughout an admission. The nursing process will be discussed in a step-by-step fashion.

STEP 1: Assessment (Gathering the Data)

An assessment involves gathering both objective and subjective data. Objective data is measurable, such as vital signs, and subjective data are derived from patient or family responses to open- or closed-ended questions or their own statements. The collection of these data points is performed in a systematic fashion using critical thinking skills. The data collected should include not only physiological data, but also the social, cultural, psychological, economic, and life-style factors. Data collected is generally from a nursing perspective in conjunction with medical findings and diagnostic studies. Additionally, the nurse should include the components of the patient's story using open-ended questions which helps facilitate this process. Current data related to the cause of the admission or current health problem are included. Also, historical data existing prior to the current problem are included.

In the nursing process, the nursing assessment is the foundation upon which the rest of the steps are built. It is essential to determine nursing diagnoses which are responsive to nursing interventions. Additionally, actual, and potential problems and strengths are determined in this step.

STEP 2: Diagnosis (Analyzing the Data)

Diagnosis involves the use of the data collected to develop a nursing diagnosis. In order that a patient is managed holistically, the nurse will cluster and organize data from the patient's story, objective and subjective data collected and form an evaluative judgment. Generally, nursing diagnoses are clinical judgments made based on an individual, family, or group's response to certain health conditions or life processes, or their vulnerability to those responses. Incorporating Maslow's hierarchy of needs into the nursing diagnosis helps nurses prioritize and plan nursing care.

The nursing diagnosis is the basis for the nurse's care plan. It is dependent on the accuracy of the nursing assessment and requires updating when there is a change in patient status. The nursing diagnosis is different from the medical diagnosis. It changes according to the patients progress or conclusion of condition.

Formulating the nursing diagnosis consists of a three-part diagnostic statement: Problem, Etiology, and Symptoms.

- **Problem:** Term that represents the problem; it is the nursing diagnosis taken from The North American Nursing Diagnosis Association International (NANDA-I) list.
- **Etiology** is related to phrase; related to factor or contributor to the problem, it is not the medical diagnosis.
- **Symptoms:** The symptoms identified by the nurse during the assessment of the patient.

Types of Nursing Diagnoses

1. ***Risk Nursing Diagnosis:*** A clinical judgment regarding the risk that an individual, family group, or community may develop an unfavorable human response to health circumstances or life processes.

   The following must be present for a Risk Nursing Diagnosis:
   a. *Risk factors*: Contribute to increased vulnerability. There are no related factors (etiological factors).
   b. Example: Risk for falls (diagnosis) as evidenced by impaired mobility (risk factor).
2. ***Problem Focused Diagnosis:*** A clinical judgment regarding an unfavorable response to health circumstances or life processes that is present in an individual, family, group, or community. It is an actual diagnosis, a prob-

lem that is present based on signs and symptoms.

The following must be present for a problem-focused diagnosis:

a. *Defining characteristics*: The observable signs and symptoms (subjective and objective data) or inferences that cluster as manifestations of the nursing diagnosis. Anything a nurse can observe, hear, touch or information provided by the patient or the patient's family. Phrased by: "as evidenced by" or "manifested by" in the nursing diagnosis.
b. *Related to factors:* Which are the etiological factors. Related to factors either contribute to, are related to, is a preceding condition or cause of the diagnosis. Related factors should not be the medical diagnosis. Phrased by "R/T" or "related to" in the nursing diagnosis.
c. Example: Ineffective breathing pattern (diagnosis) related to pain (etiological factor) as evidenced by shortness of breath and nasal flaring (defining characteristics).

3. ***Health Promotion Diagnosis***: A clinical judgment about motivation and the desire to achieve better health and well-being, expressed by a patient's readiness to improve specific health behaviors.

   The following must be present for a health-promotion diagnosis:

   a. *Defining characteristics:* phrased by "as evidenced by."
   b. Example: Readiness for enhanced comfort.

4. ***Syndrome Diagnosis:*** A clinical judgment concerning a particular group of nursing diagnoses that occur together and that should be addressed together, through similar nursing interventions.

   The following must be present for a syndrome diagnosis:

   a. Diagnostic label.
   b. *Defining characteristics*: two or more nursing diagnoses.
   c. *Related to factors:* are not required, however may be utilized to add clarity.
   d. Example: Frail elderly syndrome.

STEP 3: Planning (Formulating Goals, Outcomes, and Interventions)

The planning stage is where the desired patient specific goals and outcomes are established, and priorities are formed. At this point, nursing interventions are also planned. The patient's goals should be specific, clear, detailed, and measurable. Both short-and long-term goals should be included. After identifying the goals(s) or outcomes(s), the nurse will develop nursing interventions that need to be performed in order for the patient to reach these endpoints.

Nursing interventions should be prioritized based on urgency of need. Maslow's hierarchy of needs can be used to determine the highest priority as well as the use of ABC (airway, breathing, and circulation) and safety. Nursing interventions should be clear, specific and indicate what the nurse is expected to accomplish. Nurses should review their patient's goals and outcomes during each shift to assess the usefulness and relevance of the treatement plan as well as to determine if goals need modification based on the patient's updated status.

STEP 4: Implementation

Implementation is the execution of the nursing interventions outlined in the plan of care. That is, it involves putting the plan into action. The process begins with understanding the NCP for goals or outcomes that are to be evaluated during the time the patient is under their care or for their shift to ensure the nursing interventions necessary are initiated and remain aligned.

STEP 5: Evaluation

In the last stage, the nurse evaluates the patient to determine if the desired outcome was achieved. The nurse monitors the patient's response to the nursing interventions and documents them in the patient record. In cases where the outcome was not achieved, the nurse needs to reassess the patient and change the plan according to the current situation. The nursing process is cyclic; however, it must follow the continuum of the patients progression through a hospital course. To address patients evolving needs and or unmet goals and outcomes, the nurse will continously assess their patient and begin the nursing process from the primary step when needed.

Implementing the Nursing Care Plan for the Geriatric Patient

The geriatric population is a vulnerable one and even more so the geriatric surgical patient undergoing intervention in an acute and unplanned scenario has needs that are exceptionally different from other patient groups. The nursing process provides a systematic approach to facilitate the planning of an individualized plan of care that addresses the various health concerns of the geriatric patient.

In many cases, acute care hospitals are the entry point of geriatric patients into the healthcare system. Nursing care may begin in the emergency room and be transferred just as the patient is to a surgical or critical care unit. Regardless of the location or timing of care being provided, the goal is to restore the geriatric patient to an optimal level of functioning and prevent complications.

A nurse's role in caring for the geriatric acute surgery patient is unique in relation to other patient populations. There is a greater demand for understanding the holistic existence of the patient prior to hospitalization including physical, social, mental, emotional, and spiritual needs. Furthermore, there are physiologic and cognitive changes with aging that may affect geriatric patients undergoing surgery. It is of the utmost importance that nurses are aware of this and include interventions in their NCPs specific to this population to avoid any potential complications and optimize outcomes. The NCP should be developed upon admission to the hospital and regularly revised allowing for updates according to changes in a patient's condition until the patient is discharged.

Special Considerations for Implementing the Nursing Care Plan for the Geriatric Patient

The nurse should use an age-specific approach to assess the geriatric patient. A comprehensive assessment of physical and psychosocial function is vital. This assessment may result in a nurse needing to modify the environment for sensory and musculoskeletal changes. The nurse should be prepared to provide an adequate amount of time and focus allowing the patient time to respond to questions, in a comfortable, private setting with limited distractions. Geriatric patients may have long histories, when completing the health history and interviewing the patient, it may be beneficial to structure the interview, collaborate with the patient and use a goal-directed interviewing process to obtain pertinent information.

The physical assessment of the geriatric patient usually comes after the health history and interview. The nurse should use a systematic approach to perform the physical assessment and take into consideration: explaining the process and each step in simple terms, provide privacy, use a sequence that minimizes position change, warn of potential pain, and encourage questions. The nurse should include an assessment of the functional, cognitive, affective, social, and mobility assessment. Measures such as the frailty index can be incorporated to provide objectivity to the data collected.

- **Functional assessment:** Should include the measurement of the patient's ability to perform activities for independent living and basic self-care tasks. Due to polypharmacy, delirium, urinary incontinence, falls, lack of exercise, insufficient nutritional intake, iatrogenic infection, loss of function and self-care ability, advanced age, comorbidities, and other risk factors associated with the acute care setting, a geriatric patient would benefit from a functional assessment.
- **Cognitive assessment:** Should include a mental status assessment that is used to determine the patient's level of cognitive function.

- **Affective assessment:** To differentiate low moods to depression.
- **Social assessment:** May provide information about the patient's ability to handle physical impairments and their support network.
- **Frailty index assessment:** Patients older than 70 years old should be screened for risks associated with frailty.
- **Mobility assessment:** Assess the patient's ability to move, strength, limitations, and/or equipment or aids required.

Risks of Hospitalization for the Geriatric Patient

Risks of hospitalization of the geriatric patient include the following: adverse drug reactions, falls, infections, immobility, functional decline, malnutrition, impaired skin integrity, sleep disturbance, polypharmacy, incontinence, and delirium. The NCP should address these potential risks for the geriatric patient, and nursing interventions should be used to help prevent any iatrogenic complications. Additionally, the NCP should address actual problems or at-risk problems related to the patient's surgical procedure or postoperative care. Some of the common risks of hospitalization for the geriatric patient will be discussed next.

Implementation of Nursing Care Plans for the Geriatric Patient Status Post-Acute Surgery Would Include the Following Common Risks (Would Require Prioritization Based on Patient Needs and Assessment)

Immobility

Assessment:

- Assess the patient's baseline and current mobility status.
- Perform a comprehensive mobility assessment.

Diagnosis: Select a NANDA-I diagnosis for actual or at-risk nursing diagnoses.

Outcome/Goal: Patient is free from complications of immobility.

Plan: Formulate goals/outcomes and select appropriate nursing interventions to help the patient achieve goals/outcomes such as targeted exercise programs, physical therapy, and functional mobility programs.

Implementation: Nursing Interventions Aimed at Promoting Mobility Include (Not Limited to) Interventions Must Be Prioritized Based on the Patient's Assessment

- Provide non-skid footwear.
- Perform active or passive range of motion exercises.
- Utilize appropriate mobility devices to facilitate patient getting out of bed and ambulating.
- Schedule time for ambulating and getting patient out of bed to a chair.
- Utilize appropriate mobility devices or aids.

Evaluate: Reassess patient to check if nursing interventions helped the patient meet the desired goal/outcome. If the goals/outcome were not met, reassess, make changes, and start the nursing process over.

Falls

Assessment:

- Assess the patient's risk factors for falls.
- Assess patient room for risk factors and institute corrective action.
- Perform a comprehensive fall risk assessment.

Diagnosis: Select a NANDA-I diagnosis for actual or at-risk nursing diagnoses.

Outcome/Goal: Absence of falls, reduce preventable falls and injury.

Plan: Formulate goals/outcomes and select appropriate nursing interventions for implementation to help achieve goals/outcomes.

Implementation: Nursing Interventions Aimed at Preventing Falls Include (Not Limited to). Interventions Must Be Prioritized Based on the Patient's Assessment

- Implement fall protocol used at facility.
- Promote mobility.
- Implement safety measures: bed in lowest position, chair in lowest position and brake used, call bell in reach always, bed and/or chair exit alarms used, use chairs with armrests, handrails, grab bars in the toilet and shower, frequent bedside rounding by staff, use of nonskid slippers, nightlights, nonskid floor, eyeglasses, and hearing aids used if required, place all required items within reach, use a whiteboard in the patient's room to display important information in large print, assessment of medications, cognitive assessment, and implementing a toileting schedule.

Evaluate: Reassess patient to check if nursing interventions helped the patient meet the desired goal/outcome. If the goals/outcome were not met, reassess, make changes, and start the nursing process over.

Infection

Assessment:

- Assess for signs and symptoms of an infection.
- Assess the patient's risk factors for infections.
- Assess vital signs.
- Assess laboratory values indicative of infection.
- Assess for sepsis and SIRS criteria.
- Assess characteristics of urine (geriatric patients are at risk for urinary infections).
- Assess any tubes, drains or intravenous access, urinary catheters, and the need for them.
- Assess surgical site or wound for appearance and drainage.

Diagnosis: Select a NANDA-I diagnosis for actual or at-risk nursing diagnoses.

Outcome/Goal: Absence of infection.

Plan: Formulate goals/outcomes and select appropriate nursing interventions for implementation to help achieve goals/outcomes.

Implementation: Nursing Interventions Aimed at Preventing Infections (Not Limited to). Interventions Must Be Prioritized Based on the Patient's Assessment

- Perform hand hygiene before contact with patient, before aseptic procedure, after touching the patient or patient surroundings, and before application and after removal of gloves and any time deemed necessary.
- Maintain strict asepsis for wound care and dressing changes and report abnormal appearance of the surgical site or any abnormal drainage from the surgical site to the health care provider.
- Encourage coughing, deep breathing, and use of the incentive spirometer (pulmonary hygiene).
- Encourage ambulation and mobility.
- Provide oral hygiene.
- Encourage fluid intake if not contraindicated and nutritional intake.
- Review the need for any tube, line, drains daily at multidisciplinary rounds.
- Removal of tubes, drains, indwelling catheters as soon as appropriate according to the health care provider.
- Use universal and contact precaution protocol.

Evaluate: Reassess patient to check if nursing interventions helped the patient meet the desired goal/outcome. If the goals/outcome were not met, reassess, make changes, and start the nursing process over.

rium

essment:

- Assess the patient's baseline and current cognitive status.
- Assess medication usage (especially psychoactive agents, narcotic analgesics, and medications with anticholinergic effects) and polypharmacy.
- Assess for acute pain, infection, immobilization, use of restraints, urinary catheterization, dehydration, environmental factors, and psychosocial factors.
- Assess for risk factors of delirium.
- Perform a comprehensive cognitive assessment.

Diagnosis: Select a NANDA-I diagnosis for actual or at-risk nursing diagnoses.

Outcome/Goal: Absence of delirium.

Plan: Formulate goals/outcomes and select appropriate nursing interventions for implementation to help achieve goals/outcomes.

Implementation: Nursing Interventions Aimed at Preventing Delirium (Not Limited to). Interventions Must Be Prioritized Based on the Patient's Assessment

- Reorientation.
- Cognitive stimulation.
- Mobilize the patient (ambulation and exercise throughout day).
- Hearing aid and glasses in place.
- Facilitate adequate sleep (noise reduction at night, quiet room and avoid waking the patient if possible).
- Maintenance of nutrition and hydration.
- Involve family and or significant other and family visitation.
- Try nonpharmacological approaches for anxiety and pain.
- Pain control.
- Avoid restraint use if possible.

Evaluate: Reassess patient to check if nursing interventions helped the patient meet the desired goal/outcome. If the goals/outcome were not met, reassess, make changes, and start the nursing process over.

Impaired Skin Integrity/Pressure Injuries

Assessment:

- Perform a comprehensive skin integrity assessment (including assessment of bony prominences and assessing under and around medical devices whenever possible).
- Assess skin integrity and risk factors (use a valid tool).
- Assess nutritional status.
- Assess for urinary/fecal incontinence.
- Assess mobility status.

Diagnosis: Select a NANDA-I diagnosis for actual or at-risk nursing diagnoses.

Outcome/Goal: Absence of pressure ulcers and skin breakdown.

Plan: Formulate goals/outcomes and select appropriate nursing interventions for implementation to help achieve goals/outcomes.

Implementation: Nursing Interventions Aimed at Preventing Pressure Ulcers and Skin Breakdown (Not Limited to). Interventions Must Be Prioritized Based on the Patient's Assessment

- Minimize shearing and friction.
- Initiate turning and repositioning protocol.
- Mobilize patient.
- Apply redistribution mattresses.
- Use support surfaces to reduce pressure.
- Use barrier products and protect skin from moisture.
- Raise heels off the bed mattress.

- Use devices to assist with transferring and lifting.
- Encourage adequate hydration and nutrition.
- Educate the patient and family about methods to maintain skin integrity.
- Minimize pressure on bony prominences.

Acute Pain

Assessment:

- Assess pain with vital signs, during hourly rounding and the required time interval after pain medication administration.
- Use the pain assessment tool according to your organization (assess pain location, onset, intensity, quality, and duration).
- Perform a comprehensive pain assessment.

Diagnosis: Select a NANDA-I diagnosis for actual or at-risk nursing diagnoses.

Outcome/Goals: Absence of pain. Patient has acceptable pain control level.

Plan: Formulate goals/outcomes and select appropriate nursing interventions for implementation to help achieve goals/outcomes.

Implementation: Nursing Interventions Aimed at Acute Pain (Not Limited to). Interventions Must Be Prioritized Based on the Patient's Assessment

- Provide pain relief measures before severe onset.
- Provide non-pharmacologic methods of pain.
- Administer analgesics nonopioids as ordered by the health care provider based on the order for type of pain.
- Administer opioids as ordered by the health care provider based on the order for the type of pain (be aware of the side effects and challenges/risks/benefits of using these types of medications with the geriatric patient).
- Perform nursing tasks during the peak effect of analgesics to prevent pain.

Implementation of the Nursing Care Plan for the Geriatric Patient Status Post-Acute Surgical Procedure

Geriatric patients have unique nursing care needs in addition to general postoperative nursing care when hospitalized for an acute surgical procedure. A NCP for a geriatric patient should consider the risks of hospitalization, individualized nursing needs, and general postoperative nursing care. Through the NCP, a patient-centered plan of care can be developed to facilitate a collaborative, effective, and synergistic team effort to improve patient outcomes.

References

1. American Nurses Association. The nursing process. n.d.. https://www.nursingworld.org/practice-policy/workforce/what-is-nursing/the-nursing-process/.
2. Bashaw M, Scott DN. Surgical risk factors in geriatric perioperative patients. AORN. 2012;96(1):58–74. https://doi.org/10.1016/j.aorn.2011.05.025.
3. Doenges M, Moorhouse MF, Murr AC. Nursing care plans for individualizing client care across the life span. 10th ed. Philadelphia: F.A. Davis Company; 2014.
4. Eliopoulos C. Fast facts for the gerontology nurse: a nursing care guide in a nutshell. New York: Springer; 2014.
5. Ladwig GB, Makic MB, Martinez-Kratz M. Nursing process, clinical reasoning, nursing diagnosis, and evidence-based nursing. In: Ackley BJ, Ladwig GB, Makic MB, Martinez-Kratz M, Zanotti M, editors. Nursing diagnosis handbook. Philadelphia: Elsevier; 2022.
6. Meiner SE. Gerontologic nursing. Maryland Heights: Mosby; 2015.
7. NANDA. Glossary of terms. 2022. https://nanda.org/publications-resources/resources/glossary-of-terms/.
8. Newfield SA, Hinz MD, Scott-Tilley D, Sridaromont KL, Maramba PJ. Cox's clinical applications of nursing diagnosis: adult, child, women's, mental health, gerontic, and home health considerations. Philadelphia: F.A. Davis Company; 2007.

9. Pérez-Ros P, Martínez-Arnau F. Delirium assessment in older people in emergency departments. A literature review. Disease. 2019;7(14):1–12. https://doi.org/10.3390/disease7010014.
10. Toney-Butler TJ, Thayer JM. Nursing process. Treasure Island: Stat Pearls; 2022.
11. Tullman DF, Blevins C, Fletcher K. Delirium, prevention, early recognition, and treatment. In: Boltz M, Capezuti E, Fulmer T, Zwicker D, editors. Evidence-based geriatric nursing protocols for best practice. 5th ed. New York: Springer; 2016. p. 251–2.

Nursing and Polypharmacy

60

Barbara M. Brathwaite

Introduction

As the population in the United States continues to age, there has been an increase in the number of older adults, those at least 65 years of age, with complex medical conditions and chronic illnesses. Many older adults have multiple chronic conditions (MCC), defined as two or more chronic illnesses, and include asthma, chronic obstructive pulmonary disease, cardiovascular disease, depression, anxiety, diabetes, and osteoarthritis, resulting in the need for multiple medications. Multiple medications may be appropriate for older adults with chronic conditions however, without proper oversight and guidance, polypharmacy, and/or the use of potentially inappropriate medicines (PIMs), may result in serious adverse outcomes and even mortality.

In the absence of a universal definition, polypharmacy is defined as the regular use of five or more medications which include those that are prescribed and nonprescribed, vitamins, herbal, or dietary supplements, and includes the presence of the risk of at least one serious drug interaction. Excessive polypharmacy is defined as the concurrent use of ten or more medications.

B. M. Brathwaite (✉)
Stony Brook University School of Nursing, Stony Brook, New York, USA
e-mail: barbara.brathwaite@stonybrook.edu

Polypharmacy is widespread among older adults and is associated with increased utilization of PIMs. Potentially inappropriate medications include medications that may be ineffective, or of minimal benefit, and medications that can potentially interfere with desired health outcomes and contribute to medication related harm. Polypharmacy is a serious health concern among older adults. While it is important to take vitamins and supplements especially with aging, it should be done under the guidance and supervision of a medical provider.

Statistics

Adults aged 65 years and older are inclined to take more medications than any other age group because of the occurrence of multiple coexisting chronic illnesses. Managing multiple medications, taken concurrently, can be particularly challenging, complicated, expensive, and difficult to track. Polypharmacy, particularly with respect to prescribed medications, creates a significant burden for patients and their families who need to understand the reasons for each medication, ensure they take the medication as prescribed, stop medications as ordered, obtain refills, and be alert for possible side effects. In addition, the use of multiple medications increases the risk for adverse reactions and serious drug interactions for which the patient's nurse must be made aware.

P. Petrone, C. E.M. Brathwaite (eds.), *Acute Care Surgery in Geriatric Patients*,
https://doi.org/10.1007/978-3-031-30651-8_60

According to a report by the Centers for Disease Control and Prevention in 2019, 83.6% of adults ages 60–79 used at least one, and 34.5% used five or more prescription medications. Use of one or more prescription medications was greater among women compared with men (72.4% compared with 65.2%). Use of five or more prescription drugs was similar between women and men (23.5% and 21.1%), respectively. As per a study in JAMA Internal Medicine, approximately 67% of older adults experience polypharmacy. In a nationwide, longitudinal study of 1.7 million older adults, almost half (44%) experienced polypharmacy, approximately one-sixth (12%) excessive polypharmacy, and one-fifth (20%) experienced polypharmacy for 1 year as noted at their follow-up appointment with their provider, which included 16.8% in those aged 65–74 years and 33.2% in those over 95 years. It is estimated that polypharmacy would result in 150,000 premature deaths and 4.6 million hospitalizations over the next 10 years.

As per the CDC's National Center for Health Statistics, the most commonly used medications among those aged 60–79 were dyslipidemia agents, 45%; hypoglycemic agents, 23.6%; beta blockers, 22.3%, antihypertensives (ACE inhibitors), 21.3%; and PPIs (proton pump inhibitors), 16.9%.

Older adults are disproportionately impacted by chronic disease. More than 85% of adults aged 65 years and over have at least one chronic illness, 60–70% have at least two, and almost one in four older adults have at least three chronic conditions. These include diabetes, cardiovascular disease, chronic obstructive pulmonary disease, asthma, cancer, and osteoarthritis.

Prevalence of Polypharmacy

Prevalence and reasons for polypharmacy vary from patient to patient and include the following: presence of multiple comorbidities; multiple providers and prescribers; personal health and cultural beliefs; insufficient health insurance and resources; inadequate medication reconciliation; and lack of deprescribing. Older adults are a vulnerable population, and therefore, at significant risk for drug related harm from inappropriate and unsafe prescribing. Drug related harm may include serious medication interactions and effects, inappropriate medication use, inadequate medical benefit, problems with medication adherence, unnecessary medication exposure, increased medication and health care costs, and the presence of side effects that can be misinterpreted as a new medical issue, leading to additional medications. For a full list of PIM use in older adults, see Table 60.1.

Nonprescription (Over the Counter) Medications, Vitamins, and Herbal Therapies

The use of nonprescription medications, vitamins, and herbal therapies is extensive. Half of patients do not classify these as "medications" and therefore, do not discuss their use with medical providers. Antihistamines, cough suppressants, laxatives, vitamins, and pain relievers (aspirin and nonsteroidal anti-inflammatory drugs) are among some of the most commonly used. There are risks and safety issues associated with these, as with prescription medications.

Adverse Outcomes

The presence of comorbid medical conditions, along with the effects of physiologic aging, frailty, and decreased physical function status, make older adults especially susceptible to harmful outcomes. Alterations in drug absorption, distribution, elimination, and hepatic and renal function may further contribute to adverse reactions and drug interactions.

The risk for adverse outcomes increases with the number of medications taken, and the more medications, the higher the risk. Statistics show there is a 10% increase per one medication, up to 50% increase with five to nine medications, and 100% increase with 20 or more medications. Patients taking more than four medications have a much greater risk of deleterious falls.

Table 60.1 2019 American Geriatrics Society Beers Criteria® for Potentially Inappropriate Medication Use in Older Adults[a]

Organ system, therapeutic category, drug(s)	Rationale	Recommendation	Quality of evidence	Strength of recommendation
Anticholinergics[b] First-generation antihistamines Brompheniramine Carbinoxamine Chlorpheniramine Clemastine Cyproheptadine Dexbrompheniramine Dexchlorpheniramine Dimenhydrinate Diphenhydramine (oral) Doxylamine Hydroxyzine Meclizine Promethazine Pyrilamine Triprolidine	Highly anticholinergic; clearance reduced with advanced age, and tolerance develops when used as hypnotic; risk of confusion, dry mouth, constipation, and other anticholinergic effects or toxicity use of diphenhydramine in situations such as acute treatment of severe allergic reaction may be appropriate	Avoid	Moderate	Strong
Antiparkinsonian agents Benztropine (oral) Trihexyphenidyl	Not recommended for prevention or treatment of extrapyramidal symptoms with antipsychotics; more effective agents available for treatment of Parkinson disease	Avoid	Moderate	Strong
Antispasmodics Atropine (excludes ophthalmic) Belladonna alkaloids Clidinium-chlordiazepoxide Dicyclomine Homatropine (excludes opthalmic) Hyoscyamine Methscopolamine Propantheline Scopolamine	Highly anticholinergic, uncertain effectiveness	Avoid	Moderate	Strong
Antithrombotics Dipyridamole, oral short acting (does not apply to the extended-release combination with aspirin)	May cause orthostatic hypotension; more effective alternatives available; IV form acceptable for use in cardiac stress testing	Avoid	Moderate	Strong
Anti-infective Nitrofurantoin	Potential for pulmonary toxicity, hepatoxicity, and peripheral neuropathy, especially with long-term use; safer alternatives available	Avoid in individuals with creatinine clearance <30 mL/min or for long-term suppression	Low	Strong

(continued)

Table 60.1 (continued)

Organ system, therapeutic category, drug(s)	Rationale	Recommendation	Quality of evidence	Strength of recommendation
Cardiovascular				
Peripheral alpha-1 blockers for Treatment of hypertension Doxazosin Prazosin Terazosin	High risk of orthostatic hypotension and associated harms, especially in older adults; not recommended as routine treatment for hypertension; alternative agents have superior risk/benefit profile	Avoid use as an antihypertensive	Moderate	Strong
Central alpha-agonists		Avoid as first-line antihypertensive	Low	Strong
Clonidine for first-line treatment of Hypertension Other CNS alpha-agonists Guanabenz Guanfacine Methyldopa Reserpine (>0.1 mg/day)	High risk of adverse CNS effects; may cause bradycardia and orthostatic hypotension; not recommended as routine treatment for hypertension	Avoid other CNS alpha-agonists as listed	Low	Strong
Disopyramide	May induce heart failure in older adults because of potent negative inotropic action; strongly anticholinergic; other antiarrhythmic drugs preferred	Avoid	Low	Strong
Dronedarone	Worse outcomes have been reported in patients taking dronedarone who have permanent atrial fibrillation or severe or recently decompensated heart failure	Avoid in individuals with permanent atrial fibrillation or severe or recently decompensated heart failure	High	Strong

Table 60.1 (continued)

Organ system, therapeutic category, drug(s)	Rationale	Recommendation	Quality of evidence	Strength of recommendation
Digoxin for first-line treatment of atrial fibrillation or of heart failure	Use in atrial fibrillation: Should not be used as a first-line agent in atrial fibrillation, because there are safer and more effective alternatives for rate control supported by high-quality evidence. Use in heart failure: Evidence for benefits and harms of digoxin is conflicting and of lower quality; most but not all of the evidence concerns use in HFrEF. There is strong evidence for other agents as first-line therapy to reduce hospitalizations and mortality in adults with HFrEF. In heart failure, higher dosages are not associated with additional benefit and may increase risk of toxicity. Decreased renal clearance of digoxin may lead to increased risk of toxic effects; further dose reduction may be necessary in those with stage 4 or 5 chronic kidney disease	Avoid this rate control agent as first-line therapy for atrial fibrillation Avoid as first-line therapy for heart failure If used for atrial fibrillation or heart failure, avoid dosages >0.125 mg/day	Atrial fibrillation: Low Heart failure: Low Dosage >0.125 mg/day: Moderate	Atrial fibrillation: Strong Heart failure: Strong Dosage >0.125 mg/day: Strong
Nifedipine, immediate release	Potential for hypotension; risk of precipitating myocardial ischemia	Avoid	High	Strong
Amiodarone	Effective for maintaining sinus rhythm but has greater toxicities than other antiarrhythmics used in atrial fibrillation; may be reasonable first-line therapy in patients with concomitant heart failure or substantial left ventricular hypertrophy if rhythm control is preferred over rate control	Avoid as first-line therapy for atrial fibrillation unless patient has heart failure or substantial left ventricular hypertrophy	High	Strong

(continued)

Table 60.1 (continued)

Organ system, therapeutic category, drug(s)	Rationale	Recommendation	Quality of evidence	Strength of recommendation
Central nervous system antidepressants, alone or in combination Amitriptyline Amoxapine Clomipramine Desipramine Doxepin >6 mg/day Imipramine Nortriptyline Paroxetine Protriptyline Trimipramine	Highly anticholinergic, sedating, and cause orthostatic hypotension; safety profile of low-dose doxepin (≤6 mg/day) comparable to that of placebo	Avoid	High	Strong
Antipsychotics, first (conventional) and second (atypical) generation	Increased risk of cerebrovascular accident (stroke) and greater rate of cognitive decline and mortality in persons with dementia. Avoid antipsychotics for behavioral problems of dementia or delirium unless nonpharmacological options (e.g., behavioral interventions) have failed or are not possible and the older adult is threatening substantial harm to self or others	Avoid, except in schizophrenia or bipolar disorder, or for short-term use as antiemetic during chemotherapy	Moderate	Strong
Barbiturates Amobarbital Butabarbital Butalbital Mephobarbital Pentobarbital Phenobarbital Secobarbital	High rate of physical dependence, tolerance to sleep benefits, greater risk of overdose at low dosages	Avoid	High	Strong

Table 60.1 (continued)

Organ system, therapeutic category, drug(s)	Rationale	Recommendation	Quality of evidence	Strength of recommendation
Benzodiazepines Short and intermediate acting: Alprazolam Estazolam Lorazepam Oxazepam Temazepam Triazolam Long acting: Chlordiazepoxide (alone or in combination with amitriptyline or clidinium) Clonazepam Clorazepate Diazepam Flurazepam Quazepam	Older adults have increased sensitivity to benzodiazepines and decreased metabolism of long-acting agents; in general, all benzodiazepines increase risk of cognitive impairment, delirium, falls, fractures, and motor vehicle crashes in older adults may be appropriate for seizure disorders, rapid eye movement sleep behavior disorder, benzodiazepine withdrawal, ethanol withdrawal, severe generalized anxiety disorder, and periprocedural anesthesia	Avoid	Moderate	Strong
Meprobamate	High rate of physical dependence; sedating	Avoid	Moderate	Strong
Nonbenzodiazepine, benzodiazepine receptor agonist hypnotics (i.e., "Z-drugs") Eszopiclone Zaleplon Zolpidem	Nonbenzodiazepine benzodiazepine receptor agonist hypnotics (i.e., Z drugs) have adverse events similar to those of benzodiazepines in older adults (e.g., delirium, falls, fractures); increased emergency room visits/ hospitalizations; motor vehicle crashes; minimal improvement in sleep latency and duration	Avoid	Moderate	Strong
Ergoloid mesylates (dehydrogenated ergot alkaloids) Isoxsuprine	Lack of efficacy	Avoid	High	Strong
Endocrine				
Androgens Methyltestosterone Testosterone	Potential for cardiac problems; contraindicated in men with prostate cancer	Avoid unless indicated for confirmed hypogonadism with clinical symptoms	Moderate	Weak
Desiccated thyroid	Concerns about cardiac effects; safer alternatives available	Avoid	Low	Strong

(continued)

Table 60.1 (continued)

Organ system, therapeutic category, drug(s)	Rationale	Recommendation	Quality of evidence	Strength of recommendation
Estrogens with or without progestins	Evidence of carcinogenic potential (breast and endometrium); lack of cardioprotective effect and cognitive protection in older women. Evidence indicates that vaginal estrogens for the treatment of vaginal dryness are safe and effective; women with a history of breast cancer who do not respond to nonhormonal therapies are advised to discuss the risks and benefits of low-dose vaginal estrogen (dosages of estradiol <25 μg twice weekly) with their healthcare provider	Avoid systemic estrogen (e.g., oral and topical patch) Vaginal cream or vaginal tablets: Acceptable to use low-dose intravaginal estrogen for management of dyspareunia, recurrent lower urinary tract infections, and other vaginal symptoms	Oral and patch: High Vaginal cream or vaginal tablets: Moderate	Oral and patch: Strong Topical vaginal cream or tablets: Weak
Growth hormone	Impact on body composition is small and associated with edema, arthralgia, carpal tunnel syndrome, gynecomastia, impaired fasting glucose	Avoid, except for patients rigorously diagnosed by evidence-based criteria with growth hormone deficiency due to an established etiology	High	Strong
Insulin, sliding scale (insulin regimens containing only short- or rapid-acting insulin dosed according to current blood glucose levels without concurrent use of basal or long acting insulin)	Higher risk of hypoglycemia without improvement in hyperglycemia management regardless of care setting. Avoid insulin regimens that include only short- or rapid-acting insulin dosed according to current blood glucose levels without concurrent use of basal or long-acting insulin. This recommendation does not apply to regimens that contain basal insulin or long-acting insulin	Avoid	Moderate	Strong
Megestrol	Minimal effect on weight; increases risk of thrombotic events and possibly death in older adults	Avoid	Moderate	Strong

Table 60.1 (continued)

Organ system, therapeutic category, drug(s)	Rationale	Recommendation	Quality of evidence	Strength of recommendation
Sulfonylureas, long acting Chlorpropamide Glimepiride Glyburide (also known as glibenclamide)	Chlorpropamide: Prolonged half-life in older adults; can cause prolonged hypoglycemia; causes SIADH glimepiride and glyburide: Higher risk of severe prolonged hypoglycemia in older adults	Avoid	High	Strong
Gastrointestinal				
Metoclopramide	Can cause extrapyramidal effects, including tardive dyskinesia; risk may be greater in frail older adults and with prolonged exposure	Avoid, unless for gastroparesis with duration of use not to exceed 12 weeks except in rare cases	Moderate	Strong
Mineral oil, given orally	Potential for aspiration and adverse effects; safer alternatives available	Avoid	Moderate	Strong
Proton pump inhibitors	Risk of Clostridium difficile infection and bone loss and fractures	Avoid scheduled use for >8 weeks unless for high-risk patients (e.g., oral corticosteroids or chronic NSAID use), erosive esophagitis, Barrett esophagitis, pathological hypersecretory condition, or demonstrated need for maintenance treatment (e.g., because of failure of drug discontinuation trial or H2-receptor antagonists)	High	Strong
Pain medications				
Meperidine	Oral analgesic not effective in dosages commonly used; may have higher risk of neurotoxicity, including delirium, than other opioids; safer alternatives available	Avoid	Moderate	Strong

(continued)

Table 60.1 (continued)

Organ system, therapeutic category, drug(s)	Rationale	Recommendation	Quality of evidence	Strength of recommendation
Non-cyclooxygenase-selective NSAIDs, oral: Aspirin >325 mg/day Diclofenac Diflunisal Etodolac Fenoprofen Ibuprofen Ketoprofen Meclofenamate Mefenamic acid Meloxicam Nabumetone Naproxen Oxaprozin Piroxicam Sulindac Tolmetin	Increased risk of gastrointestinal bleeding or peptic ulcer disease in high-risk groups, including those >75 years or taking oral or parenteral corticosteroids, anticoagulants, or antiplatelet agents; use of proton pump inhibitor or misoprostol reduces but does not eliminate risk. Upper gastrointestinal ulcers, gross bleeding, or perforation caused by NSAIDs occur in ~1% of patients treated for 3–6 months and in ~2–4% of patients treated for 1 year; these trends continue with longer duration of use. Also, can increase blood pressure and induce kidney injury. Risks are dose related	Avoid chronic use, unless other alternatives are not effective, and patient can take gastroprotective agent (proton pump inhibitor or misoprostol)	Moderate	Strong
Indomethacin Ketorolac, includes parenteral	Increased risk of gastrointestinal bleeding/ peptic ulcer disease and acute kidney injury in older adults indomethacin is more likely than other NSAIDs to have adverse CNS effects. Of all the NSAIDs, indomethacin has the most adverse effects	Avoid	Moderate	Strong
Skeletal muscle relaxants Carisoprodol Chlorzoxazone Cyclobenzaprine Metaxalone Methocarbamol Orphenadrine	Most muscle relaxants poorly tolerated by older adults because some have anticholinergic adverse effects, sedation, increased risk of fractures; effectiveness at dosages tolerated by older adults questionable	Avoid	Moderate	Strong

Table 60.1 (continued)

Organ system, therapeutic category, drug(s)	Rationale	Recommendation	Quality of evidence	Strength of recommendation
Genitourinary				
Desmopressin	High risk of hyponatremia; safer alternative treatments	Avoid for treatment of nocturia or nocturnal polyuria	Moderate	Strong

CNS central nervous system, *HFrEF* heart failure with reduced ejection fraction, *NSAID* nonsteroidal anti-inflammatory drug, *SIADH* syndrome of inappropriate antidiuretic hormone secretion

[a]The primary target audience is the practicing clinician. The intentions of the criteria include (1) improving the selection of prescription drugs by clinicians and patients; (2) evaluating patterns of drug use within populations; (3) educating clinicians and patients on proper drug usage; and (4) evaluating health outcome, quality of care, cost, and utilization data

[b]See also criterion on highly anticholinergic antidepressants

The 2019 American Geriatrics Society Beers Criteria® Update Expert Panel. The 2019 American Geriatrics Society Beers Criteria® for potentially inappropriate medication use in older adults. J Am Geriatr Soc. 2019:67(4)674–694. doi.org/10.1111/jgs.15767

Furthermore, the type of medication has been shown to significantly influence the fall risk.

Non-adherence can result when patients are prescribed multiple medications. Negative experiences and financial burdens can impact health beliefs and health behaviors and result in non-adherence and poor health outcomes.

While it may be clinically appropriate and medically necessary, and not specifically a sign of improper treatment, the use of multiple medications in the older patient is related to a rise in morbidity, mortality, harmful drug incidents and interactions, decreased quality of life, delirium, disability, falls and accidents, impaired mobility issues, fractures, orthostatic hypotension, pneumonia, malnutrition, diminished functional capacity and functional decline, renal failure, gastrointestinal and intracranial bleeding, increased hospital length of stay, increased rates of readmissions, long-term care placement, and increased use of the health care system including urgent care visits, emergency department visits, and hospitalizations. Adverse reactions are often unrecognized in patients with complicated histories because of competing comorbidities and poor awareness and communication among medical providers. Medications commonly associated with adverse outcomes or adverse drug effects include diuretics, antidepressants, central nervous system agents, antibiotics, cardiovascular drugs (antihypertensives), anticoagulants, hypoglycemics, steroids, opioids, anticholinergics, and nonsteroidal anti-inflammatory drugs (NSAIDS).

Adverse Drug Event/Adverse Drug Reactions

An adverse drug event (ADE) refers to an injury or harm experienced by a patient as a result of the appropriate or inappropriate use of a drug and includes adverse drug reactions, overdoses, and impairment from the use of the drug including dose alterations and dose discontinuations. An adverse drug reaction (ADR) is a response to a drug which is unpleasant and unintended and caused by use of a drug at regular dosages during normal use. It is estimated that ADEs are responsible for up to one-fourth of all acute geriatric admissions. Adverse drug events are avoidable, are one of the most dangerous consequences of polypharmacy, and are higher in the geriatric patient due to age-related changes. Risk factors for ADEs include polypharmacy, multiple comorbidities, prior adverse medication reactions, cognitive impairment, and dementia. For a list of PIMs in older adults due to drug–disease or drug–syndrome interactions that may exacerbate the disease or syndrome, see Table 60.2. For a list of PIMs that should be used with caution in older adults, see Table 60.3.

Table 60.2 2019 American Geriatrics Society Beers Criteria® for potentially inappropriate medication in older adults due to drug–disease or drug–syndrome interactions that may exacerbate the disease or syndrome[a]

Disease or syndrome	Drug(s)	Rationale	Recommendation	Quality of evidence	Strength of recommendation
Cardiovascular					
Heart failure	Avoid: Cilostazol Avoid in heart failure with reduced ejection fraction: Nondihydropyridine CCBs (diltiazem, verapamil) Use with caution in patients with heart failure who are asymptomatic; avoid in patients with symptomatic heart failure: NSAIDs and COX-2 inhibitors thiazolidinediones, (pioglitazone, rosiglitazone) dronedarone	Potential to promote fluid retention and/or exacerbate heart failure (NSAIDs and COX-2 inhibitors, nondihydropyridine CCBs, thiazolidinediones); potential to increase mortality in older adults with heart failure (cilostazol and dronedarone)	As noted, avoid, or use with caution	Cilostazol: Low Nondihydropyridine CCBs: Moderate NSAIDs: Moderate COX-2 inhibitors: Low Thiazolidinediones: High Dronedarone: High	Cilostazol: Strong Nondihydropyridine CCBs: Strong NSAIDs: Strong COX-2 inhibitors: Strong Thiazolidinediones: Strong Dronedarone: Strong
Syncope	AChEIs Nonselective peripheral alpha-1 blockers (i.e., doxazosin, prazosin, terazosin) Tertiary TCAs Antipsychotics: Chlorpromazine Thioridazine Olanzapine	AChEIs cause bradycardia and should be avoided in older adults whose syncope may be due to bradycardia. Nonselective peripheral alpha-1 blockers cause orthostatic blood pressure changes and should be avoided in older adults whose syncope may be due to orthostatic hypotension. Tertiary TCAs and the antipsychotics listed increase the risk of orthostatic hypotension or bradycardia	Avoid	AChEIs, TCAs, and antipsychotics: High Nonselective peripheral alpha-1 blockers: High	AChEIs and TCAs: Strong Nonselective peripheral alpha-1 blockers and antipsychotics: Weak

Central nervous system					
Delirium	Anticholinergics (see table 7 and full criteria available on www. geriatricscareonline. org.) Antipsychotics[b] Benzodiazepines corticosteroids (oral and parenteral)[c] H2-receptor antagonists Cimetidine Famotidine Nizatidine Ranitidine Meperidine Nonbenzodiazepine, benzodiazepine Receptor agonist hypnotics: Eszopiclone, zaleplon, zolpidem	Avoid in older adults with or at high risk of delirium because of potential of inducing or worsening delirium Avoid antipsychotics for behavioral problems of dementia and/or delirium unless nonpharmacological options (e.g., behavioral interventions) have failed or are not possible and the older adult is threatening substantial harm to self or others. Antipsychotics are associated with greater risk of cerebrovascular accident (stroke) and mortality in persons with dementia	Avoid	H2-receptor antagonists: Low All others: Moderate	Strong
Dementia or cognitive impairment	Anticholinergics (see table 7 and full criteria available on www. geriatricscareonline. org) Benzodiazepines Nonbenzodiazepine, benzodiazepine receptor agonist hypnotics Eszopiclone Zaleplon Zolpidem Antipsychotics, chronic and as needed use[b]	Avoid because of adverse CNS effects Avoid antipsychotics for behavioral problems of dementia and/or delirium unless nonpharmacological options (e.g., behavioral interventions) have failed or are not possible and the older adult is threatening substantial harm to self or others. Antipsychotics are associated with greater risk of cerebrovascular accident (stroke) and mortality in persons with dementia	Avoid	Moderate	Strong

(continued)

Table 60.2 (continued)

Disease or syndrome	Drug(s)	Rationale	Recommendation	Quality of evidence	Strength of recommendation
History of falls or fractures	Antiepileptics Antipsychotics[b] benzodiazepines nonbenzodiazepine, benzodiazepine receptor agonist hypnotics Eszopiclone Zaleplon Zolpidem Antidepressants TCAs SSRIs SNRIs Opioids	May cause ataxia, impaired psychomotor function, syncope, additional falls; shorter-acting benzodiazepines are not safer than long-acting ones. If one of the drugs must be used, consider reducing use of other CNS-active medications that increase risk of falls and fractures (i.e., antiepileptics, opioid-receptor agonists, antipsychotics, antidepressants, nonbenzodiazepine and benzodiazepine receptor agonist hypnotics, other sedatives/hypnotics) and implement other strategies to reduce fall risk. Data for antidepressants are mixed but no compelling evidence that certain antidepressants confer less fall risk than others	Avoid unless safer alternatives are not available; avoid antiepileptics except for seizure and mood disorders Opioids: Avoid except for pain management in the setting of severe acute pain (e.g., recent fractures or joint replacement)	Opioids: Moderate All others: High	Strong
Parkinson disease	Antiemetics Metoclopramide Prochlorperazine Promethazine All antipsychotics (except quetiapine, clozapine, pimavanserin)	Dopamine-receptor antagonists with potential to worsen parkinsonian symptoms Exceptions: Pimavanserin and clozapine appear to be less likely to precipitate worsening of Parkinson disease. Quetiapine has only been studied in low-quality clinical trials with efficacy comparable to that of placebo in five trials and to that of clozapine in two others	Avoid	Moderate	Strong

Gastrointestinal					
History of gastric or duodenal ulcers	Aspirin >325 mg/day non–COX-2–selective NSAIDs	May exacerbate existing ulcers or cause new/additional ulcers	Avoid unless other alternatives are not effective, and patient can take gastroprotective agent (i.e., proton pump inhibitor or misoprostol)	Moderate	Strong
Kidney/urinary tract					
Chronic kidney disease stage 4 or higher (creatinine clearance <30 mL/min)	NSAIDs (non-COX and COX selective, oral and parenteral, nonacetylated salicylates)	May increase risk of acute kidney injury and further decline of renal function	Avoid	Moderate	Strong
Urinary incontinence (all types) in women	Estrogen oral and transdermal (excludes intravaginal estrogen) Peripheral alpha-1 blockers Doxazosin Prazosin Terazosin	Lack of efficacy (oral estrogen) and aggravation of incontinence (alpha-1 blockers)	Avoid in women	Estrogen: High Peripheral alpha-1 blockers: Moderate	Estrogen: Strong Peripheral alpha-1 blockers: Strong

(continued)

Table 60.2 (continued)

Disease or syndrome	Drug(s)	Rationale	Recommendation	Quality of evidence	Strength of recommendation
Lower urinary tract symptoms, benign prostatic hyperplasia	Strongly anticholinergic drugs, except antimuscarinics for urinary incontinence (see Table 7 and full criteria available on www.geriatricscareonline.org)	May decrease urinary flow and cause urinary retention	Avoid in men	Moderate	Strong

AChEI acetylcholinesterase inhibitor, *CCB* calcium channel blocker, *CNS* central nervous system, *COX* cyclooxygenase, *NSAID* nonsteroidal anti-inflammatory drug, *SNRI* serotonin norepinephrine reuptake inhibitor, *SSRI* selective serotonin reuptake inhibitor, *TCA* tricyclic antidepressant

[a] The primary target audience is the practicing clinician. The intentions of the criteria include (1) improving the selection of prescription drugs by clinicians and patients; (2) evaluating patterns of drug use within populations; (3) educating clinicians and patients on proper drug usage; and (4) evaluating health outcome, quality of care, cost, and utilization data

[b] May be required to treat concurrent schizophrenia, bipolar disorder, and other selected mental health conditions but should be prescribed in the lowest effective dose and shortest possible duration

[c] Excludes inhaled and topical forms. Oral and parenteral corticosteroids may be required for conditions such as exacerbation of chronic obstructive pulmonary disease but should be prescribed in the lowest effective dose and for the shortest possible duration

The 2019 American Geriatrics Society Beers Criteria® Update Expert Panel. The 2019 American Geriatrics Society Beers Criteria® for potentially inappropriate medication use in older adults. J Am Geriatr Soc. 2019:67(4)674–694. doi.org/10.1111/jgs.15767

ble 60.3 2019 American Geriatrics Society Beers Criteria® for Potentially inappropriate medications: drugs to be d with caution in older adults[a]

rug(s)	Rationale	Recommendation	Quality of evidence	Strength of recommendation
spirin for primary evention of rdiovascular disease d colorectal cancer	Risk of major bleeding from aspirin increases markedly in older age. Several studies suggest lack of net benefit when used for primary prevention in older adult with cardiovascular risk factors, but evidence is not conclusive. Aspirin is generally indicated for secondary prevention in older adults with established cardiovascular disease	Use with caution in adults ≥70 years	Moderate	Strong
Dabigatran Rivaroxaban	Increased risk of gastrointestinal bleeding compared with warfarin and reported rates with other direct oral anticoagulants when used for long-term treatment of VTE or atrial fibrillation in adults ≥75 years	Use with caution for treatment of VTE or atrial fibrillation in adults ≥75 years	Moderate	Strong
Prasugrel	Increased risk of bleeding in older adults; benefit in highest-risk older adults (e.g., those with prior myocardial infarction or diabetes mellitus) may offset risk when used for its approved indication of acute coronary syndrome to be managed with percutaneous coronary intervention	Use with caution in adults ≥75 years	Moderate	Weak
Antipsychotics Carbamazepine Diuretics Mirtazapine Oxcarbazepine SNRIs SSRIs TCAs Tramadol	May exacerbate or cause SIADH or hyponatremia; monitor sodium level closely when starting or changing dosages in older adults	Use with caution	Moderate	Strong
Dextromethorphan/ quinidine	Limited efficacy in patients with behavioral symptoms of dementia (does not apply to treatment of PBA). May increase risk of falls and concerns with clinically significant drug interactions. Does not apply to treatment of pseudobulbar affect	Use with caution	Moderate	Strong

(continued)

Table 60.3 (continued)

Drug(s)	Rationale	Recommendation	Quality of evidence	Strength of recommendatio
Trimethoprim-sulfamethoxazole	Increased risk of hyperkalemia when used concurrently with an ACEI or ARB in presence of decreased creatinine clearance	Use with caution in patients on ACEI or ARB and decreased creatinine clearance	Low	Strong

ACEI angiotensin-converting enzyme inhibitor, *ARB* angiotensin receptor blocker, *PBA* pseudobulbar affect, *SIAD* syndrome of inappropriate antidiuretic hormone secretion, *SNRI* serotonin norepinephrine reuptake inhibitor, *SSI* selective serotonin reuptake inhibitor, *TCA* tricyclic antidepressant, *VTE* venous thromboembolism

[a]The primary target audience is the practicing clinician. The intentions of the criteria include (1) improving the selectio of prescription drugs by clinicians and patients; (2) evaluating patterns of drug use within populations; (3) educatin clinicians and patients on proper drug usage; and (4) evaluating health outcome, quality of care, cost, and utilizatio data

The 2019 American Geriatrics Society Beers Criteria® Update Expert Panel. The 2019 American Geriatrics Societ Beers Criteria® for potentially inappropriate medication use in older adults. J Am Geriatr Soc. 2019:67(4)674–694. doi org/10.1111/jgs.15767

Reproduced with Permission

Drug–Drug Interactions

The use of multiple medications increases the chances for potential drug–drug interactions, and the more medications taken, the greater the risk. A drug–drug interaction is the pharmacologic or clinical response to a drug combination that differs from the known effects of each of the two drugs individually. Drug interactions may lead to an increase or decrease in the adverse or beneficial effects of the drugs. Antimicrobial and cardiovascular drugs are most commonly involved in drug–drug interactions. The most common adverse events are delirium, heart and acute renal failure, and orthostatic hypotension. Table 60.4 contains potentially clinically important drug–drug interactions to be avoided in older adults. For a list of medications that should be avoided or have their dosage reduced based on renal function, see Table 60.5.

Medical Interventions

In order to decrease harmful adverse reactions and reduce the impact on multiple organ systems, healthcare prescribers should frequently monitor and evaluate their patient's medications and deprescribe whenever possible. Minimizing the number of prescribed medications, limiting the number of medication changes, adjusting medications down to the minimum effective dosage, simplifying the dosing plan, or stopping them when a patient's health status changes, in addition to being aware of prescribing guidelines and potentially inappropriate medications, are vital.

Deprescribing

While polypharmacy is associated with risks to health, wellness, and well-being, prescribers should be careful, and should not arbitrarily reduce the number of multiple medications in older adults. Endeavors must essentially focus on deprescribing. Researchers are studying guidelines for deprescribing, with the goal to decrease or stop medications that may no longer be effective or may be causing harm. Deprescribing would occur at an individual level and would result in safer alternatives which would reduce the risk, improve outcomes, and would make the management of prescriptions less of a burden for patients and their families.

Resource to Assist Prescribers

There is no single resource that has been shown to be exceptional in improving patient health outcomes and decreasing polypharmacy risks. However, the following tools are used to assist in

Table 60.4 2019 American Geriatrics Society Beers Criteria® for potentially clinically important drug-drug interactions that shoul

Object drug and class	Interacting drug and class	Risk rationale	Recommendation	Quality of evidence	Strength of recommendation
RAS inhibitor (ACEIs, ARBs, aliskiren) or potassium-sparing diuretics (amiloride, triamterene)	Another RAS inhibitor (ACEIs, ARBs, aliskiren)	Increased risk of hyperkalemia	Avoid routine use in those with chronic kidney disease stage 3a or higher	Moderate	Strong
Opioids	Benzodiazepines	Increased risk of overdose	Avoid	Moderate	Strong
Opioids	Gabapentin, pregabalin	Increased risk of severe sedation-related adverse events, including respiratory depression and death	Avoid; exceptions are when transitioning from opioid therapy to gabapentin or pregabalin, or when using gabapentinoids to reduce opioid dose, although caution should be used in all circumstances	Moderate	Strong
Anticholinergic	Anticholinergic	Increased risk of cognitive decline	Avoid; minimize number of anticholinergic drugs (see Table 7 available on www.geriatricscareonline.org)	Moderate	Strong
Antidepressants (TCAs, SSRIs, and SNRIs) antipsychotics Antiepileptics benzodiazepines and nonbenzodiazepine, benzodiazepine receptor agonist hypnotics (i.e., "Z-drugs") Opioids	Any combination of three or more of these CNS-active drugs[a]	Increased risk of falls (all) and of fracture (benzodiazepines and nonbenzodiazepine, benzodiazepine receptor agonist hypnotics)	Avoid total of three or more CNS-active drugs[a]; minimize number of CNS-active drugs	Combinations including benzodiazepines and nonbenzodiazepine, benzodiazepine receptor agonist hypnotics or opioids: High All other combinations: Moderate	Strong
Corticosteroids, oral or parenteral	NSAIDs	Increased risk of peptic ulcer disease or gastrointestinal bleeding	Avoid; if not possible, provide gastrointestinal protection	Moderate	Strong
Lithium	ACEIs	Increased risk of lithium toxicity	Avoid; monitor lithium concentrations	Moderate	Strong
Lithium	Loop diuretics	Increased risk of lithium toxicity	Avoid; monitor lithium concentrations	Moderate	Strong
Peripheral α-1 blockers	Loop diuretics	Increased risk of urinary incontinence in older women	Avoid in older women, unless conditions warrant both drugs	Moderate	Strong

(continued)

Table 60.4 (continued)

Object drug and class	Interacting drug and class	Risk rationale	Recommendation	Quality of evidence	Strength of recommendation
Phenytoin	Trimethoprim-sulfamethoxazole	Increased risk of phenytoin toxicity	Avoid	Moderate	Strong
Theophylline	Cimetidine	Increased risk of theophylline toxicity	Avoid	Moderate	Strong
Theophylline	Ciprofloxacin	Increased risk of theophylline toxicity	Avoid	Moderate	Strong
Warfarin	Amiodarone	Increased risk of bleeding	Avoid when possible; if used together, monitor INR closely	Moderate	Strong
Warfarin	Ciprofloxacin	Increased risk of bleeding	Avoid when possible; if used together, monitor INR closely	Moderate	Strong
Warfarin	Macrolides (excluding azithromycin)	Increased risk of bleeding	Avoid when possible; if used together, monitor INR closely	Moderate	Strong
Warfarin	Trimethoprim-sulfamethoxazole	Increased risk of bleeding	Avoid when possible; if used together, monitor INR closely	Moderate	Strong
Warfarin	NSAIDs	Increased risk of bleeding	Avoid when possible; if used together, monitor closely for bleeding	High	Strong

ACEI angiotensin-converting enzyme inhibitor, *ARB* angiotensin receptor blocker, *CNS* central nervous system, *INR* international normalized ratio, *NSAID* nonsteroidal anti-inflammatory drug, *RAS* renin-angiotensin system, *SNRI* serotonin norepinephrine reuptake inhibitor, *SSRI* selective serotonin reuptake inhibitor, *TCA* tricyclic antidepressant
[a]CNS-active drugs: antiepileptics; antipsychotics; benzodiazepines; nonbenzodiazepine, benzodiazepine receptor agonist hypnotics; TCAs; SSRIs; SNRIs; and opioids
The 2019 American Geriatrics Society Beers Criteria® Update Expert Panel. The 2019 American Geriatrics Society Beers Criteria® for potentially inappropriate medication use in older adults. J Am Geriatr Soc. 2019:67(4)674–694. doi.org/10.1111/jgs.15767

le 60.5 2019 American Geriatrics Society Beers Criteria® for medications that should be avoided or have their age reduced with varying levels of kidney function in older adults

edication class d medication	Creatinine clearance at which action required, mL/min	Rationale	Recommendation	Quality of evidence	Strength of recommendation
nti-infective					
iprofloxacin	<30	Increased risk of CNS effects (e.g., seizures, confusion) and tendon rupture	Doses used to treat common infections typically require reduction when CrCl <30 mL/min	Moderate	Strong
rimethoprim-ulfamethoxazole	<30	Increased risk of worsening of renal function and hyperkalemia	Reduce dose if CrCl 15–29 mL/min avoid if CrCl <15 mL/min	Moderate	Strong
Cardiovascular or hemostasis					
Amiloride	<30	Increased potassium and decreased sodium	Avoid	Moderate	Strong
Apixaban	<25	Lack of evidence for efficacy and safety in patients with a CrCl <25 mL/min	Avoid	Moderate	Strong
Dabigatran	<30	Lack of evidence for efficacy and safety in individuals with a CrCl <30 mL/min. Label dose for patients with a CrCl 15–30 mL/min based on pharmacokinetic data	Avoid; dose adjustment advised when CrCl >30 mL/min in the presence of drug-drug interactions	Moderate	Strong
Dofetilide	<60	QTc prolongation and torsade de pointes	Reduce dose if CrCl 20–59 mL/min avoid if CrCl <20 mL/min	Moderate	Strong
Edoxaban	15–50 < 15 or > 95	Lack of evidence of efficacy or safety in patients with a CrCl <30 mL/min	Reduce dose if CrCl 15–50 mL/min avoid if CrCl <15 or > 95 mL/min	Moderate	Strong
Enoxaparin	<30	Increased risk of bleeding	Reduce dose	Moderate	Strong
Fondaparinux	<30	Increased risk of bleeding	Avoid	Moderate	Strong
Rivaroxaban	<50	Lack of efficacy or safety evidence in patients with a CrCl <30 mL/min	Nonvalvular atrial fibrillation: Reduce dose if CrCl 15–50 mL/min; avoid if CrCl <15 mL/min venous thromboembolism treatment and for VTE prophylaxis with hip or knee replacement: Avoid if CrCl <30 mL/min	Moderate	Strong

(continued)

Table 60.5 (continued)

Medication class and medication	Creatinine clearance at which action required, mL/min	Rationale	Recommendation	Quality of evidence	Strength of recommendatio
Spironolactone	<30	Increased potassium	Avoid	Moderate	Strong
Triamterene	<30	Increased potassium and decreased sodium	Avoid	Moderate	Strong
Central nervous system and analgesics					
Duloxetine	<30	Increased gastrointestinal adverse effects (nausea, diarrhea)	Avoid	Moderate	Weak
Gabapentin	<60	CNS adverse effects	Reduce dose	Moderate	Strong
Levetiracetam	≤80	CNS adverse effects	Reduce dose	Moderate	Strong
Pregabalin	<60	CNS adverse effects	Reduce dose	Moderate	Strong
Tramadol	<30	CNS adverse effects	Immediate release: Reduce dose Extended release: Avoid	Low	Weak
Gastrointestinal					
Cimetidine	<50	Mental status changes	Reduce dose	Moderate	Strong
Famotidine	<50	Mental status changes	Reduce dose	Moderate	Strong
Nizatidine	<50	Mental status changes	Reduce dose	Moderate	Strong
Ranitidine	<50	Mental status changes	Reduce dose	Moderate	Strong
Hyperuricemia					
Colchicine	<30	Gastrointestinal, neuromuscular, bone marrow toxicity	Reduce dose; monitor for adverse effects	Moderate	Strong
Probenecid	<30	Loss of effectiveness	Avoid	Moderate	Strong

CNS central nervous system, *CrCl* creatinine clearance, *QTc* corrected QT interval, *VTE* venous thromboembolism
The 2019 American Geriatrics Society Beers Criteria® Update Expert Panel. The 2019 American Geriatrics Society Beers Criteria® for potentially inappropriate medication use in older adults. J Am Geriatr Soc. 2019:67(4)674–694. doi.org/10.1111/jgs.15767
Reproduced with Permission

identifying potentially inappropriate medication use: the American Geriatrics Society (AGS) called the AGS Beers Criteria® for Potentially Inappropriate Medication Use in Older Adults, STOPP (Screening Tool of Older People's Prescriptions), and START criteria, and the Medication Appropriateness Index. Choosing the best treatments to improve inappropriate polypharmacy and achieve better outcomes is necessary, and this field is growing. Such recommendations assist providers to consider deprescribing and can reassure that deprescribing medications is based on sound medical evidence.

American Geriatrics Society

Medical providers employ guidelines in order to prescribe medications safely to older adults. These updated guidelines from the American Geriatrics Society and called the AGS 2019 Updated Beers Criteria® is designed to decrease the problems associated with medication by developing the criteria to improve medication choice; educate providers and patients; decrease adverse drug events; and serve as a means for evaluating quality of care, cost, and drug use of older adults. The criteria consist of particular medications, and over-the-counter medications, based on evidence, that one should avoid or use with caution. For a full list of PIM use in older adults, see Table 60.1. Potentially inappropriate medications that may exacerbate the disease or syndrome in older adults due to drug–disease or drug–syndrome interactions, are listed in Table 60.2. For a list of PIMs that should be used with caution in older adults, see Table 60.3. Table 60.4 contains potentially clinically important drug–drug interactions to be avoided in older adults. For a list of medications that should be avoided or have their dosage reduced based on renal function, see Table 60.5.

Nursing Interventions/Implications

The nurse is often the first to evaluate the patient whether during the hospital stay, other inpatient facility, or the outpatient arena. Avoidance of patient harm and enhanced patient experience begin with this encounter.

Health History

The nurse should obtain a thorough health history including past and present medical history, previous surgical history, and current medications. Does the patient have any sight, sensory, or swallowing/speech impairments? Do they use glasses, contact lenses, hearing aids? Do they have any prosthetic devices and/or dentures? Are there any learning or language barriers? Are there any socioeconomic issues that could affect care? Answers to these questions establish social determinants of health, identify issues regarding medication adherence, and help to evaluate if patients understand their medication regimen. Communicating with the patient by speaking calmly in a reassuring manner establishes a therapeutic environment of mutual respect. Questions should be presented slowly, in a nonthreatening, nonjudgmental manner.

Chart Review

The nurse should review preoperative information carefully with attention to detail including the history and physical examination, medication history, laboratory results, cardiac consult and EKG, other consultation reports, and all relevant information.

Medication Reconciliation

This is a sound, evidence-based practice to identify and predict adverse reactions in vulnerable older adults including detailed documentation, monitoring, and a regular review of all medications through medication reconciliation.

The nurse should communicate with patients and families to determine an accurate list of all medications, including prescription, over the counter, vitamins, and herbal remedies. This not only includes the name of the medication, but also the dosage, frequency, route, and reasons for taking it. Ask the patient the method they use to remember to take their medication. Do they use a calendar, pill sorter, or a seven-day organizer? Knowing their method can determine whether it needs to be modified to improve adherence and safety. The staff should encourage the caregiver to bring the patient's medications to the hospital, including over-the-counter medications, vitamins, and herbal remedies.

The clinical staff should assess that prescriptions have been ordered correctly, and that, if needed, a patient has stopped taking a medication when replaced with another medication. Multiple prescribers may have prescribed medications for the same condition, and the patient may continue to take them all. It is important to make sure the patient and family are aware and understand why the medication is being stopped.

Through the admission process, the nurse should obtain a complete up-to-date list of medications and identify possible challenges regarding adherence and medication costs. Perioperatively and upon discharge as well medication reviews should be conducted regularly. Ideally, medication lists should be monitored by the nurse and an interdisciplinary team.

Medication Adherence Assessment

Polypharmacy can lead to problems with medication adherence in older adults, especially if associated with age-related issues, and can result in serious outcomes. The health and medication beliefs of the patient and caregiver should be assessed. Priority should be given to understand the patient's beliefs regarding their need for medication. Including the caregiver in these conversations can help to facilitate shared decision-making, improve adherence, and hopefully, reduce risk. Once this is done, medication adherence recommendations can be implemented.

During hospitalization and upon discharge, it is important that nurse and the patient discuss the patient's concerns and challenges related to their medications. The patient should be evaluated for potential barriers to adherence such as financial and insurance issues, use of multiple providers and pharmacies, complex medication regimen, cognitive, hearing and/or visual impairment, mobility issues, and oral health and/or swallowing problems. Problems with adherence may be due to lack of understanding, confusion, or forgetfulness. Some patients may experience unpleasant side effects to a medication and decrease the dosage or stop taking the drug, on their own. Those with visual difficulties may have problems reading prescription labels. Patients with financial problems may decide not to fill a prescription or decide to decrease their dosages to extend their supply.

Interventions to help improve adherence can consist of a combination of educational and behavioral strategies. It is important to discuss the barriers with the patient's provider and the pharmacy. Possibly simplifying the medication regimen by decreasing the number of dosages may help. Improving communication among the patient, caregiver, and multidisciplinary team, and educating the patient and caregivers are the most important areas to help increase adherence. Studies show face-to-face motivational approaches, that include the patient's involvement in the plan, are effective. Polypharmacy and medication adherence present a unique challenge for the older adult, their family, caregiver, and the healthcare team.

Symptom Identification

The early detection and recognition of clinically important adverse events and reactions are crucial in identifying patients who are at higher risk for such outcomes. Nurses are in a unique position to recognize and possibly reduce the adverse effects of multiple medications by being alert and considering that some symptoms may be caused by certain medications. Often most challenging is to differentiate the symptom as a drug response, from a symptom as a sign of their underlying disease.

By identifying patients who are at risk for inappropriate polypharmacy, nurses can educate patients, families, and caregivers about the dangers and educate on preventive tactics. Education should include that a medication may be stopped, or a dosage altered, if it is no longer beneficial, or is causing harm. Special emphasis must be made that patients should never stop taking medications without their doctor's instruction.

Patient Safety

Comorbidities and Falls

Multiple comorbidities and falls are serious health problems for older adults and are a growing health concern. The presence of comorbidities and polypharmacy, in addition to the age-related decline in functional capacity and muscle strength and flexibility, increases the risk for falls. Half of patients over 80 years of age fall once a year, and of those, there is a higher risk of subsequent falls. Risk factors for falls include a sedentary lifestyle, impaired cognitive function, impaired vision, frailty, malnutrition, alcohol abuse, and polypharmacy The consequences of falls can be catastrophic, resulting in disability and long-term care placement, loss of quality of life, fear of falling, depression, and lack of self-confidence and independence. Falls are the leading cause of traumatic brain injury and mortality among older adults.

Acute Care Issues

Many patients admitted to a general surgical unit are taking medicines for conditions unrelated to surgery. Polypharmacy is present in the majority of older adults having surgery and is associated with increased postoperative mortality, increased adverse events, and higher health cost utilization.

As adults continue to age, there is an increasing probability they may be hospitalized for acute issues requiring surgery. Older patients may develop cognitive impairment and delirium in acute care settings, exacerbated by hospital stimuli, considerable noise and light, and unfamiliar surroundings. Hospital acquired delirium is a temporary but serious condition, presenting as emotional and cognitive impairment, but can result in longer hospitalizations and negative outcomes. A high percentage of hospitalized patients 70 years old and above experience delirium, and the rate is much higher for those undergoing surgery or in intensive care. Polypharmacy can exacerbate this problem by contributing to impaired cognition, confusion, anemia, and delirium.

Polypharmacy is a growing health problem in older adults when they present to the emergency department for a variety of reasons, and it has the potential to create adverse medication events and interactions. The greater the number of concurrent medications, the presence of comorbidities, and physiologic changes related to aging can affect drug metabolism and decrease therapeutic effects. The risk of potential adverse medication events and interactions can occur when given new medications in the emergency department.

Obtaining an accurate history and up-to-date medication list, and then a thorough examination of the medication list of older adults presenting to an emergency department is vital. Polypharmacy and excessive polypharmacy are independent risk factors for adverse health outcomes after an emergency visit.

Medications Used Preoperatively, Perioperatively, Postoperatively

Medications that may be given in the preoperative, perioperative, and postoperative settings include anesthetic agents, benzodiazepines, antibiotics, analgesics, anticoagulants, and anti-inflammatory agents. The effects of opioids and benzodiazepines together with the actions of the patient's regular medications are likely to produce adverse effects. When using these medications, older adults require a much lower dosage.

Nurses working in perioperative areas should be aware of a patient's preoperative medications and the medications that have been prescribed in the perioperative setting. A structured medication review can help prevent dangerous consequences. It has been reported that a critically ill patient may be given as many as 10–20 medications in a perioperative setting. As medication interactions increase significantly with the number of medications, the most significant nursing intervention is a thorough and accurate assessment of the patient. Early recognition of potentially harmful medication effects is critical.

Patient Education

Education must involve good communication. Meeting with the patient and caregiver facilitates trust and open dialogue. Educating the patient and their caregiver is one of the most important ways to improve adherence. One should discuss the importance of keeping an updated, accurate list of all medications, prescribed and over the counter, vitamins, and herbal products. Include the dosage, frequency, and reasons for the medication. The list should include the names and numbers of all providers, and name and number of their pharmacy.

The patient and caregiver should be educated about each medication including the reasons for it, side effects, and the importance of taking as prescribed. Review the potential adverse and drug related problems that may develop, and that serious adverse effects are a cause for emergency care. Explain that they should contact their provider with any questions or concerns, especially if their health changes. Remind them to never stop taking a drug without consulting their provider. Also, if appropriate, help patients set up memory aids such as pill boxes, use of color-coded charts, automatic dispensers, or telephone or message services to remind them to take their medication. Always verify that the patient understands and agrees with the instructions. Ask them to repeat the instructions back to you.

Conclusion

The goal of older adults as they age is to ensure or maintain good health, which means independence, productivity, and security. Unfortunately, older adults are disproportionately affected by chronic disease, which can lead to emotional, behavioral, and physical health issues. Chronic disease is also associated with the risk of polypharmacy. Patients with several comorbidities, in addition to the increase in variety of medications and herbal remedies available, contribute to the adverse effects of polypharmacy.

Given the risks and burdens of polypharmacy and potentially inappropriate medications, nurses must be vigilant in assessing their patients, conscientious in reviewing patient medication lists, thorough in monitoring patient medications, detailed in providing education to patients and caregivers about adherence and risk reduction, and creative in applying evidence-based strategies to treat basic symptoms with the goal to optimize wellness and quality of life.

References

1. By the 2019 American Geriatrics Society Beers Criteria® Update Expert Panel. American Geriatrics Society 2019 updated AGS beers criteria® for potentially inappropriate medication use in older adults. J Am Geriatr Soc. 2019;67(4):674–94. https://doi.org/10.1111/jgs.15767.
2. Hales CM, Servais J, Martin CB, Kohen D. Prescription drug use among adults aged 40-79 in the United States and Canada. NCHS Data Brief. 2019;(347):1–8.
3. Halli-Tierney AD, Scarbrough C, Carroll D. Polypharmacy: evaluating risks and deprescribing. Am Fam Physician. 2019;100(1):32–8.
4. Gjorgjievski M, Ristevski B. Postoperative management considerations of the elderly patient undergoing orthopaedic surgery. Injury. 2020;51(Suppl 2):S23–7. https://doi.org/10.1016/j.injury.2019.12.027.
5. Lavan AH, Gallagher P. Predicting risk of adverse drug reactions in older adults. Ther Adv Drug Saf. 2016;7:11–22. https://doi.org/10.1177/2042098615615472.
6. Maher RL, Hanlon J, Hajjar ER. Clinical consequences of polypharmacy in elderly. Expert Opin Drug Saf. 2014;13(1):57–65. https://doi.org/10.1517/14740338.2013.827660.
7. Mamaril ME. Nursing considerations in the geriatric surgical patient: the perioperative continuum of care. Nurs Clin North Am. 2006;41(2):313–28, vii. https://doi.org/10.1016/j.cnur.2006.01.001.
8. Morin L, Johnell K, Laroche ML, Fastbom J, Wastesson JW. The epidemiology of polypharmacy in older adults: register-based prospective cohort study. Clin Epidemiol. 2018;10:289–98. https://doi.org/10.2147/CLEP.S153458.
9. NCOA. National Council on Aging. Get the facts on healthy aging center for healthy aging for professionals. https://www.ncoa.org/article/get-the-facts-on-healthy-aging.
10. NIH NIA. National Institute on Aging. The dangers of polypharmacy and the case for deprescribing in older adults. 2021. https://www.nia.nih.gov/news/dangers-polypharmacy-and-case-deprescribing-older-adults.
11. Nixdorff N, Hustey F, Brady A, Vaji K, Leonard M, Messinger-Rapport BJ. Potentially inappropriate medications and adverse drug effects in elders in the ED. Am J Emerg Med. 2008;26(6):697–700. https://doi.org/10.1016/j.ajem.2007.12.007.
12. Oktora M, Alfian S, Bos J, et al. Trends in polypharmacy and potentially inappropriate medication (PIM) in older and middle-aged people treated for diabetes. Br J Clin Pharmacol. 2021;87(7):2807–17. https://doi.org/10.1111/bcp.14685.

13. Qato DM, Wilder J, Schumm LP, Gillet V, Alexander GC. Changes in prescription and over-the-counter medication and dietary supplement use among older adults in the United States, 2005 vs 2011. JAMA Intern Med. 2016;176(4):473–82. https://doi.org/10.1001/jamainternmed.2015.8581.
14. Rankin A, Cadogan CA, Patterson SM, Kerse N, Cardwell CR, Bradley MC, Ryan C, Hughes C. Interventions to improve the appropriate use of polypharmacy for older people. Cochrane Database Syst Rev. 2018;9(9):CD008165. https://doi.org/10.1002/14651858.CD008165.pub4.
15. Uchmanowicz I, Jankowska-Polańska B, Wleklik M, Lisiak M, Gobbens R. Frailty syndrome: nursing interventions. SAGE Open Nurs. 2018;4:2377960818759449. https://doi.org/10.1177/2377960818759449.

Outcomes in Geriatric Trauma and Emergency General Surgery

61

Franchesca Hwang, Leslie S. Tyrie, and Nicole Goulet

Introduction

Individuals are living longer due to lifestyle improvements and advances in medical care. Therefore, it is not surprising that we are now encountering an increasing number of geriatric trauma and emergency surgical patients. There is a growing surgical field devoted to the care and management of this population. Different management pathways are developed to address the specific set of challenges in elderly trauma and surgical patients as their in-hospital, post-discharge, and long-term outcomes vary from their younger counterparts.

Geriatric Trauma

Geriatric trauma has been defined as starting at the age of 55 years old. For the purposes of our discussion, we define elder and/or geriatric trauma as occurring in patients over the age of 65. The burden of geriatric trauma continues to expand. Just under one quarter of all trauma admissions are elderly; this is estimated to become 40% by 2050. Trauma represents the fifth leading cause of death in all geriatric patients. Morbidity and mortality after trauma are higher than their younger cohorts when adjusted for injury severity. With increasing injury severity (ISS), mortality in the elderly steeply increases especially with every 5-year age increase after 70 years. Up to one-third of elderly trauma patients with an ISS greater than 16 will die in the hospital.

The distribution and mechanism of elderly trauma are different from those under the age of 65. By a large majority, the mechanism of injury in elderly patients is falls, and of these, most are ground level falls. Additionally, ISS is lower overall in elderly trauma. In one study of injured elderly patients across all trauma systems, they found 47% had an ISS less than 9 and 97% an ISS less than 16. Despite the low ISS overall, because of comorbid conditions and physiologic changes that occur as we age, elderly persons account for a disproportionate number of deaths due to injury. In-hospital case-fatality for geriatric trauma is up to four times greater than their younger counterparts. However, geriatric patients who survive their traumatic injuries should gain some meaningful functional outcome and a return to independent living. These results are age dependent as patients older than 80 have worse functional outcomes than those aged 65–80. Nonetheless, elderly brain injured patients, while taking longer and additional resources, can eventually reach the same rehabilitation goals as younger matched patients.

F. Hwang · L. S. Tyrie · N. Goulet (✉)
NYU Grossman School of Medicine, NYU Langone Health Brooklyn, Brooklyn, NY, USA
e-mail: Franchesca.Hwang@nyulangone.org

P. Petrone, C. E.M. Brathwaite (eds.), *Acute Care Surgery in Geriatric Patients*,
https://doi.org/10.1007/978-3-031-30651-8_61

In-Hospital and Post-Injury Mortality

Crude morality rates for geriatric trauma patients in large population studies appear to range from 2 to 5%. Mortality increases with higher injury severity scores—most particularly when ISS is greater than 16—and with age greater than 70. It is suggested that preexisting comorbidities are a risk factor for mortality.

One study compared the survival of elderly trauma patients to non-injured cohorts. In this study, the in-hospital mortality was 4.1%. Hospital case-fatality steeply increased in the moderately and severely injured group. Those with ISS over 25 had a 56% in-hospital mortality, and those with ISS between 16 and 24 had 13% mortality. On the other hand, mortality steeply dropped with ISS less than 16 (4% in ISS 9–15; 3% in ISS <9). While early mortality post injury was most common, risk of death persisted even after discharge from the hospital. Overall, 5-year risk of death could be again stratified by ISS. Injury severity score up to 24 conferred a relative risk of death within 5 years of 1.6–1.8, compared to the non-injured; whereas relative risk of death increased to 5.8 if ISS was greater than 25.

Age was also a factor in relative risk of death within 5 years post injury. This risk increased as age increased starting at the age bracket of 72–76 (relative risk of death = 1.5) and increasing up to 2 times per 5 years of age until age 97–100 (relative risk of death = 9.5). These findings suggest that the oldest of the old are truly at a higher risk of dying from traumatic injuries, even when adjusting for the injury severity. Intensive monitoring as well as early goals-of-care discussion need to be initiated as soon as possible to improve outcomes and to provide patient-centered care in those at the extremes of age.

Preexisting illness also correlated to adverse outcome; persons with a lower Charleston index 1–3 had a two-fold relative risk of death while a higher Charleston index 10–13 had a greater than eight-fold increase in the risk of death.

Premorbid conditions (PMCs) exist in one-third of trauma patients aged over 75 years compared to 3.5% in the young. Studies have suggested that PMCs may lead to worse outcomes when compared to patients without. The PMCs that may affect morbidity and/or mortality include:

- Peripheral arterial occlusive disease (stage IV)
- Heart disease
- Hepatitis/liver cirrhosis
- Carcinoma/malignant disease
- Coagulation disorder
- Obesity
- Steroid use/immunosuppression
- Obstructive pulmonary disease
- Diabetes
- Renal disorder

It is suggested the comorbidities that lead to the highest risk of mortality include hepatic disease, renal disease, and preinjury cancer. However, the data is conflicting, and additional studies refute the finding that PMCs contribute to mortality. Premorbid conditions may play a greater role in less severely injured patients as critically injured patients most likely die from the burden of traumatic injuries, and the PMCs do not contribute to the immediate care of patients who die of their trauma.

Additionally, mortality can be stratified based on injury. A National Trauma Data Bank (NTDB) retrospective study compared blunt traumatic injury in the elderly (age > 65) vs. the non-geriatric (age 18–65). Thirty-one percent of the study population were > 65 years of age, and the mean age was 78. The geriatric population was more often white (85% vs 68%) and female (58% vs 31%). The most common presenting mechanism was fall (79%) with 82% from ground level. Motor vehicle crash (MVC) was the second most common mechanism (12%). Pedestrian struck (3%), assault (2%), motorcycle crash (1%), and other accounted for the remaining 3%. Overall, geriatric patients had a higher presenting systolic blood pressure and a lower heart rate and were less likely to present with signs of shock, highlighting the need for higher suspicion for presence of injuries in geriatric trauma even when their vital signs appear to be normal. The ISS was lower overall for geriatric vs. non-geriatric (NG) patients and in each body region except for the

Table 61.1 Mortality Data

Mechanism	Geriatric mortality rate (%)	Non-geriatric mortality rate (%)	Age > 65 as independent risk factor for mortality (odds ratio)
Ground level falls	4.2	1.9	2.3
Motor vehicle crash	5.6	1.9	4.3
Pedestrian struck	7.8	3.3	3.0
Assaults	3.3	0.7	3.4
Motorcycle crash	4.6	2.7	2.1

Adapted from Brown et al. A Comprehensive Investigation of Comorbidities, Mechanisms, Injury Patterns, and Outcomes in Geriatric Blunt Trauma Patients. *Am Surg*. 2016;82 (11):1055–1062

head and lower extremity. Twenty-four percent of head abbreviated injury scale (AIS) was greater than 3 in geriatric patients vs. 18% in NG, and lower extremity AIS greater than 3 was observed in 24% of geriatric vs. 8% of NG. The most common injuries in the elderly after a ground level fall were traumatic brain injury (23%), hip fracture (21%), and lower extremity fracture (33%). Also common were upper extremity fracture, thoracic/rib injuries, pelvic fracture, and spine fracture. Abdominal injuries were uncommon. The incidence of rib/thoracic, pelvis and spine fractures increased with mechanisms such as motor vehicle crash, pedestrian struck, and motorcycle crash. Mortality rates for different mechanisms of injury are shown in Table 61.1.

Incidence of Morbidity and Common Causes of Death Following Blunt Injury

In-hospital complications in geriatric trauma include infections (pneumonia, urinary tract infection, sepsis), thromboembolic events, and organ failure with lungs being the most commonly affected organ (85%). Geriatric patients have an overall higher incidence of multiple organ dysfunction syndrome (MODS) when compared to the young. The elderly experiences a higher incidence of late trauma deaths; these are primarily due to MODS (up to 50% of elderly deaths).

In one single institution study, over 1000 geriatric patients admitted following blunt trauma to a single level 1 center were reviewed, and morbidity and mortality outcomes were examined. The mean age was 79 years. Falls accounted for 88% of injuries, followed by MVC and pedestrian struck. Most commonly observed injuries were orthopedic and head trauma. Ten percent of patients had rib fractures. The majority (67%) of patients had an ISS between 9 and 14. The median length of stay was 7 days. The authors found that 21% of survivors had in-hospital complications. The most common were sepsis (7%) and pneumonia (7%). Surgical site infection occurred in 5% of patients and venous thromboembolism in 2% of patients. Overall mortality was 3%: 63% died of severe TBI, 20% from sepsis and/or MODS, 14% with severe multisystem trauma with hemorrhagic shock, and 3% from high spinal cord injury. More than half of the mortality was in patients older than 86 years. Older age, ISS, and comorbidities were independent predictors of mortality (older age: aOR = 1.1, ISS aOR = 2.5, and comorbidities aOR = 1.3). Comorbidities associated with in-hospital mortality were coronary artery disease, renal failure, dementia, and warfarin use. Warfarin use in other studies has been shown to have no effect on outcomes except in traumatic brain injury.

Penetrating Injury and Severe Hemorrhage

The incidence of penetrating trauma in the elderly is low. In United States, some estimates of the incidence are reported to be as high as 10%; other studies suggest that the incidence is less than 4%. European data has shown that only 4% of all geriatric trauma deaths result from a penetrating trauma mechanism. In the literature, there is an association between penetrating trauma and worse outcomes in the elderly. Mortality estimates are as high as 55%. Blood transfusion, elevated shock index, lactic acidosis, hemorrhagic shock, and age over 75 have been associated with higher mortality. However, there is also literature suggesting that older patients with penetrating trauma do not have increased complication rates compared to their younger counterparts and recommend aggressive care. The age distribution, severity of injury, and comorbid conditions in each study likely account for many of these observed differences. Additionally, there are differences in the mechanism of penetrating trauma in elderly patients. When examining rates of firearm injuries, there is an increasing incidence of self-inflicted injuries in elderly males as part of attempted suicides. These account for 46% of gunshot injuries in those aged between 65 and 75 and 56% of gunshot injuries in those over the age of 75. Older patients with firearm injuries have a higher incidence of head trauma and a higher mortality. Although it is a small subset of trauma population, more studies are needed to better understand outcomes of penetrating geriatric trauma given the high mortality.

Post-Discharge Outcomes and Readmission

As elderly trauma patients have a high risk of in-hospital morbidity and mortality upon admission, they similarly have a high risk of morbidity and mortality upon discharge with 86% of elderly trauma patient deaths occurring after leaving the hospital. Elderly ground level fall patients have a 1-year mortality of 24% when they are discharged alive. Many post-discharge outcomes are shown to be associated with disposition locations: home vs. skilled nursing facility (SNF) vs. inpatient rehab facility (IRF). The ideal outcome for any patient, and elderly trauma patients are no different, is a discharge destination of home with premorbid functional status. Elderly patients have been shown to have a higher rate of discharge to IRFs and SNFs than younger patients, but overall, studies suggest that approximately two-thirds of geriatric trauma patients are discharged home and the remaining to nursing and rehab facilities. Several population and hospital-based cohort studies have demonstrated worse survival for patients discharged to SNF as they have a risk of death 1.6–3.9 times greater than those discharged home. More specifically, elderly trauma patients who sustained a ground level fall and were discharged to SNFs had a three times greater risk of 1-year mortality compared with patients who were discharged home with no assistance. Significant predictors of 1-year mortality were increasing age, transfer to another acute care facility, ICU admission, longer hospital length of stay, and Charleston comorbidity score of greater than 2.

Discharge planning is an integral process for all trauma centers but especially important for those centers with a predominantly geriatric population. Decisions are based on age, functional ability, social support, insurance coverage along with many other factors. Increased age, ICU length of stay, ISS, total number of injuries (with extremity and pelvis being most contributory), number of comorbidities, and having Medicare insurance were all found to be predictors of adverse discharge disposition (IRF/SNF) in trauma patients presenting after a fall. Much work has been done to examine factors that might predict which elderly patients will need rehab in order to start the disposition process sooner. This earlier knowledge of who benefits from rehab would lead to improved coordination among the providers, consultants, social workers, patients, and their families resulting in more efficient transition of care, decreased hospital length of stay, decreased costs, and decreased associated risks.

Readmissions can lead to higher rates of morbidity and mortality and increased costs. They also lead to decreased reimbursement based on the Hospital Readmissions Reduction Program instituted in 2012, allowing the Centers for Medicare and Medicaid Services to reduce payments to hospitals with excess disease-specific and hospital-wide readmissions. Geriatric trauma patients have been shown to be particularly susceptible to readmissions due both to their comorbidities, but also from repeat falls and complications of injury. Even a low mechanism of injury such as a ground level fall can result in a high ISS and even admission to the ICU. Elderly patients who sustain a ground level fall have been shown to have a readmission rate of 45% within 1 year of injury, and on average, they were dmitted 1.7 times. Additionally, patients nitted to the ICU initially were at the highest k for readmission (twice as likely to be readted within 30 days). As was discussed previsly, geriatric trauma patients discharged to IFs have been shown to have higher mortality d morbidity, and the same has been shown for admissions. There is growing research showing creased readmission rates of elderly trauma tients who have been discharged to any facility her than home. Ayoung-Chee et al. demonrated nearly a 51% readmission rate of elderly ound level fall patients discharged to a SNF ith 16% at 30 days and 38% within 1 year. trosberg et al. found slightly different results ith a 30-day readmission rate of geriatric trauma atients from rehab being the highest at 16%, folowed by extended care facility (ECF), which ncludes SNF and acute care facilities (13%), compared to home (6%). One of the most imporant findings in their study was that only discharge destination was independently associated with readmission, and no other factors were found to be predictive of readmission: ISS, comorbidity-polypharmacy score, LOS, pretrauma location (home vs ECF), age, or preinjury functional status.

Frailty in Trauma

Although discussed elsewhere in this book, one cannot fail to mention how frailty contributes to not only in-hospital outcomes but also postdischarge outcomes, such as readmission, repeat falls, increased morbidity, and mortality in the elderly. Various frailty scores have been developed and reported in trauma literature, but one prospective study by Joseph et al. developed and validated the trauma-specific frailty index (TSFI), which stratified patients as frail, prefrail, and nonfrail. Not only were the frail patients more likely to develop hospital complications with urinary tract infections and pneumonia at the highest rates compared to the nonfrail and prefrail but also more likely to be discharged to SNFs compared to the other two groups (nonfrail 8%, prefrail 18%, frail 47%). Frailty was shown to correlate with increased rate of readmission due to a new traumatic injury (motor vehicle crash and fall most common), compared to nonfrail elderly patients at 6 months (40% vs. 4%). Additionally, frail patients were not only more likely to have recurrent falls within 6 months compared to nonfrail patients (65% vs 5%), but they were more likely to have a higher number of falls.

Geriatric Emergency General Surgery

Nearly one million older patients are admitted to hospitals for emergency general surgery (EGS) conditions every year in the United States. EGS is associated with high mortality and morbidity in geriatric patients. Older patients undergoing emergency laparotomy represent a very high-risk patient population. The 1-year mortality is over 50% among patients over the age of 85 who underwent an emergency major abdominal surgery.

The age cutoff for geriatric EGS is usually considered to be at or above 65. However, the population is becoming increasingly older worldwide, and many older patients at extreme age undergo emergency general surgery. Therefore, some studies in literature focusing on geriatric EGS set their age cutoff to be higher than 65. For the purpose of discussion for this geriatric EGS section, we will be using various age groups over the age of 65. Many of the most common geriatric emergent abdominal surgical procedures studied in literature are the following: appendectomy, cholecystectomy, colectomy, laparotomy, abdominal hernia repair, adhesiolysis, and gastric procedures. The most common indications for emergency laparotomy are bowel obstruction and/or bowel perforation including perforated appendicitis.

Emergency Laparotomy and Damage Control Laparotomy

The in-hospital mortality ranges from 9% to 22% in older patients undergoing emergency laparotomy; however, the highest mortality was observed in those who had bowel ischemia and/

or bowel perforation (38–50%). Once geriatric patients develop complications from emergency laparotomy, mortality increases up to three times. Major morbidity that requires surgical, endoscopic, or radiological interventions was 14%, and the delay in surgery for more than 24 hours was an independent predictor for major morbidity with the adjusted odds ratio of 13. Diabetes mellitus was found to be an independent risk factor to surgical delay over 24 hours most likely as it blunted physiological response and contributed to atypical presentation in older patients. These findings highlight the need for a high index of suspicion in those with diabetes and to expedite surgical care when indicated in geriatric patients with EGS diagnoses. In addition, preventing complications initially and recognizing and treating any complications promptly could substantially decrease their mortality and morbidity.

The 30-day mortality rate for older patients presenting with emergency general surgical diagnoses such as bowel obstruction, bowel ischemia, bowel perforation, or gastrointestinal ulcers undergoing major abdominal surgery ranges from 10 to 30%. The long-term outcomes for these patients are worse. One-year mortality ranges from 15 to 40%, and one-year readmission rates are over 40% among those who underwent emergency laparotomy.

Damage control laparotomy has been increasingly utilized in emergency general surgery as it has been widely adopted in trauma care. There was one retrospective study assessing if damage control laparotomy in geriatric patients is associated with higher adverse outcomes compared to younger counterparts. This study found no significant difference in the rates of primary abdominal closure after index procedure, time to primary closure, mortality, hospital and ICU length of stay, and incidence of intrabdominal abscess. Expectedly, the mortality was high at 42%, but this mortality was not significantly higher than that of non-geriatric patients. This study suggests that age alone should not be a contraindication for performing damage control laparotomy, and it can be safely utilized in geriatric EGS patients.

Appendicitis

Even for one of the most commonly performed procedures, appendectomy, it carries significant morbidity in older patients. Conversion from laparoscopy to open appendectomy was significantly higher in patients over the age of 75 (17% vs. 3% in younger counterparts), and the percentage of perforated appendicitis was over 50% in this group with the 30-day mortality as high as 6%, which was 30 times higher than those younger than 75 (0.2%). The very high incidence of perforation and hence significant morbidity associated with appendicitis could be explained by multiple factors: the presence of malignancy such as adenocarcinoma in older patients and delay in operative treatment during the hospital course. The surgical delay due to incorrect diagnoses or due to hesitation of surgeons to operate on older patients when surgery is indicated is a modifiable component in geriatric surgical care that could potentially improve their mortality and morbidity.

Biliary Disease

Biliary diseases in older patients are associated with adverse outcomes due to comorbidities and reduced physiological reserves. High-risk patients presenting with acute cholecystitis are sometimes treated with antibiotics or percutaneous drainage instead of cholecystectomy. A systematic review assessed the outcomes of early cholecystectomy in geriatric patients over the age of 70 with acute cholecystitis. This review reported perioperative mortality rate of 3.5%; causes of death were pulmonary or cardiac complications predominantly. Given the frequent adverse outcomes associated with cholecystectomy in high-risk patients such as older patients, non-operative management of acute cholecystitis has been utilized. The CHOCOLATE trial, a randomized controlled multicenter study, however, suggests that percutaneous drainage is not associated with reduced mortality compared to laparoscopic cholecystectomy. Percutaneous drainage is, in fact, associated with increased major complications and longer hospital length of stay in high-risk patients. One systematic review similarly reported that almost half of the patients treated with percutaneous drainage undergo cholecystectomy eventually, and patients managed with antibiotics alone are still at risk of biliary sepsis requiring emergency surgery. Another study of patients with acute cholecystitis over the age of 80 demonstrated that although the 30-day mortality is higher for the cholecystectomy group compared to non-operative group (12% vs. 10%), the cholecystectomy group had a reduced 1-year mortality of 21% vs. 27%, again suggesting potential benefits of surgical treatment in the very old patients. Among those patients managed non-operatively with antibiotics, readmission rates for biliary related disease were as high as 55% compared to 17% for those who had undergone surgery. Those who had percutaneous cholecystostomy tubes had the highest 30-day and 1-year mortality of 13% and 35%, respectively, which can be due to selection bias as the higher mortality is not completely related to the management themselves but rather related to patient characteristics. Nonetheless, a more definitive surgical treatment in older patients with acute cholecystitis should be considered with optimized perioperative care in a multidisciplinary approach.

Small Bowel Obstruction

Another surgical dilemma when caring for geriatric patients is deciding whether or not to take patients presenting with bowel obstruction to the operating room, and once the decision has been made, when to do so. Bowel obstruction is one of the most common indications for laparotomy as stated previously. As the population is growing older overall, and the chance of having abdominal surgery increases with age, small bowel obstruction (SBO) is a surgical diagnosis commonly seen in geriatric patients. SBO management in the setting of adhesive disease is mostly non-operative with nothing by mouth, bowel rest, and/or nasogastric tube decompression unless there are signs of threatened bowel or peritonitis. However, this approach requires a surgeon to be able to assess if the patient is having bowel function and to obtain reliable abdominal exams, which may be challenging in older patients who may have preexisting dementia or are more likely to develop in-hospital delirium. Another factor may be the surgeon's reluctance to operate on elderly patients unless they develop obvious indications for surgery, at which time the surgical intervention may be too delayed. Delay in surgery is associated with more frequent need to perform bowel resection in geriatric patients. In addition, malnutrition is highly prevalent in older adults, and most patients presenting with bowel obstruction have not had adequate nutrition even in the pre-hospital setting. This factor should also be taken into account when deciding the optimal timing to operate as malnutrition is a known risk factor for adverse outcomes in abdominal surgery. Outcomes can be improved in older patients with bowel obstruction if surgery is expedited as soon as patients show any signs of failure of non-operative management of SBO.

Stratification and Prognostication

When it comes to risk stratification and prognostication in geriatric surgical patients, numerous tools exist. Many agree that chronological age alone does not predict outcomes; thus, frailty score or index is often used to predict postoperative morbidity and mortality. The limited use of some frailty scores in the setting of emergency general surgery is due to the impracticality of some tools, which tend to be extremely comprehensive with too many factors and because they require objective functional tests, such as grip strength or gait speed, which are almost impossible to obtain in patients with an acute illness. One example of frailty index used to predict postoperative complications in geriatric patients is modified frailty index (MFI), which include these 11 variables: history of diabetes mellitus, congestive heart failure, hypertension, cerebrovascular accident with or without neurological deficit, myocardial infarction, peripheral vascular disease, COPD, prior coronary revascularization, or impaired sensorium, and non-independent functional status. The MFI score was more predictive of postoperative morbidity and mortality in EGS patients over the age of 60 than increasing age or American Society of Anesthesiologists (ASA) class. Based on the multivariate logistic regression for 30-day mortality, frailty was associated with the odds ratio of 12 for adverse postoperative outcomes.

A more recent study looked at the association between frailty and 30-day mortality, stratified by high- and low-risk EGS procedures in medicare beneficiaries. The high-risk procedures included excision of small intestine, excision of large intestine, peptic ulcer repair, lysis of peritoneal adhesions, and laparotomy; the low-risk procedures included appendectomy and cholecystectomy. Among the patients who underwent EGS procedures, frailty was independently associated with mortality in both high-risk and low-risk procedures after adjusting for patient and hospital characteristics. Interestingly, frailty was associated with 2 times the risk of mortality in low-risk procedures compared to 1.5 times in high-risk procedures, regardless of operative approaches of laparoscopic versus open. This finding again highlights the need for more comprehensive, thoughtful strategies even in more common, "low-risk" procedures such as appendectomy and cholecystectomy, when caring for older patients, especially the frail. Additionally, regardless of which frailty score or index one chooses to use, they need to be able to assess risks of each patient expeditiously and offer the most patient-oriented treatment option through early goals-of-care discussions.

Geriatric Specific Care in EGS

Literature supports better outcomes for geriatric trauma patients in high-volume trauma centers with geriatric support; similarly, patients operated by high-volume surgeons performing 8 or more EGS procedures/year have reduced mortality and failure-to-rescue. Those operated by low-volume surgeons are 1.9 times more likely to have in-hospital mortality and 1.7 times more likely to have failure-to-rescue compared to their higher-volume counterparts after adjusting for all patients and hospital factors. This finding underscores the need for geriatric specific care in emergency general surgery and prompts more thoughtful decision-making in all aspects of perioperative care: preoperative, whether or not to operate, as well as intraoperative and postoperative. In terms of postoperative care, postoperative complications during the index hospitalization were the strongest predictors of death at 30, 180, and 365-days when adjusting for age and comorbidities. Hypervigilance to prevent postoperative complications may result in higher survival for this vulnerable patient population.

Conclusion

Outcomes after geriatric trauma and emergency surgery vary widely but overall have been shown to have worse morbidity and mortality rates, especially in those who are frail, severely injured, and at increased age. Although frailty rather than age alone has been shown to correlate with outcomes, mortality increases for every 5–10 years of life, and every decade matters especially for geriatric trauma patients. In addition, ISS does predict adverse outcomes with a dramatic increase in mortality for ISS over 16. In emergency general surgery, even common procedures, such as appendectomy and cholecystectomy, have high morbidity especially for those older patients with multiple comorbidities which at times may lead to a delay in surgical care. Many factors are difficult to change such as increasing age and number of comorbidities. However, there are many other controllable factors that can mitigate poor outcomes. Elderly patients may in fact benefit from earlier definitive operations for source control. High-volume centers that can provide multidisciplinary care and appropriate resources and are familiar with the challenges specific to older patients have demonstrated improved outcomes. Disposition planning should start early in geriatric trauma and emergency general surgery patients. This should focus as much as possible on home discharge with home health services or acute rehab facilities as these discharge destinations have been associated with better long-term outcomes. Although higher mortality rates are seen in elderly trauma patients, when they do survive, there is an increasing body of literature to suggest they regain reasonable functional status. As the population continues to grow and age, so should our focused care on their special surgical and traumatic needs.

References

1. Ayoung-Chee P, McIntyre L, Ebel BE, et al. Long-term outcomes of ground-level falls in the elderly. J Trauma Acute Care Surg. 2014;76(2):498–503. https://doi.org/10.1097/TA.0000000000000102.
2. Bonne S, Schuerer DJ. Trauma in the older adult: epidemiology and evolving geriatric trauma principles. Clin Geriatr Med. 2013;29(1):137–50. https://doi.org/10.1016/j.cger.2012.10.008.
3. Brown CV, Rix K, Klein AL, et al. A comprehensive investigation of comorbidities, mechanisms, injury patterns, and outcomes in geriatric blunt trauma patients. Am Surg. 2016;82(11):1055–62.
4. Castillo-Angeles M, Cooper Z, Jarman M, et al. Association of frailty with morbidity and mortality in emergency general surgery by procedural risk level. JAMA Surg. 2021;156(1):68–74. https://doi.org/10.1001/jamasurg.2020.5397.
5. Cooper Z, Mitchell SL, Gorges RJ, et al. Predictors of mortality up to 1 year after emergency major abdominal surgery in older adults. J Am Geriatr Soc. 2015;63(12):2572–9. https://doi.org/10.1111/jgs.13785.
6. Gubler KD, Davis R, Koepsell T, et al. Long-term survival of elderly trauma patients. Arch Surg. 1997;132(9):1010–4. https://doi.org/10.1001/archsurg.1997.01430330076013.
7. Hakkarainen TW, Ayoung-Chee P, Alfonso R, et al. Structure, process, and outcomes in skilled nursing facilities: understanding what happens to surgical patients when they cannot go home. A systematic review. J Surg Res. 2015;193(2):772–80. https://doi.org/10.1016/j.jss.2014.06.002.
8. Hildebrand F, Pape HC, Horst K, et al. Impact of age on the clinical outcomes of major trauma. Eur J Trauma Emerg Surg. 2016;42(3):317–32. https://doi.org/10.1007/s00068-015-0557-1.
9. James MK, Robitsek RJ, Saghir SM, et al. Clinical and non-clinical factors that predict discharge disposition after a fall. Injury. 2018;49(5):975–82. https://doi.org/10.1016/j.injury.2018.02.014.
10. Joseph B, Orouji Jokar T, Hassan A, et al. Redefining the association between old age and poor outcomes after trauma: the impact of frailty syndrome. J Trauma Acute Care Surg. 2017;82(3):575–81. https://doi.org/10.1097/TA.0000000000001329.
11. Kirshenbom D, Ben-Zaken Z, Albilya N, et al. Older age, comorbid illnesses, and injury severity affect immediate outcome in elderly trauma patients. J Emerg Trauma Shock. 2017;10(3):146–50. https://doi.org/10.4103/JETS.JETS_62_16.
12. Loozen CS, van Ramshorst B, van Santvoort HC, et al. Early cholecystectomy for acute cholecystitis in the elderly population: a systematic review and meta-analysis. Dig Surg. 2017;34(5):371–9. https://doi.org/10.1159/000455241.
13. Mehta A, Dultz LA, Joseph B, et al. Emergency general surgery in geriatric patients: a statewide analysis of surgeon and hospital volume with outcomes. J Trauma Acute Care Surg. 2018;84(6):864–75. https://doi.org/10.1097/TA.0000000000001829.
14. Strosberg DS, Housley BC, Vazquez D, et al. Discharge destination and readmission rates in older trauma patients. J Surg Res. 2017;207:27–32. https://doi.org/10.1016/j.jss.2016.07.015.
15. Vilches-Moraga A, Rowley M, Fox J, et al. Emergency laparotomy in the older patient: factors predictive of 12-month mortality–Salford-POPS-GS. An observational study. Aging Clin Exp Res. 2020;32(11):2367–73. https://doi.org/10.1007/s40520-020-01578-0.

The Elderly and Pandemics: COVID-19 and Others

62

Conrado J. Estol, Verónica Lacal, and Sebastián Nuñez

Life Expectancy

For the first time in history, life expectancy significantly exceeds health expectancy. This means that people live longer but in many cases with poor health. The challenge is then to improve prevention and medical management of non-communicable and communicable diseases causing the largest burden of disease worldwide. In the year 1900, the average life expectancy was 32 years, while in 2019 it reached 73 years.

Myocardial infarction, stroke, and dementia represent the first, fourth, and sixth causes of death in the US and are also the main cause of disability limiting quality of life due to neurological sequelae, cognitive deficits, congestive heart failure, and other complications. The immediate goal should be for people to turn 90 or 100 years of age with a body and brain that are fully functional. Even in high-income countries, a large proportion of people in the eighth decade and beyond have a significantly limited quality of life in activities of daily living due to the aforementioned diseases. In people aged 65 and older, infections in general, and pneumonia and influenza in particular, are a very important cause of death. By the early twentieth century, infections accounted for the top three causes of death in adults: influenza/pneumonia, tuberculosis, and gastroenteritis caused 30% of mortality in the US. The appearance of the SARS-CoV-2 pandemic has highlighted the vulnerability of the population in general and particularly in the segment with advanced age.

C. J. Estol (✉)
BREYNA, Heart and Brain Medicine, BREYNA, Buenos Aires, Argentina

Stroke Unit, Sanatorio Güemes, Buenos Aires, Argentina
e-mail: Conrado.estol@stat-research.com

V. Lacal
Infectious Disease Department, Sanatorio Güemes, Buenos Aires, Argentina

S. Nuñez
Epidemiological Research Department, Fundacion Sanatorio Güemes, Buenos Aires, Argentina
e-mail: snunez@fsg.edu.ar

The SARS-CoV-2 Pandemic and the Elderly

In 2019, the novel virus SARS-CoV-2 was reported in Wuhan, China. The virus initially spread in the Hubei province and by February 2020 it was present in various countries worldwide.

By May 2022, the SARS-CoV-2 pandemic infected 500 million people worldwide although the real number is probably 5–10 times those that have been confirmed through testing. Deaths have reached six million, but the true number may be closer to 15 million. Men have been affected more severely compared to women, and

P. Petrone, C. E.M. Brathwaite (eds.), *Acute Care Surgery in Geriatric Patients*,
https://doi.org/10.1007/978-3-031-30651-8_62

low socio-economic groups—African American and Hispanic in the USA—have disproportionally suffered higher rates of hospitalizations and deaths. The group most vulnerable to the infection has been that of people above 70 years of age, especially those with cardiovascular disease and obesity as comorbidities.

Once it became clear that the elderly had higher rates of infection, hospitalization, and death, it was recommended that older people kept 2-week supplies of essential foods and medicines, avoided public gatherings and requested help to get groceries. A survey in the United States during 2021 showed that the elderly was not only more vulnerable to the infection with SARS-CoV-2 but also suffered from limited access to health care and had a greater burden of economic and social loss. The data was obtained from 18,000 individuals 65 years of age and older in 11 high-income countries. Although economic hardship, job losses, and decreased health care access were observed widely, it was more significant in the USA. Economic difficulties were experienced by 19% of the elderly in the USA versus 15% in Canada, 14% in Australia, 8% in France, and 3% in Germany, among others. Also, the USA had the largest proportion of older individuals that did not plan to get the COVID-19 vaccine.

Death from COVID-19 was compared to 65 causes of death in the US. Deaths by age were also analyzed in 27 different countries compared to those in Israel. Death from COVID-19 increased exponentially with age at a rate near the median for other age-related causes of death but it was 3–8 times higher than pneumonia and influenza deaths. Mortality (deaths from COVID compared to all deaths) and fatality (deaths among patients with COVID-19) varied significantly among countries probably due to differences in the capacity of the various health systems evaluated.

Why Are the Elderly more Vulnerable?

The main reason of this greater vulnerability could be immunosenescence which is the decline in the immune system effectiveness associated with increasing age. This occurs as a result of an autoimmune response generated by autoantibodies produced by age-related changes in the thymus. Also, the so-called inflammaging promotes the development of abnormal pro-inflammatory phenotypes that result in chronic inflammation and responses to infection that increase organ damage due to an exacerbated production of inflammatory cytokines, reactive oxygen species, and acute phase reactants. Age affects both the adaptive and innate immune responses. In the latter, changes occur in epithelial barriers, antimicrobial peptides and mucus, as well as macrophages, neutrophils, natural killer cells, natural killer T cells, dendritic cells, and complement proteins. Moreover, the response to treatments with monoclonal antibodies, other medications and the effect of all vaccines have been proven to be diminished in older people.

This process probably starts around 60 years of age and is marked by age 70. Immunosenescence leads to a greater vulnerability from infections—flu and other infection death rates are greater in elderly patients-, autoimmune diseases and for the risk of developing cancer. The major changes occur with senescent and decreased numbers of peripheral T and B cells. Also, DNA age associated damage probably had a role in the greater severity of COVID-19 in the elderly.

Another mechanism for the greater susceptibility to infection in the elderly are the Angiotensin Converting Enzyme 2 receptors (ACE2). These receptors have been key as binding sites that allow the infection of cells by the SARS-CoV-2 virus. A high expression of ACE2 receptors in the lungs and upper airway explains the rapid capacity of the virus to infect individuals through the respiratory system and result in the lung damage observed in most. The presence of ACE2 receptors is diminished in the elderly what is contradictory with their higher susceptibility to get infected. The explanation is that the ACE2 enzyme has an important role regulating the immune and inflammatory responses. Various studies have shown that the ACE2 enzyme provides significant protection against different ctions. Therefore, the reduction of this yme in the elderly may in part explain their r response to COVID-19 disease.

An additional mechanism of damage could be itrophils which normally are part of infection itrol but in the elderly their activity becomes iormal and cause tissue injury. Statins have en shown to block the enzyme that alters utrophil function and thus have a regulatory ect in the immune system, which is indepen-nt from their cholesterol lowering activity. One iall study at the University of Birmingham in ople with pneumonia aged 68–90 years, ran-omized half the patients to receive simvastatin r 7 days. At 30 days, 20% of the patients who d not take the statin died compared to 6% of iose in the group treated with the statin. One udy on 14,000 patients at Wuhan University uring the COVID pandemic showed a lower eath rate in the group that was receiving statins rior to the infection.

For all the above reasons, it has been curious o see patients in their 80s, 90s and beyond that developed COVID-19 and were minimally symp-tomatic or even asymptomatic. A French nun who was probably the oldest person infected with SARS-CoV-2, tested positive for the virus at age 116 and remained completely asymptomatic. In fact, the usual scenario has been that even mild infections proved to be deadly in the elderly.

The Effects of the Pandemic in Different Scenarios

In Europe and United States, nursing homes were devastated by the effects of COVID-19 disease. Spread of COVID-19 started at a faster rate in resident homes after the virus was disseminated. Because of variables such as age, sex, infection risk, disabilities, and comorbidities, mortality was up to 130 times higher in nursing homes compared to the elderly living in their homes. These facilities were also commonly the source of super-spreader events.

In February 2020, Italy was the first and most severely affected country outside of China. At this time, when nobody knew how deadly this pandemic would be, the northern parts of Italy (Lombardia, Veneto) and other large cities around the world were ravaged by the virus. The elderly was most affected.

The significant impact in Italy probably had to do with the fact that it is the country with the old-est population in Europe and the second oldest people in the world after Japan. The median age at death in Italy was 80 years during the first year of the pandemic. Interestingly, the city of Vo, also in the north of Italy, implemented an aggressive testing program among all its citizens and could extinguish the pandemic early becoming an exception to the significant devastation that occurred in the region. It can be speculated that because the winter of 2020 had fewer cases and deaths from influenza, this left a larger pool of susceptible elderly people for infection with SARS-COv-2 the so-called, dry tinder effect. In a similar way, strict and prolonged lockdowns could have also increased the susceptibility of elderly people to infection with the virus. Also, Sweden and other countries with a high life expectancy had their elderly care facilities more severely affected. Another factor that played an important role in propagating the pandemic was a significant employee cross-work that carried the virus among different nursing homes. The USA reached one million recorded deaths by mid-May 2022. The majority of Americans who died from COVID were over 65 years of age. By the above date, 252,612 people older than 85 died from COVID in the USA. In the 75–84 years group 254,328 deaths occurred, and in the 65–74 years range, 226,809 people died. In comparison, 65,757 people died in the 45–54 years of age group and 2600 in the 15–24 years old segment. Importantly enough, COVID was also the fourth leading cause of death in people 15–24 years and the second cause of death in those 25–44 years old. In the 45–54 years of age group, COVID was the number one cause of death in 2021.

In the US, the Navajo population was severely affected despite living in areas that were not as densely populated like other severely affected regions such as New York, Florida, and others. However, contagion spread among the Navajo people to the point that so many of the elderly died that there was fear that the Navajo language could be lost because it was spoken mostly by older people. Across all states, mortality for native Americans was disproportionally higher than that for African Americans and Hispanics despite belonging to similarly low socio-economic groups. Native Americans living in reservations were most severely affected. On the other extreme, New Zealand's Prime Minister Jacinda Arden decided to order a strict, limited lockdown of 7 weeks. At the time, the country had less than 200 cases and soon after the lockdown the cases and hospitalizations progressively decreased. The only person that died was an elderly woman. With this strategy, New Zealand maintained a good control of the pandemic throughout its course.

It soon became clear that the elderly had to be especially protected and, in many cases, from their own younger family members that could be the vectors of infection. This strategy led to a long period of isolation for this vulnerable subgroup especially before vaccines became available. The negative impact of these measures in the mental health of the elderly has been of great magnitude.

The Omicron Surge and Vaccination

With the Omicron surge at the end of 2021, a booster was proven necessary to have what could be considered a completed vaccination. A study from Israel published in the New England Journal of Medicine proved that the boosted elderly had significantly lower rates of severe disease and death. Interestingly, boosters decreased hospitalizations across all age groups. In fact, by April 2022 Pfizer requested approval for a booster dose in the 5–11-year-old group. By June 2022, both the Pfizer and Moderna vaccines were approved for the 6 months to 5 years of age population. It has been quite a surprise that more than a year after the vaccination campaign was initiated, the US had a quite slow vaccination campaign and had not reached 80% of the population with two doses and held the 57th position among countries that administered a first booster. This has occurred despite President Biden and Rochelle Walensky, CDC director, strongly encouraging all people to get boosted.

An additional complication was that the Omicron surge during the winter occurred at the time when flu is most frequent. The data showed that having COVID-19 and the flu at the same time doubled the chances of death and quadrupled the need for a respirator. However, despite the low efficacy of flu vaccines which was approximately 16%, the number of flu cases was not severe during the 2022 winter. This was explained by the so-called viral interference in which two competing viruses—COVID-19 and influenza—can decrease the severity of the illness caused by one of them.

Following the experience in Israel, most countries decided to apply a second booster at 4 months from the first booster mostly based on age criteria and for the immunocompromised. In Israel, the fourth dose is applied to everyone above 60 years, the UK indicated a second booster beyond 75 years of age, and in the US this booster is offered to those older than 50 years. Israeli data from March 2022 revealed that antibodies waned at 4 weeks following the second booster.

When the B.A.2 Omicron variant emerged, various parts of Asia had the most significant increase in infections seen during the pandemic and experienced an increase in death rates. One reason is that a strict and successful zero COVID strategy resulted in a general population that had not been exposed to the COVID-19 virus and thus did not have effective immune defenses. In Hong Kong because of a slow vaccination campaign, in part due to lack of trust from the citizens in the government, 50% of people above 75 years of age had not received the full 3 doses necessary to avoid severe disease from the Omicron variant. The exact opposite occurred, for example, in most regions of Africa where the average age is 27, a large proportion of the population had been infected and the vaccination campaign was focused in the elderly population.

The appearance of multiple Omicron variants has changed the pandemic's toll. These variants are highly contagious and include the European

BA2, the BA4 and 5, accounting for the fifth wave in South Africa, and the BA2.12 that was dominant in New York. During the January and February of 2022 Omicron outbreak, the vaccinated accounted for 40% of deaths compared to 23% during the September Delta wave. Two-thirds of the deaths occurred in people over the age of 75 compared to 30% during the Delta surge. This increased in deaths among the vaccinated is explained by a less effective and rapidly waning effect of the vaccines in the elderly. Most of the hospitalizations and deaths occurred among elderly people who did not have boosters.

As an example of the effect of infections in older people despite being vaccinated, the CDC page from March 2022 showed that the hospitalization rate for patients up to 50 years of age was increased by 2 compared to the group older than 75 years which was increased by 8. Death increased by 10 for the group younger than 50 years of age and by 140 for those older than 75 years. All the rates were relative to the 18–29 years old range category.

Important lessons regarding management in elderly individuals emerged as a result of the SARS-CoV-2 pandemic. First, because of a less effective immune system, people above 60 years of age should be the first group to receive vaccinations, probably starting with those older than 80 years. Those who live in residences with other individuals and care takers should be put under strict protocols to prevent contagion. Economic support should be available for the advanced age group and they should have priority for health care consults to decrease the risk of treatment discontinuation for cardiovascular and other diseases. These measures could decrease or avoid the enormous toll that the COVID-19 pandemic caused in this vulnerable segment of the population.

The Argentinean Experience at the Main COVID-19 Referral Hospital

With 600 beds, Sanatorio Guemes (SG) was the largest private clinic in Argentina and was selected as the main COVID-19 referral center in the city of Buenos Aires—population three million. Twenty three percent of all COVID-19 patients diagnosed in the city were hospitalized at the SG. By September 2021, a total of 34.375 patients were admitted to SG and 1.427 patients were admitted to the ICU. The average length of stay was 9 days. Overall mortality was 41%. 499 (35%) patients were older than 70 years of age and they accounted for the majority of deaths. A total of 838 patients required intubation, there average length of stay was 12 days and mortality for this group was 51%. Only 20 patients received tocilizumab. The SG participated in six international trials of different treatments for COVID-19.

With 130,000 deaths, Argentina ranked 24 worldwide for mortality per million people. Reasons for these results include a low performance of PCR diagnostics tests throughout the pandemic, no access to rapid antigen tests, a slow vaccination campaign with extensive use of Sinopharm and Sputnik vaccines with the latter having significant delays in delivery of the second and different dose. Pfizer and Moderna were available late in the pandemic and mostly as boosters. A prolonged but limited lockdown was ineffective to control dissemination of the virus but caused a major GDP fall. The above issues and a health system with chronic deficiencies explain Argentina's limited performance facing the pandemic. Other emerging countries such as our neighbors Uruguay and Chile had successful performances for both testing and vaccination.

Other Pandemics and the Elderly

The first pandemic for which rigorous epidemiological and clinical data are available was the influenza pandemic in 1918. Since then, three other influenza pandemics have occurred (1957, 1968, and 2009). In the 80s, the human immunodeficiency virus (HIV) was detected and by 2022 this pandemic has generated more than 50 million deaths.

Influenza

The *Orthomyxoviridae* family includes Influenza A and B species, among others. Influenza A virus is a single-stranded negative-sense RNA virus encoding eight major genes, including two major surface antigens: hemagglutinin (HA) (having 18 subtypes) and neuraminidase (NA) (11 subtypes). The natural host for influenza A is wild waterfowl. It is important to consider that domestic poultry and pigs can also be hosts, creating potential for genetic recombination of strains of avian and porcine origin. Influenza B almost exclusively affects humans, and since it has a lower rate of mutations, it has not been associated with pandemics.

Seasonal flu is more prevalent in the elderly, children under 2 years of age and people with chronic disease, with the highest mortality rate occurring in older patients. In contrast, during epidemic or pandemic periods, the greatest mortality rate occurs in populations under 65 years of age.

The first major pandemic occurred in 1918 and was caused by the H1N1 subtype. It was called the flu or Spanish influenza, although the virus did not originate in Spain. It probably began on March 11, 1918 at Fort Riley, Kansas, United States, and from there it rapidly spread worldwide. By the end of 1919, the Spanish flu had killed millions of people around the world and its impact was such that in 1 year it caused more deaths than World War I which had just finished. In February 1957, the second pandemic called Asian Influenza occurred, producing approximately four million deaths. The causative virus was H2N2. In early 1968, the third pandemic was caused by the H3N2 virus, causing almost two million deaths and was called Hong Kong influenza. In March 2009, an outbreak of swine flu began in Mexico, declaring an alert in April of the same year.

Influenza Pandemic in 1918

The 1918–19 influenza pandemic remains the world's largest single mortality event for which there are detailed records. More than half of the world's population was infected. Three waves of the so-called Spanish influenza in the period 1918–1919 killed more than 50 million people worldwide in the course of a few years. Young adults (particularly those in their early 20s), pregnant women, and isolated populations accounted for a disproportionate share of mortality. Researchers thought the elderly were spared due to prior exposure to other viruses, giving them immunity to the disseminated viral strains.

Some epidemiologists hypothesized that the 1890 birth cohort was more likely immunologically primed by exposure to the 1890 influenza pandemic, the last pandemic prior to 1918. An individual's infection/immune history is important for the influenza virus and has been variably referred to as "original antigenic sin" or "antigenic antiquity."

Influenza Pandemic in 2009

In March 2009, a new influenza A virus was detected. This new virus, named (H1N1) pdm09, contained a combination of influenza genes not previously identified in animals or humans. It had two genes from influenza viruses that normally circulate in pigs in Europe and Asia, three genes that normally circulate in North American pigs, as well as genes from avian and human influenza viruses. Between April 2009 and April 2010, the CDC in the United States and other groups estimated that 284,400 (range 151,700–575,400) people died worldwide from the infection. Severe cases occurred in young people between 20 and 49 years of age, as well as in patients with risk factors (immunosuppression, pregnancy, obesity, COPD, and a smoking history).

Globally, it was estimated that 80% of deaths related to the (H1N1) pdm09 virus occurred in people under the age of 65. This differs from typical seasonal influenza epidemics, during which an estimated 70–90% of deaths occur in people ≥65 years of age.

HIV Pandemic

In the United States in the early 80s, acquired immunodeficiency syndrome (AIDS) was described for the first time. With more than 50 million deaths, it ranks next to the 1918 influenza pandemic and the bubonic plague of the fourteenth century in terms of mortality. The epidemic has reached all regions and has been particularly alarming in countries with limited resources, especially in sub-Saharan Africa and Southeast Asia, as well as populations in Eastern Europe, Latin America and the Caribbean. At the end of 2019, statistics on the global burden of HIV reported that 36.2 million adults and 1.8 million children (<15 years) were living with HIV/AIDS. Among adults, 1.5 million were newly infected with HIV and 600,000 deaths were registered that year. However, since the introduction of antiretroviral therapy, the clinical and epidemiological characteristics of HIV infection changed dramatically: it went from being subacute and fatal to become a chronic disease in which other age-related conditions are also emerging among this population such as geriatric syndromes, including frailty, falls, and cognitive decline.

Along with this different disease pattern, a few new concepts have emerged such as "Aging" people with HIV, "Aged" people with HIV, and "accelerated aging" in young adults living with HIV. "Aging" people with HIV refers to those patients who survived the initial HIV epidemic and now live well into their 60s, 70s, and beyond. The Centers for Disease Control estimates that nearly 50% of people with HIV in the US are 50 years of age and older. Estimates from some European countries predict a "silver tsunami" within the HIV community, with people aged 50 and over accounting for almost 70% of people with HIV in the coming years. Currently, more than two-thirds of deaths among people with HIV are attributable to non-HIV-associated illnesses. Approximately, 83% of people with HIV aged 50 years or older and 63% aged 18–49 years have at least one comorbidity other than HIV. By the eighth decade, all patients have at least one comorbidity in addition to HIV, and more than two-thirds have multi-morbidities.

Along with these long-term survivors, many people were diagnosed at an older age—"Aged" people with HIV—after the advent of effective ART. With the pandemic having spread beyond the initial risk groups, one factor that contributes to new infections in older adults is that not only patients, but also health systems, often do not perceive older adults to be at risk of contracting HIV. In addition, age-related health conditions may mislead physicians to not consider HIV as a possible differential diagnosis. All this may contribute to delaying the diagnosis of HIV and consequently achieve poorer outcomes. It is also known that in this population, immune recovery, measured as an increase in the number and percentage of CD4 cells, is slower and less significant. All these factors make the elderly a real challenge for HIV care professionals.

One study that compared 404 patients with aging HIV (patients were seropositive for HIV for 20.6 years) and 404 aged HIV patients (<11.3 years of seropositivity) with 2424 healthy controls, found that patients with HIV had a higher number of comorbidities (defined as at least 2 comorbidities) than controls but also that aging patients with HIV tended to have higher comorbidities than those diagnosed at an older age. Probably, a longer exposure to chronic inflammation and immune activation induces immunosenescence in aging people with HIV, which can partially explain these observations. At the molecular level, evidence has been found for early shortening of telomeres and increased accumulation of amyloid plaques in the brain at a younger age in HIV-positive patients.

In conclusion, only in the last years of the pandemic we have begun to recognize older adults with HIV as a complex and increasingly growing population. Knowing their characteristics is essential to face the challenge that this group represents and to be able to offer them better health care.

References

1. https://www.who.int/data/gho/data/indicators/indicator-details/GHO/life-expectancy-at-birth-(years)
2. Sahyoun NR, Lentzner H, Hoyert D, Robinson KN. Trends in causes of death among the elderly. Aging trends (Hyattsville, Md). 2001;1:1–10. https://doi.org/10.1037/e620692007-001.
3. Santesmasses D, Castro JP, Zenin AA, Shindyapina AV, Gerashchenko MV, Zhang B, et al. COVID-19

is an emergent disease of aging. Aging Cell. 2020;19:e13230. https://doi.org/10.1111/acel.13230.
4. Sasson I. Age and COVID-19 mortality: a comparison of Gompertz doubling time across countries and causes of death. Demogr Res. 2021;44:379–96.
5. Pawelec G. Age and immunity: what is “immunosenescence”? Exp Gerontol. 2018;105:4–9.
6. Nikolich-Zugich J, Knox KS, Rios CT, Natt B, Bhattacharya D, Fain MJSARS. CoV-2 and COVID-19 in older adults: what we may expect regarding pathogenesis, immune responses, and outcomes. Geroscience. 2020;42:505–14. https://doi.org/10.1007/s11357-020-00186-0.
7. Sapey E, Greenwood H, Walton G, et al. Phosphoinositide 3-kinase inhibition restores neutrophil accuracy in the elderly: toward targeted treatments for immunosenescence. Blood. 2014;123(2):239–48. https://doi.org/10.1182/blood-2013-08-519520.
8. Sapey E, Patel JM, Greenwood H, et al. Simvastatin improves neutrophil function and clinical outcomes in pneumonia a pilot randomized controlled clinical trial. Am J Respir Crit Care Med. 2019;200:1282–93.
9. Livingston E, Bucher K. Coronavirus disease 2019 (COVID-19) in Italy. JAMA. 2020;323:1335.
10. Bar-On YM, Goldberg Y, Mandel M, et al. Protection by a fourth dose of BNT162b2 against omicron in Israel. N Engl J Med. 2022;386:1712–20.
11. Shanks GD. COVID-19 versus the 1918 influenza pandemic: different virus, different age mortality patterns. J Travel Med. 2020;27(5):taaa086. https://doi.org/10.1093/jtm/taaa086.
12. Dawood FS, Iuliano AD, Reed C, Meltzer MI, Shay DK, Cheng PY, Bandaranayakc D, Breiman RF, Brooks WA, et al. Estimated global mortality associated with the first 12 months of 2009 pandemic influenza a H1N1 virus circulation: a modelling study. Lancet Infect Dis. 2012;12(9):687–95. https://doi.org/10.1016/S1473-3099(12)70121-4.
13. UNAIDS. Global AIDS update —seizing the moment—tackling entrenched inequalities to end epidemics. 2020.
14. Erlandson KM, Karris MY. HIV and aging: reconsidering the approach to Management of Comorbidities. Infect Dis Clin N Am. 2019;33(3):769–86. https://doi.org/10.1016/j.idc.2019.04.005.
15. Guaraldi G, Zona S, Brothers TD, Carli F, Stentarelli C, Dolci G, Santoro A, Beghetto B, Menozzi M, Mussini C, Falutz J. Aging with HIV vs. HIV seroconversion at older age: a diverse population with distinct comorbidity profiles. PLoS One. 2015;10(4):e0118531. https://doi.org/10.1371/journal.pone.0118531.

Index

P. Petrone, C. E. M. Brathwaite (eds.), *Acute Care Surgery in Geriatric Patients*,
https://doi.org/10.1007/978-3-031-30651-8

M

N

O

P

T

U

GPSR Compliance

The European Union's (EU) General Product Safety Regulation (GPSR) is a set of rules that requires consumer products to be safe and our obligations to ensure this.

If you have any concerns about our products, you can contact us on ProductSafety@springernature.com

In case Publisher is established outside the EU, the EU authorized representative is:

Springer Nature Customer Service Center GmbH
Europaplatz 3
69115 Heidelberg, Germany

Batch number: 10731391

Printed by Printforce, the Netherlands